Eric Lindeman
6906 N.W. Blair Rd
Kansas City, MO 64152

Oral Diagnosis/
Oral Medicine

Oral Diagnosis/
Oral Medicine

DAVID F. MITCHELL, B.S., D.D.S., Ph.D.

The Late Professor and Chairman, Department of Oral Diagnosis/Oral Medicine, Indiana University School of Dentistry, Indianapolis, Indiana

S. MILES STANDISH, D.D.S., M.S.

Professor of Oral Pathology and Chairman, Department of Oral Diagnosis/Oral Medicine, Indiana University School of Dentistry, Indianapolis, Indiana

THOMAS B. FAST, D.D.S., M.S.D.

Professor, Department of Oral Medicine, College of Dentistry, University of Florida, Gainesville, Florida

THIRD EDITION

Lea & Febiger · Philadelphia · 1978

Library of Congress Cataloging in Publication Data

Mitchell, David F
  Oral diagnosis.

  Includes index.

  1. Teeth–Diseases–Diagnosis. 2. Mouth–Diseases–Diagnosis. I. Standish, S. Miles, 1923– joint author. II. Fast, Thomas B, joint author. III. Title [DNLM: 1. **Diagnosis,** Oral. 2. Mouth diseases. WU141 M6810]
RK308.M57   1977   616.3'1   76-30670

ISBN 0-8121-0590-7

Published in Great Britain by HENRY KIMPTON PUBLISHERS, LONDON

Print number: 5 4 3 2 1

PRINTED IN THE UNITED STATES OF AMERICA

Dedicated to the memory

of the late

Dr. David F. Mitchell

Preface

Oral diagnosis/oral medicine is the foundation upon which the dental curriculum as well as dental practice rests. It represents the application of the basic biologic sciences to daily practice. Although the subject stands as an entity in the conventional dental curriculum, it is an integral part of each clinical discipline. Oral diagnosis and oral medicine involve the recognition of the disease and subsequent management of the patient.

To the beginning student, *the* diagnosis becomes an all too elusive and frustrating objective of the initial examination. In Section I a logical, systematic approach to diagnosis is outlined, permitting the novice to conduct an adequate examination early in his clinical training and to advance as rapidly as his program permits. The introduction to radiographic interpretation is especially designed to prompt early interest in this field.

The experienced dentist may find that Section I furnishes a useful review, or he may wish to proceed directly to subsequent sections on more advanced concepts of diagnosis and patient care. A working knowledge of the basic biologic sciences is assumed, since this is fundamental to the recognition and management of oral disease. Throughout the book, clinical signs and symptoms are correlated with basic concepts of disease.

Section II gives attention to important epidemiologic and genetic considerations which guide one toward correlation of the past history of the patient with the presenting physical findings. The physical examination proceeds in an orderly fashion through anatomic regions, and appropriate diagnostic techniques and instruments are discussed. Common, easily recognized diseases which occur in each region are illustrated. A comprehensive compilation of diagnostic tests available in oral and clinical pathology laboratories may be used by the reader in accordance with his training and experience.

After extensive consideration of the diagnosis and emergency management of painful conditions occurring in dental patients, Section III deals with the recognition of specific diseases, and conditions of increasing complexity which involve the various anatomic regions. Special emphasis is placed on the approach to clinical diagnosis. Detection of the lesion, determination of the primary tissue affected and the probable basic pathologic process involved, represent sequential steps leading to a differential (or definitive) diagnosis. Cross references both to text and illustrations in other chapters allow the reader to consider a subject item from various aspects.

In Section IV, analysis of diagnostic findings, treatment planning, and hospital dentistry are discussed. Chapter 18 deals with legal implications related to dental practice and offers an introduction to forensic dentistry. Chapter 19 covers the diagnosis and management of medical emergencies which may be encountered in the dental office.

Indianapolis, Indiana   S. MILES STANDISH
Gainesville, Florida   THOMAS B FAST

Acknowledgments

We wish to acknowledge the expertise of Dr. Charles E. Tomich who prepared the epidemiologic material, and that of Drs. Gerald H. Prescott and David Bixler for the chapter on dental genetics. Dr. Abdel El-Kafrawy provided especially valuable counsel in his review of numerous sections of the textual material and assisted in the preparation of the appendix and index.

Our gratitude is extended to the following: Harvey Sarner, Paul Fast, and Forrest Bowman, Jr., for their assistance on legal matters; Rolando De Castro, D.M.D., for his excellent art work; Mr. Richard Scott and Mrs. Alana Fears for photographic assistance; Miss Shirley Shazer, research assistant, for exceptional laboratory technological assistance, which made much of the supporting research possible; and Mrs. Jane Powell and Ms. Willa Howard for superb secretarial assistance.

Thanks are due to the many former graduate students and esteemed colleagues who furnished information and illustrations, and to Professor Paul Barton, A.B., M.A., for conscientious correction and refreshing condensation of the manuscript.

For tolerating, encouraging, and supporting this activity, we particularly thank Dean Ralph E. McDonald, Indiana University School of Dentistry, and Dean Donald L. Allen, University of Florida College of Dentistry.

We humbly and respectfully acknowledge the guidance and leadership of the late Dr. David F. Mitchell to whom this edition is dedicated.

S.M.S.
T.B F.

Contents

Section I

Introduction to
Oral Diagnosis/Oral Medicine

This section is directed primarily to the student or the dentist seeking an overview of the parameters of oral diagnosis/oral medicine as well as a concise working knowledge of the procedures to be followed in the oral examination. Specifically, this section is designed to: (1) review the interrelationships of local and systemic disease and the clinical manifestations of the fundamental disease processes (Chap. 1), and (2) outline a systematic approach to the oral physical examination and radiographic interpretation (Chap. 2).

Oral diagnosis is the art of using scientific knowledge to identify oral disease processes and to distinguish one disease from another. *Oral medicine* is concerned with diagnosis and treatment, with consultation and referral and other phases of patient management; it deals especially with the relationship between oral and systemic diseases.

This field of *oral diagnosis/oral medicine* is fundamental to the practice of dentistry. Through effective diagnosis and patient care the dentist gains the respect of patients and colleagues alike, and receives the primary reward for any practitioner of the health professions—the knowledge that he is helping people.

Rapport should be established during the first contact. This implies a pleasant relationship with a ready exchange of information between patient and practitioner. The matter of rapport is equally important if the patient is first met by auxiliary personnel. Emphasis must be placed on cleanliness, and when instruments are involved, on sterility.

If auxiliary personnel are used, their duties must be defined and limited in accordance with the particular state dental practice laws. The practitioner or student overseeing them must be recognized as the responsible person.

Whether findings are written or dictated, they should be recorded in ink or by typewriter for permanence and medicolegal purposes. Accuracy is all-important. Patients should not be allowed to review their own records at any time.

Following are the basic components of diagnosis as practiced by any member of the health science team.

Anamnesis—the previous medical and dental history obtained from the patient during systematic interrogation.

Subjective symptoms and signs—as recognized and reported by the patient, *e.g.* pain, paresthesia, anesthesia, nausea, past occurrence of bleeding or swelling.

Objective findings—as detected by the examiner, *e.g.* hemorrhage, discoloration of teeth or soft tissues, swelling, and abnormal consistency of a part.

Technical aid—any technique, special test or instrument used to help establish a

1

diagnosis, such as the radiograph, pulp testing procedures, biopsy and the therapeutic trial.

If these four methods of obtaining information are used properly, with or without the aid of another opinion or reference to the literature, a diagnosis usually can be established.

Other terms commonly used in this field are described below.

Tentative diagnosis—a preliminary "educated guess" as to the nature of a condition before all diagnostic data are assembled. Sometimes treatment or therapeutic trial may be instituted on the basis of such a "working" or provisional diagnosis.

Differential diagnosis—when a condition may be due to two or more different diseases or forms of abnormality, the careful consideration and listing of these possibilities.

Definitive diagnosis—the final diagnosis based on a demonstrably accurate appraisal of all available data.

The process of making a final (definitive) diagnosis is essentially problem solving and as such lends itself to standard problem-solving techniques. An organized and orderly approach to data collection, testing, and analysis of findings is essential in order to obtain a high incidence of success in an efficient manner, as diagrammed below.

Prognosis—a forecast as to the outcome of a disease, made with or without therapy.

Consultation—obtaining the advice of others on the diagnosis of a specific oral condition, or on the management of a patient having some additional condition not directly related to the oral complaint. If the oral diagnostician recognizes the many possible systemic afflictions that may manifest themselves in the tissues apparent to him, and if he will conscientiously strive to detect them, categorize them in some way and seek effective consultation, he will render his patients an invaluable service. Thus, in any given case, the advice of another general practitioner of dentistry, the patient's physician, or a specialist in any field of dentistry or medicine might be sought.

When medical consultation is needed, it usually is wise to work with the patient's family physician, who in turn may refer the patient to a specialist of his choice. Nonetheless, it is ethical for the dentist to refer the patient to any specialist.

Referral—sending a patient to another person for consultation and/or treatment. This is best done by letter but may be accomplished in person or by telephone. If one receives a patient by referral, it is a matter of courtesy to acknowledge the fact and the outcome, again preferably in writing.

The recognized specialties of dentistry and medicine are listed below as an aid in referral.

Subjective Symptoms
Objective Signs
Cerebration
Test
―――――――――――
Differential Diagnosis

Differential Diagnosis
Tests
Cerebration
―――――――――――
Final Diagnosis

Final Diagnosis
Treatment Plan
Treatment
―――――――――――
SUCCESS

American Specialty Boards (1969)

Dentistry

Endodontics
Oral Pathology
Oral Surgery
Orthodontics
Pedodontics
Periodontics
Prosthodontics
Public Health

Medicine

Anesthesiology
Colon and Rectal Surgery

Dermatology
Family Practice
Internal Medicine
a. Allergy
b. Cardiovascular Disease
c. Gastroenterology
d. Pulmonary Disease
Neurologic Surgery
Obstetrics and Gynecology
Ophthalmology
Orthopedic Surgery
Otolaryngology
Pathology
Pediatrics
a. Allergy and Cardiology
Physical Medicine and Rehabilitation
Plastic Surgery
Preventive Medicine
Psychiatry and Neurology
a. Child Psychiatry
Radiology
Surgery
Thoracic Surgery
Urology

Chapter 1

Fundamental Disease Processes and their Clinical Characteristics

THE APPROACH TO CLINICAL DIAGNOSIS

The recognition of oral disease of either local or systemic origin is accomplished by *observation, interrogation, physical examination* and *interpretation*. From the information collected and recorded (which may include radiographic and laboratory studies), the fundamental disease process (*e.g.* inflammation) is first established and the specific disease entity (*e.g.* marginal gingivitis) is then identified.

While a great many oral diseases are easily recognized by their typical features, others require a more systematic approach for interpretation.

DETECTION OF ABNORMALITY

There is a wide, grey, unknown area (Fig. 1-1) between normalcy and abnormality which narrows as more is learned from the diagnostic findings, and as the skills of the examiner improve.

It is wise to develop a systematic approach to the problem-solving task of making a diagnosis—particularly in the more difficult situations. Without an organized approach, the data collected often are meaningless. Thus, the first step is to identify the symptoms suggestive of abnormality (subjective):

1. Pain and sensitivity
2. Paresthesia
3. Abnormal smells and tastes
4. Abnormal sounds
5. Hallucinations
6. A feeling of pressure or tension

Next, identify the signs of abnormality (objective):

1. Changes in morphology of a tissue, organ, or structure
2. Change in consistency of a tissue, organ, or structure
3. Change in color of a tissue, organ, or structure
4. Change in mobility of a tissue, organ, or structure
5. Change in function of a tissue, organ, or structure
6. Change in temperature of a tissue, organ or structure

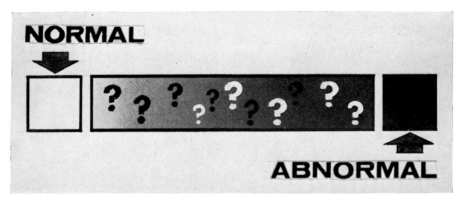

Fig. 1-1. Wide grey area separating the normal from the abnormal.

With this information, it is usually possible to identify several fundamental disease processes which are producing the sign/symptom complex. Once accomplished, testing procedures may be used to develop a differential and then a final diagnosis.

Basic Fundamental Disease Processes
1. Developmental Disturbances
    Disturbances in growth and development
    Hereditary disorders
    Familial diseases
    Congenital defects
2. Degenerative and Reactive Processes
    Atrophy
    Necrosis
    Hypertrophy
    Hyperplasia
3. Physical and Chemical Injuries
    Traumatic injury
    Iatrogenic disease
    Factitial injury
4. Inflammatory and Infectious Diseases
    Acute, chronic inflammation
    Bacterial, viral and mycotic infections
    Immunologic disturbances
    Hypersensitivity and drug reactions
5. Neoplasia
    Benign neoplasms
    Malignant neoplasms
6. Blood Dyscrasias
7. Metabolic Disturbances
8. Dermatoses
9. Neural, Neuromuscular and Psychogenic Disorders

In the study of diseases per se, it is helpful to have a system of classification. Oral pathologists use various systems, some based upon regional locations (*i.e.* diseases of lips, palate, and tongue) and some on appearance (*i.e.* red lesions, white lesions, and ulcers). A common method for categorizing disease is based primarily upon underlying fundamental disease processes, hence the category headings read very similarly to the list of fundamental disease processes. It is at this point where the traditional study of clinical diagnosis and that of academic oral pathology interface and become a continuum.

Categories of Disease
1. Congenital—Developmental
2. Infectious—Inflammatory
3. Neoplastic
4. Arthritic
5. Neurogenic—Psychogenic
6. Degenerative
7. Traumatic
8. Other

The astute oral diagnostician first identifies the symptoms and signs and then attempts to determine the basic disease processes acting to produce the findings.

Whether establishing a tentative, differential, or definitive diagnosis, the experienced examiner then mentally reviews the broad categories of disease and, by exclusion, eliminates the more unlikely possibilities. Since the presenting signs and symptoms are reflections of the underlying basic pathologic processes, knowledge of the associated clinical features of a disease serves as the basis for diagnosis.

This chapter will consider some interrelationships of local and systemic disease and clinical manifestations of the fundamental disease processes.

INTERRELATIONSHIPS AND MULTIPLE ORIGINS OF DISEASE

Whenever an abnormality is detected in a patient, the alert practitioner should search diligently for other related abnormalities; this search must sometimes extend to other members of the patient's family, or even to his social or occupational contacts.

Developmental abnormalities often are bilateral, so if a dental anomaly is detected on one side its counterpart should be suspected on the other. Further, certain dental and oral anomalies are associated with developmental defects of other bodily parts and systems, often with serious connotations. An example is the bifid rib-multiple jaw cysts-basal cell nevus syndrome (Fig. 4–4). Dentinogenesis imperfecta or amelogenesis imperfecta encountered in a patient should prompt an investigation of other mesodermal or ectodermal structures, respectively, both of the patient and other members of his family.

One endocrine imbalance may be associated with another. By virtue of the "master gland" role of the anterior pituitary in relation to the other endocrine glands, complex interrelationships of endocrinopathies may occur. For example, between 30 and 40 percent of patients with acromegaly, if untreated, become diabetic and develop the associated cardiovascular, retinopathic and neuropathic complications characteristic of the latter disease.

Because of the delicate physiologic interrelationships of the many constituents of blood, a deficiency or oversufficiency of one factor or cell often results in an imbalance of others. For example, the overgrowth of leukemia cells in the bone marrow typically crowds out megakaryocytes, thus resulting in a secondary thrombocytopenia with its associated bleeding problems.

A patient who has had one malignant tumor is more likely to have another than is a similar patient who has not had cancer. Benign neoplasms (e.g. neurofibroma) are also sometimes multiple in origin as in von Recklinghausen's disease of skin (multiple neurofibromatosis) (Fig. 14–60).

Nutritional deficiencies likewise are multiple more often than not. The emotionally disturbed individual may develop injurious habits which lead to new symptoms and further reinforce his anxiety and potentiate the development of cancerphobia. Arthritis of a temporomandibular joint obviously may be a reflection of other joint involvement, just as stomatitis may often be associated with dermatitis. A patient known to be hypersensitive to some food or medicament is likely to have or to develop other allergies or idiosyncrasies. Even contagious diseases may overlap one another. Thus, a patient known to have one venereal disease is a likely candidate for another.

ORAL MANIFESTATIONS OF LOCAL AND SYSTEMIC DISEASES

The vast majority of diagnostic problems encountered by the dentist are of "local" origin, i.e. they arise primarily from the teeth, periodontium, oral mucosa, bone or other oral and contiguous structures. However, the oral findings in some generalized or systemic diseases may simulate oral disease of local origin. The concept of total or comprehensive patient care requires that the dentist be alert to the patient's general health problems and knowledgeable about the oral manifestations of systemic disease.

A surprisingly large number of systemic diseases are known to present signs and symptoms that may be detected by the dentist. While he is not expected to be familiar with all of these, he is expected to detect abnormality, to suspect possible cause or causes, and to obtain such aid as necessary from others so that an early diagnosis can be established and adequate treatment instituted. For example, acute lymphocytic leukemia in children diagnosed and treated early with combinations of chemotherapy and radiation has responded very favorably in recent times. This "borderline" between dentistry and medicine is broad, intangible, and of particular importance to patient care by both professional groups.

Once the basic pathologic process is identified, regardless of whether the disease is of "local" or "systemic" origin, it is logical next to identify, usually by exclusion, the broad category of disease involved. In this manner, it is possible to determine management of the patient with some authority and to select such additional diagnostic procedures (*e.g.* biopsy, aspiration, therapeutic trial) as may be necessary to establish a definitive diagnosis.

Developmental Disturbances

Disturbances in growth and development may be manifested clinically by *aplasia* or failure of formation (*e.g.* anodontia, facial or oral clefts, aplasia of salivary glands); *hypoplasia* or incomplete formation (*e.g.* microdontia, microglossia); *dysplasia,* with abnormal arrangement of tissues and organs (Fig. 1–2); *hamartomas* (*e.g.* hemangioma, supernumerary teeth, exostoses) (Figs. 1–3, 7–27); and generalized under- or overdevelopment of body tissues and structures (*e.g.* hemiatrophy, hemihypertrophy) (Fig. 11–1). The clinician detects most developmental abnormalities by gross and radiographic observations.

Hereditary disorders refer to abnormalities which tend to follow a genetic or inherited pattern (see Chap. 4). *Familial diseases* are those which tend to run in families and are probably hereditary, even though the mode of inheritance is not clearly established. *Congenital disturbances* are those which are present at birth but are not necessarily of hereditary origin. Some congenital diseases may actually be present at birth

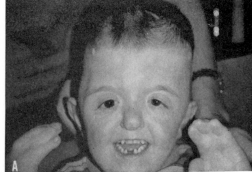
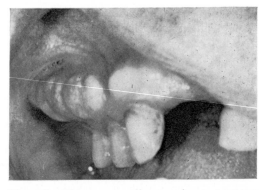

Fig. 1-2. *A,* Apert's syndrome or acrocephalo-syndactyly. Craniofacial changes shown include antimongoloid slant of eyes, low-set ears, bulbous nose and tooth loss. *B,* Radiograph of hands showing syndactyly.

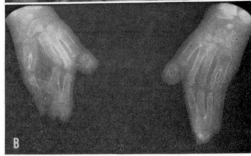

Fig. 1-3. These unusually prominent exostoses are very hard and white to yellow beneath the thin mucosa. They are bilateral and unimportant except in patients needing prostheses.

but not become clinically evident until later in life, such as certain of the inborn errors of metabolism. Congenital defects range in severity from the grossly deformed monster to lesser variations and anomalies.

Hereditary ectodermal dysplasia may be

accompanied by deficiencies of teeth and major and minor salivary glands (Fig. 4–17). Severe periodontal disease may develop in a child as a part of the hereditary syndrome of Papillon-LeFevre (Fig. 4–18). Congenital syphilis may be associated with malformed permanent incisors and molars afflicted by the disease during the morpho-

genic and appositional stages of their development.

The history of a lesion or condition dating back to the birth of the patient, or the occurrence of similar lesions in other members of his family, is most important in categorizing such conditions (Fig. 1–4).

The developmental cysts are very common in the jawbones and oral region. A cyst,

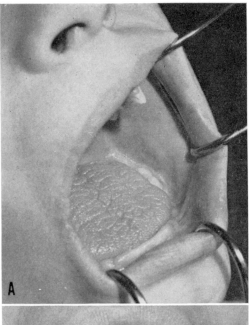

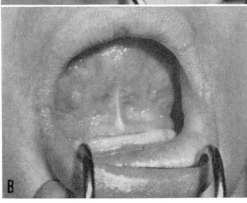

Fig. 1-4. *A*, This 16-year-old boy has lost nearly all of his teeth from rampant caries. The mouth was quite dry and the orifices of the major salivary gland ducts could not be found. Notice the unusual surface of the tongue and the absence of the left parotid papilla. *B*, The edentulous ridge of the anterior mandible is shown and the absence of the sublingual papillae is apparent. (Wood and Mitchell, Oral Surg. Oral Med. Oral Path., *15*, 1075, 1962.)

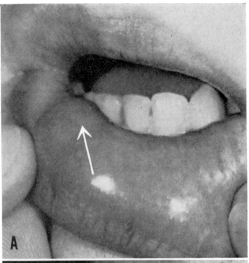

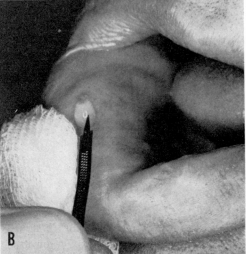

Fig. 1-5. *A*, Mucocele of lower right lip. The mucosa over this deeply situated lesion is of normal color. If the lesion were more superficial, the color would be lighter. *B*, A mucocele has been lanced and a clear, mucoid material is emitted. While this procedure aids in establishing the diagnosis, appropriate treatment is complete excision.

defined as a pathologic epithelial-lined cavity filled with fluid or caseous material, can arise only in the presence of epithelium. By the nature of the embryonic development of the maxillae, with the palatal and alveolar lines of closure (sites of clefts) and the nasopalatine ducts, many epithelial (ectodermal) inclusions occur. Add to those of the maxillae and the mandible the fifty-two anlagen of the deciduous and permanent teeth, and their respective "epithelial rests of Malassez," and it is understandable that many cysts occur in these bones. In addition, retention cysts may occur in relation to major or minor salivary glands (Fig. 1–5).

Thus, developmental cysts of inexact etiology may occur, or, more commonly, a traumatic or infectious stimulation of these epithelia may result in inflammatory cyst formation. In either case, collections of a fluid not unlike serum may be palpated if near a surface, and on aspiration may be found to be straw-colored or colorless. The most common cyst of inflammatory origin is the apical periodontal cyst associated with a tooth with a necrotic, infected pulp.

Degenerative and Reactive Processes

Living tissues may respond to noxious stimuli in several ways depending upon the severity of the injury and the tissues involved. For example, abrasion, attrition, erosion or chronic caries of the teeth may induce sclerosis of the primary dentin and stimulate secondary dentin formation. Acute caries, on the other hand, will soon involve the dental pulp, causing necrosis. Hyaline degeneration may be found in scar tissue and in the gingival arterioles of diabetics.

Atrophy, reduction in size of an organ or tissue, may occur in a rare, unexplainable form such as hemifacial atrophy, or more commonly in the alveolar process of the edentulous person. Masticatory muscles and jawbones may atrophy and weaken owing to decrease in function after paralysis or to ankylosis of the temporomandibular joint (disuse atrophy). Some atrophy of major

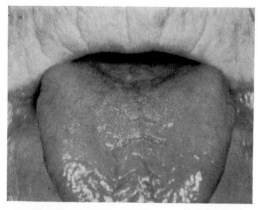

Fig. 1-6.   An elderly female as evidenced by the wrinkled upper lip and the barely detectable vermilion border. Note the smooth, bald tongue and the cheilitis at the corners of the mouth. These signs are suggestive of nutritional deficiency.

and minor salivary glands with decrease in function is seen as a physiologic effect of aging (physiologic or senile atrophy). Likewise, mucous membranes become pale, thin and fragile in appearance with age; comparable changes with wrinkling are also seen in the lips and skin of the elderly (senile atrophy). The dorsum of the tongue may exhibit atrophic change due to nutritional deficiency with the filiform papillae becoming indistinct (Fig. 1–6).

Hypertrophy of the masticatory muscles may occur in patients with jaw-clenching or tooth-grinding habits (bruxism). True hypertrophy, an increase in size of an organ without an increase of unit cellular constituents, is difficult to demonstrate in tissues other than muscle (Fig. 1–7).

Hyperplasia, an increase in size due to an increase in number of cells, is a common pathologic process, and the word is frequently, though inaccurately, used interchangeably with hypertrophy. The *keloid* is an example of hyperplastic scar tissue while the *pyogenic granuloma* represents exuberant granulation tissue growth in response to a local irritant (Fig. 1–8). Inflammatory fibrous hyperplasia of the oral mucous membranes is commonly seen in the tissues adjacent to ill-fitting dentures.

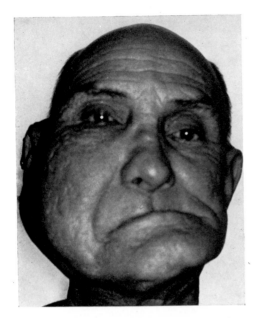

Fig. 1-7. Elderly man with progressive enlargement of half of the middle third of his face, including the mandible. This represents a rare case of hemifacial hypertrophy or hyperplasia of unknown etiology.

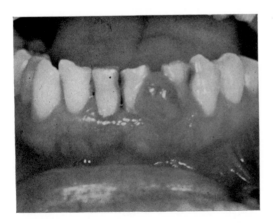

Fig. 1-8. Gingival pyogenic granuloma. This is the most common localized inflammatory lesion of the gingiva. It is a vascular mass of chronically inflamed, hyperplastic connective tissue. Lack of contact between the associated teeth probably predisposed to food impaction and the inflammatory response.

Physical and Chemical Injuries

Physical injuries are commonly encountered in the oral tissues and include not only actual physical disruption of tissue conti-nuity but thermal and electrical burns, cold, ultraviolet radiation and x-irradiation injury as well. Thus, physical injuries range from minor cuts and abrasions of the mucosa to the more severe traumatic ulcers, fractured teeth, and fractured jaws. Ultraviolet (sunlight) damage to the lips and skin of the face is commonly found in older patients, some of whom may develop carcinomas. Patients who have received therapeutic radiation may show postradiation dermatitis and stomatitis, pigmentation changes, loss of skin appendages and salivary gland function, "radiation caries," incomplete tooth development, osteoradionecrosis and/or carcinoma, depending upon the circumstances of the treatment.

Chemical injuries are produced in oral tissues by reaction of the agent directly with the oral tissues (*e.g.* acids, alkalies, sclerosing agents), by modification of cell metabolism or enzyme systems by drugs or other chemicals (*e.g.* chemotherapeutic agents which inhibit cell mitosis, aspirin medications which may modify blood platelet function), or by the physical presence of the agent (*e.g.* heavy metal poisons). Caustic agents such as acids and bases induce necrosis and sloughing of the mucosa (*e.g.* aspirin, silver nitrate, trichloroacetic acid, phenol burns) (Figs. 14–27, 14–28). Therapeutic agents at the appropriate dosage are effective in controlling or curing disease, yet in excess create tissue damage. The deposition of heavy metals such as bismuth or amalgam in the connective tissues generally induces little or no damage. However, the deposits appear as discolored areas which must be differentiated from physiologic and pathologic pigmentations, nevi and malignant melanomas.

Iatrogenic disease is injury inflicted by the physician (*iatro*), literally, or by the dentist or other member of the health science team. It may take many forms. Antibiotic agents prescribed to combat infection may cause skin rash, stomatitis, or neuromuscular symptoms. The tetracycline antibiotics

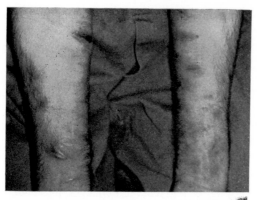

Fig. 1-9. Factitial injuries on the inner surfaces of the forearms of a seated patient are shown. He is mentally retarded and disturbed and the scars and wounds were self-inflicted.

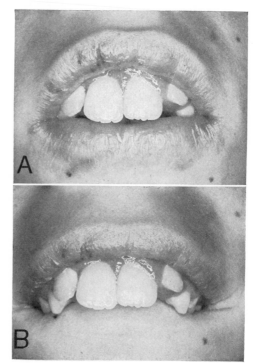

Fig. 1-10. Factitial injury. *A,* The cracked upper lip is due to mouth-breathing. However, the cause of the excoriated and ecchymotic lesions of the lower lip and adjacent skin was not immediately obvious, *B,* By observation of the patient the cause of the self-induced (factitial) injury was determined.

may induce intrinsic staining of developing teeth with a characteristic yellow fluorescence under ultraviolet light (Fig. 7–59). An ill-fitting denture may cause an inflammatory hyperplasia of underlying epithelial and connective tissues. Subcutaneous emphysema may follow the injudicious use of the air syringe in deep periodontal pockets or extraction wounds and is characterized by soft, non-inflammatory swelling and crepitus of the subcutaneous tissues of the face or temple.

Factitial injury represents damage inflicted either deliberately or unknowingly by the patient (Figs. 1–9, 1–10). Cheek biting (pathomimia, morsicatio buccarum), the use of snuff and smoking may induce characteristic white (hyperkeratotic) mucosal lesions. Ulceration and necrosis may occur when a patient suffering pain applies aspirin or a cauterizing solution such as lemon extract to his gingivae to relieve a toothache. Toothbrush injuries and "fingernail habits" cause marked local gingival recession.

Inflammatory and Infectious Diseases

The cardinal signs of inflammation are *rubor* (erythema or redness), *tumor* (swelling), *calor* (heat), and *dolor* (pain).

The inflammatory reaction of tissue to injury may be due to physical, chemical and biologic factors such as trauma, heat, radiation, chemical cauterization or hypersensitivity, or to bacterial, viral and mycotic invasion (Fig. 1–8). The vascular, cellular and biochemical phases of this protective and reparative reaction include leukocytic infiltration, vasodilatation, edema and occasionally necrosis. Endothelial and fibroblastic proliferation (granulation tissue) predominates in the repair phase of the inflammatory process.

Thus, inflammation may appear grossly on a surface as an erythematous but intact area or adjacent to an area of necrosis (ulceration). Chronic inflammatory hyperplasia of connective tissues is the basis for many intraoral overgrowths; this form of tumefaction is seen in the common gingival pyogenic granuloma (Fig. 1–8), the hyper-

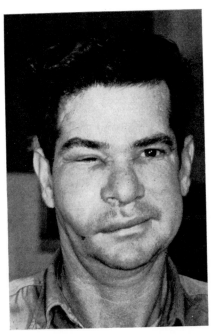

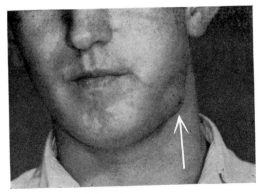

Fig. 1-12. Chronic facial cellulitis and fistula from an abscessed lower left molar. The red swelling of several weeks' duration is indurated and was said to drain periodically.

Fig. 1-11. Acute, severe right facial cellulitis associated with an abscess of an upper bicuspid. When the right eye was forcibly opened, it was bloodshot. (Mitchell, in *Endodontics,* ed. by Healey, courtesy of the C. V. Mosby Co.)

plasia of the pulp polyp, denture injury hyperplasia, and hyperplastic gingivitis.

Pain is generally associated with acute and subacute inflammatory reactions whereas it is not a feature of chronic inflammation such as periodontitis. Painless pulpitis, for example, commonly leads to pulp necrosis and periapical pathosis and yet may be completely asymptomatic.

In *acute inflammation,* the swelling is usually diffuse and firm. After severe sunburn, the swelling is caused by vasodilatation, increased capillary permeability, leukocytic infiltration and edema. After acute trauma, vessel rupture with hematoma (bruise) formation is an added cause.

Chronic inflammation, as in long-standing infections, often results in an indurated swelling owing to marked infiltration of tissues with many lymphocytes and plasma cells, plus the proliferation of endothelial cells and fibroblasts (Fig. 1-12). The common periapical granuloma represents such a response to low-grade infection or by-products of tissue injury from a non-vital tooth pulp. Less commonly seen, the specific granulomatous infections (*e.g.* tuberculosis) are characterized by the exuberant overgrowth of granulation tissue.

An accumulation of pus, which consists largely of dead or dying polymorphonuclear leukocytes surrounded by an inflamed wall of living, vascular connective tissue, represents an *abscess.* It may be acute, that is, of recent origin and severe in nature, or chronic and relatively asymptomatic. If the lesion is near a surface, the "rebound" effect of a fluid-filled sac may be palpated. Aspiration by means of a needle and syringe of grey or blood-tinged suppurative material is incontrovertible evidence of abscess. A "pointing" abscess exhibits a shiny white or yellow point on the swollen, reddened surface of overlying mucosa or skin, indicating an optimum site for incision to establish drainage (Fig. 2-15).

The abscess may be relieved by lancing, either by incision through soft tissue or by bur through tooth to pulp chamber. Frequently the acute abscess is relieved and converted to a more chronic lesion by spontaneous drainage through a natural or developing fistulous tract. In such cases (as in a chronic parotitis or osteomyelitis), diagnostic evidence of pus may be seen upon palpating the involved region and observing the flow of pus from the tract opening.

Oral manifestations of both local and systemic *bacterial, viral,* and *mycotic infections* are frequently seen, particularly the exanthematous diseases of childhood. The skin lesions of chickenpox (Fig. 1–13) and the

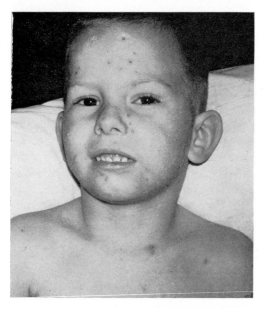

Fig. 1-13. The skin lesions of chickenpox (varicella) are seen on the face and chest. These multiple, raised vesicles usually subside without scar formation. This child also had a single lesion on the soft palate which resembled an aphthous ulcer.

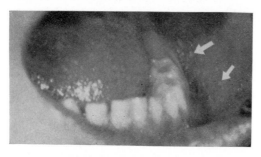

Fig. 1-14. Koplik's spots are seen on the left buccal mucosa of this child who is suffering with measles (rubeola). These indistinct white to bluish spots are about a millimeter in diameter and are considered to be prodromal signs often apparent before the skin rash occurs.

mucous membrane lesions of measles are shown (Fig. 1–14). The circumoral pallor and so-called strawberry tongue of scarlet fever and the swollen parotid glands of mumps are other examples. The *granulomatous diseases* including syphilis, tuberculosis and actinomycosis may present primary or secondary lesions in and about the mouth.

Immunologic disturbances, including allergies and autoimmune diseases, present special diagnostic problems since the etiologic factor is often obscure. Allergic reactions may be of the immediate type (*e.g.* angioneurotic edema, anaphylaxis) or the delayed type (*e.g.* agranulocytosis secondary to drug idiosyncrasy) (Fig. 14–50).

Hypersensitivity and drug reactions may cause considerable difficulty in diagnosis since these can take a variety of forms (pp. 25, 104). Contact allergenic stomatitis from foods, cosmetics and dentifrices has been described. Xerostomia occurs as a reaction to amphetamines, antihistamines and other drugs. Generalized gingival hyperplasia due to Dilantin therapy for epileptic seizure is common.

Neoplasia

True tumors or neoplasms typically occur as localized, single, purposeless and autonomous overgrowths of one or more tissues. Occasionally multiple neoplasms occur, as in neurofibromatosis and carcinomatosis. The etiology of neoplasms is essentially unknown. They seldom if ever regress, and malignant forms may invade widely and metastasize. The surface configuration (Fig. 1–15) and the color and consistency of the lesion may suggest the primary tissue origin and the tentative diagnosis. For example, the lipoma appears yellow and is of a soft, fatty consistency; the hemangioma may be red or purple, soft in consistency, and will blanch under pressure.

Clinical characteristics of benign tumors include: localization, encapsulation, pedunculation, color and consistency characteristic of the tissues of which they are composed,

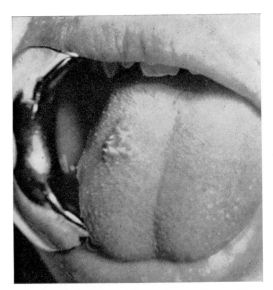

Fig. 1-15. Papilloma of the tongue. The papillary projections which are of the same color as the surrounding mucosa suggest the diagnosis.

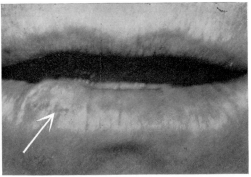

Fig. 1-17. Early squamous cell carcinoma on the lower lip of a young adult male. The lesion is ulcerated, tumefied (note the raised, rolled border), indurated and has been present for several weeks (four cardinal signs of cancer). Wide excision was performed.

lymph nodes (which in turn become enlarged and indurated) or to distant sites by way of the blood stream.

The terminology used to designate benign tumors identifies the specific tissue with a stem, such as *aden-, fibr-* and *neur-,* which is combined with the suffix *-oma* meaning tumor (Fig. 1–18). Benign neoplasias may involve epithelium (papilloma, adenoma), fibrous connective tissue (fibroma), neural tissue (neuroma, neurofibroma, neurilemmoma), vascular tissues (hemangioma, lymphangioma), bone (osteoma), fat (lipoma) and muscle (myoma).

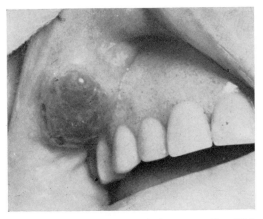

Fig. 1-16. Hemangioma of the upper lip. This blue, raised mass has been present as long as the patient can remember. Although it had created no problem for the patient, she was advised to have it treated by injections of a sclerosing solution, or to have it removed surgically. Some such lesions may respond to irradiation.

and slow, painless and expansile growth without regression or metastasis (Fig. 1–16).

In contrast, malignant lesions may present the four cardinal signs of cancer: tumefaction, induration, ulceration and chronicity (Fig. 1–17). They usually grow rapidly, are invasive and tend to metastasize to regional

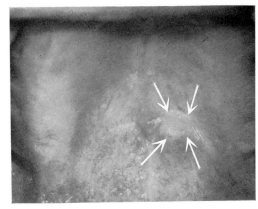

Fig. 1-18. The round, slightly raised lesion at the junction between the hard and soft palate on the left side proved to be a pleomorphic adenoma after excision.

When malignant tumors of these tissues are involved, the stem is given a suffix of *carcinoma* for epithelial lesions (adeno*carcinoma*), and sarcoma for most other connective tissues (fibro*sarcoma,* neuro*sarcoma,* lipo*sarcoma,* leiomyo*sarcoma*).

Certain neoplasms may appear simultaneously in many sites, some of them within the mouth (*e.g.* neurofibromatosis, papillomatosis, carcinomatosis). Further, malignant lesions of other parts of the body may metastasize to the jaws and neighboring structures and a few have been demonstrated in the dental pulp.

Usually tumors are identified by microscopic study of the tissue and then eradicated by surgery, x-radiation or chemotherapy. In general the dentist treats benign tumors of the mouth by conservative surgical excision. Once diagnosed, malignant lesions usually are treated by surgeons or radiation therapists, frequently in teaching and research hospitals or special cancer treatment centers.

The dentist with special interest or training in prosthetics may play an important role in the rehabilitation of such patients by fashioning appliances (somatoprostheses) to restore the normal appearance and function of the face and jaws (Fig. 1–19).

An important phase of the differential diagnosis of suspected neoplastic lesions is the judicious use of a working knowledge of the relative incidence, common sites of occurrence, epidemiology and natural history of neoplasms of the oral and paraoral regions (see Chaps. 11, 15). For example, the most common cancer that the dentist is likely to encounter is the squamous cell (epidermoid) carcinoma occurring on the lower lip of the elderly Caucasian male (Fig. 1–17). The dentist clearly has the best opportunity of any of the health professionals to detect and diagnose oral and paraoral neoplastic disease in its early stages.

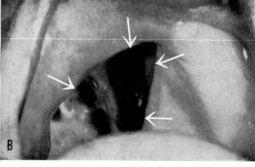

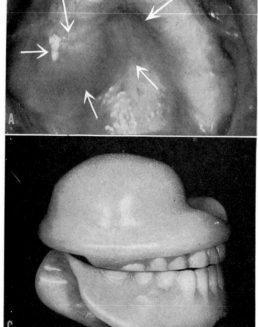

Fig. 1-19. *A,* This elderly male sought dentures. The large, red and somewhat soft mass of the right alveolar process of the maxilla was of no concern to him. After radiographs, biopsy revealed the presence of epidermoid carcinoma of the maxillary sinus. The lesion and surrounding tissues were excised. (Shafer, Hine and Levy, *Oral Pathology,* courtesy of W. B. Saunders Co.) *B,* This is the postoperative defect several weeks later. *C,* The prosthetic appliance served the patient well. The obturator portion is hollow to reduce weight. (Courtesy of Dr. Joseph White.)

Blood Dyscrasias

The leukemias, many anemias, and disturbances of the platelets as well as other components of the blood may exhibit a defective clotting mechanism and exhibit clinical findings of spontaneous gingival hemorrhage, petechiae, ecchymoses and generalized gingival hyperplasia (Fig. 1–20). Pallor, prolonged bleeding after oral surgery, severe destruction of alveolar bone without obvious reason, and lack of resistance to infection are other signs of such diseases of the blood (pp. 405–408).

Metabolic Disturbances

Disturbances in metabolism characteristically involve many body tissues and organ systems. Because of their protean nature, they may simulate a number of other diseases. Among the metabolic disturbances of interest to the dentist are the endocrinopathies, nutritional disturbances, the lipid and non-lipid reticuloendothelioses, the collagen diseases, autoimmune diseases, inborn errors of metabolism and certain metabolic diseases of bone such as Paget's disease, osteopetrosis, and infantile cortical hyperostosis.

The *endocrinopathies* frequently show associated oral changes, most notably in diabetes mellitus, hyperparathyroidism (von Recklinghausen's disease of bone), hypopi-

tuitarism, hypothyroidism (cretinism, myxedema) and hyperpituitarism (giantism, acromegaly). The formation, eruption and physiologic exfoliation of teeth and growth of jaws are intimately related to all other bodily growth processes, and are particularly affected by insufficiency or excess of the growth-affecting hormones of the pituitary and thyroid glands (Fig. 1–21). Uncon-

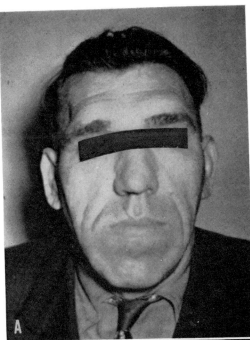

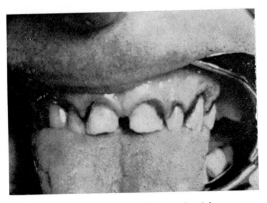

Fig. 1-20. This 45-year-old truck driver complained of nose bleeds and bleeding gums. Notice the gingival hemorrhage which was spontaneous. A routine hemogram revealed leukemia, and the patient died a few months later.

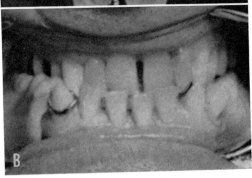

Fig. 1-21. *A,* Acromegaly. Notice the accentuated frontal bosses and the thick features emphasizing the nose and ears. The lower lip appears to be overfull. *B,* Mandibular protrusion gradually developed after the onset of acromegaly during the third decade of life. This change was due to the persistent activity of the condylar growth centers of the mandible.

Table 1-1.   Diseases of Inexact Etiology Showing Oral Manifestations

Connective Tissue Diseases

Scleroderma
Dermatomyositis
Periarteritis nodosa
Rheumatic fever
Disseminated lupus erythematosus
Rheumatoid arthritis
Sjögren's syndrome

Heritable Disorders of Connective Tissue

Marfan syndrome
Ehlers-Danlos syndrome
Osteogenesis imperfecta
Homocystinuria
Mucopolysaccharidosis
Vitamin D-resistant rickets
Other skeletal dysplasias

Inborn Errors of Metabolism

Albinism
Maple syrup urine disease
Alkaptonuria
Cystinuria
Tyrosinemia
Homocystinuria
Phenylketonuria
Hypophosphatasia (hypophosphatasemia)
Hypophosphatemia (vitamin D-resistant rickets)

Autoimmune Diseases

Benign lymphoepithelial lesion
   Mikulicz's disease
   Sjögren's syndrome
Hashimoto's struma
   (chronic thyroiditis)
Rheumatoid arthritis
Idiopathic thrombocytopenic purpura
Myasthenia gravis
Acquired hemolytic anemia

Reticuloendothelioses

Non-lipid reticuloendotheliosis
   Letterer-Siwe disease
   Hand-Schüller-Christian disease
   Eosinophilic granuloma

Lipid reticuloendotheliosis
   Niemann-Pick disease
   Gaucher's disease
   Amaurotic familial idiocy
   Familial leucodystrophy
   Xanthomas

trolled diabetes (pp. 245–249) may predispose to xerostomia, glossodynia and an increase in severity of periodontal disease. The melanotic pigmentation of Addison's disease (pp. 255, 382) may be seen intraorally as well as on the skin.

In addition to the endocrinopathies, whole groups of diseases of unknown or inexact etiology with oral manifestations have been described in recent years, such as the reticuloendothelioses, inborn errors of metabolism, "collagen diseases," and autoimmune diseases. Examples of diseases commonly included in each of these groups are listed in Table 1–1. It should be noted, however, that a growing body of evidence suggests

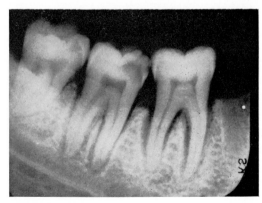

Fig. 1-22.   This periapical radiograph illustrates the wide periodontal ligament space around the molars of a patient with scleroderma.

that certain of the so-called collagen diseases are in fact examples of autoimmune diseases or hypersensitivity states.

Certain of the connective tissue diseases in particular present oral manifestations or special dental problems, notably scleroderma and rheumatic fever. Scleroderma may present radiographic evidence of a thickened periodontal ligament (Fig. 1–22). Many other conditions of unknown etiology, such as Paget's disease and the histiocytosis X diseases, typically involve the oral regions.

Classical oral signs of *nutritional imbalance* such as bleeding gums and exfoliation of the teeth (scurvy), cheilosis (riboflavin deficiency), and glossitis (pellagra) are rarely encountered in clinical practice except in alcoholics, in food faddists or in

patients with gastrointestinal disturbances (*e.g.* steatorrhea, sprue, pernicious anemia). Hypervitaminosis A and D also may occur.

Vitamin C deficiency has been caused by an overzealous parent who boiled a child's orange juice, thereby destroying the vitamin C. Vitamin D deficiency in the infant or child may result in enamel hypoplasia as well as the classical bone changes. Atrophic changes in mucous membranes and the skin may be signs of deficiency of some of the B vitamins. The protective effect of a proper intake of fluoride against dental caries is well

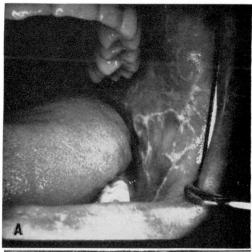

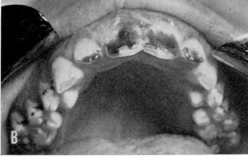

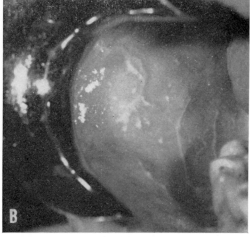

Fig. 1-23. *A,* Dental fluorosis or mild mottled enamel, varying from opaque white to mottled brown, as seen in the teeth of a dentist native to Colorado Springs. Note the absence of caries. *B,* Severe dental fluorosis in a girl from the northwest. The family well water was found to contain 11 ppm of fluoride.

Fig. 1-24. Lichen planus. *A,* Striae of Wickham are shown on the inner surface of the left cheek. *B,* Another case showing similar features. Note the interlacing, slightly raised Wickham's lines.

known; contrarily, an excess may cause fluorosis with mottling of the enamel (Fig. 1–23) and modifications of bone.

Dermatoses

A large number of dermatologic diseases may involve oral mucous membranes, and in some conditions the appearance of intraoral lesions may precede involvement of the skin, as in the various forms of lichen planus (Fig. 1–24), pemphigus, and erythema multiforme (see Chap. 11).

Neural, Neuromuscular, and Psychogenic Disorders

The neural and neuromuscular disorders encompass a broad spectrum of disease entities which may arise in the several anatomic components of the peripheral and central nervous systems. Their clinical manifestations are a varied and often confusing array of signs and symptoms which range from altered functions of the Aristotlean senses (vision, taste, smelling, hearing, touch) or subsenses (deep touch, temperature, pain, stretch, proprioception) to spasticity and paralysis of the voluntary muscles. These conditions may thus involve the sensory, motor, or autonomic systems, central neurons of the brain or spinal cord, or the muscle proper.

Table 1-2. Neuralgias and Other Sensory Neuropathies

Trigeminal neuralgia
Paratrigeminal syndrome
Sphenopalatine neuralgia
Glossodynia
Glossopharyngeal neuralgia
Atypical facial neuralgia
Causalgia
Periodic migrainous neuralgia
Trotter's syndrome
Ramsey-Hunt syndrome
Crocodile-tears syndrome
Temporal arteritis
Horner's syndrome

Table 1-3. Myopathies and Other Neuromuscular Disorders

Muscular Dystrophies
  Generalized familial muscular dystrophy
  Facioscapulohumeral muscular dystrophy
  Oculopharyngeal muscular dystrophy
  Ocular myopathy
  Limb-girdle myopathy
  Late distal muscular dystrophy
  Myotonic dystrophy

Myotonias
  Congenital myotonia
  Myotonic dystrophy
  Paramyotonia congenita

Hypotonias
  Tay-Sachs disease
  Infantile muscular atrophy
  Acute infectious polyneuritis (Guillain-Barré syndrome)
  Benign congenital hypotonia

Myasthenias
  Myasthenia gravis

Myositis
  Functional myositis
  Infectious myositis
  Traumatic myositis
  Myositis ossificans
  Dermatomyositis

Other Neuromuscular Disorders
  Bell's palsy
  Melkersson-Rosenthal syndrome
  Marcus-Gunn phenomenon
  Inverted Marcus-Gunn syndrome
  Bilateral facial palsy
  Congenital facial diplegia
  Unilateral vagal paralysis
  Hypoglossal paralysis
  Pseudobulbar palsy
  Cerebral palsy
  Orofacial dyskinesia
  Multiple sclerosis
  Parkinson's disease
  Epilepsy
  Progressive muscular atrophy
  Progressive bulbar palsy
  Amyotrophic lateral sclerosis

Sensory function disorders of the cranial nerves pose special problems in diagnosis of the underlying pathologic process. Pain is the most common symptom encountered and is usually associated with an inflammatory/infectious process of dental origin (neuritis). In the neuralgias, however, no organic lesion of the nerve can be identified (Table 1–2). Other aberrant sensations reflecting sensory disturbances are lost or altered taste, smell or other sensory functions; hypesthesia, paresthesia or anesthesia; and hypersensitivity, including hyperalgesia and hyperacusis.

Motor function disorders may be centered in the central motor nuclei, the motor nerve, the myoneural junction or the muscle itself as a primary myopathy. Modified reflexes; muscular spasm, tremor or fasciculation; hypotonia, myotonia or myasthenia; muscle paralysis and atrophy; and dysphagia or dysphonia are expected signs and symptoms of motor function disease (Table 1–3).

Autonomic nervous system signs commonly accompany the atypical neuralgias. These may be salivation, lacrimation, nasal congestion, sweating, flushing, diplopia, miosis or ptosis.

Emotional and psychogenic disorders are common among patients of dentists and physicians. These may appear clinically as psychosomatic disorders, self-induced (factitial) injuries, atypical facial pain, cancerphobia, and hysteria or other overt antisocial behavior. It is recognized that lichen planus, benign migratory glossitis, atypical neuralgia and the temporomandibular joint-pain-dysfunction syndrome have a strong psychogenic component, as do a number of the common oral habits such as bruxism, thumb-sucking, lip biting, etc. While a certain degree of anxiety is to be expected in the average dental patient, his complaints cannot be summarily dismissed as neurotic if a logical explanation is not immediately apparent. Rather, the dentist is obligated to carry out a thorough investigation of the patient's signs and symptoms to confirm or rule out the presence of obscure or incipient disease.

2

Chapter 2

Techniques of Initial Examination

OBSERVATION OF PHYSICAL CONDITION

Ordinarily, the receptionist records certain minimal information about the patient in advance of the examination. A review of this information before meeting the patient will be helpful in establishing rapport. In the case of a returning patient, the record of previous visits and treatment should be reviewed.

The patient tends to judge the office *decor* and the auxiliary personnel as well as the dentist. The new patient's judgment may be influenced by considerable apprehension. Common courtesy and a sincere interest in his problems are essential by all during this critical introductory period.

Thus, the dentist may elect to greet the patient in the waiting room to create a "first impression" away from the somewhat colder, clinical atmosphere of the examining room. For the same reason, interrogation may be conducted in the dentist's private office rather than in the operating room.

This first contact with the patient constitutes an essential part of the examination, even if the patient is not aware that he is under observation (Fig. 2–1*A* and *B*). A general evaluation may be made of his movements, manner of dress and of speaking, the mental attitude, as well as the characteristics of his hair, skin and eyes.

INTERROGATION AND RECORDING

The examiner notes the name, age, race, occupation, address and home and office phone numbers of the patient. A questionnaire may be useful to help guide the discussion. It may be completed by the patient and auxiliary prior to the examination, or by the dentist at the time of interrogation. In either case it should be reviewed by the dentist with the patient. Usually the questionnaire contains information concerning the patient's dental and medical history. Reasons for recording this information are obvious or will become more apparent later. For example, certain forms of pathoses may

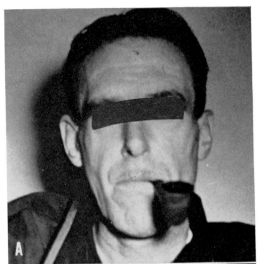

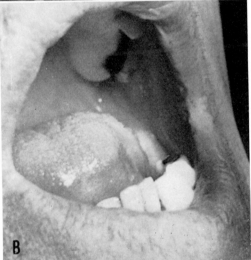

Fig. 2-1. *A,* Patient smoking his pipe in the waiting room prior to the dental appointment. *B,* The slightly raised, adherent white patch of hyperkeratosis on the lip is associated with pipe position. Note the tobacco-stained upper molar.

to an increased susceptibility to dental caries. Certain wind instruments may influence the occlusion of the musician. The dentist, physician, pharmacist, veterinarian or their auxiliary personnel who have access to drugs may take many medications which can influence oral and general health.

The approximate date of the last visit to a dentist should be recorded with a brief notation of services obtained. Any difficulties encountered during previous dental care such as excessive hemorrhage after extractions, or dissatisfaction with the care received, should be noted. These will help to establish the "dental I.Q." of the patient and indicate the need for patient education. In the interest of radiation safety, the date and type of previous diagnostic or therapeutic x-radiation may be important.

The patient's problem (chief complaint) is briefly recorded more or less in his words as the reason for his presence at this time. He may have been recalled for examination. If not, and he states that he is here for a "checkup," this reason should not be accepted initially. Further questioning often reveals why he desires the checkup—perhaps a vague pain has occurred recently, or some other sign or symptom has been recognized, prompting him to appear. If so, this is the item to be recorded. If the patient has been referred by another member of the health professions, it is proper to record the name and address of the referring person, and to acknowledge such referral.

PAST MEDICAL HISTORY

A major objective of the initial examination is to assess the general health of the patient. It is not a substitute for an examination by the patient's physician. If he has not been examined by his physician for some time, and particularly if there is any doubt as to his general health, it is proper and advisable to refer him for such appraisal.

The patient should be asked if he is under the care of a physician for any reason, and the date of his last visit should be recorded

be more or less common among persons with certain occupations; also this information might help in identifying the patient or his record.

Interrogation may begin with the determination or discussion of the *occupation* of the patient. The importance of occupation may be illustrated by the case of the baker who works in an atmosphere of sugar and starch and frequently tastes his products—leading

with the name and address of the physician and the reason for the visit. When indicated, the patient's physician should be consulted to confirm or deny the presence of serious illness that might endanger the patient during dental care or that might endanger the dentist or his auxiliary personnel and other patients through contagion.

Orderly progress through a series of carefully prepared questions is suggested. If at any time a positive or questionable reply is evoked, it should be noted on the record whether it appears to be significant at that time or not, and additional pertinent questions should be asked. Following are some *examples* of questions that may be asked, which briefly survey the major systems of the body. (A more thorough discussion of this topic is given in Chapter 5.) They are worded in a fashion understandable to most patients. Obviously they may be modified depending on such factors as age, education and sex of the patient.

1. Have you suffered any serious illness recently?
2. Have you ever been seriously ill—sufficient to require hospitalization?
3. Have you had any heart disease; or high or low blood pressure; or any disease of the blood?
4. Do you have frequent "colds" or coughing spells?
5. Do you have any difficulty in breathing?
6. Do you have any stomach or intestinal complaints?
7. Have you had any glandular problems such as diabetes or thyroid disease?
8. Have you had any kidney trouble or urinary bladder infections?
9. Do you suffer from fainting spells?
10. Have you ever fainted?
11. Are you taking medicine regularly?
12. Have you ever taken any medicine?
13. Are you allergic to anything?
14. Have you taken penicillin previously?
15. Did it cause trouble in any way?

If most of the replies thus far obtained have been negative, it may be useful to ask at this point: "How is your general health?

How do you feel now?" By this stage of the interview, the patient may feel sufficiently confident to reveal the existence of signs or symptoms that have not been brought out by previous questions. If all appears to be well, at least you may be sure by this time that you have conscientiously tried to detect the presence of general health problems. The permanent record of this fact could provide important diagnostic information and even medicolegal protection for you at a later date.

The significance of the replies clearly entered on the patient's permanent record

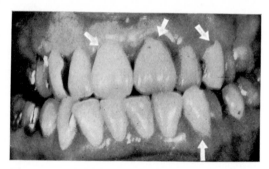

Fig. 2-2. This 35-year-old woman returned with more than 20 new carious lesions. More than a year previously, all of her necessary dental care had been completed. One year previously, accidental brain injury caused narcolepsy. Large doses of amphetamine sulfate were prescribed. Xerostomia and rampant caries resulted.

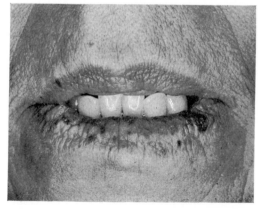

Fig. 2-3. This woman had suffered emotional illness for which a tranquilizer (Thorazine) was prescribed. The resulting xerostomia caused her to lick her lower lip repeatedly, resulting in the cheilitis. Small red ulcers and scabs are present.

becomes increasingly apparent as one progresses in the technique of obtaining the history (Figs. 2–2 and 2–3). Even in the absence of positive replies, it will have been determined whether or not the patient considers himself to be well or ill, and the examiner may reach his own conclusion in this regard also.

The significance of positive replies must be determined. For example, if the patient says he has "high blood pressure," it may be best to discuss the condition with the patient's physician before proceeding with definitive treatment. It is important to determine and record the patient's resting blood pressure in the dental office. Similarly, if he admits to a tendency to bleed excessively following dental extractions, simple tests to determine the bleeding or clotting time can be conducted in the dental office. If these are abnormally prolonged, consultation is necessary. The *techniques* for and *limitations* of such tests will be discussed later.

A history of a respiratory ailment could be of clinical significance, particularly if general anesthesia is planned. Respiratory infections or conditions such as tuberculosis, emphysema and even the common cold constitute a rather substantial risk. The danger of contagion of any unrecognized infection is obvious (Fig. 2–4A and B).

Some commonly voiced complaints of the laity can be useful in establishing the patient's general health or emotional status even though they may have no direct bearing on the diagnosis of an oral condition. For example, a "stomach ailment" might suggest anxiety in some instances, and "female trouble" could have many connotations. Such complaints could be of clinical significance and require further evaluation to determine their importance.

The matter of medications (including self-medication and home remedies) is extremely important. In this day and age, with more than 50,000 prescription items available, careful attention to medications taken by patients is essential. *The Physicians' Desk*

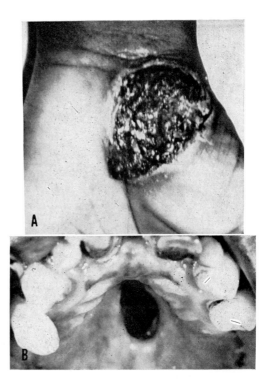

Fig. 2-4. *A*, Gumma of the palm of a patient with syphilis. (Courtesy of Dr. Niles R. Hansen.) *B*, Residual palatal perforation due to a healed gumma in another patient.

Reference and some publications from pharmaceutical firms have color guides which help identify standard drugs by their appearance, whether tablet or capsule.

In a recent year it was estimated that more than two hundred deaths in this country were due to anaphylactic shock brought on by administering penicillin to previously sensitized patients. The increasing use of systemic steroid therapy (administration of cortisone or corticoids such as prednisolone) is gaining importance. A patient who has been taking such drugs can be induced into a state of shock called an adrenal crisis by stress alone. The patient who has suffered from a "stroke" or "heart attack" may be taking anticoagulant therapy such as Dicumarol regularly. If this fact has not been established and the necessary precautions taken, surgery may result in excessive and unexpected hemorrhage thereby endangering the health of the patient.

In summary, the primary purposes of a thorough interrogation and clinical examination are: (1) to detect any oral disease which the dentist will be called upon to treat; (2) to detect any oral signs of systemic diseases which may require consultation with a physician, and thus establish early treatment for the patient; (3) to recognize the patient who may be a poor surgical risk; (4) to protect the dentist, his other patients, and auxiliary personnel against possible contagion; and (5) to allow the examiner to assess the education and attitude of the patient, which may serve as a guide in establishing an effective treatment plan. Through sympathetic questioning, rapport is established and some insight into the educational and socioeconomic status of the patient is gained.

DETECTION OF ABNORMALITY

Once the symptoms have been identified, the focus should be placed on detection of abnormality via the signs noted in the examination. Be alert to any detectable variations in: (1) *morphology*—an increase or decrease in the size, or a change in shape of an anatomic region; (2) *consistency*—a

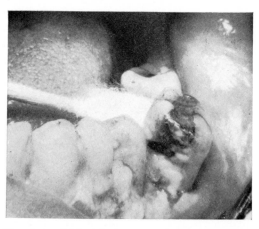

Fig. 2-6. This 81-year-old woman complained of toothache. The excessive mobility of the lower first molar is illustrated. The regional gingival tissue is hyperkeratotic and indurated, and periodontal bone destruction has resulted from this invasive squamous cell carcinoma.

part may feel softer or harder than expected (Fig. 2–5); (3) *color*—intensification, lessening, or change; (4) *mobility*—an exceptionally loose tooth (Fig. 2–6), or limitation of movement of the jaws or tongue; (5) *function*—an increase or decrease in the salivary flow, or a change in speech pattern; (6) *temperature*—an elevation or decrease in body temperature or that of a localized part.

The examiner must use his senses with acuity to detect these signs of abnormality. Even the sense of smell may help one detect the "acetone breath" of the diabetic or the odor of the alcoholic.

THE PHYSICAL ORAL EXAMINATION

The *gait* of the approaching patient, the exposed *skin* (Fig. 2–7) of the face and neck, hands and legs may yield important findings. The *hair* and *eyes* should be observed. Enlarged or painful *lymph nodes* detected by sight, palpation or through the patient's complaint must be noted (Fig. 2–8).

In examining the oral cavity the dentist is entitled, indeed obligated, to have a clear field for observation. The patient should be

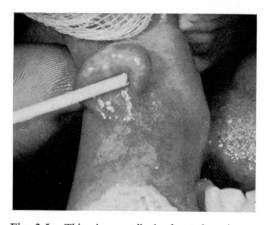

Fig. 2-5. This circumscribed, elevated, pedunculated, soft lesion in the corner of the mouth is characteristic of a fibroma. The normal color of the overlying mucosa and the soft consistency of the lesion are illustrated.

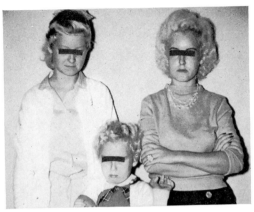

Fig. 2-7. These blond sisters with blue eyes suffered from amelogenesis imperfecta. This illustrates familial ectodermal similarities.

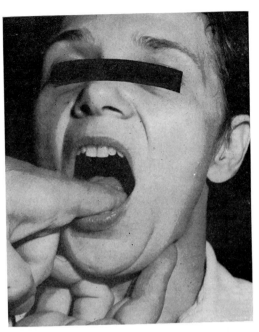

Fig. 2-9. Bimanual palpation for the submaxillary salivary gland. (Fast and Forest, Dent. Clin. North America, March, 1968.)

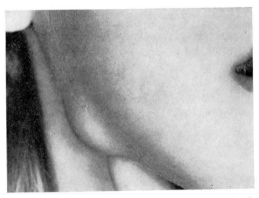

Fig. 2-8. A large submaxillary lymph node is revealed by displacement during palpation.

seated comfortably with proper head support and draping. Adequate lighting is essential. Instruments for the routine examination include a mouth mirror, dental explorer and periodontal pocket probe. If these are supplied in a sterile package which is opened before the patient, this show of cleanliness will reassure him. Adequate visualization also requires that the mouth be free of gross debris. While it is seldom required, the examiner should not hesitate to have the patient rinse the mouth or even use a toothbrush prior to detailed examination. It may be useful to spray the mouth with a cleansing solution.

The regions of the parotid, the submaxillary and sublingual major *salivary glands* should be palpated for enlargement or change in consistency. If they are normal, only the submaxillary salivary glands will be palpable in most instances.

Since the range of normality in a large number of patients is great, constant practice with bimanual, intra- and extraoral palpation (Fig. 2–9) is required to prepare one to recognize minor variations of abnormality. Any unusual findings should be described in some detail in the record.

The examiner should take and record body temperature, blood pressure, and respiratory rates so that occasional deviations from normal will be detected.

Speech defects detected in the course of conversation may provide a clue to the presence of malocclusion, cleft palate, ankyloglossia or a defective prosthetic appliance. Speech may be altered in a person who has suffered a cerebrovascular accident or other neurologic disease.

Observing for abnormal *mandibular movements* during opening and closing of the jaws,

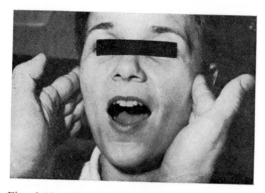

Fig. 2-10. Bilateral palpation of the temporo-mandibular joints. (Fast and Forest, Dent. Clin. North America, March, 1968.)

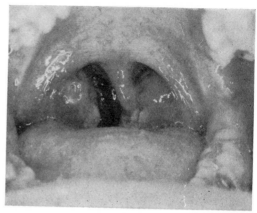

Fig. 2-11. Note the enlarged tonsils behind the anterior palatine pillars. The roughened white surfaces are ulcerated due to Vincent's angina. Dysphagia is a prominent symptom.

and for abnormal lateral and protrusive excursions during simulated chewing, is an important step in the examination. Palpation of the *mandibular condyles* (Fig. 2–10) in front of the ears permits evaluation of excessive or restricted condylar movements and "clicking" of the joints. Any malocclusion observed and the jaw relationship (Angle classifications I to III) should be recorded.

The lips and buccal mucosa are retracted for an unobstructed visual examination and careful, deep palpation is used to detect changes in consistency. Should cursory examination of the soft tissue reveal a suspicious ulcer it might be well to wear a finger cot or rubber glove while palpating the lesion; direct transmission of infection in this way is extremely uncommon, but it is possible.

The inner surface of the lower lip should be dried and examined for a moment or two until the multiple emissions of tiny beads of saliva from the *minor salivary glands* are seen. Secretion of saliva from the orifice of *Stensen's duct* may be induced by gentle massage of the gland anterior to the tragus of the ear.

The soft palate should be examined at rest and in function, and the hard and soft palate should be palpated deftly. Likewise, by depressing the tongue and pulling it forward with a tongue blade or mouth mirror, the examiner may see the *oropharynx* (Fig.

2–11). In a patient with an acute upper respiratory infection, redness of this region may be noted or nasal or sinus drainage may be apparent on the posterior wall of the pharynx (postnasal drip).

The *tongue* at rest may be observed for unusual tremor or surface abnormality. Then it may be grasped with a piece of gauze, gently pulled forward and laterally and its hidden surfaces examined with the aid of the mirror. Palpation of the tongue, especially of the posterolateral borders, should be done. These are common sites for carcinoma and are not easily observed. At this time the *floor of the mouth* may be inspected visually and with bimanual palpation. The submaxillary and sublingual glands should be palpated and the flow of saliva from the orifices of Wharton's ducts observed.

A cursory examination of the *teeth, gingiva* and *alveolar mucosa* is made to detect gross abnormalities, but detailed evaluation of these tissues might better be deferred until full-mouth radiographs have been obtained.

EXAMINATION OF THE TEETH AND PERIODONTIUM

Of the several methods used to designate teeth diagrammatically, none has gained

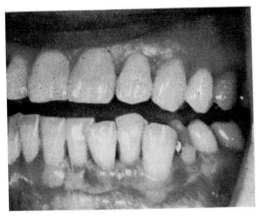

Fig. 2-12. Develop the habit of counting teeth. Note the supernumerary lower anterior tooth.

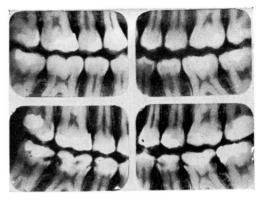

Fig. 2-13. These bite-wing films of an 18-year-old female illustrate the remarkable progress of dental caries from December to the following July. Just after the top radiographs were made, she moved from her home to an apartment and changed many of her eating habits. (Mitchell, in *Oral Hygiene*, ed. by Bunting, Lea & Febiger.)

complete acceptance by the profession. Because the Universal System appears to be the most widely used, it is described here. This system of marking teeth uses the numbers 1 to 32, beginning with the upper right third molar (#1) and progressing around the arch to the upper left third molar (#16) to the lower left third molar (#17) and around the arch to the lower right third molar (#32). The teeth should be examined in numerical sequence, and careful inspection of each tooth surface and the adjacent periodontium is most important (Fig. 2–12). Visual inspection of the teeth and gingiva should be correlated with the commonly used 16-film radiographic survey placed on a viewbox beside the patient. *The films are mounted so that the convexity of the dot on the films is toward the viewer.* Thus the films depict the teeth of the patient that the examiner sees as he faces the patient, and he may readily refer to the films, the teeth and the patient's chart. It should be recognized that the radiograph is simply one additional diagnostic aid and not a substitute for the carefully conducted clinical examination. The radiograph does not accurately demonstrate occlusal surface caries, or periodontal bone loss on the lingual or buccal surfaces of tooth roots. Bite-wing films enhance the study of proxi-

mal surfaces of adjacent teeth and the crest of the alveolar bone (Fig. 2–13).

Each tooth is examined by probing rather forcefully with the point of the sharp explorer in the pits and grooves of the occlusal, buccal and lingual surfaces. The interproximal surfaces are explored to detect hidden carious lesions, cracks, overhanging restorations and calculus. A carious lesion or deep fissure prone to caries is present if the sharp explorer point can be forced into a groove and "sticks" even when the handle is not supported. The marginal ridges of posterior teeth and proximal surfaces of anteriors may show subtle changes in color with direct or reflected light from the dental mirror, revealing the presence of underlying caries. Interproximal decay or a defective restoration sometimes may be detected by passing dental floss between the teeth. If the floss becomes frayed, this may indicate a sharp margin. Compressed air should be used routinely to cleanse and dry the teeth so they may be seen better.

Percussion (tapping the tooth with an instrument such as the handle of the mirror) may induce abnormal movement, pain or a change in sound. The color of the individual tooth and of the teeth in general should be noted.

Compressed air (Fig. 2–14) is used to force away the marginal gingivae and reveal the presence of a deep gingival sulcus or a periodontal pocket and calculus. The gingival crevice around all teeth should be explored gently with the periodontal pocket probe (Fig. 2–15) and unusual findings should be recorded. If heavy calculus, plaque

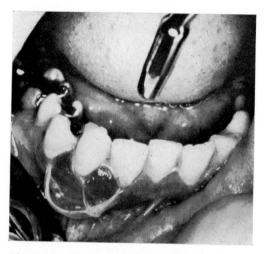

Fig. 2-14. Compressed air on the gingiva of a patient with chronic desquamative gingivitis results in the ballooning of the desquamating layer of the gingival mucosa. (Courtesy of Dr. Stephen F. Dachi.)

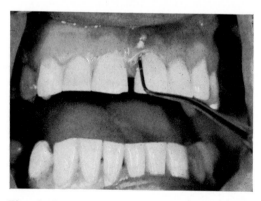

Fig. 2-15. The calibrated periodontal pocket probe is inserted 6 mm subgingivally to the depths of a pointing lateral abscess. The pulp of the associated tooth was vital. (Mitchell, Practical Dental Monographs, Jan. 1965, courtesy of Year Book Medical Publishers Inc.)

or stain is present, a prophylaxis may be necessary before the teeth and root surfaces can be thoroughly examined. Plaque may be demonstrated to the patient by means of a disclosing solution.

Some charting systems call for descriptions of restorations. Although this is very useful in the armed forces since the need for dental identification must be anticipated, this much detail is seldom called for in private practice. Should "dental identification" be necessary for forensic reasons, the records described here and the routine radiographs usually suffice.

INTRODUCTION TO RADIOGRAPHIC INTERPRETATION

Used properly and with discretion, the radiograph is a valuable adjunct in diagnosis. Like all diagnostic aids, however, it is seldom the final answer and remains only an adjunct. Its value is limited to what can be seen on a two-dimensional sheet of translucent material. As with any diagnostic test, mismanagement in the performance and misinterpretation of the results must be avoided.

Orientation

Whether viewing a film or a print of a film in this book, consider that you are viewing the teeth and jaws of the patient looking from the outside into his mouth. Once this stipulation is made, one can determine quickly whether the film represents the right or left side of an upper or lower jaw. For details on the technique of orientation, see Chapter 8.

Anatomy and Age

Note the anatomy of the lamina dura and the trabecular pattern of the periodontal bone. Observe the morphology of the crowns and roots of the teeth, the outline of a maxillary sinus, a foramen or other landmarks. Form the habit of counting teeth. The presence of the deciduous, mixed or permanent dentition will furnish obvious clues as to the age of the patient. The degree of occlusal or incisal wear and the size of pulp chambers are also indicative of age.

Limitations of Interpretation

You are looking at a two-dimensional picture and you cannot read the third dimension into it. Do not try to interpret depth from one film. All you see are shadows of structures of relative radiopacity which lie somewhere between the source of x rays and the film in the mouth. Note the relative density of enamel, dentin and bone. In reference to bone, all one can see is the amount of it; that is, the radiopacity of the bone depends on the thickness of the cortical plates and the numbers and size of the trabeculae. The circumscribed radiolucency denoting periapical lesions is due to the relative absence of bone tissue in the periapical region and the thinness of the overlying cortices.

Radiodense structures include metallic restorative materials, calculus and unusual amounts of bone, as in the torus mandibularis or in productive osseous neoplasms. One cannot determine the chemical or physical properties of bone tissue by routine radiographic examination.

Many factors which occur during exposure and processing of the film may influence interpretation. The amount of exposure, angulation of the rays to the film face, speed of the film, developing and fixation times and temperature and the many possibilities of superimposition of anatomic and foreign structures should be kept in mind. Because of these many factors, the technique of positioning the patient, the film packet, and the tube, and the darkroom procedures are standardized as much as possible so that films processed anywhere will be meaningful to interpreters everywhere.

Foreign bodies which may appear to be embedded in bone actually may be objects loose within the tube of the machine, or resting in the hair on the side of a patient's face, or embedded in soft tissue over the bone.

With these principles in mind and after viewing many radiographs of patients of all ages, one is prepared to detect developmental or acquired defects of teeth and bone. Subsequently, regional perioral structures may be studied through radiography of the temporomandibular joint, major salivary glands, maxillary and other sinuses, and the soft tissues of the cheeks, tongue and floor of the mouth.

EXERCISE IN RADIOGRAPHIC INTERPRETATION

Figure 2–16A illustrates the maxilla of a fetus stillborn 6 months *in utero,* and Figure 2–16B the maxilla of a stillborn at full term. The jaws were disassociated from surrounding structures and occlusal views were made on the table top. In the jaw of the fetus, note that the incisal edges of the deciduous upper central incisors have been calcified, and presumably the morphodifferentiation stage of these and the other primary tooth germs have established the future morphology of the crowns. Identify the nasal septum and out-

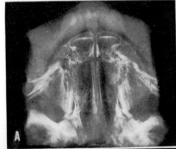

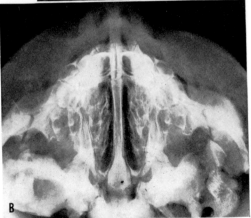

Fig. 2-16.

line of the nose. Note the midline suture and the relative radiolucency on either side of the nasal septum showing the thin palatal bone in this region, in contrast to the thicker alveolar bone around the developing teeth. Compare the structures described above with those seen at birth in the lower picture, 2–16B. Here the outlines of the coronal portions of all the deciduous teeth are apparent. There is an overall increase in size of the jaw with the development of the teeth during the last trimester of pregnancy.

Figure 2–17A and B illustrates the mandibles of the two stillborn. The midline suture is wide in the 6-month fetus. Note the early calcification of some of the teeth and the positions of the follicles of others. The mandible of the full-term infant shows a tendency toward closure of the midline suture and increasing development of the 10 deciduous teeth. There is a space for the follicle of

the first permanent molar. Notice how the body of the mandible is rather fully occupied with these few small teeth, and give thought to the amount of growth that must take place during the next several years so that the jaws may accommodate 16 larger permanent teeth.

The midline suture of the mandible should close sometime during the first year of life. Viewing a conventional periapical film of the lower centrals of a 6-month-old infant has resulted in misinterpretation by examiners who considered this line to be a fracture.

Using the principles outlined thus far, study the following figures carefully. Remember orientation, anatomy and age, limitations of interpretation, and the possible occurrence of technical artifact. *After you have answered the related questions, refer to page 41 et seq. and compare answers.*

Figure 2–18. Which side of the maxilla is portrayed? How old is the patient? Do you see signs of disease or other abnormality?

Figure 2–19A–D shows periapical views of one individual. The patient's right side is on your left. How old is the patient? What is wrong, if anything? What is the prognosis?

Figure 2–20 shows a bite-wing film of which side? What is the patient's age? What is wrong, if anything? Note the anatomy of the crowns of the maxillary teeth.

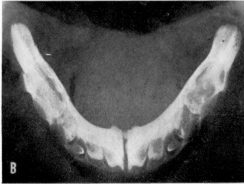

Fig. 2-17.

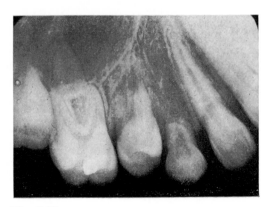

Fig. 2-18.

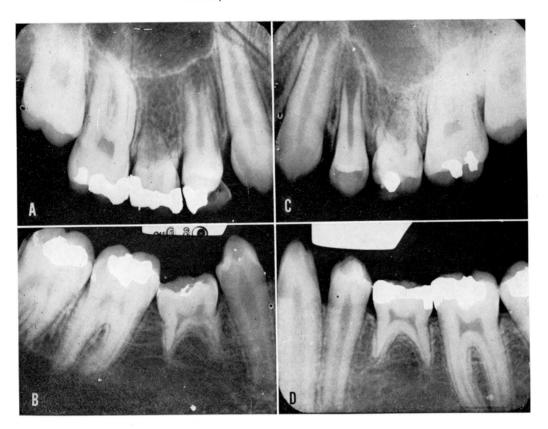

Fig. 2-19.

Figure 2–21A and B is of the lower anterior region, and the canine and bicuspid of which side? In the conventional (labiolingual) view of the canine, note that the pulp resembles a rather straight string. In the midline view, however, the morphology is entirely different (a mesiodistal portrayal due to position of the edge of the film and direction of the beam). This should be kept in mind during restorative procedures. One cannot see the three-dimensional anatomy in a single radiograph. Near the neck of the canine on the distal surface in Figure 2–21A is a radiolucent area. Is this a carious lesion? Note the size and morphology of the pulps of the incisors. What is the circular radiopacity with the central radiolucency well below the apices of the incisors?

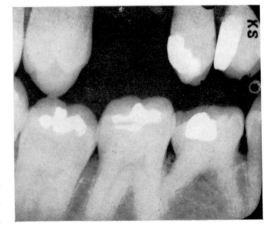

Fig. 2-20.

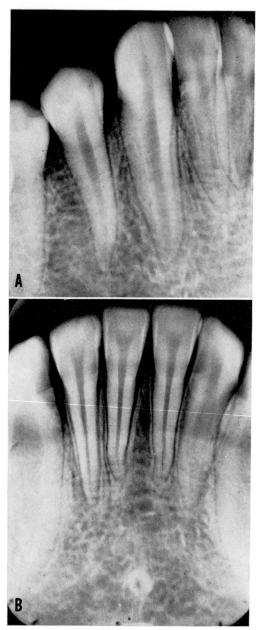

Fig. 2-21.

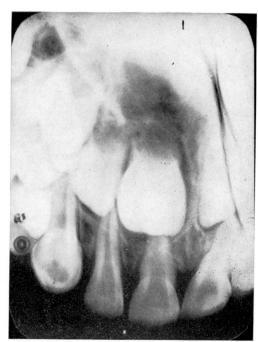

Fig. 2-22.

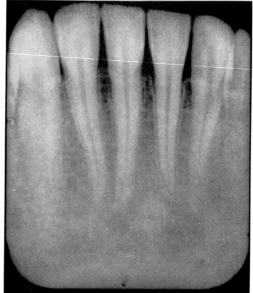

Fig. 2-23.

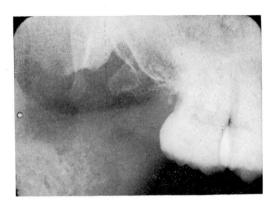

Fig. 2-24.

Figure 2–22. How old is this patient? What artifact is apparent? Are the diastemas normal? Is there evidence of abnormality?

Figure 2–23. How old is the patient? What is the circular radiopacity just beneath the apices of the centrals?

Figure 2–24. After orientation, name the structures illustrated and look for pathosis.

Figure 2–25. Why did this patient lose his central incisors? What are the two radiolucent vertical lines in the alveolar process?

Figure 2–26. Which side of the mandible is shown?

Figure 2–27. This shows the lower right second or third molar and in the lower cor-

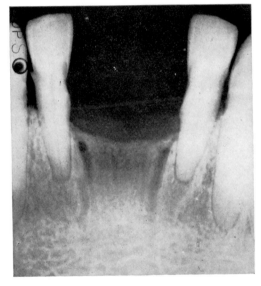

Fig. 2-25.

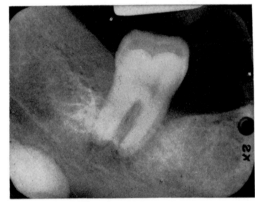

Fig. 2-27.

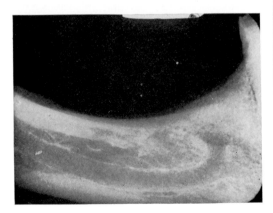

Fig. 2-26.

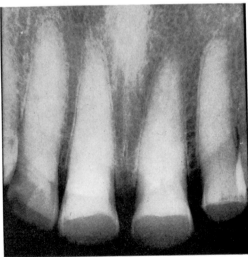

Fig. 2-28.

ner of the film a radiopaque object is seen; note its morphology. The apices of the molar tooth are surrounded by a radiolucent area.

Figure 2–28. Orient yourself. Study the teeth and periodontium. What is the age of the patient? Is there any obvious pathosis or periodontal bone loss? *Refer to page 43 and compare answers.*

Figure 2–29. This is a conventional periapical view. Can you orient yourself and explain why this looks so different from the previous views of the upper anterior region?

Figure 2–30. This is a conventional view of the lower incisor region of the same patient (above). What is the relatively radiopaque extension in the center of the film?

Figure 2–31. How old is the patient? Are the diastemas of importance? Is there undue crowding of the permanent incisors?

Figure 2–32*A* and *B*. What is the age of this patient? Is developmental or other abnormality apparent? The crowns of the lateral incisors suggest abnormality that could be interpreted as *dens in dente.*

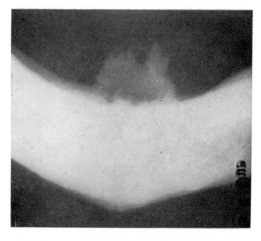

Fig. 2-30.

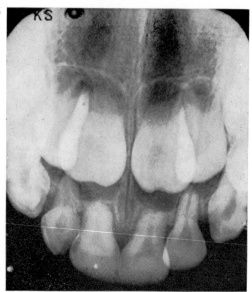

Fig. 2-31.

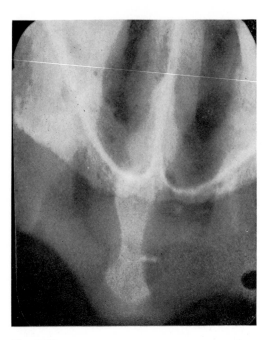

Fig. 2-29.

Figure 2–33. This is an extraoral view of the left mandible of an 18-year-old male. Note the phase of development and lack of eruption of the lower third molar. The patient was asymptomatic and the pulps of the first and second permanent molars were vital. The radiolucency around the apices of the first permanent molar is continuous with the extensive radiolucency seen further poste-

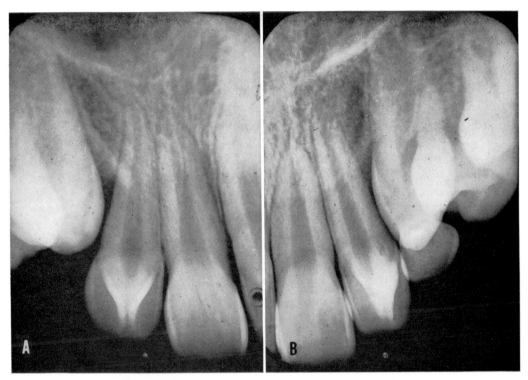

Fig. 2-32.

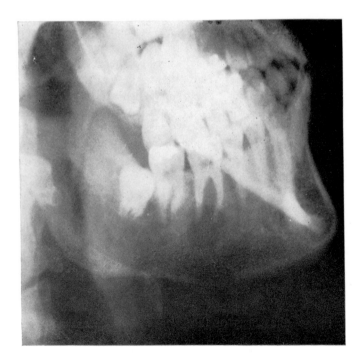

Fig. 2-33.

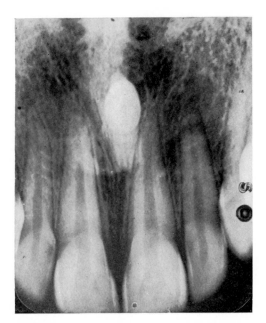

Fig. 2-34.

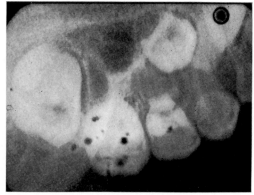

Fig. 2-35.

riorly. With this information at hand, and viewing this radiograph, how many conditions could you name that the radiolucency might represent?

Figure 2–34. This illustration serves as an introduction to treatment planning. How old is the patient? What is the radiopaque structure in the middle of the picture? What treatment do you recommend? Why?

Artifacts

A few of the many artifacts which may occur due to positioning, exposure, processing, and interpretation of films are illustrated here.

Figure 2–35. This is a portion of a routine pedodontic survey wherein a conventional adult periapical film was used to obtain an occlusal view of the maxilla. The patient was asked to hold the film gently in place with his teeth but he bit it instead. Note that the "radiolucent" dots due to biting pressure correspond to the tips of the cusps of the deciduous molars.

Figure 2–36. In the composite illustration (A, B and C), the periapical film to your

upper right shows a radiopacity of unusual shape near the apex of the upper left central incisor. This radiograph was taken of a patient in an institution for the mentally retarded. After the results were seen, a second radiograph was taken, using the same machine, as depicted on your upper left. The angulation of the rays was varied and the object apparently "moved," so calculations were made to determine whether the foreign body was nearer the labial than the palatal surface. The results were not conclusive, so the occlusal view at the bottom of the figure was made. Notice that the foreign body again appears next to the upper left central as in the original radiograph. Plans were made for surgical exploration and removal of the foreign body.

Fortunately, a consultant was aware of the circumstances and the fact that the x-ray machine had been modified the day before, taking steps necessary to make the machine safer. The machine was used irregularly in this population because of the difficulty of obtaining routine full-mouth radiographs on many of the retarded patients. Practice exposures with the same machine using films lying on the bracket table, revealed this same foreign body on subsequently developed films.

The final diagnosis was a periapical radiolucency of the non-vital (by pulp test) upper

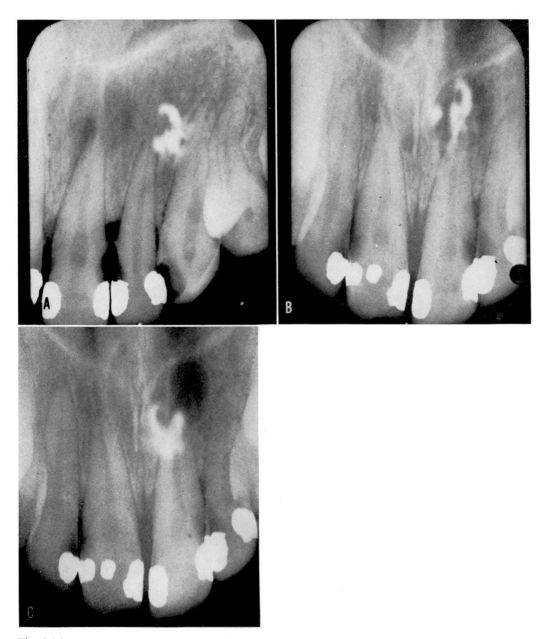

Fig. 2-36.

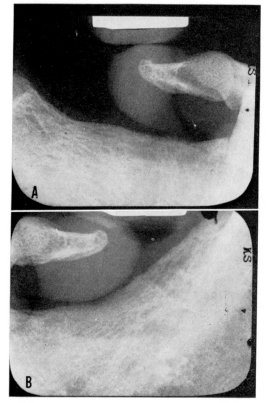

left central incisor—and the presence of an elusive metallic filing within the x-ray tube.

Figure 2–37*A* and *B*. These radiographs illustrate the mandible of a partially edentulous patient. Note that the two films were not placed as deeply as they could have been, and there are two peculiar "lesions" above the posterior alveolar ridges. The similarity of these "lesions" is undeniable. The diagnosis was bilateral "phalangiomas."

Fig. 2-37.

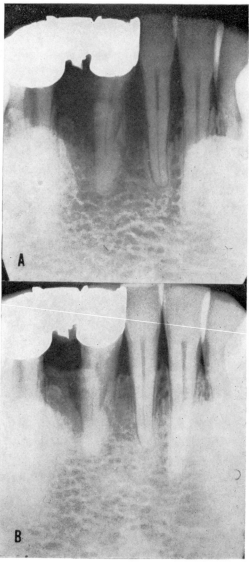

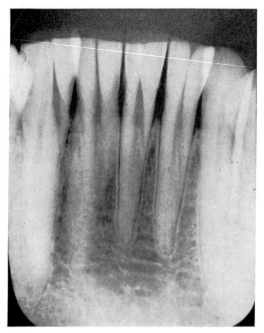

Fig. 2-38.   Fig. 2-39.

Figure 2–38. Look carefully at this illustration (and avoid the mistake of double exposure in the future)!

Figures 2–39*A* and *B*. This shows two different views of the same region of a patient. The top picture, *A*, might suggest severe periodontal disease, whereas the one below, *B*, would not. This is an example of inadequate exposure time in *A* above, and normal exposure time below, *B*. The bilateral radiopacities are mandibular tori.

Figure 2–40. Artifacts also occur during film processing. Notice the fingerprint and the dark spots resulting from contamination of the film in the darkroom by the dental

hygienist who had just given the patient a prophylaxis and a stannous fluoride treatment.

Figure 2–41. Whereas the radiolucency in the region of the upper lateral incisor and canine might suggest to the uninitiated that it is a globulomaxillary cyst, a water spot on the drying film created this illusion.

Answers to Questions in Exercise

Figure 2–18. Upper right bicuspid region. Eleven years old. Based on the radiograph alone, one would have to say "plus or minus a year." Root formation and eruption of the second molar have only begun. Note the extent of root formation of the bicuspid. Did you count the teeth and note their morphology? The deciduous canine is partially resorbed although there is no succedaneous tooth above it. It is not possible to say precisely why resorption took place or whether it will continue. The permanent canine and a bicuspid are congenitally missing. Since we can see two roots on the bicuspid, the odds would suggest that this is a first bicuspid and that the second is missing. Note the diastemas.

Figure 2–19. The patient is probably 11 or 12 years of age. The lower "12-year molars" are in position with considerable root formation; however, the upper second molars have not entirely erupted, and the roots of the upper bicuspids and cuspids are incompletely formed. Four second deciduous molars are retained and there are no permanent successors. The upper right first deciduous molar, with a disto-occlusal restoration in it, is retained by gingival attachment although the root has been resorbed. This loose crown may well have been the cause of discomfort that occasioned the visit. Notice the mesial tipping of the lower right first and second permanent molars, impacting the second deciduous molar. The lamina dura around this deciduous tooth suggests the possibility of ankylosis. To determine this, do not rely on the radiograph alone, but tap the tooth and listen to the sound. Ankylosed

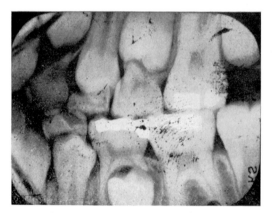

Fig. 2-40.

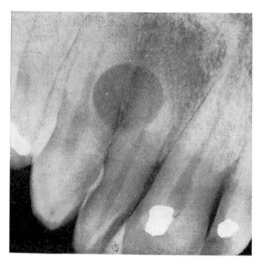

Fig. 2-41.

teeth have a "ring" while healthy periodontal ligaments yield a dull, "muffled" sound when percussed because of the cushioning effect of the ligament. In any case, deciduous "space maintainers" are in place, and may or may not be shed. Watchful waiting during this developmental period is recommended. The bilaterality of developmental anomalies is demonstrated.

Figure 2–20. Right side. Missing upper first permanent molar. Retained lower deciduous second molar. The patient is 63 years of age, as suggested by the abrasion apparent as a radiolucent area on the occlusal surface of the lower first molar, and by the diminished pulp size in all of the teeth. Figure 2–20*A* shown here is the bite-wing film of the opposite side. Note that the abnormality is bilateral—often the case with developmental defects. See the wide-spread roots of the retained deciduous tooth. If a permanent bicuspid had been present, as it erupted the roots of the deciduous tooth might have been resorbed in their coronal one-half and the tips could have been left intact. Indeed, it is in the lower bicuspid region that retained deciduous root tips are seen most frequently in later life. These are of no consequence unless they are connected with the mouth, symptomatic, or surrounded by radiolucency.

Figure 2–21*A* and *B*. The midline and the right side of the mandible are shown.

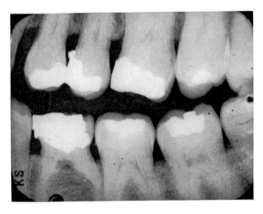

Fig. 2-20A.

Since the roots are fully formed and all teeth are erupted, the patient must be at least 14 or 15 years of age, because root formation usually is complete within a year or so after eruption. This patient is 16 years old as revealed by the large pulp size and lack of occlusal wear. The radiolucency on the distocervical surface of the cuspid is "adumbration" (umbra—shadow), an artifact of anatomy. In dental anatomy you learned that the distal surface of the root of this tooth was concave. The x rays pass through this and the small amount of bone near the cervix more readily, creating the illusion of a cavity. If it were a carious lesion, it would be at or just below the contact, and *not* subgingival.

Figure 2–22. Since the deciduous teeth are in position, the patient must be over 2 years of age; the fact that the developing crowns of the permanent teeth are nearly complete and root formation is beginning would suggest that he is 4 or 5 years of age. The linear black lines were caused by creasing the film when the large film packet was placed in the small mouth of the child. More diastemal space will be needed before clinical eruption of the larger crowns of the permanent teeth can take place. Compare the size of the permanent and deciduous central incisors and recognize that growth and development will allow the 32 large permanent teeth to succeed the 20 small deciduous ones. No pathosis is apparent.

Figure 2–23. All roots are fully formed and the pulps are rather small. Incisal attrition is mild. The age can only be estimated as a young to middle-aged adult. The circular radiopacity represents the bony canal around the so-called lingual foramen. It is not always present as a distinct entity. It is on the lingual surface in the region of the genial tubercles. The inferior border of the chin is very radiopaque. (Feel your chin.) Adumbration is seen on the distal side of the lower right lateral incisor.

Figure 2–24. This represents the upper right posterior region. Note the coronoid process which is *not* "behind" the upper third molar as it may appear. One cannot read the third dimension. Remember how this film was placed in the patient's mouth and the direction from which the x-ray beam came. Note the posterior tuberosity and the bony extension posteriorly which represents an exostosis. See the hamular process springing down from the superimposed pterygoid plates. Actually this film was made on a skull. It would be difficult to place the film so far posteriorly in the mouth of a living patient because of the soft palate and posterior pharyngeal wall.

Figure 2–25. Periodontal disease undoubtedly caused the loss of the central incisors. Note the calculus on the rounded mesial aspects of the roots of the laterals, and the spicule at the cervix of the right lateral. The height of the alveolar bone is decreased. The radiolucent lines represent nutrient canals which are normally present but seldom visualized as well. When the teeth are lost and the alveolar process shrinks, it not only decreases in height but also becomes thinner in a labiolingual direction. The prosthodontic patient with this remodeling is said to have a "knife-edge ridge." In this patient, with thinner cortices and less marrow space, and no superimposing teeth, the nutrient canals are readily apparent. Such canals are between all the teeth, but are seldom seen.

Figure 2–26. You may have thought the ascending radiopacity to your right was the ascending ramus, and that this represented the lower left posterior portion of the mandible. If so, you were wrong. It is a canine tooth with some incisal abrasion. The periodontal membrane space is not very marked, but it is apparent. Thus, this is the lower right side. Notice the mandibular canal opening to the mental foramen. The teeth of the patient have been missing for some time; hence the decrease in height of the alveolar process. In general, bone is created for the body where it is needed, and it is withdrawn when it is not.

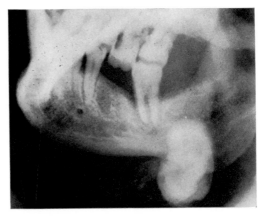

Fig. 2-27A.

Figure 2–27. Another radiograph of the same patient, Figure 2–27*A* is shown here to explain the previous one. In this view, note that the relationship of the molar tooth to the radiopaque object has been reversed due to the fact that this is an extraoral view, and the film was held against the side of the face (instead of in the mouth) and the x rays were directed through the right mandible in an oblique direction. The radiopacity now clearly is not a third or "fourth molar" and probably is not within bone. Indeed it is a large sialolith which occupies almost the entire right submaxillary salivary gland. Note also the mental foramen and coronoid process.

Figure 2–28. The patient is elderly (77 years old) as suggested by the extreme amount of abrasion. Although contact points have been lost due to the wear, the periodontal bone is of a good height and the relative radiopacity is unusually marked. This patient chewed tobacco and introduced much abrasive material into his mouth with the leaf.

Figure 2–29. The patient was edentulous and had worn no dentures for many years. As a consequence, there was very little alveolar process behind which an incisal view film could be placed. The film, therefore, had to be placed almost horizontal, parallel to the flat palate. Then, in order for the x-ray beam to approach the desirable 90-

degree angle to the film, the tube had to be placed above the nose and the rays directed downward in an "occlusal" direction. Note the extremely thin alveolar process, the cartilaginous nasal septum, outline of the nose, and internal nasal passages.

Figure 2–30. For the same reasons, film position was that of an occlusal view and the x rays were directed upward from beneath the chin. The genial tubercles, which often become elongated with age (as do other bony prominences at sites of muscle attachments), are apparent. Such a mass can be palpated on the lingual surface of the mandible, at the sites of attachment of the geniohyoid and genioglossus muscles in older patients.

Figure 2–31. This 4- or 5-year-old child has a deciduous dentition with roots beginning to resorb. Hopefully, additional diastemas will occur in time for the eruption of the larger permanent incisors. If you neglected to study the morphology of the developing central incisors, you may not have noted that the incisal edges are notched and the crowns are screwdriver-shaped. These are typical Hutchinsonian incisors. It was suspected from the gross appearance that this child might have congenital syphilis. Such a history was denied by the parent. This view corroborated the diagnosis.

Figure 2–32A and B. Did you note the retained crown of the patient's left deciduous cuspid? He is approximately 10 or 11 years old. See Figure 2–32C, which shows a cast of the teeth of this patient. Note the unusual cingulum on each lateral incisor, and again observe that one cannot interpret the third dimension in the previous films. This is an exophytic bulging of the enamel, rather than an endodontic invagination. Note the retained deciduous crown and the space for the permanent tooth on the opposite side. The second permanent molar has erupted on one side, but not on the other. Except for a somewhat narrow anterior arch, and the unusually formed lateral incisors, developmental anatomy is within the range of normality.

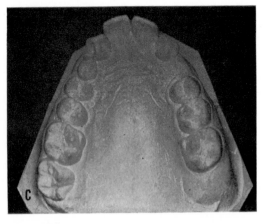

Fig. 2-32C.

Figure 2–33. A multilocular radiolucent lesion near the angle of the mandible in a young male should immediately suggest the possibility of ameloblastoma. In the differential diagnosis, other benign neoplasms should be considered. "Osteitis fibrosa cystica" of hyperparathyroidism could be represented here with a gross "brown tumor" consisting microscopically of many giant cells and vascular connective tissue. Multiple myeloma, histiocytosis X, the xanthomatoses, lymphosarcoma, metastatic carcinoma or sarcoma, and a host of other conditions could be on your list.

By aspiration, 5 ml of blood were obtained. The lesion was surgically explored (cautiously), and a then empty cavity with no distinct lining was seen. The wound was closed and it healed uneventfully. A diagnosis of traumatic hemorrhagic cyst was made.

Figure 2–34. This is an exercise dealing with *treatment planning*. The patient is a young adult. The central object is an inverted mesiodens. Note the enamel of the crown, the dentin of the remainder of the tooth, including the complete root formation and the pulp chamber. Before you elect to remove this supernumerary tooth, or before you elect to leave it alone, consider the consequences. If this is a "captive patient" whom you have known and can expect to be able to follow regularly, this may affect your point of view. On the other hand, if this is a new patient, perhaps a man who has orders to go overseas with the armed forces in three days, this will affect your judgment.

Assuming that you can neither see the mesiodens intraorally nor palpate it, the next step would be to locate it by use of an occlusal view radiograph. Let us say that it is found to be centrally located within bone. If you elect to remove it surgically, simply because it does not belong there, might you endanger the vitality of one central incisor, or both? Would immediate endodontics be required during or following removal? Could a postoperative infection trouble your patient in the immediate future?

If you elect to leave the mesiodens alone, what might occur? Could eruptive forces endanger either central incisor? This is entirely unlikely because of the direction in which the tooth is pointing. Eruption, like growth, takes place during tooth formation, and active eruption ceases once the root is developed. Even if active eruption should occur, the tooth would move nasally away from the apices of the permanent teeth. A supernumerary tooth is a hamartoma which has no continuous growth potential like a true neoplasm.

Observe the radiolucent region immediately around the crown of the supernumerary tooth. What tissues are present? Certainly epithelial tissue and fibrous connective tissue are present. The epithelium is the remnant of the ameloblasts which were derived from the inner-enamel epithelium, and this could give rise to the development of a dentigerous (follicular) cyst. As you know, the dentigerous cyst can develop the benign yet dangerous ameloblastoma within its wall. The usual treatment for ameloblastoma is less than conservative, and in this case might mean a partial maxillectomy. Should this be the fate of your soldier patient abroad under dire circumstance? Now, what is your decision?

Recognize that the mesiodens is uncom-mon, the inverted mesiodens is less common, and the dentigerous cyst around the crown of the inverted mesiodens is exceedingly rare. The occurrence of an ameloblastoma in this position around an inverted mesiodens is almost unheard of. Therefore, with due consideration and careful playing of the odds, you might well decide to leave the condition as it is, advise the patient and give him a copy of the radiograph, and suggest that he advise the first dental officer he encounters as well as those he may meet later. Should any problem arise, it is most unlikely to be of an immediate nature, and conservative surgical removal could be done later if necessary. Obviously if the patient were elderly, a similar decision could have been made very easily.

INTRODUCTION TO TREATMENT PLANNING

Treatment planning for a dental patient is done after a thorough examination has been made, including evaluation of the patient's mental attitude toward dentistry, educational background, his emotional, sociologic, and financial status, age and general health. These factors are as important as the intraoral findings in planning treatment, and because of this fact a final plan often may not be made until late in the treatment phase. For example, a removable prosthesis might not be indicated in a patient with seizures or severe ataxia, or with a history of therapeutic radiation around the mouth.

The following is an *example* of a sequence that could be used to plan treatment for many routine patients. Since all patients differ, deviations from this framework will be necessary.

Initial Phase

1. Evaluate systemic factors which might alter the actual method of treatment. For example, patients with a history of rheumatic fever may need prophylactic antibiotics before certain treatment, those with hypertension or who are excessively

apprehensive may need sedation, and patients with hemorrhagic tendencies may need transfusions prior to or following surgery. Consultation would be indicated in such cases.

2. Detect, control and/or eradicate any neoplasia, hemorrhage, pain or other problems of an emergency nature. Techniques used might include cytologic smears, biopsy, special radiographs, hemograms, and exploration. Treatment might vary from excision or pulp capping to incision and drainage, or referral.

3. Control beginning pathosis. Perform gross scaling and temporarily restore large carious lesions. Determine caries susceptibility and advise patients of preventive measures. Correct damaging habits, accomplish occlusal analysis and design fixed or removable restorations.

Treatment Phase

4. Prophylaxis, subgingival curettage, or other periodontal therapy. Endodontic care. Interceptive orthodontics.

5. Permanent restoration of carious and missing teeth and restoration of functional occlusion and proper esthetics. For example, this phase might entail the placement of an amalgam restoration in a patient with only one cavity; or the extensive operative, fixed and removable prosthetic care necessary in a patient with many missing teeth and a high degree of caries susceptibility; or a post-mandibulectomy somatoprosthesis.

Maintenance Phase

6. Post-reconstruction home care advice and recall. Patients should be advised of good home care of periodontal and dental tissues, how to care for dentures, partials, and how to clean under pontics. They should also be advised to return for periodic examinations at 6-month intervals. (See Fig. 7–36.)

BIBLIOGRAPHY

Burket, L. W.: *Oral Medicine. Diagnosis and Treatment,* 6th Ed., Philadelphia, J. B. Lippincott Co., 1971.

Cecil and Loeb Textbook of Medicine: Paul B. Beeson and Walsh McDermott, editors, 11th Ed., Philadelphia, W. B. Saunders Co., 1963.

Cheraskin, E.: Roentgenographic manifestations of osseous changes in the jaws, Oral Surg., *12,* 442, 1959.

Colby, R. A., Kerr, D. A. and Robinson, H. B. G.: *Color Atlas of Oral Pathology,* 2d Ed., Philadelphia, J. B. Lippincott Co., 1961.

Dent. Clin. North America, Oral Medicine Symposium, David F. Mitchell, consulting editor, March, 1968.

Drinnan, A. J. and Fischman, S. L.: Medical-dental relationships, Dent. Clin. North America, March, 1968.

Ennis, L. M., Berry, H. M., and Phillips, J. E.: *Dental Roentgenology,* 6th Ed., Philadelphia, Lea & Febiger, 1967.

Ghadimi, H.: Diagnosis of inborn errors of amino acid metabolism, Amer. J. Dis. Child, *114,* 433, 1967.

Gorlin, R. J. and Pindborg, J. J.: *Syndromes of the Head and Neck,* New York, McGraw-Hill Book Co., 1964.

Harrison, T. R., Adams, R. D., Bennett, L. L., Jr., Resnik, W. H., Thorn, G. W. and Wintrobe, M. M.: *Principles of Internal Medicine,* 5th Ed., New York, McGraw-Hill Book Co., 1966.

Hayduk, S., Bennett, C. R., and Monheim, L. M.: Subcutaneous emphysema after operative dentistry: report of a case, J. Amer. Dent. Ass., *80,* 1362, 1970.

Identification guide for solid dosage forms, J.A.M.A., *182,* 1145, 1962.

Kerr, D. A., Ash, M., Jr. and Millard, H. D.: *Oral Diagnosis,* 3rd Ed., St. Louis, C. V. Mosby Co., 1970.

McCarthy, P. L. and Shklar, Gerald: *Diseases of the Oral Mucosa,* New York, McGraw-Hill Book Co., 1964.

Myers, H. M., Dumas, M. and Bullhorn, H. B.: Dental manifestations of phenylketonuria, J. Amer. Dent. Ass., *77,* 586, 1968.

Nizel, A. E.: *The Science of Nutrition and Its Application in Clinical Dentistry,* Philadelphia, W. B. Saunders Co., 1966.

Physicians' Desk Reference: Product Identification Section, 30th Ed., Oradell, N. J., Medical Economics, Inc., 1976.

Shafer, W. G., Hine, M. K. and Levy, B. H.: *A Textbook of Oral Pathology,* 3rd Ed., Philadelphia, W. B. Saunders Co., 1974.

Stafne, E. C.: *Oral Roentgenographic Diagnosis,* 3rd Ed., Philadelphia, W. B. Saunders Co., 1969.

Section II

Comprehensive Clinical Oral Diagnosis

This section is designed to:

1. reinforce the background knowledge of the reader in the genetics and epidemiology of oral disease (Chaps. 3, 4)

2. describe the utilization of the health history and diagnostic techniques and procedures available for the clinical demonstration of disease processes (Chaps. 5, 6)

3. describe the more common conditions typically encountered at the various oral and extraoral sites under the purview of the dentist (Chap. 7)

4. review the methods for routine and special radiographic examination and interpretation (Chap. 8) and

5. survey oral and clinical laboratory methods and their application in the diagnosis of oral and systemic disease states (Chap. 9).

Chapter 3

Epidemiologic Considerations*

A complete understanding of the anamnesis, the collected data concerning a patient, is mandatory; and a basic knowledge of epidemiology helps to bring it about.

The very term *epidemiology* seems to cause an aversion in some dental practitioners. For them it connotes field work, voluminous reports, complicated statistics, and even more complicated results. They feel that this is work for public health officials and need not concern the clinician. However, epidemiologic methods help the clinician to gather and interpret facts relevant to his patient's medical history, present condition and prognosis.

* Contributed by Charles E. Tomich, D.D.S., M.S.D., *Associate Professor, Department of Oral Pathology, School of Dentistry, Indiana University—Purdue University at Indianapolis.*

DEFINITION OF EPIDEMIOLOGY

Epidemiology, a broad and complex discipline, was defined at a meeting of American epidemiologists in 1952 as the study of all factors and combinations of factors that affect health and disease in a population. Etymologically, the word is derived from the Greek *epi,* upon, and *demos,* people. Thus, it is the study of diseases which occur "upon the people."

Frost (cited by Rogers) defined epidemiology as "the science of the mass phenomena of diseases." Although one invariably thinks of epidemics of contagious diseases in relation to epidemiology, this is only part of the epidemiologist's area of inquiry. His investigations are not limited to communicable diseases; rather, epidemiology is the study of *all diseases and all health concerns* of human groups in relation to total environment. Its principles are applied to cardiovascular problems, cancer, malnutrition, mental illness, hereditary and congenital diseases, and even to accidents.

Epidemiology is no newcomer to medical science. Naturally, diseases which affected vast portions of the population were the early targets of epidemiologic investigations. Perhaps the earliest disease to be scrutinized, mentioned in Biblical times, was leprosy.

Some believe that many cases called leprosy at that time were, in fact, psoriasis.

While the scope is broader, the epidemiologic method used today—namely, *observe, record* and *reflect*—is not essentially different from the method used in the school of Hippocrates. After Hippocrates, epidemiology was at a standstill until the time of Galen, who renewed the interest in it and did much to revive the teachings of Hippocrates. After Galen, interest in epidemiology (and in science as a whole) again declined until the sixteenth century. At that time, a biologist, Fracastorius, wrote on contagion and contagious diseases. He studied and named syphilis. Gordon credits him with laying the foundation for modern epidemiology.

The epidemiologist may start with a number of cases and use them as a reference to a population, or he may start with a population and find cases of disease in it. He must be constantly aware of variations which exist in human traits, and must understand how the environment may affect the group under investigation. His objective is a better understanding of the nature of disease and an identification of any predisposing factors. Populations with a high rate of a certain disease and, conversely, those with a low rate of the disease, are studied with the hope that the cause and associated factors may be identified. By identifying these factors, epidemiology can teach people how to avoid disease and live healthy lives.

RELEVANT AREAS OF EPIDEMIOLOGIC INVESTIGATION

As a method of learning about disease and health, epidemiology is important to all members of the health services. The dentist is especially concerned with epidemiologic studies of oral diseases and conditions, and certain related medical problems.

Cardiovascular Disease

Cardiovascular disease is the primary threat to existence and is responsible for over 720,000 deaths (38 percent) yearly in the United States. Statistics by the American Heart Association indicate that more than 14.5 million adults between 18 and 79 years of age have heart disease.

Rheumatic Fever and Rheumatic Heart Disease

Rheumatic fever is an infectious, febrile disease which occurs as a delayed result of infection (usually upper respiratory) with group A hemolytic streptococci. It is characterized by inflammatory changes in the joints and the heart. *Rheumatic heart disease* is a result of rheumatic fever, and is essentially a pancarditis although the endocardium is usually most critically involved. The endocardium covering the valves becomes thickened and later scarred. This causes stenosis of the valve opening and "heart murmurs" often result.

Epidemiologists disagree about the influence of such factors as constitution, climate, geography, diet, urbanization and household conditions. Morton and co-workers collected epidemiologic data on more than 17,000 Colorado school children, and found a prevalence rate of 1.7 cases of rheumatic heart disease per 1000. The prevalence rates appeared to be higher in children from lower socioeconomic levels. This seems to be borne out by other investigators, who found the highest incidence rate among teen-agers, possibly because older children are more likely to be exposed to streptococcal infection. These investigators felt that apparent ethnic differences were probably due to socioeconomic factors.

Rheumatic fever is encountered much more often in the northern states than in the southern. The greater prevalence in lower economic strata probably is due to poverty and associated malnutrition, overcrowding and substandard housing, all of which may predispose to increased incidence of streptococcal disease. In addition, there is some evidence for a hereditary predisposition to the disease.

Only one-third of the patients with rheumatic fever recover completely with no evidence of cardiac disease. Thus, the history of rheumatic fever and/or rheumatic heart disease is of considerable importance to the dentist. It has been estimated that a million people in the United States have rheumatic heart disease.

A patient with a history of rheumatic fever or rheumatic heart disease poses a special problem to the dental practitioner. Dental prophylaxis, periodontal surgery and other oral surgical procedures could endanger such a patient by creating a bacteremia which could lead to the life-threatening disease *subacute bacterial endocarditis,* with bacterial vegetations on the already scarred valves. A large retrospective study of 60 patients with bacterial endocarditis who were seen at the University of Michigan Hospital during a 10-year period has been reported by Mostaghim and Millard. It was shown that some dental procedures were responsible for the development of bacterial endocarditis; however, oral infections such as pericoronitis and periapical abscesses were shown to be precipitating factors. For this reason, the American Heart Association recommends treatment with penicillin (or other antibiotics in penicillin-sensitive individuals) starting 1 to 2 hours before the procedure and continuing for 2 days thereafter.

Congenital Heart Disease

Congenital heart disease includes a group of pathologic conditions due to faulty development of the heart and great vessels during embryonic life. It is the cause of approximately 2 percent of all deaths, but clinically accounts for approximately 5 percent of all cardiovascular diseases, and over half of all heart diseases in children. Between 30,000 and 40,000 children are born annually in the United States with heart defects. Approximately half of these children die during childhood. On the other hand, modern diagnostic and cardiac surgical methods are enabling a greater number of afflicted children to live normal or near-normal lives.

Congenital heart defects, as with all congenital defects, may be due to genetic or environmental factors. A positive family history is good evidence for genetic factors. Consanguinity predisposes to congenital defects, and has been implicated in congenital heart disease. Higgins, however, feels that although this factor may account for an increased incidence, it is not important in the etiology of congenital heart disease. The high incidence of congenital heart defects in patients with Down's disease (mongolism) has long been known.

Radiation, anoxia, certain drugs (*e.g.* thalidomide, cortisone) and maternal rubella infection during early pregnancy may predispose to developmental defects. A disconcerting fact, however, is that in most cases of congenital heart disease neither genetic nor environmental factors can be implicated.

Morton and Huhn found a prevalence rate of 4.6 cases per 1000 school children. Atrial septal defects and valvular pulmonic stenosis were the defects encountered most frequently. Similar studies showed prevalence rates ranging from 1.5 cases per 1000 individuals in Chicago to 6.0 cases per 1000 in Miami.

It is not at all unlikely that the dentist will be confronted with such a patient. The same precautions (prevention and control of bacteremia) must be taken for a victim of congenital heart disease that are taken for those afflicted with rheumatic heart disease to prevent subacute bacterial endocarditis.

Coronary Heart Disease

Coronary heart disease is important to the dentist because he, as an important member of the health team, must be familiar with the leading cause of death of adults in the United States. Furthermore, coronary heart disease is the leading cause of death among dentists themselves. The death rate because of occlusive coronary heart disease has increased steadily during the past two decades.

One-third of all deaths among males between 1 and 65 years of age are due to this cardiovascular disease. The vast majority of fatal cases are in the over-45 groups, accounting for over one-half of the deaths among those people.

Clinical methods are relatively insensitive in detecting early coronary heart disease. However, autopsies of young soldiers killed during the Korean War revealed atheromatous plaques occluding one-half or more of the lumen of some coronary arteries in 15 percent of those autopsied. A similar study on accident victims revealed atheromatous plaques in 17 percent of males aged 10 to 19 years and 45 percent of those aged 20 to 29 years.

Most epidemiologic studies concerning patients with coronary heart disease have shown that four "major risk factors" are involved. These are the levels of serum lipids (cholesterol and triglycerides), obesity, hypertension, and cigarette smoking. Other risk factors cited are genetic factors, sex and racial predisposition, lack of physical activity, and certain metabolic diseases such as diabetes mellitus.

Diabetes Mellitus

Diabetes mellitus is a disorder of carbohydrate metabolism characterized by hyperglycemia and glycosuria associated with a lack of insulin production. Sharkey has estimated that over 4 million people in the United States have diabetes and that only half of them have been diagnosed. McDonald and Fisher state that "at a minimum, . . . 1.6 million cases could be diagnosed today if physicians examined their patients for the disease." A national rate of 8.1 unknown cases of diabetes per 1000 was first published by Remein in 1959.

Diabetes may occur at any age, but the incidence curve reaches its peak in the fifth and sixth decades. Women are more frequently affected (3:2) than males. In Japan, however, diabetes was "two or three times" more common in men than in women. This was explained on the basis that Oriental women in their forties and fifties are, on the whole, less obese than their western counterparts (Blackard et al.).

The etiology of diabetes is undetermined in the majority of cases. Obesity occurs in from 50 to 77 percent of diabetic patients, while 8 to less than 1 percent are underweight at the onset of their disease. It seems probable that other endocrine glands are related to faulty carbohydrate metabolism. The pituitary, adrenal and thyroid glands are likewise important in carbohydrate metabolism.

The hereditary nature of diabetes is indicated by the increased incidence in patients with a family history of diabetes. White implies that 100 percent of the offspring of conjugal diabetics would develop the disease if the etiology of diabetes in both parents were the same. The predisposition to diabetes is inherited as a non-sex-linked Mendelian recessive. Host factors such as obesity, age (above 40), female sex, and multiparity appear to be predisposing factors also but are difficult to document.

A dental patient with diabetes or with a family history of diabetes demands special care. Should a practitioner suspect that an individual has undiagnosed diabetes, he may use various screening tests. If he is reluctant to perform these procedures, however, or mistrusts their accuracy, he must refer the patient to a physician.

The following procedures are recommended for the diabetic patient:

1. Frequent dental prophylaxis and personal oral hygiene instruction. The systemic insult of uncontrolled diabetes intensifies periodontal disease caused by local factors, and infection anywhere intensifies the diabetes.
2. Medical consultation prior to oral surgical or protracted restorative procedures to be sure that optimum control of the disease is being maintained.
3. Careful use of vasoconstrictors in local anesthetics. These agents are capable of increasing the level of sugar in the blood.

4. Antibiotic administration prior to extensive oral surgical procedures. Diabetics are often prone to infection due to an impaired vascular system.
5. Impressing the patient with the importance of an adequate dietary regimen.

Tuberculosis

Within the past century, beginning with Koch's discovery of the *Mycobacterium tuberculosis,* much has been learned concerning this chronic granulomatous disease. Within the past generation, significant strides have been made in the chemotherapeutic treatment of tuberculosis. Many have been spared from incapacitation and death. However, tuberculosis is still a public health problem. In 1974, there were 14.3 new active cases per 100,000 population in the United States. Although the death rate due to tuberculosis has dropped dramatically to slightly less than 2 per 100,000 population at the present time, the incidence and prevalence have not declined so rapidly. In addition to the new cases occurring each year, over 300,000 cases of tuberculosis are currently under medical care.

The fact that tuberculous lesions may occur intraorally makes the disease especially important to the dentist. Usually the oral lesions are secondary to pulmonary lesions and the patient is aware of the disease. However, there are still many undiagnosed cases since the disease may have an insidious onset and the patient may be unaware of its presence. Since primary and secondary lesions may occur in the mouth, careful clinical evaluation of chronic ulcerations is mandatory.

Venereal Diseases

Venereal disease has plagued man since before recorded history. In recorded history, the "great pox," or "syphilis," ravaged an entire continent, killing and crippling countless people. The advent of penicillin in the 1940s seemed to herald the eradication of venereal disease. Unfortunately, this has not materialized.

Syphilis

It was not until the twentieth century that Schaudinn and Hoffman discovered the causative organism, *Treponema pallidum.* August von Wassermann introduced the complement fixation test shortly after the identification of the spirochete. The so-called breakthrough in the treatment of syphilis was the use of penicillin. From 100,000 reported cases in 1947, syphilis dropped to a low of 6,251 reported cases in the United States in 1957. It seemed as though penicillin and rigid epidemiologic supervision by the armed forces had succeeded in making syphilis only a minor health problem. Consequently, syphilology was deemphasized in medical school, the requirement of premarital serologic tests was abandoned, and federal venereal disease control programs were reduced virtually to non-existence.

This relaxation was short-lived, however, for in 1962, only 5 years after an all-time low incidence rate, there were 20,000 reported cases. In reality, it is probable that 100,000 unreported cases were treated during 1962. A nationwide survey in 1963 of 131,000 physicians disclosed that they were reporting 1 of approximately 10 privately treated cases of syphilis (Brown). It was estimated that there were possibly 1 million cases of syphilis in the United States in 1965 (Shapiro).

A U.S.P.H.S. report in 1962 stated that ". . . there may be more than 200,000 cases of infectious venereal disease occurring among teenagers every year." For example, among the reported cases of syphilis in Indiana in 1975 (1,128), approximately half (47 percent) were in the 15 to 24 age group.

Since the three stages of syphilis may involve the oral regions, it behooves the dentist to be aware of this increasing problem. The chancre may occur on the lips, tongue, buccal mucosa, tonsil or other intraoral site. It is virtually impossible to diagnose such a lesion on the basis of appearance alone. At one stage or another, on the lip, the chancre may simulate herpes labialis; on the tonsil,

3

it may resemble the necrotizing ulceration of Vincent's angina (Fig. 2–11); and the mucous patch of the secondary stage may resemble the aphthous ulcer. The lesions of the primary and secondary stages are those most likely to be seen by the dentist. It is not common to see the gumma of the tertiary stage without other signs or symptoms to make one suspect syphilis. At present, it is said that only about one-third of the *untreated* syphilitic patients ever develop lesions of the tertiary stage.

It must be remembered that, in the primary stage, a serologic test may be negative. In the secondary stage it will be positive. These two stages, especially the secondary stage, are highly infectious and the lesions are teeming with spirochetes. A rapid test has been devised for office use to detect suspected cases of syphilis. Again, if one is reluctant to perform such a test or mistrusts the accuracy of the test, referral to a physician is indicated.

This discussion is not intended to imply that luetic lesions in the oral cavity are common. Rather, it is an attempt to arouse the practitioner's suspicion and to put an end to any false sense of security with regard to the incidence of syphilis. The "great imitator" is still with us.

Gonorrhea

Gonorrhea is caused by a gram-negative diplococcus, *Neisseria gonorrhoeae,* and is characterized by a purulent urethritis. Galen is responsible for the name "gonorrhea" which means "flow of seed." The organism was identified by Neisser in 1879. Although it is an ancient disease, adequate treatment evolved slowly. The advent of the sulfonamides in the 1930s was important, but resistant strains developed before long. Penicillin proved to be very effective and the incidence of gonorrhea declined. Again, complacency was a mistake. Today conservative estimates put the number of new cases in the United States at 2.5 million a year. The increased rate among teen-agers

is contributing to this ever-increasing rate. Again, the many unreported cases, perhaps 15 to 20 for each reported case, hinder the venereal disease control personnel in locating contacts.

While intraoral manifestations of a gonococcal infection are not common, they do exist. Gonococcal stomatitis may occur if the oral tissues are exposed to the organism. This may be seen in the newborn of a contaminated mother as well as in the adult. Since this condition manifests no pathognomonic clinical appearance, it is difficult to diagnose. Most cases manifest themselves as multiple areas of ulceration, often mimicking erythema multiforme. Minute pustules may be evident superimposed upon or adjacent to the ulcerated and erythematous mucosa. Virtually any area of the oral mucosa may be involved. A high index of suspicion is a prerequisite to diagnosis. Dentists can transmit the disease from one patient to another and can become infected themselves by caring for the patient. Cutaneous gonococcal infections are rare, but the unsuspecting dentist could become infected by finger contact with the patient. Obviously, surgical gloves should be used in suspected cases.

The practitioner should be aware of public health reports concerning the incidence of venereal disease within his state. Such reports are easily obtainable; usually they receive newspaper coverage. It is not at all unlikely for some patients seen in the average dental practice to be afflicted with venereal disease. It must be remembered that it is possible to encounter a patient with syphilis and gonorrhea simultaneously.

Viral Hepatitis

Viral hepatitis is an acute infectious disease which manifests in two forms—*hepatitis A* (infectious hepatitis) and *hepatitis B* (serum hepatitis). The two forms are immunologically distinct but morphologically similar. Viral particles have been identified ultrastructurally in the serum of patients with hepatitis B; however, the virus has not been isolated and grown in tissue culture. In 1965, immunologic studies discovered an antigen associated with viral hepatitis. This antigen, found in the serum of an Australian aborigine, came to be known as the *Australia antigen*. This antigen was later named *hepatitis associated antigen* (HAA) and is presently known as *hepatitis B surface antigen* (HB$_s$AG), since evidence suggests that it is associated with the hepatitis virus and may in fact be on the virus. By identifying this antigen in serum, it is possible to differentiate hepatitis B from hepatitis A.

For all practical purposes, the clinical picture of patients with serum hepatitis is identical to that of patients with infectious hepatitis. Malaise, fatigue, headache, nausea, vomiting, dark urine, jaundice, and upper abdominal pain are the most frequent symptoms. Liver function tests are often necessary to evaluate the extent of liver damage.

Next to measles, viral hepatitis is the most prevalent viral disease reportable to public health authorities. It was first considered reportable in 1952. An incidence peak was reported in 1954, and another in 1961, when more than 72,000 cases appeared. Reported cases declined to approximately 37,000 in 1964. Subclinical carriers of the virus do exist, conceivably 20 to 40 for every clinical case.

The principal method of dissemination of infectious hepatitis is person-to-person contact through a fecal-oral route, usually by ingestion of contaminated food and water. The importance of close personal contact with carriers is exemplified by the recurrence of epidemics among institutionalized, handicapped persons. Hepatitis B exists only in blood and even minute amounts of the contaminated blood are infectious if injected. Transmission usually occurs after blood or plasma transfusion (hence, the term "serum hepatitis") but is also seen after injection with contaminated needles and after surgical procedures with contaminated instruments.

A study of 119 cases of viral hepatitis was reported by Sultz. He gathered a control group of 119 persons of similar age, race, sex and neighborhood. The results showed a significant relationship between earlier tissue penetration by physicians and the ensuing disease. Tissue penetration by dentists and auxiliary hospital personnel was not found to be a significant factor, but the report should prompt concern regarding this possibility.

Dentists can aid in preventing this infectious disease and must take care against contracting the disease themselves. Personal hygiene and the effective use of germicidal soap can virtually reduce to zero the possibility of cross-infection by personal contact. In controlling serum hepatitis, the use of properly sterilized needles and instruments is obligatory. Sterilized, disposable needles are recommended. Surgical gloves should be worn during all oral surgical procedures.

Malignant Disease

The terms "malignancy" and "cancer" are quite familiar to the American public. Perhaps no other disease entity, with the possible exception of cardiovascular diseases, is receiving as much attention from epidemiologists and other investigators.

The American Cancer Society consistently publishes pertinent data concerning the incidence of cancer and the cancer death rate. For example, the number of *new* cases of cancer in 1976 is 675,000 and the estimated death rate is 370,000.

Pulmonary cancer is responsible for more deaths in the United States than any other single malignancy. The death rate for cancer of the lung almost doubled between 1950 and 1964 when it rose from 12.2 deaths per 100,000 population to 24 deaths per 100,000. During this 15-year period, more than 467,000 Americans died of lung cancer. Recently, the American Cancer Society predicted that 83,800 persons in the United States will die of lung cancer during 1976. This would account for over 22 percent of all deaths due to cancer.

The Surgeon General's Report (*Smoking*

and Health) of 1964 causally related lung cancer to cigarette smoking, and a brief decline in cigarette consumption ensued. Now, however, cigarette consumption per capita in the United States equals the rate noted before the report.

Cancer of the large bowel is second only to pulmonary cancer in the number of deaths attributable to a single malignancy in the United States. It is estimated that nearly 39,000 Americans will die of this cancer during 1976. This figure accounts for over 10 percent of all deaths due to cancer. Some of the epidemiologic factors cited are race, socioeconomic status, dietary pattern, body weight, smoking and chronic constipation. A dietary pattern which includes a high intake of fat seems to show the best correlation. Chronic constipation has been implicated to a somewhat lesser degree.

Levy presented an excellent review and evaluation of the evidence that viruses may cause leukemia and other malignant diseases in man. Within the present century, and especially since 1932, a remarkable number of virus-induced tumors in man and especially in animals have been reported. Notable reports include the sarcoma of the fowl reported by Rous, mammary carcinoma in the mouse and the "milk-factor" described by Bittner, and the fibroma and papilloma in the rabbit described by Shope.

There is some presumptive evidence implicating viruses in human cancer but there is no unequivocal evidence. Epidemiologic studies have given some presumptive evidence that viruses are capable of producing leukemia in man. Heath and Hasterlik studied leukemic children in an Illinois community. The incidence of leukemia in a group of 8 children was quite interesting for 7 of the 8 attended the same school and lived in the same residential area. However, other epidemiologic data on "leukemic clusters" are needed before conclusions can be reached.

Certainly there is no conclusive evidence implicating viruses as *the* cause of cancer.

However, it is possible that viruses carry some tumor-producing agent at the molecular level, or that the viruses themselves act as co-carcinogens. Levy stated that only 20 years ago scientists gave slight consideration to the premise that viruses are capable of causing human cancer. Today it is plausible. Tomorrow it may become fact. When the breakthrough occurs, epidemiology will have played an important part.

Although epidemiologic factors in oral cancer (q.v.) are most pertinent to the dentist, the astute practitioner should be aware of malignancy occurring in other areas of the body. This is necessary if only because of metastatic lesions which may involve oral structures. Among the more common lesions which may metastasize to the oral regions are carcinoma of the breast, kidney, lung, prostate, cervix and gastrointestinal tract. Cash and co-workers studied all cases seen at the Mayo Clinic during a 46-year period in which malignant lesions metastasized to the jaws. The primary sites of the 20 confirmed cases are shown in Table 3–1.

The Department of Oral Pathology of the Indiana University School of Dentistry has in its files 42 metastatic lesions to the jaws excluding those of the lip, face or tongue. The most common location of the known primary lesion was the breast, accounting

Table 3-1. Metastatic Lesions to the Jaws

Primary	No. of Cases
Kidney	5
Lip	5
Colon (including the sigmoid)	3
Breast	2
Skin (of the face and nose)	2
Prostate	1
Rectum	1
Tongue	1

Data from: Cash, C. D., Royer, R. Q. and Dahlin, D. C.: Metastatic tumors of the jaws. Oral Surg. 14, 897, 1961.

for 17 of the 42 lesions. In contrast to the Mayo series, only one lesion was from the kidney. The mandible is the usual site of metastasis with pain and/or paresthesia being the most common presenting symptoms. Sudden numbness of the chin has been called a most alarming signal of such metastasis.

IMPORTANT AREAS OF DENTAL EPIDEMIOLOGY

Important advances have been made in dentistry through epidemiologic studies. Oral diseases are particularly suited for study by epidemiologic methods because they are easily observed and accurate identification can be made.

Dental Caries

Dental caries is the most prevalent chronic disease affecting mankind. Once calcified tooth structure is lost, it can never form again. Thus, the manifestation of caries persists throughout the life of the affected tooth. This fact is epidemiologically important, for it forms the basis of the study of caries incidence. The epidemiologist is able to perform DMF (decayed, missing, filled) studies of teeth (DMFT) or tooth surfaces (DMFS). This one simple example of the epidemiologic method—observe, record, and reflect—has led the way in the study of dental caries, and the result has been an effective method of prevention. This is, of course, the use of fluoride compounds in preventing dental caries.

Incidence

Prehistoric man rarely suffered from dental caries. Dental caries has not been found in anthropologic studies of skulls from before the Neolithic or New Stone age. Even in the Neolithic period, caries incidence was low and was probably due to food impaction between teeth. The normal self-cleansing dental and gingival architecture was lost because of attrition and periodontal disease. The coarse diet and absence of refined carbohydrates in the diet were not conducive

to caries. Carious lesions have been found rather frequently in Egyptian mummies. At this early time, caries plagued man frequently enough so that crude attempts were made to restore teeth. Caries incidence increased as civilization advanced.

Today, there are more than 700 million carious teeth in the United States: an average of more than 3 per person. Approximately 98 percent of all Americans have dental decay at some time during their lives. The common occurrence of dental caries has led to a sense of indifference and inevitability. Many people feel that teeth are simply temporary anatomic blocks of enamel which are meant to decay and then be removed.

Fortunately, as Englander so aptly stated, oral diseases (including caries) are admirably suited for epidemiologic studies because they are more readily accessible and identifiable than most chronic diseases. One of the first large studies on caries incidence was done by Brekhus at the University of Minnesota. He examined 10,455 incoming freshmen and found a mean rate of DMFT of 10.2. Later, Healey and Cheyne compared 3,234 Indiana University students to 4,348 of their counterparts at the University of Minnesota. The mean DMFT was 10.12 and 11.08 respectively. Another study of college students was reported by Hadjimarkos and Storvick, who found a mean DMFT of 14.12 and a mean DMFS of 33.4. These epidemiologic field studies are best performed on large groups of persons in similar environments (such as schools) or on a large group of persons from various locales but present at a central area (such as a military recruit training center).

The military establishments have at hand many men within a small age group. Many caries incidence studies have been performed at these facilities and have provided much needed base-line information for the researcher. Massler and his associates examined 4,043 Naval recruits and recorded a mean DMFT of 11.3 and a DMFS of 25.2. Hellman and co-workers, in a vast study of 183,000 Naval and Marine recruits, found that the average recruit needed 6.16 restorations. More recently, Shannon and his colleagues examined 5,298 enlistees in the United States Air Force. Subjects came from every portion of the United States. Excluding third molars from the study, they found that the dental status of the average enlistee could be expressed as: number of teeth present, 26.7; carious teeth, 6.8; carious surfaces, 11.2; filled teeth, 6.5; filled surfaces, 12.8; and DMFS, 27.9. Essentially, this study was in agreement with the study of Szmyd and McCall, who reported that the average Air Force enlistee required 6.77 restorations.

Host Factors

While the incidence of dental caries is important, it is more interesting to view caries incidence with regard to the person who contracts caries. These are, to an epidemiologist, the *host factors*. Only the most pertinent will be discussed.

Age. In the past, it was generally believed that dental caries was a "childhood" disease and that the caries rate declined in the post-pubertal years after reaching a peak in the 15 to 19 age group (Fig. 3–1). Dunning,

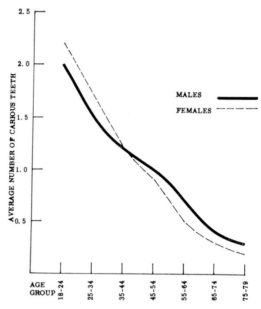

Fig. 3-2. Average adult caries experience by sex and age: United States, 1960–62. (Data from Public Health Service Publication No. 1000-Series 11-No. 7. Selected Dental Findings in Adults by Age, Race, and Sex: United States—1960–1962.)

however, feels that this peak represents accumulated needs and not necessarily current needs or dental caries incidence. Citing two studies, he believes that caries incidence shows a straight-line increase, thereby implying a uniform increase in caries experience. It does seem likely that caries incidence is lower in the early post-eruption years since time is needed for carious lesions to develop. A Public Health Service study of dental disease showed that in adults the highest caries rates were recorded in the 18 to 24 age group with a constant decline thereafter (Fig. 3–2). Some studies show a second peak of caries incidence in ages over 60 when patients experience cervical caries following gingival recession.

Sex. Many studies have been made to detect variation in caries incidence between the sexes. Studies have shown that the female has a higher caries rate in the permanent teeth than a male of the same age. The difference is slight, and in many studies is of no

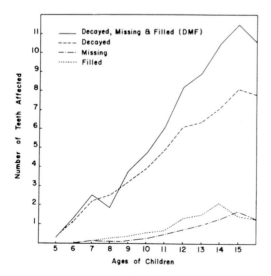

Fig. 3-1. A compilation of results of surveys demonstrating the relative incidence of dental caries according to age.

statistical significance. The 1962 Public Health Service study showed an average DMFT of 19.6 for all men and 21.1 for all women. However, the number of decayed teeth in the average woman was 1.1, slightly less than the 1.2 rate recorded for men.

The popular belief of the past that pregnancy accelerates caries incidence in the female has not been substantiated. There is no known mechanism by which a developing fetus could withdraw calcium from the teeth or cause a predisposition to decay in the mother.

Race. There are definite differences in caries incidence between racial groups. The Public Health Service study showed a significantly lower DMF in the black adult than in the Caucasian adult. The average number of decayed teeth per Caucasian adult was lower (1.1) than in the black (1.8). The greatest difference was noted in filled teeth. The average Caucasian adult had nearly 5 times as many restored teeth as the black adult. While socioeconomic differences may explain some of these findings, there is evidence which indicates a lower caries incidence in blacks.

The English are said to have notoriously bad teeth. The Irish also have been shown to have a high incidence of dental caries. Conversely, the Chinese and Russians have relatively low incidence rates of caries.

Environmental Factors

Dunning discussed environmental factors in dental caries and compared such variables as amount of sunshine, rainfall, humidity, water hardness and urbanization. He concluded that geographic factors do play a role in caries experience. Abundant sunshine and low relative humidity seemed to be associated with low caries incidence. However, this climate is commonly found in the southwestern United States, an area abundantly endowed with naturally occurring fluorides in the water. This latter factor has proven to be of major importance and, through epidemiologic studies, has provided what is per-

haps the most important finding in dental history.

Prevention

Caries prevention occupies much of the time spent by dental investigators. Epidemiology stimulated much of this interest and resulted in the discovery of the role of fluoride in preventing dental caries. Prevention without the use of fluorides is important as well. Bibby states that overoptimism about the preventive effects of fluorides could lead to the tragic neglect of other preventive measures.

Dean states that mottled enamel was first mentioned in 1901 in Eager's report of observations made in and near Naples, Italy. In the United States, a page from the 1908 minutes of the Colorado Springs (Colorado) Dental Society, then known as the El Paso County Odontological Society, contained the first mention of mottled enamel. It referred to "Colorado Stain," a brown stain which occurred frequently in children's teeth in the Colorado Springs area. A committee was appointed to investigate the condition, and McKay was one of the members.

Black and McKay discussed in detail "mottled teeth" which had been sent to Black for study from dentists in the Rocky Mountain area of the United States. Black noticed the absence of dental decay when he visited an endemic area and later McKay discussed the relation of mottled enamel to caries incidence. At this time (1908), the cause of mottled enamel was unknown. However, McKay speculated that ". . . water borne influence . . . must be considered." Thus, McKay did feel that some substance in the water caused mottled enamel. As McKay continued his extensive investigation, water supplies were analyzed. At one time, low calcium content was considered to be an etiologic factor, as was the lime content of the water.

The first person to suspect fluorine as the causative agent was not a dentist but an industrial chemist, H. V. Churchill, who publicly expressed his views at a session of the American Chemical Society in 1931 and later reported his findings. McKay argued against this premise but later, based on Dean's studies, fluorine was definitely established as the causative agent.

In the 1930s Dean directed a monumental epidemiologic study of dental fluorosis in 235 areas in the United States. His "mottled enamel index" and "mottled enamel index of a community" are still used today. Even at this early time he stated that amounts of fluoride in domestic water supplies not exceeding 1 part per million (ppm) were *probably* of no deleterious public health significance.

Since then, the literature contains numerous reports of investigations demonstrating the value of fluorides in caries prevention, and the safety with which they may be used. It may be said that the epidemiologic method was responsible for this achievement in preventive dentistry.

Cleft Lip and Cleft Palate

Of the developmental disturbances with which the dentist is associated, the most important are *cleft lip* and/or *cleft palate*. Although the two are actually developmental defects of two separate oral structures, they are commonly discussed together. Greene, however, feels that the two entities should be studied separately, whenever possible.

Etiology

The etiology of cleft lip and cleft palate presents a complex picture of theories and possible predisposing factors. Perhaps the reason many epidemiologic studies have been undertaken is because there is doubt concerning the etiology as well as the many possible predisposing factors. Since it is possible for the cleft lip and cleft palate to occur separately, it is even possible for the etiologic agents to differ.

There are two main theories of the pathogenesis of cleft lip. The first suggests that the defect results from a failure of proper mersion of the globular portion of the median nasal process with the lateral nasal and maxillary processes. The second theory, called the *theory of mesodermal penetration,* suggests that the defect is caused by the failure of mesoderm to penetrate the ectodermal "hood" which forms the lip.

The proponents of both theories generally agree on the pathogenesis of cleft palate formation, namely, the lack of mersion of the two palatal processes with each other or with the frontonasal process.

Heredity. Heredity is one of the most important factors in the etiology of cleft lip and cleft palate. Clinical studies have shown that up to 45 percent of cases of cleft lip and/or cleft palate were the offspring of similarly afflicted parents. It has been estimated that the child of one affected parent has a 5-percent chance of being similarly malformed; when both a parent and a sibling are affected, the risk increases to 15 percent in succeeding children.

Experimental Cleft Lip and Cleft Palate. Many investigators have been successful in experimentally producing clefts in laboratory animals. Clefts have been produced by diets either excessively high or deficient in vitamin content; by administration of cortisone, barbiturates and tranquilizers; by stress, radiation and certain infectious diseases. While these defects have been produced experimentally by such means, there is no concrete evidence of the same cause-effect relationships in humans. On the other hand, teratogens such as thalidomide and maternal rubella infection undoubtedly are capable of causing cleft lip and/or cleft palate (among other birth defects) in humans. Greene and his colleagues have stressed the coexistence of other congenital anomalies with cleft lip and cleft palate.

Incidence

It has been estimated that more than 250,000 persons in the United States have cleft lip and/or palate and that the incidence is approximately 6,000 yearly.

Two vast epidemiologic studies have been reported by Greene and his co-workers and by Donahue. In both investigations birth certificates were used as sources of information. Milham states that the incidence of cleft lip and cleft palate may be higher than some surveys indicate because of incomplete information on birth certificates. The birth certificates of 143 cleft lip-cleft palate cases were examined and on 39 (27.2 percent) of the certificates the defects were not noted. In another attempt to determine under-reporting, it was found that only 817 (62.7 percent) of 1,301 patients being treated for the condition had the defect recorded on their birth certificates. Greene recognized this problem but still felt that such records could be useful in epidemiologic studies.

Donahue divided the variables pertaining to incidence into three groups: (1) *Variables determined at conception.* These include sex, color, plurality, maternal age, birth order and maternal nativity. (2) *Variables related to gestation.* These include length of pregnancy, associated anomalies, classification of cleft, complications of pregnancy and prenatal care. (3) *Variables related to birth.* These include geographical location, urban-rural environment, legitimacy, month of birth, weight and presence of an attendant.

His findings were based on 6,070 infants with cleft lip and/or cleft palate derived from an examination of nearly six million birth certificates from 17 states. In two separate reports based on an examination of five million birth certificates, Greene and his colleagues presented data on more than 6,000 cases with clefts. The following generalities are based on these and similar studies.

Race. Blacks have the lowest incidence of clefts (1:1821) while Japanese have a relatively high incidence rate (1:674). It has been speculated that, in the early uncivilized tribes of Africa, the practice of destroying all deformed infants had a depressive effect on the propagation of clefts. This premise tends to support the hereditary role in etiology.

Geographical Distribution. The mean incidence rate in the United States is in the vicinity of 1:900 births. The highest incidence rate in the United States is in Montana (1:624) and lowest in South Carolina (1:1681). A high incidence rate has been noted in Montana Indians and was the basis for an interesting report by Tretsven. The low incidence in South Carolina (and other southern states) is probably due to a proportionately higher incidence of black births. On the other hand, this region had the highest number of births attended by non-medical personnel and lack of recognition may have been a factor.

Sex. Males are more frequently affected than females. Ratios have varied from 51:49 to 2:1. Many studies have reported clefts of the lip, with or without associated palatal clefts, to be more common in males; cleft palate alone to be more common in females; and, considering all types of clefts together, males are more frequently affected. This has led to such explanations as one which holds that the conditions are sex-linked with male dominance and another which theorizes that environmental insults have a selective action on the male in utero.

Parental Age and Birth Order. The highest rate of children born with clefts occurs among mothers in the 20 to 24 age group. This is the most fertile age category for all women. Some have suggested that the increased incidence of clefts is in direct proportion to advanced maternal and/or paternal age; others have shown either non-significant or non-existent differences. Therefore, the role of parental age remains unclear.

The importance of the order of birth also is controversial. At this time, it is generally believed that birth order is not related to the occurrence of clefts.

Associated Anomalies. Greene and co-workers noted a strong positive relationship between clefts and associated developmental anomalies. Twenty-seven percent of babies with cleft palate alone, and 14 percent of those with both cleft lip and cleft palate, had other congenital malformations. The most frequently encountered defects are positional foot defects, polydactyly, circulatory defects, deformed ears and anomalous limbs.

Management

The management of affected patients necessarily involves many areas of dentistry and medicine. A combined effort using the knowledge and abilities of surgeons, orthodontists, speech therapists and the general dentist provides the most effective management of such patients, sometimes with the aid of psychologists, sociologists and others.

Periodontal Disease

There is little doubt that most periodontal disease is due primarily to poor oral hygiene which results in the accumulation of bacterial plaque and calculus. These local factors incite an inflammatory response in the periodontal tissues which results in gingivitis and, if allowed to progress, in periodontitis.

Investigators have attempted to prove that factors other than local can *cause* periodontal disease. Nutritional deficiency, stress, endocrine imbalances and other systemic diseases, to name a few, have been mentioned as important factors in the etiology of periodontal disease. None has yielded unequivocal results. However, it is generally believed that systemic factors, superimposed upon preexisting local factors, may lead to more rapid progression of periodontal disease. An example of this is seen in uncontrolled diabetics. Markedly advanced periodontal disease is not uncommon even in young adults with this condition; however, local factors are invariably present. It is interesting, however, that Shklar and colleagues reported severe periodontal disease in a strain of diabetic Chinese hamsters in the absence of apparent local factors.

Occlusal traumatism has been mentioned as a cause of periodontal disease by numerous investigators. It is difficult to imagine traumatogenic occlusion producing anything in a healthy periodontium other than migration or attrition of the teeth. Again, in a person with preexisting periodontal disease, the process may be accelerated. Bhaskar and Frisch recently discussed occlusal trauma as it relates to the biologic and clinical aspects of periodontal disease. Waerhaug has stated, "There is no evidence that trauma from occlusion causes gingivitis or periodontitis, nor that trauma is a predisposing factor."

Incidence

The epidemiologic interest in periodontal disease has been primarily in its incidence. The epidemiologist's goal is to determine effective means of control and prevention after analyzing incidence rates in relation to various locales, racial groups and other environmental factors.

The prevalence of periodontal disease in the United States has been estimated at 90 million cases. This figure represents *advanced* periodontal disease. The results of the Public Health Service study for the prevalence of periodontal disease in the United States is depicted graphically in Figure 3–3. The study showed that 70 percent of the average Caucasians above the age of 20 had periodontal disease. In the average black, more than 8 of 10 had periodontal disease. Concurrent calculus indices were consistently higher in the blacks and, in virtually all cases, lack of oral hygiene corresponded to the severity of the disease.

The Periodontal Index (PI) and the Simplified Oral Hygiene Index (OHI)

A *Periodontal Index* for measuring the prevalence and severity of periodontal disease has been devised and used extensively by Russell. By visual clinical examination, all teeth are appraised with regard to the condition of the supporting tissues. Scores for each tooth are numerical, ranging from "0"

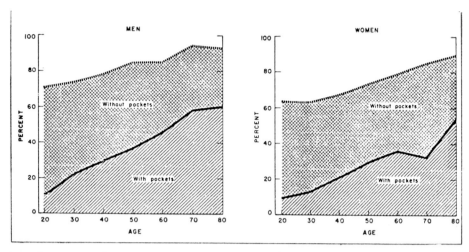

Fig. 3-3. Percentage of men and women with periodontal disease, with and without pockets, by age: United States, 1960–62. (Data from Public Health Service Publication No. 1000-Series 11-No. 7. Selected Dental Findings in Adults by Age, Race, and Sex: United States—1960–1962.)

(no evidence of periodontal disease) to "8" (advanced destruction with loss of masticatory function). The average of the teeth scored is an individual's periodontal index or PI. This index was designed primarily for epidemiologic field work in the prevalence of periodontal disease. Invariably this method is used in major population studies, and so the dentist should be aware of it. Its use in a private practice is not warranted because the scores must be "calibrated." That is, in a given patient, all examiners must report scores which concur closely; since the scores are given on a subjective basis, the results would be invalid if the examiners did not agree on what actually constitutes a certain score. The index could be of value to periodontists in private practice for comparison among patients.

Greene and Vermillion have devised an excellent method for classifying the oral hygiene status of a population. It is known as the *Simplified Oral Hygiene Index* (*OHI–S*) and has two components, the *Debris Index* (*DI*) and the *Calculus Index* (*CI*). In the anterior area, the labial surfaces of the maxillary right central incisor and the mandibular left central incisor are scored. In the posterior maxillary area, the buccal surfaces of the first fully erupted molar pos-

terior to the second bicuspid on the left and right sides are scored. Usually, this is the first molar but may be the second or third if the others are missing. In the posterior mandibular area, the lingual surfaces of the first fully erupted molar posterior to the second bicuspid on both sides are scored. Thus, in a normal dentition, selected surfaces of 6 teeth are scored. Should no molars exist in one quadrant, only 5 teeth are scored. Likewise, should *both* central incisors in an arch be missing, only 5 teeth are scored. If only one central incisor is present in an arch, it is scored.

The examining and scoring are quite simple and after a few "practice" examinations, can be performed accurately and rapidly. The following criteria are used to determine the debris score which ranges from "0" to "3":

0–No debris or stain present.
1–Soft debris covering not more than one-third of the tooth surface being examined, or the presence of extrinsic stains without debris, regardless of surface area covered.
2–Soft debris covering more than one-third but not more than two-thirds of the exposed tooth surface.
3–Soft debris covering more than two-thirds of the exposed tooth surface.

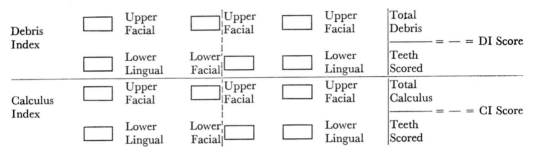

Fig. 3-4. A simple form for recording debris and calculus indices.

The criteria for the calculus score are similar:

0–No calculus present.
1–Supragingival calculus covering not more than one-third of the exposed tooth surface being examined.
2–Supragingival calculus covering more than one-third but not more than two-thirds of the exposed tooth surface, *or* the presence of individual flecks of subgingival calculus around the cervical portion of the tooth.
3–Supragingival calculus covering more than two-thirds of the exposed tooth surface *or* a continuous heavy band of subgingival calculus around the cervical portion of the tooth.

An explorer and a mirror are the only instruments necessary. After the scores are recorded, the total is divided by the number of teeth examined. The quotient denotes the debris and calculus indices. Together they constitute the oral hygiene index. At *least two surfaces* must have been scored—such would be the case of an individual with an edentulous maxilla and no molars in one quadrant—to perform a valid index. The DI and CI values may range between "0" and "3." The OHI–S (the sum of the DI and CI) would have a value which ranges from "0" to "6." The scores may be recorded on a convenient form similar to the one shown in Figure 3–4.

This simple index could easily be used in the office of any practitioner, and it would be most valuable in follow-up observations and periodic recalls. With practice, no more than 1 minute would be necessary. This can be done just before charting of caries and can be a part of the patient's permanent record. In this way the dentist uses the epidemiologic method and in only a few moments stores beneficial information.

Epidemiology

Information on the epidemiology of periodontal disease has been accumulating recently, although the first studies were started only a few years ago. Prior to the mid-1950s, little was known of the incidence and prevalence of periodontal disease. Hine expressed his views concerning the need for epidemiologic studies and felt that preventive periodontics could not be established until "base lines" were established.

Subsequently many epidemiologic field studies have been conducted. The World Health Organization sponsored Ramfjord's studies in India, and the U.S. Public Health Service sponsored Greene. A W.H.O. Expert Committee on Periodontal Diseases recommended further studies. Nevitt performed extensive work in Egypt, Iran, Syria and the Sudan. He found an exceedingly low prevalence rate of periodontal disease in the Sudan as compared to other Middle East countries. Later, Emslie confirmed Nevitt's findings and speculated that the low prevalence might be due to frequent oral cleansing as a part of a religious rite. Likewise, low caries and high fluorosis rates existed among the Sudanese.

In all studies, the most widespread finding in periodontal disease is the presence of local irritating factors. Waerhaug reported that in Ceylon not one case of periodontosis— that is, severe bone loss without gingivitis and the presence of local irritating factors— was seen in 10,000 persons examined. A consistent finding was the positive correlation between poor oral hygiene and the severity of periodontal disease. An association between increasing age and increased severity of disease is also noted frequently. In some studies, however, marked periodontal disease was observed in young populations. This has been observed in India by Ramfjord and in Jewish refugees in Lebanon by the Interdepartmental Committee on Nutrition for National Defense (ICNND).

Russell has discussed the progress of epidemiologic studies pertaining to periodontal disease. Although much has been done, many questions remain unanswered. Meanwhile, a vigorous preventive program is essential, and this is the responsibility of all practitioners. The effective removal of irritation and the proper motivation of patients can prevent or control most periodontal disease.

Oral Cancer

Of all malignant diseases, none is as important to the dentist as oral cancer. Approximately 8,300 people are expected to die in 1976 in the United States as a result of primary oral cancer. Earlier detection, diagnosis and treatment could prevent many such deaths.

Incidence

Approximately 675,000 new cases of cancer of all types are expected to occur in the United States during 1976. The American Cancer Society predicts that 3.5 percent or 23,800 of these cases will be primary within the oral cavity or on the lips.

Epidermoid (squamous cell) carcinoma accounts for the majority of cases of oral malignancy, estimates being 90 to 95 percent. Carcinoma of the lip, which is the most common, has an excellent prognosis; the overall survival rate is about 85 percent.

Small lesions of the lip that are treated early have an even better prognosis; reports show 5-year survival rates of nearly 95 percent. After the lip, the most common location is the tongue, but unfortunately a malignant tumor in this area of the mouth has the poorest prognosis.

It is not unlikely that the average practitioner will have the opportunity to perform diagnostic procedures in patients with intraoral cancer. As the dentist increases his observation of perioral structures such as the salivary glands, maxillary sinuses, temporomandibular joints, the oropharynx and other regions of the head and neck, he increases his capacity to detect abnormality and refer for therapy many other cases of cancer. The astute practitioner will recognize the clinical signs coupled with the patient's presenting symptoms, if any. In this manner, early therapy will be obtained and his patients will benefit.

Etiology and Predisposing Factors

Although the cause of cancer is unknown, certain factors are seen in association with oral cancer more frequently than could occur by chance alone.

Sex. Males are more frequently afflicted than females at a ratio of approximately 5:1. This might be explained by hormonal differences; however, the male preponderance is decreasing, which suggests another explanation: namely, the increased use of tobacco and alcoholic beverages by females.

Race and Culture. Ethnic factors appear to be important in the incidence of oral cancer. The highest incidence and mortality rates of oral cancer occur in India. Oral cancer is the most common malignancy affecting East Indians today. Many of them habitually use a "quid" composed of betel nut, slaked lime, tobacco and sometimes spices. This is held in the mouth for prolonged periods of time, often during sleep. Recently, Hirayama obtained strong supportive evidence that the disease is often associated with this habit.

Tobacco. An association between the use of tobacco and oral cancer has been suspected for many years. Virtually all epidemiologics studies have shown an association of this nature. Oral cancer occurs significantly less often in non-users of tobacco than in users.

Many authorities believe that tobacco acts as a co-carcinogen rather than as a carcinogen. The basis for this is that tobacco and tobacco smoke *per se* are not capable of inducing experimental carcinoma in laboratory animals. Hirayama stated that the incidence of carcinoma is not particularly high in areas of Asia where tobacco alone is chewed. In his opinion the tobacco-lime combination plays the most important role in oral cancer, and he said that future study will be needed to determine which plays the major role.

Among patients who habitually use tobacco, the practitioner should be especially wary of persistent white lesions of the oral cavity, especially those occurring in the floor of the mouth and on the ventral and lateral surfaces of the tongue. Persistent hoarseness in an older, cigar-smoking patient should alert the dentist to the possibility of laryngeal carcinoma.

Alcohol. Many investigators feel that there is a definite correlation between alcohol consumption and oral cancer. Trieger and associates reviewed the records of all patients at the Massachusetts General Hospital with a diagnosis of carcinoma of the tongue. During a 9-year period, 198 cases were diagnosed. Of these, 108 records were sufficiently complete to deduce the presence of certain predisposing factors. Eighty-two (75.9 percent) admitted to excessive alcohol consumption. Forty-eight (44.4 percent) had unequivocal evidence of hepatic cirrhosis.

Since virtually all heavy drinkers are smokers, the combination may present an important dual factor in the incidence of oral cancer. Trieger's study showed that 97 cases (89.8 percent) were smokers. Again, the possible importance of co-carcinogens cannot be denied.

Syphilis. In earlier studies, patients afflicted with carcinoma of the tongue were reported to have syphilis in 20 to 40 percent of the cases. In the study by Trieger and colleagues 20 patients (18.5 percent) had a positive history, physical finding or serologic test for syphilis. Nineteen of these lesions were in the anterior two-thirds of the tongue. Thus, the investigators stated that syphilis was not important in lesions of the posterior one-third and base of the tongue. Keller studied oral cancer (including malignancy of the lip and pharynx) in 2,177 men. He found no association between oral cancer and syphilis.

Nevertheless, many other authorities agree that there is a positive correlation between a history of syphilis and the incidence of oral cancer, especially carcinoma of the tongue.

Plummer-Vinson Syndrome. The Plummer-Vinson syndrome is a symptom complex characterized by iron deficiency anemia, dysphagia, and atrophic oral mucous membranes. Achlorhydria, koilonychia and splenomegaly also are seen at times. The syndrome is most commonly seen in Scandinavian women. The atrophic mucosa apparently predisposes to carcinoma. Females account for about 30 percent of oral cancer cases in the United States, and about 40 percent in Scandinavian countries.

Viruses. As in all malignant disease, viruses have never been positively linked with the etiology of oral cancer. However, the possibility remains. One interesting lesion, possibly of viral origin and termed the *African lymphoma,* was first reported by Burkitt. Most often seen in the mandible, this lesion was originally found in children living in a narrow zone of central Africa limited to elevations of less than 5,000 feet and with an annual rainfall of over 200 inches. The temperature in these regions did not fall below 60°F. For this reason, Burkitt considered the possibility of a viral disease with the mosquito being a possible insect vector. More recently the lesion has been found in other areas, including North America. However, the tumor is endemic in Africa and New Guinea. Burkitt's epidemiologic investigations concerning this interestof epidemiologic field work. With only pencil and paper, he ventured into the bush gathering valuable information which he later published. For this reason, the tumor has been given the eponyms "Burkitt tumor," "Burkitt sarcoma," and "Burkitt lymphoma." Virologic investigations concerning this interesting tumor continue at the present time. Recently the Epstein-Barr virus (EBV) has been isolated and implicated in the pathogenesis of this lesion.

Experimental Oral Cancer

Salley was one of the first to produce oral cancer experimentally in a laboratory animal. A polycyclic hydrocarbon was repeatedly applied to the mucosa of the cheek pouch of the hamster, which induced the experimental carcinoma. Many others have since reproduced Salley's results. The most frequently used carcinogens have been the type used by Salley. Viruses have not as yet been found capable of inducing oral cancer in laboratory animals.

Epidemiologic Studies

A global epidemiologic study for the classification of all malignant lesions, including those occurring in the oral cavity, has been undertaken under the auspices of the World Health Organization. Certain strategically located *reference centres* have been established to collect and classify these lesions and to clarify all facts concerning them. It is hoped that diversity in nomenclature and all aspects of doubt will be eliminated through this worldwide study. Chaves has stated that these epidemiologic studies will lead to better teaching of oral diagnosis and oral pathology and will enable dentists to obtain an excellent preparation in oral medicine.

Kreshover has stressed the importance

of epidemiologic investigation in cancer research:

"Unquestionably, in the complex field of cancer research today we are approaching a horizon of considerably more light than there was in earlier scientific pursuits—this light, interestingly enough, being provided in large measure by an application of the nonsophisticated tools of classical epidemiology. It is simplicity of reasoning to conclude that until we learn all that we can about the natural history of a disease, whatever its nature, in the laboratory of populations, there is indeed a nonstable base for the bench scientist to approach relevant problems."

BIBLIOGRAPHY

General

Christen, A. G. and Jendresen, M. D.: Military oral medicine, Dent. Clin. North America, March, 1968.
Council on Dental Therapeutics: Type B (serum) hepatitis and dental practice, J. Amer. Dent. Ass., *92,* 153, 1976.
Gordon, J. E.: *The Epidemiology of Health,* New York, New York Academy of Medicine, p. 14, 1953.
Greenberg, Morris: *Studies in Epidemiology,* New York, G. P. Putnam's Sons, p. 4, 1965.
Rogers, F. B.: *Epidemiology and Communicable Disease Control,* New York, Grune & Stratton, p. 2, 1963.
Sultz, H. A.: A study of the role of tissue penetration in the transmission of viral hepatitis, Amer. J. Public Health, *54,* 1263, 1964.
Thomson, D. R.: Tuberculosis as a world problem: the current epidemiological position, Trop. Doct., *4* 154, 1974.
Tomich, C. E.: The anamnesis and epidemiology, Dent. Clin. North America, March, 1968.

Cardiovascular Disease

Epstein, F. H.: The epidemiology of coronary heart disease, J. Chronic Dis., *18,* 735, 1965.
Higgins, I. T. T.: The epidemiology of congenital heart disease, J. Chronic Dis., *18,* 699, 1965.
Morton, W. E. and Huhn, L. A.: Epidemiology of congenital heart disease, J.A.M.A., *195,* 1107, 1966.
Morton, W. E., Huhn, L. A. and Litchy, J. A.: Rheumatic heart disease epidemiology: observations in 17,336 Denver school children, J. A. M. A., *199,* 879, 1967.
Mostaghim, D. and Millard, H. D.: Bacterial endocarditis: a retrospective study, Oral Surg., *40,* 219, 1975.

Sackett, D. L. and Winkelstein, W., Jr.: The epidemiology of aortic and peripheral atherosclerosis, J. Chronic Dis., *18*, 775, 1965.

Schweitzer, M. D., Gearing, F. R. and Perera, G. A.: The epidemiology of primary hypertension, J. Chronic Dis., *18*, 847, 1965.

Stamler, J.: Cardiovascular disease in the United States, Amer. J. Cardiol., *10*, 319, 1962.

Diabetes Mellitus

Blackard, W. G., Omori, Y. and Freeman, L. R.: Epidemiology of diabetes in Japan, J. Chronic Dis., *18*, 415, 1965.

Levin, H. L.: Some dental aspects of endocrine diseases, Oral Surg., *19*, 466, 1965.

McDonald, G. W. and Fisher, G. F.: Diabetes prevalence in the United States, Public Health Rep., *82*, 334, 1967.

Remein, Q. R.: A current estimate of the prevalence of diabetes in the United States, Ann. N. Y. Acad. Sci., *82*, 229, 1959.

Sharkey, T. P.: Diabetes mellitus: present problems and new research. I. Prevalence in the United States, J. Amer. Diet. Ass., *58*, 201, 1971.

White, P.: The incidence of diabetes, Med. Clin. North America, *49*, 957, 1965.

Venereal Disease

Brown, W. J.: Reports by physicians called key to eradication of VD, J.A.M.A., *190*, 12, 1964.

Chue, P. W. Y.: Gonorrhea—its natural history, oral manifestations, diagnosis, treatment and prevention, J. Amer. Dent. Ass., *90*, 1297, 1975.

Curtis, A. C.: National survey of venereal disease treatment, J.A.M.A., *186*, 46, 1963.

Feldman, W. H.: Yesterday's triumphs: today's problems, J.A.M.A., *194*, 33, 1965.

Shapiro, M. I.: Teen-agers and venereal disease, J.A.M.A., *194*, 617, 1965.

U.S. Public Health Service: The eradication of syphilis, Pub. 918, 2nd printing, March, 1962.

Malignant Disease

Bittner, J. J.: Some possible effects of nursing on the mammary gland tumor incidence in mice, Science, *84*, 162, 1937.

Cash, C. D., Royer, R. Q. and Dahlin, D. C.: Metastatic tumors of the jaws, Oral Surg., 14, 897, 1961.

Heath, C. W. and Hasterlik, R. J.: Leukemia among children in a suburban community, Amer. J. Med., *34*, 796, 1963.

Levy, B. M.: Viruses as carcinogenic agents, J. Dent. Res., *45*, 528, 1966.

Rous, P. A.: A sarcoma of the fowl transmissible by an agent separable from the tumor cells, J. Exp. Med., *13*, 397, 1911.

Shope, R. E.: A filterable virus causing a tumor-like condition in rabbits and its relationship to virus myxomatosum, J. Exp. Med., *56*, 803, 1932.

————: Infectious papillomatosis of rabbits, J. Exp. Med., *58*, 607, 1933.

U.S. Public Health Service, Mortality from diseases associated with smoking: United States, 1950–64, Pub. 1000, 1966.

Wynder, E. L., and Shigematsu, T.: Environmental factors of cancer of the colon and rectum, Cancer, *2*, 1520, 1967.

Dental Caries

Bibby, B. G.: Caries prevention without fluorides, Dent. Clin. North America, July, 1962.

Black, G. V. and McKay, F. S.: Mottled teeth—an endemic developmental imperfection of the enamel of the teeth heretofore unknown in the literature of dentistry, D. Cosmos, *58*, 129, 1916.

Brekhus, P. J.: A report on dental caries in 10,455 university students, J. Amer. Dent. Ass., *18*, 1350, 1931.

Churchill, H. V.: Occurrence of fluorides in some waters of the United States, J. Int. Eng. Chem., *23*, 996, 1931.

Dean, H. T.: A summary of the epidemiology of chronic endemic dental fluorosis (mottled enamel), Texas Dent. J., *55*, 86, 1937.

Dunning, J. M.: Incidence and distribution of dental caries in the United States, Dent. Clin. North America, July, 1962.

Englander, H. R.: Epidemiology: a fundamental discipline in dental research, J. Amer. Dent. Ass., *65*, 755, 1962.

Hadjimarkos, D. M. and Storvik, C. A.: The incidence of dental caries among freshmen students at Oregon State College, J. Dent. Res., *27*, 299, 1948.

Healey, H. J. and Cheyne, V. D.: Comparison of caries prevalence between freshmen students in two midwestern universities, J. Amer. Dent. Ass., *30*, 692, 1943.

Hellman, L. P., Ludwick, W. E. and Oesterling, B. J.: Naval dental needs and treatment, J. Amer. Dent. Ass., *55*, 828, 1957.

Massler, M., Ludwick, W. E. and Schour, I.: Dental caries and gingivitis in males 17 to 20 years old at the Great Lakes Naval Training Center, J. Dent. Res., *31*, 319, 1952.

McKay, F. S.: The relation of mottled enamel to caries, J. Amer. Dent. Ass., *15*, 1429, 1928.

Shannon, I. L., Gibson, W. A. and Terry, J. M.: Caries-experience of recruits in the U.S. Air Force, J. Pub. Health Dent., *26*, 206, 1966.

Szmyd, L. and McCall, C. M., Jr.: Restorative dentistry workload of the U.S. Air Force Dental Service, U. S. Armed Forces Med. J., *11*, 1011, 1960.

U.S. Public Health Service, Selected dental findings in adults by age, race and sex—United States 1960–1962. Vital Health Statistics, Pub. 1000.

Cleft Lip and Cleft Palate

Altemus, L. A.: Incidence of cleft lip and palate among North American Negroes, Cleft Palate J., *3*, 357, 1966.

Donahue, R. F.: Birth variables and the incidence of cleft palate: part 1, Cleft Palate J., *2*, 282, 1965.

Fujino, H., Tanaka, K. and Sanui, Y.: Genetic study of cleft lips and cleft palates based upon 2,828 Japanese cases, Kyushu J. Med. Sci., *14*, 317, 1963.

Greene, J. C.: Epidemiology of congenital clefts of the lip and palate, Public Health Rep., *78*, 589, 1963.

Greene, J. C., Vermillion, J. R. and Hay, S.: Utilization of birth certificates in epidemiologic studies of cleft lip and palate, Cleft Palate J., *2*, 141, 1965.

Greene, J. C., Vermillion, J. R., Hay, S., Gibbens, S. F. and Kerschbaum, S.: Epidemiologic study of cleft lip and cleft palate in four states, J. Amer. Dent. Ass., *68*, 387, 1964.

Milham, S., Jr.: Underreporting of incidence of cleft lip and palate, Amer. J. Dis. Child., *106*, 185, 1963.

Tretsven, V. E.: Impressions concerning clefts in Montana Indians of the past, Cleft Palate J., *2*, 229, 1965.

Periodontal Disease

Bhaskar, S. N. and Frisch, J.: Occlusion and periodontal disease, Int. Dent. J., *17* 251, 1967.

Emslie, R. D.: Report on a dental health survey in the Republic of the Sudan, World Health Organization, PA/219.65, 1965.

Greene, J. C. and Vermillion, J. R.: The simplified oral hygiene index, J. Amer. Dent. Ass., *68*, 7, 1964.

Hine, M. K.: Principles of the treatment of periodontal disease, Oral Surg., *9*, 604, 1956.

Nevitt, G. A.: Dental health in the Middle East: report of an epidemiological study, Bull. W.H.O., *25*, 263, 1961.

Ramfjord, S. P.: The periodontal status of boys 11 to 17 years old in Bombay, India, J. Periodont., *32*, 237, 1961.

Russell, A. L.: A system of classification and scoring for prevalence surveys of periodontal disease, J. Dent. Res., *35*, 350, 1956.

————: Epidemiology of periodontal disease, Int. Dent. J., *17*, 282, 1967.

Shklar, G., Cohen, M. M. and Yerganian, G.: A histopathologic study of periodontal disease in the Chinese hamster with hereditary diabetes, J. Periodont., *33*, 14, 1962.

Waerhaug, J.: Preliminary report on WHO periodontal survey in Ceylon, October-December 1960. WHO PA/175.62, 1962.

————: Current basis for prevention of periodontal disease, Int. Dent. J., *17*, 267, 1967.

Oral Cancer

Chaves, M. M.: Epidemiological studies of the World Health Organization, Int. Dent. J., *15*, 176, 1965.

Friedell, H. L. and Rosenthal, L. M.: The etiologic role of chewing tobacco in cancer of the mouth, J.A.M.A., *116*, 2130, 1941.

Hirayama, T.: An epidemiological study of oral and pharyngeal cancer in Central and South-East Asia, Bull. W.H.O., *34*, 41, 1966.

Keller, A. Z.: The epidemiology of lip, oral and pharyngeal cancers and the association with selected systemic diseases, Amer. J. Public Health, *53*, 1214, 1963.

Kreshover, S. J. and Salley, J. J.: Predisposing factors in oral cancer, J. Amer. Dent. Ass., *49*, 538, 1957.

Kreshover, S. J.: Summary—neoplasia, J. Dent. Res., *45*, 560, 1966.

Salley, J. J.: Experimental carcinogenesis in the cheek pouch of the Syrian hamster, J. Dent. Res., *33*, 253, 1954.

Stern, Diane: The influence of systemic cancer on the oral tissues, Oral Surg., *29*, 229, 1970.

Trieger, N., Ship, I. I., Taylor, G. W. and Weisberger, D.: Cirrhosis and other predisposing factors in carcinomas of the tongue, Cancer, *11*, 357, 1958.

Chapter 4

Genetics and Dental Practice[*]

A knowledge of genetics can be very useful in the diagnosis and treatment of oral diseases; and counseling of patients afflicted with hereditary entities is important to their welfare.

Genetics is defined as the study of variation. Its subspecialties are designated according to the level at which the variations take place. *Biochemical* genetics is concerned with observed variation as expressed in chemical and molecular terms and relates to specific phenotype and genotype differences. *Cytogenetics* deals primarily with the study of chromosomes. *Immunogenetics* deals

with antigens and antibodies, their reactions and inheritance in families. *Population genetics* deals with the distribution of genes in populations and families and factors that affect the frequency of these genes. *Developmental genetics* is concerned with those genetic factors which temporally coordinate cell and tissue activity during embryogenesis by production of chemical regulating factors in accord with their need. This latter area also includes the study of *congenital malformations*.

Clinical genetics is concerned with the inheritance of pathologic traits, whether innocuous or life threatening. Simply stated, genetic variation is reflected at the molecular level as specific change in protein structure, which alteration affects both the physical properties and function of the protein. Such a molecular alteration is frequently manifest to the clinician as a specific disease or syndrome.

McKusick has listed 2,336 diseases of man showing monogenic inheritance. Considering the various modes of inheritance, 1,218 are listed as dominant traits, 947 are recessive, and 171 are X-linked. Many of these disorders or diseases involve the head and neck, and are of concern to the dentist.

When hereditary disease is suspected, the recording of a pedigree frequently will con-

[*] *Contributed by* Gerald H. Prescott, D.M.D., M.S., *Associate Professor of Medical Genetics and Perinatal Medicine, Co-Director of the Prenatal Diagnosis Clinic, University of Oregon Health Sciences Center,* and David Bixler, D.D.S., Ph.D., *Professor and Chairman, Department of Oral Facial Genetics, School of Dentistry, Indiana University-Purdue University at Indianapolis.*

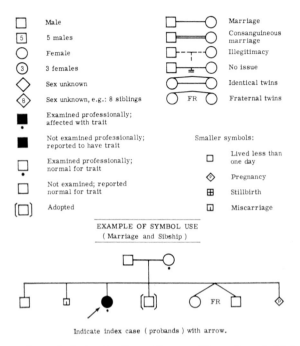

Fig. 4-1. Commonly used symbols in family pedigrees. (Prescott and Bixler, Dent. Clin. North America, March, 1968.)

firm or deny the tentative diagnosis. If the practitioner is not inclined to prepare a pedigree, he should refer the patient to a genetics consultant. Qualified genetic counselors are located in most schools of medicine and most children's hospitals have personnel knowledgeable in genetics. Many schools of dentistry are acquiring this service and can be of aid to any referring dentist.

According to Shapiro, "probably the most useful product of an adequate analysis of a genetic disease is an ability to provide empiric risk data, such as the probability that future children will be similarly affected. Furthermore, environmental familial factors may be elicited through family study." Figure 4–1 provides a list of symbols which are commonly used in constructing a pedigree for genetic analysis.

Man has 23 pairs of chromosomes, or a total of 46, which is his diploid number. One pair is the sex chromosomes which are designated the X and the Y; the human female carries two X-chromosomes, while the male has one X and one Y-chromosome. The remaining 22 pairs of chromosomes are designated autosomes (Fig. 4–2).

Genetic diseases can be divided into three classes: those produced by a single gene (monogenic trait); those produced by more than one gene (polygenic trait); those due to gross alteration in either or both chromosomal structure and number. Hemophilia is a classic example of a monogenic trait, while such human traits as height and I.Q. are polygenic in nature. Down's syndrome (mongolism) is a specific disease due to the presence of an extra chromosome in the patient's genetic complement. Individuals affected with Down's syndrome typically have 47 chromosomes rather than the normal 46 (Fig. 4–3).

DEFINITIONS

Gene—a portion of DNA coded for the synthesis of a specific protein or polypeptide chain.

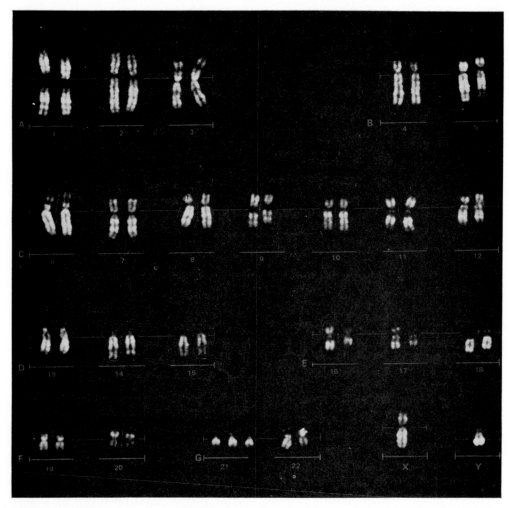

Fig. 4-2. Normal human female karyotype, showing fluorescent binding using the quinacrine technique. (Courtesy of Douglas Hepburn, U.O.H.S.C.)

Genotype—the specific set of genes carried by an individual.

Phenotype—the clinical appearance of a patient, or overt manifestation of this defect which can be seen, felt, or measured by laboratory tests.

Pleiotropy—multiple phenotypic effects produced by the same gene or gene pair.

Polygenic traits—those traits produced by many genes at different loci each with a small, additive effect. Synonyms: multifactorial or quantitative traits.

Locus—the specific site on a chromosome occupied by a particular gene.

Alleles—genes which occupy homologous loci on homologous chromosomes. Since alleles segregate at meiosis, a child receives only one allele from each parent. Only two alleles are present in any one individual at the same locus. Synonym: allelomorphs.

Dominant gene—one which expresses its phenotype in the heterozygous or single gene dose form.

Recessive gene—one which expresses its phenotype when it is present in the homozygous or double gene dose form. Such genes are not usually detectable in the heterozygote form.

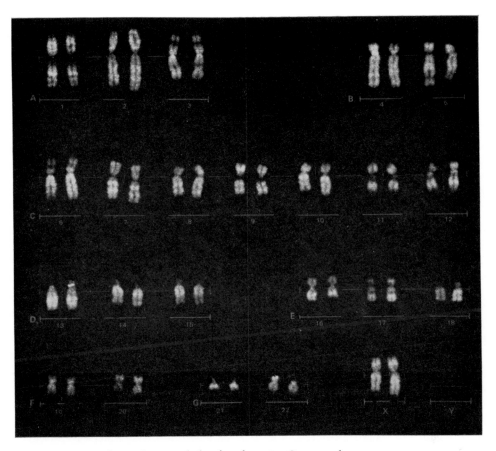

Fig. 4-3. Karyotype of a male mongol showing the extra G group chromosome.

Codominant gene—if each one of a pair of genes at the same locus is fully expressed in the heterozygote, these allelic genes are said to be codominant. Coat color in short-horned cattle provides an illustration of codominance where the homozygous dominant animals are red in color, the homozygous recessive animals are white in color, and the heterozygotes are roan (mixed red and white) in color. In humans, the ABO blood group system shows codominance.

Heterozygote—an individual whose two alleles at a given locus are different. Adjective: heterozygous.

Homozygote—an individual whose two alleles at a given locus are identical. Adjective: homozygous.

X-linked—genes on the X-chromosome; traits determined by such genes are called X-linked. Synonym: sex-linked.

Familial—occurring in different members of a family; may or may not be of genetic etiology.

Congenital—present at birth, but not necessarily genetic.

Chromosome—the nuclear structure composed of DNA which contains the units of heredity, the genes.

Autosome—any chromosome other than the sex chromosomes. Man has 22 pairs of autosomes.

Gamete—a mature germ cell (sperm or ovum) with a haploid chromosome number.

Haploid—the chromosome number of a normal gamete which contains only one member of each homologous chromosome pair. In man the haploid number is 23.

Zygote—the fertilized diploid ovum formed by the union of the haploid egg with the haploid sperm.

Penetrance—the frequency of phenotypic expression of a specific gene in a group of individuals known to carry that gene. If 80 percent of those carrying that gene show its phenotype, the trait is said to be 80 percent penetrant. Many genes in man are incompetely penetrant thereby complicating the geneticist's analysis.

Expressivity—the degree of severity of the effect of a gene in individuals with the same genotype (*i.e.* in neurofibromatosis some individuals will have skin tumors, skin pigmentation and bone changes; others will have pigmentation only).

Pedigree—a family lineage charted in a systematic manner.

Carrier—a normal-appearing individual who carries a single recessive gene (either autosomal or sex-linked) together with its normal allele (*i.e.* a normal appearing heterozygote).

Sib or sibling—brother or sister.

Proband or propositus—the index or first case in a family who is noted to have the trait in question.

Holandric—the pattern of inheritance of genes located on the Y-chromosome. Since very few genes are known to be on the Y-chromosome, the term *sex-linked* is restricted to genes on the X-chromosome.

MONOGENIC INHERITANCE

The fusion of two haploid gametes at the time of fertilization results in the formation of a diploid zygote. A zygote in which both genes for a given trait are alike (for example, T/T or t/t) is called a homozygote; one in which they are different is called a heterozygote (for example, T/t). The adjectives homozygous and heterozygous are used to describe these two conditions. A gene that shows its trait in the heterozygous condition is classically considered to be a domi-

nant factor; that which is not apparent is the recessive factor. Thus, the genotype may be T/T, T/t or t/t, while the character determined by each of these genetic combinations is the phenotype.

Actually, genes themselves are not dominant or recessive, but their action in the expression of the phenotype is referred to as dominant or recessive. Patterns followed by monogenic traits within families are determined by whether the specific trait is dominant or recessive, by whether the gene is autosomal or sex-linked, and by chance distribution of the genes from parents to children by the gametes. However, even simple monogenic patterns can be altered or obscured by factors such as pleiotropy, reduced penetrance, variable expressivity, and environmental effects. Although reduced penetrance and variable expressivity are common in autosomal dominant conditions, all of the foregoing contribute to the tremendous variability in human traits and characterize gene action in man.

Autosomal Dominant Inheritance

A hereditary trait which is governed by a single dominant autosomal allele is dentinogenesis imperfecta. In a pedigree analysis, several characteristics of autosomal dominant inheritance must be observed in order to merit that designation:

1. Every affected person has at least one affected parent.
2. Males and females are equally likely to be affected and should be capable of transmitting the trait, provided the affected gene does not cause sterility.
3. Usually there is no skipping of generations, and father-to-son and mother-to-daughter transmission should be as frequent as father-to-daughter and mother-to-son.
4. Affected persons typically transmit the trait to half their offspring.

Therefore, a dentist who has a patient with dentinogenesis imperfecta should look for additional affected individuals in the family,

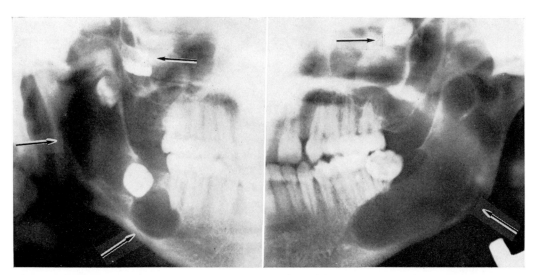

Fig. 4-4. This Panorex radiograph of a 19-year-old black girl depicts one of the principal findings in the basal cell nevus or bifid rib syndrome. Note the extremely large cysts of dental origin in all four posterior quadrants (*arrows*). Other findings in this syndrome may be bifid ribs, cutaneous nevi, calcification of the falx cerebri, medulloblastoma, and pitting of the skin on the hands and feet. This syndrome has an autosomal dominant mode of inheritance. (Prescott and Bixler, Dent. Clin. North America, March, 1968.)

and he should not overlook the counseling opportunity in regard to the risks involved in succeeding offspring. Note that all of these criteria as stated indicate 100 percent penetrance. Another autosomal dominant entity of dental interest is the bifid rib or basal cell nevus syndrome (Fig. 4–4). See Figure 4–5 for an illustration of the autosomal dominant mode of transmission.

Autosomal Recessive Inheritance

A trait transmitted as an autosomal recessive is expressed only in a person who receives the recessive gene in question from each parent; therefore, he is homozygous for

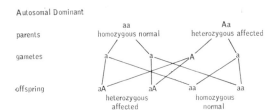

Fig. 4-5. The mechanics of the autosomal dominant mode of transmission. (Prescott and Bixler, Dent. Clin. North America, March, 1968.)

it. Often the trait appears in siblings of the proband but usually not in relatives outside the sibship, with the possible exception of first cousins. Because children affected with recessive traits usually are produced by two phenotypically normal but heterozygous carrier parents, the families which can be recognized and studied are only those in which at least one affected child has occurred. Families carrying the gene in which by chance no child is affected merge with the general population and are not diagnosed; therefore, some families carrying the gene do not have affected offspring. However, the gene may be transmitted through each generation by carriers; such a carrier will have affected children only if his or her spouse is also a carrier and the two genes meet in the zygote.

Thompson and Thompson list the criteria for autosomal recessive inheritance as: (1) The trait appears only in sibs, not in their parents, offspring or other relatives. (2) On the average, one-fourth of the sibs of the propositus are affected. (3) The parents of the affected child may be consanguineous.

Autosomal Recessive

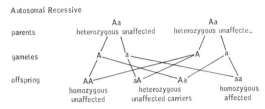

Fig. 4-6. The mode of transmission for the autosomal recessive condition. (Prescott and Bixler, Dent. Clin. North America, March, 1968.)

This is particularly true for rare recessive diseases since, if a gene is quite rare, two such genes (one in each parent) are more likely to have originated from the same individual. Hence, there would be consanguinity. (4) Males and females are equally likely to be affected (Fig. 4–6).

Some autosomal recessive diseases with dental and oral implications are: acatalasia, hypophosphatasia (Fig. 4–7), agranulocytosis, oculoauriculovertebral dysplasia syndrome, and occasionally infantile cortical hyperostosis. Figure 4–7 shows a little girl who has hypophosphatasia. This rare recessive disease was suspected by the family dentist when she lost her deciduous incisors prematurely.

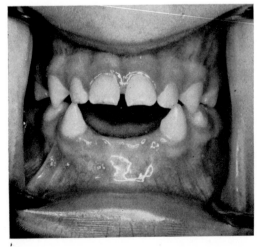

Fig. 4-7. Hypophosphatasia. This 2½-year-old child shed the lower incisors prematurely and other teeth are loose. Her identical twin has suffered similar changes. (Courtesy of Charles Poland.)

X-Linked Recessive Inheritance

A unique inheritance pattern characterizes genes on the X-chromosome. Since females have two X-chromosomes and males only have one, genes which are recessive in females behave as dominant genes in males since they are always expressed. The transmission of X-chromosomes from parents to offspring provides the basis for the pattern of X-linked (sex-linked) recessive inheritance. Affected males cannot transmit an X-linked gene to their sons since sons receive the Y-chromosome; but all daughters will receive the gene and be carriers. Father-to-son transmission of a trait rules out X-linked genes, although the possibility should always be recognized that a son may by chance have received a similar gene on the X-chromosome from his mother. Females carrying a deleterious X-linked gene may be phenotypically normal because the normal allele is dominant to the deleterious gene; however, these women transmit the deleterious gene to half of their sons, who then express the trait. These women also transmit the deleterious gene to half of their daughters who will then be carriers like their mothers. Therefore, a higher frequency of affected males with X-linked recessive traits is expected and the affected males often appear in alternate generations.

Criteria for sex-linked recessive inheritance may be listed as: (1) Incidence of the trait is much higher in males than in females. (2) The trait is transmitted by affected men to all of their daughters, who are carriers. (3) The trait cannot be transmitted from father to son. (4) The trait may be transmitted through a series of carrier females, and if so the affected males in a family are related to one another through these carrier females.

Other diseases of dental importance which are transmitted by genes on the X-chromosome are anhidrotic ectodermal dysplasia and hemophilia. One must remember that certain traits (*e.g.* supernumerary teeth, Fig. 4–8) may have different modes of transmis-

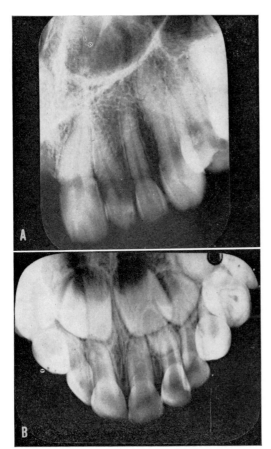

Fig. 4-8. *A,* Supernumerary upper lateral incisor in the mother. *B,* Supernumerary deciduous lateral of her daughter. Another supernumerary may be forming along with the permanent incisors.

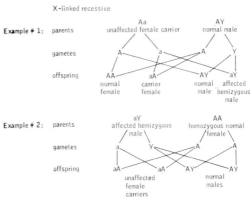

Fig. 4-9. The mechanics of the X-linked (sex-linked) recessive mode of transmission. Note that in the two examples A and a stand for the X genes. (Prescott and Bixler, Dent. Clin. North America, March, 1968.)

ever, an affected male cannot transmit the trait to his sons, but all his daughters receive his X-chromosome containing the affected gene and hence will be affected.

While this type of inheritance is uncommon, there are kindreds reported with such inheritance for the following diseases with dental implications: vitamin D resistant rickets (hypophosphatemia), the oral-facial-digital syndrome, and amelogenesis imperfecta (hypoplastic type). An illustration of the latter appears in Figure 4–10. The ex-

sion as dominant or recessive in different kindreds; however, the two different modes should not occur in the same family in order to be the same trait. See Figure 4–9 for an example of X-linked recessive inheritance.

X-Linked Dominant Inheritance

The rules for X-linked dominant inheritance are similar to those for X-linked recessive, except that in the former heterozygous females may express the condition. Since females have twice as many X-chromosomes as males, they exhibit a higher frequency of the trait. An affected female, if heterozygous, will transmit the gene to one-half of her offspring, regardless of their sex. How-

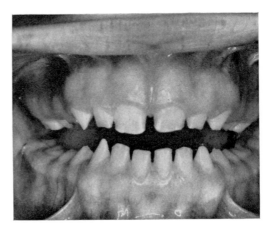

Fig. 4-10. Amelogenesis imperfecta of the hypoplastic type. The teeth are smooth and brown and a very thin layer of enamel is present.

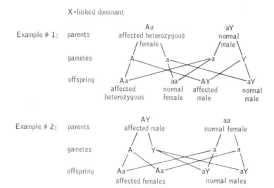

X-linked dominant

Example # 1:   parents   Aa   aY
                           affected heterozygous   normal
                                 female   male
               gametes   A   a   a   Y

               offspring   Aa   aa   AY   aY
                          affected normal   affected normal
                          heterozygous female male   male

Example # 2:   parents   AY   aa
                           affected male   normal female
               gametes   A   Y   a   a

               offspring   Aa   Aa   aY   aY
                          affected females   normal males

Fig. 4-11. The mode of transmission for the X-linked (sex-linked) dominant condition. (Prescott and Bixler, Dent. Clin. North America, March, 1968.)

amples shown in Figure 4–11 typify the X-linked dominant pattern of inheritance.

Y-Linked (Holandric) Inheritance

Y-linked inheritance should be the easiest to recognize, since every son of the affected father should be affected, and no daughter would ever be affected or transmit the trait. The Y-chromosome is remarkably free of genes since any cellular function which is required by both men and women would have to be controlled by another chromosome. Obviously, the most important function of the Y-chromosome is to determine maleness and this is most evident in unusual chromosomal aberrations where an individual receives an excess number of X-chromosomes, say 3, 4 or even 5! However, if only one Y-chromosome is present, the individual is a phenotypic male regardless of the number of X-chromosomes. See Figure 4–12 for

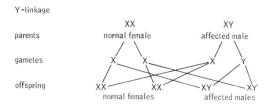

Y-linkage

parents   XX   XY
                normal female   affected male
gametes   X   X   X   Y

offspring   XX   XX   XY   XY
             normal females   affected males

Fig. 4-12. The mode of transmission for holandric (Y gene) inheritance (Prescott and Bixler, Dent. Clin. North America, March, 1968.)

an example of the holandric mode of transmission.

No specific genes on the Y-chromosome have been implicated in the etiology of a genetic disease. Apparently, the genes on the Y-chromosome are those that determine maleness.

POLYGENIC (MULTIFACTORIAL) INHERITANCE

A less well defined and more complex area of genetics is the study of those traits for which more than a single gene is responsible. Since multiple genes are involved, there is no sharp distinction between normal and abnormal phenotypes and the phenotype is continuously variable in the population. Examples in man of such continuously varying polygenic traits are stature, intelligence, tooth size, fingerprint ridge count, and skin color. This type of inheritance is based on the premise that each gene has its own effect and the sum total of all these multiple effects produces the phenotype.

A trait that can be measured quantitatively is defined as continuous (*e.g.* height). Traits that show continuous variation are difficult to study but still follow the basic concepts of Mendelian genetics. According to Sutton, "the genes involved in continuous traits are not unusual. The only special feature is that variation among several sets of genes influences one trait." These traits are then designated as exhibiting polygenic or multigenic inheritance.

A most important feature of polygenic traits is that they are very susceptible to environmental modification. A phenotype controlled by the concerted action of many genes is much more likely to be altered and modified by the existing environment than is one which is controlled by only one or even a few genes. For example, dental caries is the interaction product of three essential factors: a cariogenic diet, a caries-producing bacterial flora and a susceptible tooth. These three factors encompass a variety of biologically complicated entities such as saliva, plaque, tooth matrix formation and crystallization. It should be easy for the reader to visualize that the development of these complex elements must involve at least several genes. Environmental modification, such as properly timed systemic fluoride supplementation, produces a considerable alteration in the phenotype without changing the basic genetic constitution of the individual. By contrast, a single gene trait, such as amelogenesis imperfecta, shows very little environmental modification and routinely exhibits a characteristic phenotype in all individuals who carry the gene.

Polygenic Inheritance in the Common Dental Diseases

The practicing dentist readily recognizes among his patients a considerable variation in susceptibility to dental caries, periodontal disease and malocclusion; the former are essentially infectious diseases, whereas malocclusion is not produced by infectious organisms. Nevertheless, all three have hereditary components which are best described as *polygenic* in nature. In accord with the previous definition of polygenic disease, these diseases have the following three important features: (1) their hereditary components are produced by multiple genes, (2) environment plays a role in determining the phenotype and (3) discrete phenotypes are difficult to recognize and a continuous variation in "susceptibility" exemplifies the typical situation.

These conclusions are quite evident for the disease dental caries. Studies of human families and of twins and experimental observations with inbred rats show clearly that there is a strong, but minor, polygenic component to this disease. Environmental modification, which is the rule and not the exception in polygenic disease, is strongly evidenced by the many dietary studies, notably the Vipeholm study in Sweden, which showed the variable cariogenicity of sugars in different chemical and physical forms.

Similar findings are presumptive but not yet established for the common form of periodontal disease. Very little is known of the hereditary aspects of this disease, and it appears certain that better phenotypic description of the various types of periodontal involvement will be necessary before progress in understanding its inheritance is made. For example, periodontosis has been reported to be inherited in an X-linked dominant fashion by Melnick *et al.*

Finally, malocclusion is undoubtedly the end product of a summation of multiple developmental events such as (1) size of maxilla and mandible, (2) arch form, (3) tooth anatomy and size, and (4) tooth position in the jaws, just to name a few. All of these elements are under genetic regulation and it must be noted that the concept of occlusion involves a dynamic interrelationship of such factors. Hence, we define malocclusion as a polygenic disease. Malocclusion is uncommon in pure racial stocks, which implies that genetically homogenous populations have "normal" occlusion and genetic heterogeneity increases the incidence of jaw and occlusal discrepancies. Such findings have been demonstrated in animals by Stockard. In man, studies using twins and triplets have demonstrated that the morphology of an individual bone is under strong genetic control, but that environment plays the major role in determining how the various bony elements are combined to achieve a harmonious or disharmonious craniofacial skeleton.

Thus, the major diseases of dentistry may be polygenic in nature and thereby subject to considerable environmental modification. Admittedly, family patterns are frequently evident but the dental practitioner and the geneticist alike must be very cautious in making predictions based upon family observations because of the unknown and untested variables. It may be that the treatment plan of individuals with these diseases would be unaltered if the entire hereditary picture were known and understood. Only addi-

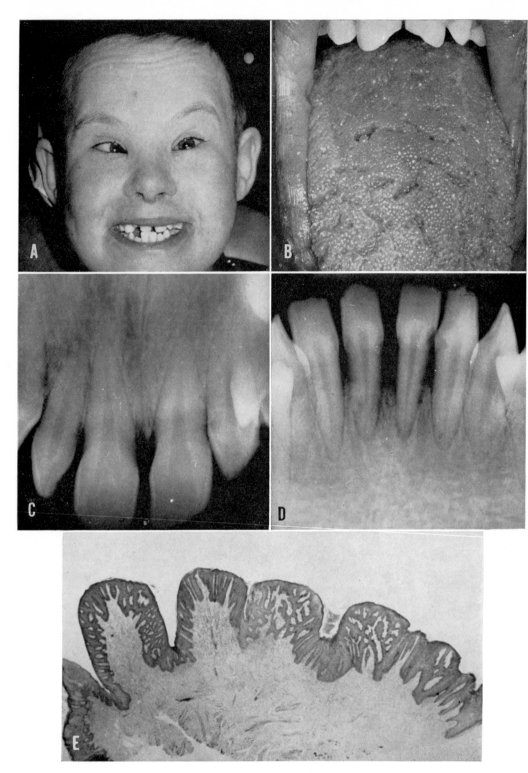

Fig. 4-13. Down's disease (mongol). *A*, Note the slant of the eyes and the strabismus. *B*, The "pebbly" tongue with fissures is characteristic of many mongoloids. Fractured anterior teeth are common among the mentally retarded. *C* and *D*, The unusual morphology of the teeth and early periodontal disease of a mongol. *E*, Photomicrograph of the tongue. Note the absence of filiform papillae.

tional research will tell us how much we may be able to regulate heredity in the control of disease.

CHROMOSOMAL ABERRATIONS

Interest in the field of cytogenetics, the study of human chromosomes, has been stimulated by the development of techniques whereby cytogeneticists can culture cells of organisms *in vitro,* and thereby examine chromosomes under the microscope for alterations in size, shape and fine structure. Typically, leukocytes from peripheral blood are used, but skin and other tissues may also be cultured. It was just such a technique of chromosome analysis, named karyotyping, that led LeJeune and Turpin in 1959 to demonstrate that the fundamental defect in mongolism (Down's syndrome) is the presence of an extra chromosome in the affected individual's karyotype. Thus, the typical mongol has 47 chromosomes with a typical facies (Fig. 4-13). Since then several human disease states have been specifically ascribed to the loss or gain of chromosomes. However, alteration in number is only one aspect of chromosome disease in man. Refined karyotyping techniques have revealed that the structure of a chromosome may be altered as well. These various structural alterations have been given the descriptive classification: (1) deletion—a piece of a chromosome is absent, (2) duplication— the insertion of an extra chromosome fragment into a chromosome from its homolog, (3) inversion—the breaking of a chromosome in two places and subsequent rejoining with the middle piece inverted, and (4) translocation—the attachment of a broken piece from one chromosome to another, but non-homologous, chromosome.

With the identification of these alterations in chromosome number and structure, a nomenclature system for the various chromosomes based upon their morphology became a necessity. The currently accepted system is called the Paris nomenclature and is primarily based upon chromosome identification by overall length and individual anatomic characteristics. Figure 4-2 shows the karyotype of a normal human female.

Each chromosome consists of thousands of genes, and it is easy to see how an extra piece—or missing piece—of a chromosome could involve many cell functions and hence result in a clinically identifiable disease state. As might be expected, disease states resulting from gross chromosomal alterations have a very complicated clinical picture involving multiple systems. This is readily apparent in Down's syndrome.

When an extra chromosome is present, that condition is spoken of as trisomy of the chromosome in question, as for example in Down's syndrome (trisomy 21) (Fig. 4-3). The extra chromosome belonging to the G group is readily apparent. Monosomy of an autosome, or a missing autosomal chromosome, had not been thought to be compatible with life until one such affected individual was recently reported with an apparent G group monosomy. On the other hand, monosomy of the sex chromosomes does occur, is compatible with life and typically affects development of both internal and external sex organs of the individual. The best known example of this is Turner's syndrome which occurs about once per 3,000 live births. These individuals are phenotypic females who are missing an X chromosome and are chromosomally designated as XO. They are typically of short stature, lacking in secondary sex characteristics and are sterile. The Turner's syndrome karyotype is shown in Figure 4-14.

Finally, after a presentation of some of the aberrant events that may occur with human chromosomes, the reader should be cognizant of the fact that only about 0.5 percent of all live births have a chromosomal abnormality.

Even though this is a relatively rare event, clinicians agree that chromosome aberrations are a significant cause of mental and physical defects.

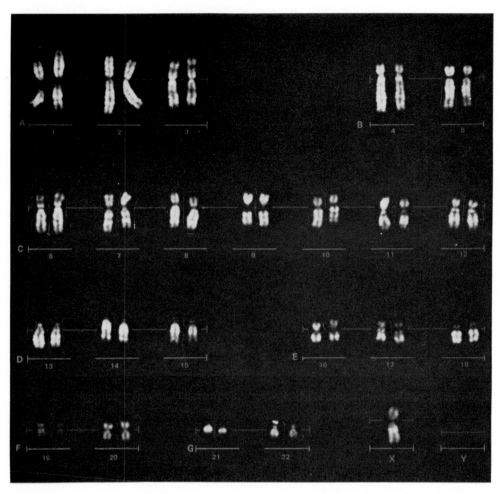

Fig. 4-14. Karyotype of a female with Turner's syndrome. Note the absence of the X-chromosome.

GENETIC COUNSELING

Information about heredity, all too often incorrect, has been provided for families to alter their reproductive behavior by friends, enemies and neighbors. The counsel of the professional geneticist should be sought. This person must have a working knowledge of human genetics and a complete understanding of genetic modes of inheritance, gene interaction in families and human populations, and chromosomal abnormalities. With this knowledge he can sort out and present facts and figures to his patients.

The geneticist must have a deep respect for the attitudes and feelings of the people he is counseling. He does not perform his function by simply making a diagnosis and presenting the bare facts. Such facts are usually presented in detail, but the framework in which they are presented is most important. Only when the patient understands these facts and they are minimally distorted by those personally involved—either consciously or unconsciously—can the counselor assume that he is performing a service. Feelings of guilt, fear, hostility and resentment are frequently encountered at the counseling table. All of the presentation and discussion must be couched in tact and sensitivity, for perhaps in no other area of

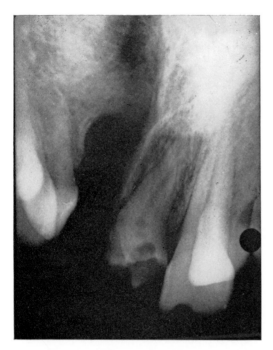

Fig. 4-15. Unilateral cleft. Hypoplastic teeth adjacent to such clefts are common and may be related to the early surgical repair.

human existence do we feel so personally responsible as in the area of conception and childbearing.

Finally, the genetic counselor must have a sincere desire to teach the truth to the full extent that it is known. By careful attention to patient responses he often can obtain the feedback necessary for evaluation of his success in communication.

Monogenic traits with complete penetrance and little variation in expressivity provide few difficulties for the genetic counselor. Unfortunately, few human hereditary problems are so well defined. Cleft lip, with or without cleft palate (CL ± CP), and isolated cleft palate (CP) provide examples of problems facing the dentist that have strong but ill-defined hereditary components (Fig. 4-15).

The dentist treating and counseling families affected with these conditions should be aware that CL ± CP is a different trait from CP alone. Since cleft lip is 3 times more common in boys than in girls, while isolated cleft palate is more common in females, a differential threshold for gene expression in the two sexes has been offered as the explanation.

Cleft lip (with or without cleft palate) affects approximately 1 child in each 1000 births (0.1 percent), and may be unilateral or bilateral. Fraser, using figures based on small and heterogeneous collections of cases, indicated that the risk of a cleft lip recurring in a family in which there is already one such child is between 4 and 7 percent if neither parent is affected, but about 11 percent when one parent is already affected (Table 4-1).

Cleft palate alone has a frequency of about 1 per 2500 (.04 percent) births in Caucasian populations. Empiric risk figures based on Robert's data indicate that, given an affected child born to normal parents

Table 4-1. Recurrence Risks for Succeeding Offspring for Cleft Lip with or without Cleft Palate (CL ± CP) and Isolated Cleft Palate (CP).

Mating Type	Normal Parents with no Affected Children	Normal Parents with One Affected Child	One Parent Affected Only	One Affected Parent with One Affected Child
Cleft lip with or without cleft palate	0.1–0.15% (1–1.5/1000)	4–7% (40–70/1000)	2% (20/1000)	10–19% (100–190/1000)
Cleft palate only	.04% (1/2500)	0.1–12% (1–120/1000)	6–7% (60–70/1000)	13–17% (130–170/1000)

Table 4-2. Some Genetic Traits Associated with the Dento-Oro-Facial Complex and their Modes of Inheritance

Genetic Trait	Frequency in Population	Mode of Inheritance
Amelogenesis imperfecta—hypocalcification type	1/20,000	AD
Amelogenesis imperfecta—local hypocalcification type	1/40,000	AD
Amelogenesis imperfecta—hypoplastic type	1/40,000	SLD
Amelogenesis imperfecta—hypomaturation type	1/40,000	SLR
Ankyloglossia	1/300	Familial (AD?)
Bifid nose (median cleft face)	rare	?
Bifid or cleft uvula	1/100 Caucasian 10/100 Indian, Japanese	AD
Cleft, median alveolar—diastema	rare	?
Cleft lip with or without cleft palate	1/800 Caucasian 1/500 Japanese 1/2500 Negro	Familial (AD?)
Cleft palate alone	1/2500 Caucasian	Familial (AD)
Darier's disease (keratosis follicularis)	rare	AD
Dentinogenesis imperfecta	1/8000	AD
Dentin dysplasia	1/50,000	AD
Ectodermal dysplasia (hypohidrotic)	rare	SLR
Fibrous dysplasia of jaws (cherubism)	rare	AD
Freckles (ephelis), susceptibility to	1/10	AD
Gingival fibromatosis, hereditary	uncommon	AD
Glossitis, median rhomboid	1/500	?
Hereditary hemorrhagic telangiectasis	1/50,000	AD
Hereditary macrocheilia	prevalent in Negro; uncommon in Caucasian	AD
Hypertrichosis	rare	AD
Hypodontia of primary dentition (usually mandibular incisor)	1/1000	?
Hypodontia of permanent dentition		
Maxillary lateral incisors	1/20	Familial (D?)
Missing premolars	1/10	Familial (D?)
Missing third molars	1/4	Familial (D?)
Ichthyosis vulgaris	uncommon	SLR
Lip, commissural pits of	1/150	AD
Lip, lower pits and fistulas of	1/25,000	AD
Micrognathia	1/500	? (Familial)
Mucosa, white folded dysplasia of	rare	AD
Papillon-Lefevre syndrome	rare	AR
Rickets, vitamin D resistant	1/20,000	SLD

Table 4-2—Continued

Genetic Trait	Frequency in Population	Mode of Inheritance
Taurodontism	rare in Caucasians, common in Eskimos, Indians and S. African natives	Familial
Teeth, fused (gemination)	1/500	AD
Tongue, fissured	1/10 (mild cases)	?
Tongue, geographic	1/50	Familial
Tongue, scrotal	as high as 1/5	AD
Torus, mandibularis	1/20	AD
Torus palatinus	as high as 1/4	AD

AD = Autosomal dominant   SLD = Sex-linked dominant

AR = Autosomal recessive   SLR = Sex-linked recessive

with no other affected first degree relatives, the chances of a subsequent cleft palate child are increased to about 1.2 percent. If such an affected child is born to normal parents in a family with an affected close relative (grandparents, parents and offspring), the recurrence risks are increased to 10 percent. Bixler *et al.* report the risk for CP offspring of a CP parent is 6 percent. The risk figures used in Table 4–1 are ranges based on several studies.

The previous paragraphs have been presented in order to give the reader perspective on the problem of genetic counseling. The question can be asked, "Is the dentist equipped to give genetic counsel?" Under certain conditions he may function quite adequately in this role. First, he must be sure of his diagnosis. Secondly, he must have information as to the hereditary aspects of the condition in question. Table 4–2 furnishes specific genetic information about some of the more common oral conditions he may observe. Finally, he must be able to communicate this information in its proper perspective to his patient or the parents. Parents frequently comment that their child's

susceptibility to tooth decay is not unexpected since their own teeth were similarly affected. The dentist must clearly delineate the roles of heredity and environment in such comments if he is to correct erroneous concepts of oral diseases that are common to the lay public.

Sometimes parents are concerned about specific dentofacial variations and may re-

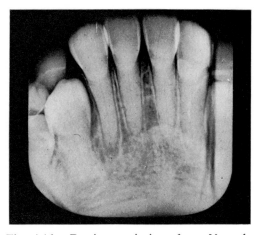

Fig. 4-16. Dentinogenesis imperfecta. Note the tendency toward obliteration of the root canals in this child. In most cases the roots are more spiked than shown here. (Courtesy of Arden G. Christen.)

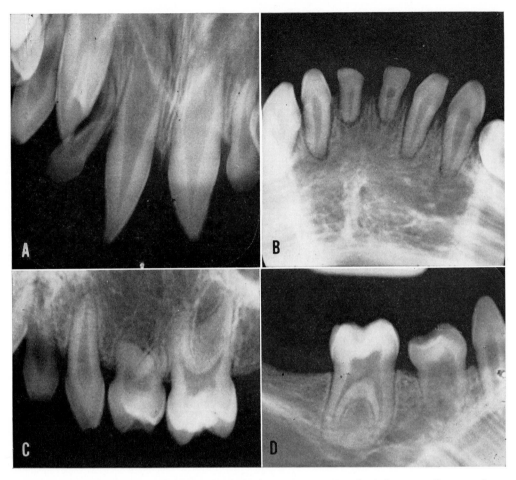

Fig. 4-17. *A–D*, Hereditary ectodermal dysplasia in an 8-year-old. The hair and nails were slow to appear and his hair is sparse. (Courtesy of Richard Haag.)

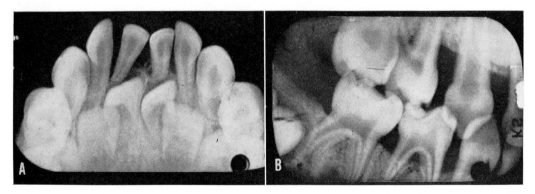

Fig. 4-18. *A*, Papillon-Lefevre syndrome. Note the loss of periodontal bone around the deciduous incisors. *B*, Bite-wing film showing bone loss in the posterior region. (Coccia, McDonald, and Mitchell, J. Periodont., *37*, 408, 1966.)

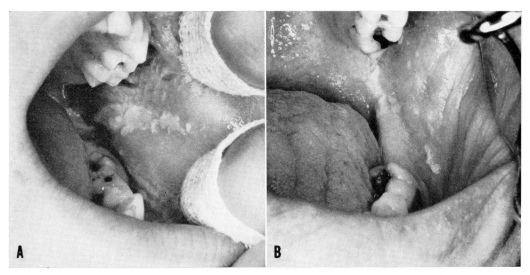

Fig. 4-19. White sponge nevus in a boy, *A,* and in his father, *B.*

quest information from the dentist. When a child has a hereditary tooth defect and the parents are so informed, they typically will be concerned about the possibility of having additional similarly affected children. If the dentist is familiar with the condition in question and can communicate easily with the family, he should do so, since he bears the professional responsibility for the oral health of this family. On the other hand, if the slightest doubt exists concerning any of the previously mentioned qualifications, he should refer the family to a genetics clinic for counseling, preferably one with a staff dentist. A great service can be performed and rapport established for future dental treatment when the patient and his family know that extra effort has been expended in the interest of their oral health.

Figures 4–16 to 4–20 illustrate some interesting cases with genetic implications.

BIBLIOGRAPHY

Bixler, D., Christian, J. G. and Gorlin, R. J.: Hypertelorism, microtia and facial clefting, Amer. J. Dis. Child., *118*, 495 1969.

Bixler, D., Fogl-Andersen, P. and Correally, P. M.: Incidence of cleft lip and palate in the offspring of cleft parents, Clin. Genet., *2*, 155, 1971.

Brookreson, K. R. and Miller, A. S.: Dentinal dysplasia: report of case, J. Amer. Dent. Ass., *77*, 608, 1968.

Chaudhry, A. P., Johnson, O. N., Mitchell, D. F., Gorlin, R. J. and Bartholdi, W. L.: Hereditary enamel dysplasia, J. Pediat., *54,* 776, 1959.

Gordon, R. R.: The indications for chromosome analysis as an aid to the clinician, Clin. Pediat., *7,* 83, 1968.

Gorlin, R. J. and Pindborg, J. J.: *Syndromes of the Head and Neck,* New York, McGraw-Hill Book Co., 1964.

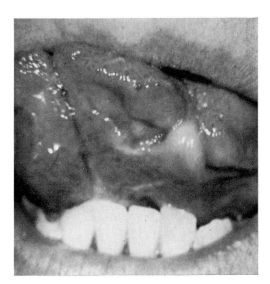

Fig. 4-20. Cleft tongue (trifid) of a mother whose daughter had the same affliction—oral facial digital dysostosis, Type I.

Johnson, O. N., Chaudhry, A. P., Gorlin, R. J.,
Mitchell, D. F. and Bartholdi, W. L.: Hereditary dentinogenesis imperfecta, J. Pediat., *54,*
786, 1959.

Lynch, H. T., Mulcahy, G. M. and Krush, A. J.:
Genetic counseling and the physician,
J.A.M.A., *211,* 647, 1970.

McCormick, J. and Ripa, L. W.: Hypophosphatasia: review and report of case, J. Amer.
Dent. Ass., *77,* 618 1968.

McKusick, V. A.: *Mendelian Inheritance in Man,*
Baltimore, The Johns Hopkins Press, 4th Ed.,
1975.

Melnick, M., Shields, E. D. and Bixler, D.: Periodontosis: a phenotypic and genetic analysis,
Oral Surg., in press.

Nance, W. E. and Engel, E.: Human cytogenetics:
A brief review and presentation of new findings, J. Bone Joint Surg., *49-A,* 1436, 1967.

Prescott, G. H. and Bixler, D.: Implications of
genetics in dental practice, Dent. Clin. North
America, March, 1968.

Reed, S. C.: *Counseling in Medical Genetics,*
Philadelphia, W. B. Saunders Co., 1963.

Srb, A. M., Owen, R. D. and Edgar, R. S.: *General Genetics,* San Francisco, W. H. Freeman,
1965.

Thompson, J. S. and Thompson, M. W.: *Genetics
in Medicine,* 2nd Ed., Philadelphia, W. B.
Saunders Co., 1973.

Witkop, C. J., Jr., Ed.: *Genetics and Dental
Health,* New York, McGraw-Hill Book Co.,
1962.

Chapter 5

Physical Evaluation for Comprehensive Care

A planned, comprehensive dental care program must include a consideration for the patient's general, oral and psychiatric health as well as his socioeconomic status, opinions and ability and desire to cooperate in treatment and post-treatment home care maintenance. A comprehensive examination includes an analysis of the patient's physical health, oral health, and attitudes. This should be determined at the first or second visit. On occasion, attitudes, the ability to cooperate and the desires of the patient cannot be assessed until some treatment has commenced, and even then the plan may not be finalized until after some treatment has been accomplished and the patient has had a chance to demonstrate his cooperation.

CHIEF COMPLAINT

After obtaining such basic information as age, sex, marital status, address, phone number and occupation, the dentist should ask the patient why he is seeking dental service at this time. Patients often fail to admit the real reason for coming to the dentist. The answer, "for a checkup," should not be too readily accepted. The patient should be induced to relate the specific signs or symptoms which prompted his coming, and they should be recorded (see questionnaire on pp. 98–101).

The dentist should gain and keep his patient's confidence and be sympathetic to his problems. Often a mere placing of a hand on the shoulder of an apprehensive patient will have a tranquilizing effect. This fact is widely recognized among practitioners of the healing arts and is referred to as the beginning of "tender loving care" (TLC).

DENTAL HISTORY

The patient should be questioned as to previous dental care, his satisfactions and dissatisfactions, attitudes toward dental treatment, and indirectly his dental I.Q. will become apparent. This helps the dentist guide him through treatment. Any reluctance regarding x-radiation can be detected and counteracted at this point. Questions 1 through 14 direct themselves specifically to the patient's dental history and attitude toward dental health and dental care (see pp. 91–93).

HEALTH INFORMATION

One of the most valuable tools in determining the patient's general physical health status and psychiatric health is the medical history.

With the increasing life expectancy today, more patients with serious health problems are ambulatory and they seek dental care. Some of these problems are unknown to the patient and some are yet undiagnosed. Special precautions often are necessary in order to care for a patient with a systemic illness; therefore, the dentist must have a thorough knowledge of the patient's health before beginning treatment. If the patient is reluctant to provide this information, a few words of explanation usually will convince him that he should do so. A complete knowledge of all medications taken by the patient, past and present, is necessary.

MEDICAL HISTORY RECORDING

There are three basic ways to obtain health information: (1) direct interrogation; (2) comprehensive questionnaire, answered by the patient; and (3) a combination of these two methods (see pp 24, 91).

Direct Interrogation

The patient is asked key questions about his health status, and the information collected is summarized. Many dental schools furnish charts with useful notes regarding the various systems to guide the student in this type of interrogation. There is a great deal of freedom in completing this type of medical history. It can vary from the extensive hospital admission-type medical history, which may be several pages long, to a mere one-sentence statement, depending on the findings and the initiative of the examiner.

Even with a patient who is perfectly healthy, however, some positive statements should be made regarding his medical history. "Past medical history, essentially negative" is not an acceptable statement, for it provides no information as to the thoroughness of the interrogation. That fact alone should tell the student that medicolegal responsibility would be neglected under such circumstances.

The patient should be questioned about signs or symptoms suggestive of abnormality in any system of the body. He should be questioned with respect to his tolerance for previous dental treatment, known allergies to medications, previous hemorrhagic tendencies, significant family history of disease, and previous operations or injuries. He should also be asked for a self-appraisal of his general health and strength. This information should be collected methodically and summarized for future reference.

The disadvantages of this method are: (1) it depends largely on the ability and experience of the dentist, and therefore in a training situation, such as the dental school, it does not provide uniform information from all patients; (2) it is easy for the questioner to forget important questions; and (3) it is time-consuming.

Health Questionnaire

This method does not involve as much of the dentist's time. A list of preselected questions is given to the patient to be answered while he is in the reception room. A quick review of positive answers provides the dentist with reasonable knowledge of the patient's health. However, this method also has its disadvantages: (1) there is less opportunity to develop rapport; (2) some patients take questionnaires of this sort too lightly and are not careful in completing the form; (3) it is difficult to select questions which cover every possibility; (4) the mental capacity of the patient (or his guardian) to comply must be considered; and (5) the tendency to allow an auxiliary person to supervise the use of the questionnaire *in toto* must be vigorously resisted.

Combination Questionnaire-Medical History

This form is an efficient means of collecting complete health information. The patient is given a questionnaire to be answered regarding his general health. Questions are asked with respect to symptoms suggestive of systemic diseases, and a place is provided for a statement of his general health. The dentist supplements this information by oral questioning regarding selected responses of the patient. In addition, a record of the patient's previous hospital admissions, injuries and the medications he has taken during the previous six months should be obtained. This information should then be correlated and summarized briefly on the record.

The dentist must be well versed in the recognition of signs and symptoms suggestive of systemic diseases. If such diseases are suspected during questioning, further investigation and/or consultation may be indicated.

Interpretation of Health Questionnaire-Medical History

1. *Have you ever been told that you have heart trouble?* A positive answer to this question might suggest a heart murmur, a previous coronary occlusion or infarction, or a history of congestive heart failure. Patients with angina pectoris or even high blood pressure might also answer "yes" to this question. Depending on the type of disorder and severity, certain precautions—*e.g.* premedication with antibiotics or sedatives, shortened appointment, and low-stress dental procedures or only minimal therapy—might be indicated.

2. *Have you ever had high or low blood pressure?* A positive answer to this question should prompt you to ask "when and how the condition was treated?" It should also prompt you to take the patient's present blood pressure and record this in the chart. Patients who are hypertensive should be referred to a physician for further diagnosis

and therapy. Those already under care might be taking drugs with side effects such as dry mouth which might, in turn, affect the caries activity. Hypotensive patients are more prone to fainting than normal patients.

3. *Do you get out of breath easily?* SOB or shortness of breath and/or dyspnea might result from a cardiac disorder such as cardiac decompensation from congestive heart failure. It might also result from a pulmonary disorder such as emphysema or asthma. Of course, it might merely indicate a patient who smokes heavily or is in poor physical condition. The importance depends on the severity, so this question alone is meaningless. Now if the patient answered this question in the affirmative and also questions 1 and 4 (he had a history of rheumatic fever), and he also had swollen ankles, you should consider a diagnosis of congestive heart failure, and refer the patient for further evaluation.

4. *Have you ever had rheumatic fever, growing pains or twitching of the limbs?* Most growing pains are thought to be caused by the long bones outgrowing the attached muscles, stretching them and causing pain, although there is some disagreement about this. Twitching of the limbs is generally considered a condition within the realm of normalcy; however, on occasion, when it becomes severe during the early years of life, it is mistakenly considered insignificant while actually it might represent an early manifestation of rheumatic fever. Today, though, with better diagnosis, children with rheumatic fever are more easily diagnosed and so they usually know if they have had rheumatic fever. The significance of rheumatic fever is that it often results in a damaged heart valve, producing a detectable heart murmur. Occasionally the heart murmur is sufficient to cause problems from valve leakage, often not; however, a damaged heart valve is of significance to the dentist. Should the patient undergo a dental procedure which causes bloodletting, a bacteremia might be produced. Pathogenic bacteria entering

the bloodstream tend to congregate on a damaged heart valve, producing bacterial endocarditis. Therefore, patients with a history of rheumatic fever should receive prophylactic antibiotics prior to any dental procedure which might produce a bacteremia.

5. *Have you fainted more than twice in your life?* The cause for the syncope is significant. It is not uncommon for a person to report that he has fainted once or twice in a lifetime, but frequent fainting or dizziness could suggest cardiovascular or neurologic disease. This being the case, proper precautions would be necessary before beginning dental treatment. Occasionally patients with epilepsy will refuse to admit that they are epileptic, but will answer positively to this question.

6. *Do you have spells of dizziness?* Patients who report that they have dizzy spells may have psychiatric problems, cardiovascular problems, or even neurologic problems, and any indication of "spells of dizziness" should be investigated very thoroughly. Usually medical consultation is indicated.

7. *Do your ankles become easily swollen?* Ankle edema is caused by congestive heart failure. It can also result from kidney disease. Any time there is inadequate return circulation to the heart from the legs, tissue fluid can collect, producing what is referred to as pitting edema. A positive answer to this question would therefore prompt you to examine the ankles for pitting edema. Remember, however, that patients can develop ankle edema from trauma or from sitting over a long period of time, especially if they have varicose veins.

8. *Do you suffer from frequent headaches?* The usual headache is the result of eyestrain, tension, or dilated, stretched cerebral blood vessels. More significant, however, are the headaches produced by hypertension and by brain tumors. Very severe headaches with occasional visual aberrations are referred to as migraine headaches. Thus, the severity and type of headache might be significant to the patient's general health and welfare. Should there be any question, referral is indicated. If the patient is taking an aspirin compound for his headache, it is important to know how often and for how long he has been taking this; the clotting mechanism can be suppressed by prolonged use of aspirin.

9. *Has a physician ever told you that you have neuritis, neuralgia or neurosis?* These three words, "neuritis, neuralgia and neurosis," are often confused by the patient as being similar, but really they are quite different. "Neuritis" refers to inflammation of a nerve or nerve sheath resulting in pain or tenderness, paresthesia or anesthesia, and it has many causes including infection and vitamin deficiencies. "Neuralgia" refers to paroxysmal pain which extends along the course of one or more nerves, and often the etiology is unknown. Some specific neuralgias (*e.g.* trigeminal neuralgia) may simulate pain of dental origin and *vice versa*. A "neurosis" is a disorder of the psychic or mental constitution and, in contrast with psychosis, is less incapacitating. Patients with neuroses frequently need sedation prior to dental treatment. If a patient indicates that he has neuritis, neuralgia, or neurosis, it is important for you to determine which of the three he has, and the additional pertinent details.

10. *Have you ever had a nervous breakdown?* The term "nervous breakdown" is a lay term for an acute emotional or psychiatric disturbance. Like patients with epilepsy, psychiatric patients often refuse to admit their problem. Because the words "nervous breakdown" seem innocuous, they are useful to detect patients who have been institutionalized or otherwise treated for psychiatric problems. Patients taking tranquilizers, mood elevators and/or antidepressants for psychiatric problems often have a depressed salivary gland flow (a side effect of the drug) with an associated increased caries rate. This question is thus important from the standpoint of caries control as well as for patient management.

The astute examiner can often detect psychiatric disorder despite denial by the patient. Habits such as rapid eyelid fluttering, puzzled facial expression, reluctance to answer questions and sometimes extreme cooperation should be viewed with suspicion. The patient who answers "yes" to virtually every question on the health questionnaire probably has some psychogenic or psychological disturbance. However, it is unwise to point this out to him. With good rapport development and a thorough understanding of the patient's problem, management for dental treatment is usually not difficult. Consultation is helpful.

11. *Has a physician ever told you that you had epilepsy?* As mentioned before, patients with epilepsy may answer "no." Epilepsy is significant in that, if a patient has a seizure during dental treatment, it would be necessary to protect him so he does not injure himself. Further, medication such as Dilantin sodium used to control epileptic seizures often causes a fibrous gingival hyperplasia which otherwise might be misdiagnosed. A clue to detection is that epileptics often have multiple scars on the face and tongue from falls and other nonfunctional activity such as chewing the tongue during a seizure. Likewise they frequently have discolored necrotic teeth from falls during a seizure. Dental care for the epileptic is quite safe providing it is known that the patient has epilepsy and proper preparation is made beforehand.

12. *Is your nose continually stuffed up?* This might indicate a chronic allergy, hypertension, or decreased resistance and a continuous cold.

13. *Do you have asthma, hay fever, sinusitis or frequent sore throats?* Asthma, hay fever and sometimes sinusitis and sore throats might be allergic in origin. Patients with one allergy are prone to have other allergies. Therefore, if an allergy is probable, the patient should be questioned as to the possibility of an allergy to penicillin, local anesthesia or other medicaments used

in dental therapy. Too, it is sometimes difficult for the allergic patient to breathe through his nose, complicating the use of rubber dams or the taking of impressions. Lastly, if the patient does have a cold or upper respiratory infection, you risk contracting this condition.

14. *Have you ever had tuberculosis?* If the patient answers "yes," you should find out when, where he was treated, and by whom, and contact the physician to make sure that the disease is not communicable. The patient treated for tuberculosis usually will not be released into society if he is infectious, but it is wise to check to be sure. Like patients with emphysema, bronchitis and severe asthma, those with advanced tuberculosis should not be given sedatives which might depress respiration further unless this is done with careful forethought.

15. *Do you suffer from stomach trouble or frequent diarrhea?* Much stomach trouble and diarrhea are nervous in origin, but can also be due to gastrointestinal infections or allergies. Patients who have gastric ulcers or gastritis frequently cannot tolerate aspirin-containing compounds and also should not be given corticosteroids. If the patient has not been examined by a physician, this should be suggested. Patients under treatment for chronic gastrointestinal upsets, particularly the very young and the very old, may have been given antiemetics such as Compazine. A side effect of this drug can produce the extrapyramidal syndrome which often simulates temporomandibular joint dysfunction syndrome.

Hopefully you are beginning to see how one question interfaces with another by now.

16. *Have you ever taken thyroid tablets?* Occasionally, thyroid tablets are given for obesity, but most properly they are given for hypothyroidism. Unless the patient is taking more than 3 gr of thyroid extract daily or its equivalent, there generally is no concern with respect to dental treatment. However, patients taking drugs to depress thyroid function should be treated only after

consultation with a physician, as a hyper-thyroid patient can go into shock following relatively minor trauma such as that which might occur during dental treatment. If this question is answered in the affirmative, therefore, be careful to determine what kind of thyroid tablets are being taken and why.

17. *Have you, or has any member of your family, ever had diabetes?* Patients who are diabetic tend to respond poorly to infections such as periodontitis. They also heal slowly following surgery. Diabetes tends to run in families; therefore, patients with a positive family history should be considered as possible diabetics. If a patient suffers from polydipsia and polyuria or if he demonstrates a lowered resistance to infection, diabetes should be suspected. Special precautions are often necessary in treating diabetics.

18. *Have you ever been told that you had kidney or bladder trouble?* Most mild kidney and bladder diseases are not significant to dental treatment. All oral foci of infection should be eliminated in patients with severe cystitis or nephritis. Long-standing nephritis of various types can cause permanent damage to the kidney and result in cardiovascular problems, so unless the patient is under the care of a physician it is wise to seek consultation before beginning dental treatment.

19. *Have you ever been treated for ear trouble or eye trouble, other than by corrective glasses?* Ask about any symptoms the patient might have if he answers this question positively and refer him to an ophthalmologist or an otolaryngologist for further diagnosis and therapy.

20. *Are you sensitive or allergic to any particular medicines?* Often patients who have allergies state that they are sensitive when they really mean they are hypersensitive. Any patient who is allergic to any known medication should be questioned very thoroughly. Often patients allergic to one medication are allergic to others, and they frequently develop additional allergies read-ily. Since aspirin and penicillin are commonly used and since many people are allergic to these two drugs, the patient should specifically be asked about any past problems with aspirin or penicillin. If the patient is allergic to any of the medications which might be used in dentistry, this should be indicated in red on the patient's chart and care should be taken not to administer these medications. Likewise, the dentist should be prepared for the increased possibility of an allergic reaction to any medication.

21. *Have you gained or lost much weight recently?* Dieting today is a fad; therefore much weight loss is due to dieting and is not significant. Unplanned weight loss however might be a sign of malignancy or other serious systemic ailment. Further, unexplained weight gain might be due to fluid retention from kidney or heart disease.

22. *Have you ever had syphilis or venereal disease?* Your patient might balk at answering this question; he might consider its significance irrelevant. Truthfully, this question is an icebreaker—it is not significant to dental treatment but is a personal question, and if the patient will answer this the chances are that he or she will be honest in some of the other personal questions. Obviously, a patient with syphilis in the secondary stage is infective to you even by contact through the oral cavity, and likewise any chronic venereal disease might lower the patient's resistance. When in doubt, wear rubber gloves.

23. *Have you ever had an operation?* Types and details of any recent operations should be investigated and listed. Uneventful recovery from recent major surgery can be helpful in predicting the successful, uneventful outcome of dental treatment. Problems which occurred, if any, should be thoroughly analyzed prior to oral surgery.

24. *Have you ever had a series of needles, shots or injections?* Most will answer "yes" to this question but to them it might mean injections of local anesthesia or immuniza-

tion. So if they answer "yes," you should question them further to see if the series was for treatment of some chronic ailment, such as cortisone for arthritis, monthly penicillin for rheumatic fever, or cytotoxic agents for a neoplasm. Such treatment would be significant.

25. *Have you ever been told that you have a tumor or cancer?* If the answer is "yes" then you will want to determine the type of tumor, whether it was benign or malignant, if it has been successfully treated, and its location, as this would influence your examination procedures later.

26. *Have you ever had anesthesia, local or general?* Often patients will answer "no" and if so they should be questioned further. If they answer "yes," make sure they know what local and general anesthesia mean, and that they have had no difficulty with anesthesia.

27. *Have you been told not to take Novocain or any other medication?* If the answer is "yes," the types of medications and reasons for prohibition should be determined and listed. They should be included in the summary of the medical history, with good documentation.

28. *Are you taking any medications or receiving any treatment by a physician?* If so, you should determine for what conditions, the name of the physician giving the treatment and the medication.

29. *Have you ever had anemia?* Patients who have anemia often are weak and have oral mucosal pallor or paleness. Occasionally they bleed excessively following oral surgery or prophylaxis and they tend to faint more readily than the average individual because of the decreased circulating hemoglobin in the bloodstream. The type of anemia is important, as anemia occurs in patients with leukemia as well as in patients with iron deficiencies, abnormal gastrointestinal absorption, and chronic bleeding.

30. *Have you ever had excessive bleeding following tooth removal or cuts, or do you have frequent nosebleeds?* Patients with a history of frequent nosebleeds should be examined by a physician for that complaint. Spontaneous gingival bleeding is a bad sign, often of leukemia. Patients claiming excessive bleeding following tooth removal or cuts should be closely scrutinized. If they truly had excessive bleeding and not just blood mixed with saliva following a tooth extraction, for example, a careful hematologic workup is in order prior to any further treatment. A positive answer to this question thus should prompt an extensive history and follow-up.

31. *Have you ever had jaundice, liver trouble, or hepatitis?* A patient who has had or currently has hepatitis could be infectious, and treatment of this patient could be dangerous for the dentist. Chronic liver disorders can produce excessive bleeding because of insufficient prothrombin production in the liver. If the patient gives a history of hepatitis, all instruments should be carefully sterilized to prevent cross-contamination. You and your assistant should wear rubber gloves.

32. *Have you been treated for a skin disease?* If the answer is "yes," then determine the type of skin disease and the treatment. Many patients with fungal or allergic diseases of the skin are treated with corticosteroids and long-term corticosteroid therapy can cause depression of the adrenal cortex, leading to iatrogenic (doctor-induced) hypoadrenal corticism. This adrenal depression may result in pigmentation in the areas of the buccal mucosa, tongue and cheeks and even the lips, and also around newly healed skin wounds. The significance in dentistry is that, with hypofunction of the adrenal cortex, excessive stress may precipitate acute adrenal cortical insufficiency and shock. Thus the patient taking corticosteroids for dermatoses or other conditions such as arthritis should be carefully scrutinized, medical consultations should be obtained, and the patient should receive heavy doses of cortisone prior to any stressful dental procedure. Some skin diseases are

communicable and precautions for the dentist and assistant should be taken. Further, certain diseases such as senile keratosis may degenerate into basal cell carcinoma.

33. *Are your joints often painfully swollen?* Painful joints suggest arthritis, of a traumatic, rheumatoid, or degenerative type. Treatment of arthritis often includes long-term corticosteroid and aspirin therapy, and we have discussed the problems associated with prolonged use of these drugs.

34. *Have you had more than one fracture or dislocation?* Patients with a history of multiple fractures could have such disorders as hyperparathyroidism or osteopetrosis (brittle bone disease), or some other systemic disorder. Tooth extraction would therefore be risky. The reason for multiple fractures, then, should be ascertained. They could have resulted from an accident, in which event the patient might also have sustained injuries to the jaws.

35. *Do you have arthritis?* This is a direct question to determine if the patient knows if he has arthritis. We are looking at arthritic patients from the standpoint of the treatment of arthritis, and also because patients with generalized severe arthritis generally cannot be made comfortable for long periods of time in a dental chair. There is always the possibility that the temporomandibular joint could be involved.

36. *Have you often had severe toothaches?* Patients who have frequent and/or severe toothaches should be questioned as to the length of time they are in pain and the severity of the pain. Toothache to a patient usually means pain in the jaw region. This should help you in your examination to determine the exact etiology. Obviously, the pain might be the result of periodontal disease or deep carious lesions or a multitude of other things including trauma. This information is useful prior to examination, especially with respect to the patient's chief complaint.

37. *Have you ever had severe pain of the face and head?* A positive answer to this question should be correlated with a positive answer to the previous question. Possibly any severe pains in the face and head region might be the result of a toothache. Likewise it is possible that some neurologic problem is present. This again is good background information prior to the oral examination.

38. *Do your gums bleed when you brush your teeth?* Bleeding gums are abnormal and usually indicate some type of periodontal disease, but spontaneous bleeding of gingivae might indicate leukemia, a hemorrhagic disorder, or other serious disease of the blood. Spontaneous hemorrhage is a serious finding, whereas hemorrhage caused by minor trauma such as toothbrushing usually indicates that the patient has gingival or periodontal problems.

39. *Have you ever had gum treatments?* If so, why, and was the treatment successful in the patient's mind? We will look later to see if it was successful in our opinion.

40. *Have you ever had severe sore mouth?* A positive answer to this question would suggest Vincent's infection, acute herpetic stomatitis, stomatopyrosis (burning mouth), or glossopyrosis (burning tongue) and others. The patient should be examined for the possibility of underlying systemic diseases.

41. *Do you ever suffer from frequent cold sores or fever blisters?* This is a straightforward question designed to find out if the patient has had aphthous or herpetic lesions. Sometimes patients refer to them also as stomach ulcers.

42. *Does it hurt when you chew?* Exposed dentin in the cervical region may cause pain when eating extremely hot or cold foods or even when breathing cold air. Teeth in traumatic occlusion may be painful during mastication. Chronic granulomas, periodontal disease or periodontal abscesses also may make teeth painful and tender.

43. *Does it hurt when you open wide or take a big bite?* If the answer is "yes," it is possible that your patient has a temporomandibular joint disorder or a spasm of the

muscles associated with the temporomandibular joint.

44. *Does your jaw make noise so that it bothers you or others?* Crepitation, clicking or popping in the joint area is a sign of abnormality of the temporomandibular joint either from damage within the joint capsule or from malfunction of the muscles of mastication.

45. *Do you suffer from headaches?* This is a repeat of question #8, but it is part of a special section (questions 42 through 52) directed to ascertain the possibility of a dysfunction of the patient's stomatognathic system.

46. *Do you suffer from ear pain or pain in front of the ears?* Tenderness in the preauricular region is often a symptom of myofascial pain dysfunction syndrome or primary temporomandibular joint disorders.

47. *Do you suffer from pain in the face, jaws, eyes, throat, or neck?* A positive answer here might likewise indicate that the patient has a dysfunction of the temporomandibular joint and would trigger the need for an extensive occlusal evaluation. If the answer to this question is "yes," then questions 48 through 52 should be answered by the patient.

48. *Must you take tablets because of the above-mentioned pain or discomfort?*

49. *Does the pain or discomfort disturb your sleep?*

50. *Does the pain or discomfort interfere with your work or other activities?*

51. *Are you afraid that this is something serious?*

52. *Do you feel that you need treatment for the above problems?*

Analyzing answers to questions 47 to 52 will help determine whether an extensive occlusal analysis is indicated during the examination of the stomatognathic system.

In reviewing all of the answers to the 52 questions, a number of things should be considered. First, if there are many "yes" answers and they do not seem to correlate in terms of primary etiology, consider that

the patient might be neurotic. If a patient answers "no" to virtually all of the 52 questions, consider that he may not have taken the questionnaire seriously. Even the most healthy individual would normally answer "no" to several of the questions, and likewise many "yes" answers are not probable in a healthy patient.

At this point, then, the examiner must be directly involved. Prior to this, the patient could have filled out the questionnaire or an auxiliary might help with it, but the section entitled "To be Filled out by the Examiner" (Fig. 5–1) should be completed by the dentist.

Visits to the physician in the past six months should be indicated and dated as accurately as possible, and the reason for the visit and the findings should be recorded. *All medicines taken in the past six months* should be listed and you should then refer to the *Physician's Desk Reference* or some other reference to see why these medications were prescribed.

Thought must be given to this list as it will not only provide a clue to the patient's health state but also may shed some light on unusual oral findings. In addition, the ever-increasing problem of drug interaction must be considered.

Drug Actions and Interactions

As an example, suppose a 65-year-old male patient claims and appears to be in good health. A list of medications being taken reveals a tablet you identifiy as digitalis. With this information alone, you can surmise that he is probably under treatment for congestive heart failure, although your physical evaluation suggests he is functionally healthy. You should realize that undue stress in dental treatment could tip the scales of his delicate physiologic balance and result in cardiac decompensation. It seems logical then to sedate the patient with phenobarbital to prevent stress—*a mistake!* Phenobarbital tends to decrease the effects of digitalis and worsen the situation because of

HEALTH INFORMATION FORM

Date _____

Name: _____ Age _____

Occupation: _____

TO: Prospective Patient

Please answer the following questions by filling in the appropriate blanks. If you need help, ask the clerk. You may have several answers to each question.

1. **Chief Complaint:** What is or are your reasons for being here?
   - ☐ I am in pain
   - ☐ I am aware that I need dental treatment
   - ☐ I think I have dental or mouth infection
   - ☐ Dissatisfied with present dental appearance
   - ☐ No particular reason — just want checkup
   - ☐ Unable to chew food properly
   - ☐ Have numbness or unusual sensation
   - ☐ Think I might have a tumor or cancer

   - ☐ Other. Specify _____
   _____

   - ☐ Referred by: ☐ another dentist;   ☐ a physician   ☐ other (specify) _____
   Name & Address: _____
   _____

2. **History of Present Complaint:**
   - ☐ Recent (started within past two days)
   - ☐ Symptoms developing over long period — Specify time: _____
   _____

3. **Last Dental Visit:**
   - ☐ Within last 3 months
   - ☐ Within last 4-6 months
   - ☐ Within 7 months to 1 year
   - ☐ More than 1 but less than 5 years
   - ☐ Over 5 years
   - ☐ Never before

4. **Reason for last dental visit:**
   - ☐ Routine Exam
   - ☐ Special diagnostic and/or radiographic (x-rays)
   - ☐ Toothache
   - ☐ Tooth extractions or fractured jaw (Oral surgery)
   - ☐ Gum treatments or loose teeth (Periodontics)
   - ☐ Fillings, bridges, removable dentures, etc. (Restorations)
   - ☐ Root canal treatments (Endodontics)
   - ☐ Orthodontics (braces) or teeth straightened

   - ☐ Other, Describe _____
   _____

5. **Past dental history** (check <u>all</u> previous services received from dentist):
   - ☐ Dental exam with x-rays
   - ☐ Tooth extraction or oral surgery
   - ☐ Restorations (fillings)
   - ☐ Partial dentures (removable)
   - ☐ Crown and bridgework (fixed)
   - ☐ Special diagnostic exam — Explain: _____
   - ☐ Complete dentures
   - ☐ Periodontic treatment (gum treatments)
   - ☐ Endodontic treatment (root canal treatment)
   - ☐ Orthodontic treatment (braces)
   _____

6. **Previous dental experiences**
   - ☐ Unpleasant experience with dentist(s) in past
   - ☐ Pleased with previous dental experience
   - ☐ So-so
   - ☐ Fearful of dental treatment
   - ☐ Have had dental problems all my life
   - ☐ Have had very few dental problems in past
   - ☐ Other (Specify) _____
   _____

Fig. 5-1.   Sample form of patient questionnaire.

7. History of tooth loss

☐ Have had no permanent teeth removed
☐ Tooth loss resulting from accident
☐ Had teeth removed for orthodontics (braces) only
☐ Had teeth removed because they were loose and/or could not chew on them
☐ Other:_____

☐ Had tooth or teeth removed due to infection (abscesses) of teeth or gums
☐ Had wisdom teeth (3rd molars) removed
☐ To improve appearance
☐ Primary teeth (baby teeth) only

8. Outcome of previous extractions:

☐ Not applicable. Have never had a tooth extracted.
☐ Uneventful
☐ Dry socket or infection after extraction
☐ Excessive bleeding after extraction

☐ Healed slowly
☐ Pain after extraction
☐ Had to return to dentist after surgery for further treatment of extraction site

☐ Other: _____

9. X-rays (radiographs)

☐ I have never had tooth or jaw radiographs (x-rays) taken
☐ I have had tooth or jaw radiographs taken in past
Types taken:
☐ Single tooth films   ☐ Panoramic
☐ Bitewings   ☐ Head plates or other
☐ Full mouth series   ☐ Do not know

10. Oral Hygiene

☐ I brush after each meal
☐ I brush when I "think about it"
☐ I brush once or twice a day
☐ I never brush

☐ I use: ☐ disclosing tablets; ☐ floss; ☐ rubbertip; ☐ Stimudents; ☐ mouthwash; routinely
☐ I have had previous oral hygiene instructions.
When? _____

11. Habits

☐ Clench or "grit" teeth
☐ Grind teeth day or night
☐ Nail biting

☐ Smoking: ☐ cigarettes; ☐ cigars; ☐ pipe. Amount:_____
☐ Chew: ☐ gum; ☐ tobacco
☐ I often have tired jaws in the ☐ morning; ☐ night

☐ Other mouth, jaw or tongue habits. Specify: _____

12. Self Analysis of Oral Tissue Health

☐ Bad teeth (cavaties)
☐ Crooked teeth
☐ Bad gums
☐ Bad bite; bite feels off
☐ Frequent sores in mouth or on lips
☐ Halitosis (bad breath)
☐ Teeth painful to hot, cold, sweets (underline which)

☐ Pain or clicking in jaw joints (underline which)
☐ Bleeding mouth or gums (underline which)
☐ Swelling in mouth or jaws on occasion (underline which)
☐ Loose or drifting teeth
☐ Food catches between by teeth
☐ Bad taste

☐ Other signs or symptons. Describe: _____

13. Family Dental History

☐ One or both parents have removable dentures
☐ One or both parents had frequent dental care
☐ One or both parents take reasonable care of their mouth(s)

☐ One or both parents go to a dentist only when have problems
☐ My children have regular dental exams (once or twice per year)
☐ I have no children over 2 years of age

14. Attitudes

☐ Most people will eventually lose their teeth
☐ Good dental care can prevent the above
☐ I feel I understand how to adequately care for my mouth
☐ I want to learn more about proper home care for _myself_
☐ I want to learn more about proper home care for _my children_

☐ I am convinced that fluorides are important in the prevention of tooth decay.
☐ I am convinced that tooth brushing and the use of dental floss is important in preventing tooth decay and gum disease
☐ I am convinced that good diet prevents dental disease

Fig. 5-1—(Cont.).

15. Health Questionnaire

1. ☐ Yes ☐ No Have you ever been told that you have heart trouble?
2. ☐ Yes ☐ No Have you ever been told that you have high or low blood pressure?
3. ☐ Yes ☐ No Do you get out of breath easily?
4. ☐ Yes ☐ No Have you ever had rheumatic fever, growing pains or twitching of the limbs?
5. ☐ Yes ☐ No Have you fainted more than twice in your life?
6. ☐ Yes ☐ No Do you have spells of dizziness?
7. ☐ Yes ☐ No Do your ankles ever become easily swollen?
8. ☐ Yes ☐ No Do you suffer from frequent headaches?
9. ☐ Yes ☐ No Has a physician ever told you that you had neuritis, neuralgia or neurosis?
10. ☐ Yes ☐ No Have you ever had a nervous breakdown?
11. ☐ Yes ☐ No Has a physician ever told you that you had epilepsy?
12. ☐ Yes ☐ No Is your nose continually stuffed up?
13. ☐ Yes ☐ No Do you have asthma, hayfever, sinusitis or frequent sore throats?
14. ☐ Yes ☐ No Have you ever had tuberculosis?
15. ☐ Yes ☐ No Do you suffer from stomach trouble or frequent diarrhea?
16. ☐ Yes ☐ No Have you ever taken thyroid tablets?
17. ☐ Yes ☐ No Have you or any member of your family ever had diabetes?
18. ☐ Yes ☐ No Have you ever been told that you had kidney or bladder trouble?
19. ☐ Yes ☐ No Have you ever been treated for ear trouble or eye trouble other than corrective glasses?
20. ☐ Yes ☐ No Are you sensitive or allergic to any particular medicines (penicillin, aspirin, etc.)?
21. ☐ Yes ☐ No Have you gained or lost much weight recently?
22. ☐ Yes ☐ No Have you ever had syphilis or other venereal diseases?
23. ☐ Yes ☐ No Have you ever had an operation?
24. ☐ Yes ☐ No Have you ever had a series of "needles", "shots" or "injections"?
25. ☐ Yes ☐ No Have you ever been told that you had a tumor or cancer?
26. ☐ Yes ☐ No Have you ever had anesthesia? ☐ Local ☐ General ?
27. ☐ Yes ☐ No Have you ever been told not to take novocaine or any other medication?
28. ☐ Yes ☐ No Are you taking any medicines or receiving any treatment by any physician?
          By whom? _____
29. ☐ Yes ☐ No Have you ever had anemia?
30. ☐ Yes ☐ No Have you ever had excessive bleeding following tooth removal or cuts, or do you have frequent nose bleeds?
31. ☐ Yes ☐ No Have you ever had jaundice, liver trouble or hepatitis?
32. ☐ Yes ☐ No Have you been treated for a skin disease?
33. ☐ Yes ☐ No Are your joints often painfully swollen?
34. ☐ Yes ☐ No Have you had more than one fracture or dislocation?
35. ☐ Yes ☐ No Do you have arthritis?
36. ☐ Yes ☐ No Have you often had severe toothaches?
37. ☐ Yes ☐ No Have you ever had severe pains of the face or head?
38. ☐ Yes ☐ No Do your gums bleed when you brush your teeth?
39. ☐ Yes ☐ No Have you ever had gum treatment?
40. ☐ Yes ☐ No Have you ever had severe sore mouth?
41. ☐ Yes ☐ No Do you ever suffer from frequent "cold sores" or fever blisters?
42. ☐ Yes ☐ No Does it hurt when you chew?
43. ☐ Yes ☐ No Does it hurt when you open wide or take a big bite?
44. ☐ Yes ☐ No Does your jaw make noise so that it bothers you or others?
45. ☐ Yes ☐ No Do you suffer from headaches?
46. ☐ Yes ☐ No Do you have ear pain or pain in front of the ears?
47. ☐ Yes ☐ No Do you suffer from pain in the face, jaws, eyes, throat, neck? (If you answered "yes" to this question, please answer the next 5.)
48. ☐ Yes ☐ No Must you take tablets because of the above mentioned pain or discomfort?
49. ☐ Yes ☐ No Does the pain or discomfort disturb your sleep?
50. ☐ Yes ☐ No Does the pain or discomfort interfere with your work or other activities?
51. ☐ Yes ☐ No Are you afraid that this is something serious?
52. ☐ Yes ☐ No Do you feel that you need treatment for the above problem?

A statement of your own general health: _____

_____

Fig. 5-1—(Cont.).

TO BE FILLED OUT BY EXAMINER

SDS Score _____

Visits to Physician in Past Six Months:

Date	Reason	Findings

List all medicines taken in the past six months:

_____   _____

_____   _____

_____   _____

List all hospitalizations for any reason:

Year	City	Reason	Complications

Summarized Medical-Dental History:

Reviewed and completed by:

_____

Revised and Updated: _____   _____

_____   Date: _____

Fig. 5-1—(Cont.).

Table 5-1. Interaction of Pharmacologic Agents Commonly Used in Dentistry*

Initial Agent +	Second Agent =	Combined Effect	Initial Agent +	Second Agent =	Combined Effect
Analgesics:			**Tranquilizers:**		
Salicylates	Anticoagulant	Enhanced anticoagulation	**Chlordiazepoxide**	Antihistamine	Enhanced tranquilizing effect
	Sulfonylurea	Enhanced hypoglycemia	**or**	Alcohol	Enhanced tranquilizing effect
	Insulin	Enhanced hypoglycemia	**Diazepam**	Phenothiazine	Enhanced tranquilizing effect
	Phenformin	Enhanced hypoglycemia		Barbiturate	Enhanced tranquilizing effect
	Probenecid	Decreased uricosuria		Antihypertensive	Enhanced hypotensive effect
Acetaminophen	Anticoagulant	Enhanced anticoagulation			
Phenylbutazone	Anticoagulant	Enhanced anticoagulation	**Hypnotics:**		
	Sulfonylurea	Enhanced hypoglycemia	**Chloral hydrate**	Alcohol	Enhanced sedation
	Insulin	Enhanced hypoglycemia		Anticoagulant	Enhanced anticoagulation
	Digitalis	Decreased digitalis effects		Anticoagulant	Decreased anticoagulation effect
Oxyphenbutazone	Anticoagulant	Enhanced anticoagulation	**Barbiturate**	Corticosteroid	Decreased corticosteroid effect
	Sulfonylurea	Enhanced hypoglycemia		Digitalis	Decreased digitalis effect
	Insulin	Enhanced hypoglycemia		Alcohol	Enhanced sedation
Indomethacin	Anticoagulant	Enhanced anticoagulation		Tranquilizer	Enhanced sedation
Codeine	Tranquilizer	Enhanced analgesia		Phenothiazine	Enhanced sedation
Morphine	Tranquilizer	Enhanced analgesia	**Glutethimide**	Anticoagulant	Decreased anticoagulation effect
	Antidepressant (MAO inhibitor)	Enhanced analgesia			

Drug	Interacting Drug	Effect
Meperidine	Tranquilizer	Enhanced analgesia
	Antidepressant (MAO inhibitor)	Hypertension; or hypotension and coma
Antimicrobials:		
Penicillin	Chloramphenicol	Decreased antimicrobial effect
	Tetracycline	Decreased antimicrobial effect
	Sulfonamide	Increased antimicrobial effect
Tetracycline	Penicillin	Decreased antimicrobial effect
	Antacid	Decreased absorption
	Milk	Decreased absorption
	Anticoagulant	Enhanced anticoagulation
Chloramphenicol	Penicillin	Decreased antimicrobial effect
	Anticoagulant	Enhanced anticoagulation
	Sulfonylurea	Enhanced hypoglycemia
	Insulin	Enhanced hypoglycemia
Sulfonamide	Anticoagulant	Enhanced anticoagulation
	Sulfonylurea	Enhanced hypoglycemia
	Insulin	Enhanced hypoglycemia
	Penicillin	Increased antimicrobial effect
Anti-allergics:		
Epinephrine	Antihypertensive	Decreased hypotensive effect
	Antidepressant (MAO inhibitor)	Hypertensive crisis
	Antidepressant (tricyclic)	Enhanced antidepressant effect or increased sympathomimetic effect (Hypertensive crisis)
	Digitalis	Enhanced tendency to cardiac arrhythmias
Antihistamine	Alcohol	Enhanced sedation
	Tranquilizer	Enhanced sedation
	Phenothiazine	Enhanced sedation
Cortisosteroid	Corticosteroid	Decreased corticosteroid effect
	Barbiturate	Decreased corticosteroid effect
	Diphenylhydantoin	Decreased corticosteroid effect
	Antihistamine	Decreased corticosteroid effect

* Courtesy P. W. Y. Chue, Interaction of drugs used in dentistry, Dent. Surv., October, 1975.

Table 5-2. Possible Side Effects of Some Medications of Interest to the Dentist.*

Analgesics and sedatives	Barbiturate stomatitis, skin rash. Aspirin burn and true hypersensitivity, and excessive bleeding with heavy dose.
Anesthetics	Procaine: edema.
Antibiotics	Especially penicillin and tetracyclines: skin rash, stomatitis, superimposed candidiasis, angioneurotic edema. Tetracyclines: intrinsic stain of developing teeth. Superimposed staphylococcic infections. Streptomycin: superimposed staphylococcic infection; auditory nerve degeneration. Chloramphenicol: agranulocytosis.
Anticoagulants	Excessive bleeding.
Antidepressants	Monoamine oxidase inhibitors (MAOI) are potentiated by many drugs and even certain foods, leading to a hypertensive crisis.
Antiepileptic	Diphenylhydantoin sodium (Dilantin): gingival hyperplasia.
Antihistamines	Xerostomia, drowsiness.
Antihypertensives	Postural hypotension, syncope.
CNS stimulants	Amphetamines: xerostomia; psychic stimulation.
Corticosteroids	Delayed healing, predisposition to infection, adrenal suppression.
Heavy metals	Gingival bismuth line. Mercurial stomatitis. Argyria.
Tranquilizers	Xerostomia. Extrapyramidal syndrome (esp. phenothiazine derivatives), stomatitis.

* The more common, milder reactions are listed. Severe reactions such as anaphylactic shock and glottis edema with dyspnea occur occasionally.

drug interaction. Another sedative should be selected.

The above example merely serves to illustrate the need for an in-depth knowledge of drug actions and interactions. Recent textbooks, articles and other references must be consulted frequently to keep up-to-date on this complex and important subject. Only with a thorough knowledge of drug effects, side effects and interactions can a dentist intelligently prescribe treatment.

The simultaneous administration of several different drugs or medications can produce serious, even fatal, side effects due to: chemical incompatibility of the agents, alterations in absorption of one agent by another, interference in action at the target organ site, alterations in drug metabolism and detoxification, and interference or potentiation of drug excretion.

The subject is a large and ever-changing one and the reader is referred to several articles by Chue and by Hussar for a summary of the subject as it relates to dentistry, and to Tables 5–1 and 5–2.

List all hospitalizations for any reason. Occasionally the patient will not indicate that he has been hospitalized until we get to this section. Here then we find out if he has had a thyroidectomy or other surgery that might have some significance in dental treatment. Once this information has been collected, the dentist should review it and discuss with the patient his general dental health. A summary of all significant findings in paragraph form should be written under the section entitled *Summarized Medical/ Dental History*. The tendency with a healthy patient is to write "Past medical history essentially negative." The problem with summarizing this way is that it does not indicate the depth to which the patient's health history was investigated. Therefore, it might be wise to summarize a healthy patient's history by writing: "Patient denies any signs or symptoms suggestive of cardiovascular, respiratory, neurologic or other systems disorders and likewise denies knowledge of having any disorders in these categories. The patient is not under care of a physician for any health problems presently and has not had rheumatic fever or diabetes, and reports no allergies to previously administered drugs or anesthetics including penicillin, local anesthetics and aspirin."

Once a summary such as this has been completed, it should be referred to at future appointments since all the salient features of importance are listed. This section then should be dated as it will be valid only for several months. It will need to be updated periodically, although not in this depth. Any physical examination findings or further information regarding the patient's health should be included on the summary sheet or elsewhere in the progress record.

EVALUATION OF PSYCHIC MAKEUP

Such an evaluation is difficult to discuss briefly, but it is most important that the patient's attitude toward dentistry and his general psychic makeup be determined. The attitudes expressed about former dentists or dental treatment and difficulties with therapy should be carefully analyzed. Severe criticism of physicians or other health practitioners should provoke caution. Chronic complainers dissatisfied with everything in general should not be promised too much! The need for assessing the emotional status of dental patients is revealed by facts

such as these. More than 12 percent of American children during the ages of 5 to 19 have psychological problems severe enough to require professional attention. More than half of the physicians' patients do not have demonstrable organic disease. A psychogenic factor is frequently encountered in unruly patients, in some patients with cancerphobia or with the elusive pain symptoms of glossopyrosis and temporomandibular joint complaints. Other conditions which may involve emotional problems are lichen planus, glossitis migrans, chronic desquamative gingivitis, bruxism and xerostomia. The senile patient often suffers from amnesia and may become confused and disturbed if he is queried too much about current events; he is more comfortable discussing the good old days.

Short psychiatric questionnaires are being used by some dentists to help classify the psychic makeup and attitudes of occasional patients. Such evaluations, however, do not achieve a high degree of professional accuracy, and should be used only in collaboration with a psychologist and/or psychiatrist.

As the medical history questionnaire is completed, the dentist should have a good idea of the patient's attitudes and psychic makeup and should know whether he has or may have had psychiatric problems. Such patients should be treated with care and those who have had difficulties with previous dental treatment should not be led to expect too much, for failure may be likely.

Improper evaluation of the patient's attitude and expectations is one of the primary reasons for lawsuits against dentists. However, a little common sense and consideration can make the approach to a patient in presenting a treatment plan and providing dental treatment a rewarding experience for both. It is often important to make a note about the patient's special likes or dislikes or about a special happening in his life so that at future appointments this can be used as a point of conversation and as an aid in developing rapport.

OCCUPATION, HABITS, AND ORAL HEALTH AND DISEASE

The patient's present and past occupations should be determined. This not only creates a subject of common interest but it also may give insight as to the patient's oral health. For example, a patient who has been a baker might have a higher dental caries rate than one who has been a farmer. One who works on construction with a sand blaster might develop severe attrition. The clarinetist may displace upper incisors labially and lower incisors lingually. The watchmaker or person who works closely with fine materials is constantly under tension and may tend to have temporomandibular joint problems and factitial injuries such as lip biting. Such injuries can be quite puzzling unless the occupation is known.

SOCIOECONOMIC STATUS

Information on the patient's socioeconomic status enables the dentist to communicate better. It is improper to speak "over the head" of the patient or beneath his level of intelligence. Specific information gained here, along with what has been previously obtained, will be of value to the treatment planning. An example might be the patient with a very low income, with several missing teeth and multiple cavities. Whereas ideal therapy might be desirable, the patient's economic status might make it virtually impossible; hence, the treatment plan might not include extensive bridge work or a removable partial denture. The patient should be instructed as to the ideal treatment, and should be encouraged to plan for such final treatment at a future time.

PHYSICAL EVALUATION

Once the medical and dental history and other basic data are collected from the patient, it is important for the dentist to thoroughly evaluate the patient's general overall health. This evaluation should be done keeping in mind the relationship of oral and systemic disease and the possible effects of dental treatment on systemic health problems, and the reverse.

Although the dentist is not expected to do a complete physical examination as the physician might, a limited examination is in order. The stage has already been set by the thorough medical/dental history. The principles (*i.e.* signs-symptoms suggestive of disease, identification of fundamental disease processes and disease classifications) are identical. Likewise the techniques of inspection, palpation, percussion, auscultation, functional and laboratory tests, etc., are almost identical. Since patients visit dentists more frequently than physicians, the dentist is in a good position to detect and refer patients suspected of having significant systemic disease to a physician for final diagnosis. This is part of the dentist's role in comprehensive dental care. The dentist, likewise, can expect cooperative medical advice and care for his patients as part of his comprehensive program.

The dentist thus should be able to: (1) obtain and interpret a thorough medical/dental history, (2) perform a limited physical examination, (3) order and interpret appropriate laboratory tests, (4) evaluate findings and obtain appropriate medical consultations, if indicated.

General Observations

During the course of interrogating the patient, the dentist should remain observant, looking for signs suggesting systemic disease. It is appropriate to measure height and weight and record it in the chart, or an estimate is acceptable. General alertness or state of consciousness is another observation that might be made during initial discussions with the patient. If he appears mentally dull or groggy, an attempt should be made to determine the cause.

Nutritional status should be ascertained. If the patient appears to be emaciated or unduly obese, questions should be asked regarding diet, and an attempt should be made to determine whether the body build is based upon a systemic disorder or improper nutrition.

As this information is collected, the degree of cooperation from the patient can be further ascertained, and this information, as mentioned before, will be useful later in developing and presenting the treatment plan.

Body Size and Shape

Obviously, the size and shape of the body and body build in general should be considered. Endocrine disorders frequently affect the development of the body and body build, producing at times miniature adults and at other times giants, with various degrees in between. Generally speaking, the body is bilaterally symmetrical and any gross deviations from that symmetry should be viewed with suspicion.

Unusual posture may result from habit or from circulatory or respiratory disorders. The familiar barrel chest of the advanced asthmatic and emphysema patient, and the shortness of breath which also occurs with severe cardiac decompensation, should be recognized and further investigated.

During interrogation, slurred speech, difficulty in speaking or hoarseness should be noted and, especially if of recent occurrence, should be further investigated.

Gait

As the patient moves about the room, the nature of the gait is important to observe. Foot dragging, shuffling gait, limp, or other abnormalities of gait should prompt the examiner to question the patient further in an attempt to determine the cause, be it from accidental trauma, central nervous system disease or other.

Integument

Pointed observation of the exposed skin may reveal inflammation due to infection, hyperpigmentation due to adrenal insufficiency, pigmented moles, ulcers, macules, papules, nodules, vesicles, tumors, bullae, scaly lesions, and a multitude of other integumental abnormalities which need further investigation. Any abnormalities noted should be called to the attention of the patient and he should be further questioned. If appropriate, consultation from a physician should be obtained.

It is appropriate to palpate the skin and underlying soft tissues of the head and neck, arm and ankle regions, to determine any puffiness or generalized edema or enlargement. If this is done, a moment of explanation during the procedure is helpful to gain the patient's understanding.

Scars on exposed parts of the body should be noted and the causes determined. Jagged scars often are the result of trauma, whereas linear scars which are difficult to detect usually are surgical in nature. Thus, it is important to recognize preferred sites for surgical openings. A vertical preauricular incision is often used for condylar surgery; a curved incision in the post-auricular region is commonly used for mastoid surgery; scars on the neck may indicate previous lymph node incisions or biopsies, thyroid surgery or previous tracheostomy; a semicircular scar beneath the angle of the mandible may result from previous incision for fracture reduction.

If, during the course of the examination or the recording of the medical history, suggestions of abnormal sensation or function come forth, it is appropriate to use wisps of cotton to test the patient's ability to perceive light pressure; use a pin to test pain sensitivity over exposed parts of the body; apply heat or cold to test the sensory ability of the skin to discriminate between the two; ask the patient to move a limb and demonstrate its function and location with his eyes closed (proprioception).

Respiratory Function

If the patient has hoarseness or a chronic cough, it is appropriate to listen to the breath sounds with a stethoscope, noting any rales or abnormal gurgling sounds during breathing (inspiration or exhalation). The stethoscope might likewise be used to listen to the movement of joints which crack or pop, or function abnormally. All abnormalities should be noted in the patient's record.

A more detailed description of the examination of the head and neck will follow in a later chapter.

Vital Signs

Basic vital signs should be obtained initially from every patient; these include pulse rate, respiratory rate, temperature and blood pressure.

The respiratory rate can be easily determined without the patient's knowledge, by merely counting the number of respirations per minute. A normal non-apprehensive patient has a respiratory rate of 12 to 16 cycles per minute. Excitement, of course, increases the respiratory rate. The depth of respiration also should be noted.

The body temperature can be readily obtained by placing an oral thermometer under the tongue for three minutes, and this should be recorded initially, especially if the patient gives evidence of any systemic illness. In young children the temperature can be taken rectally or in the axillary region. Normal body temperature in the axillary region is 97.6°F, whereas rectally it is 99.6°F. The normal body temperature taken orally is 98.6°F (37°C).

Pulse and Heart Rate

The pulse rate is obtained relatively easily by placing the first finger over the patient's radial artery and counting the pulsations during a 1-min period. Normal pulse rate ranges from 60 to 80. Patients who are joggers tend to have pulse rates as low as 45 and patients who are excited or apprehensive tend to have pulse rates of 90 or above. However, a pulse rate over 100 after a period of rest should be viewed with suspicion and consultation should be obtained. A pulse rate of 120 or higher is referred to as

tachycardia and may be a sign of severe cardiovascular disease. The carotid artery may also be used for recording the pulse rate. During the course of the oral examination, as the lip is retracted, the vermilion border can be used to take the pulse rate without the patient's knowledge. Try this on yourself. Grasp your upper lip between your thumb and first finger, squeeze and then let up slowly until you feel the pulsation of the labial arteries.

Blood Pressure

Recording a base-line blood pressure is a *must* for every new dental patient. This is a very quick procedure and, with the high rate of hypertension in the population today, it is of great value. Frequently, patients become apprehensive during the course of taking a blood pressure, hence the pressure is abnormally high; it must be retaken if high. Sometimes the degree of apprehension is less if a dental auxiliary takes the blood pressure in the dentist's absence. The procedure is simple. Seat the patient in a chair with the arm flexed at about the level of the heart (you can use a dental chair). Palpate the brachial artery on the medial surface of the upper arm. Take the cuff, or sphygmomanometer, and place it so that the arrow is just over the brachial artery and it is firm but not tight. Be sure that the clothing is loosened above the cuff. Place the diaphragm of the stethoscope in the antecubital fossa just to the medial side, as shown in Figure 5–2. Elevate the pressure by squeezing the bulb to approximately 200 mm and slowly release the pressure, listening for the first sound. The first sound represents the systolic blood pressure. As the pressure in the cuff drops, the pulsations heard will suddenly lose volume. The point at which this volume suddenly decreases is referred to as the diastolic pressure. Some measure the diastolic pressure at the point at which the sound disappears totally, but there is usually no more than 5 mm difference between the two. The diastolic pres-

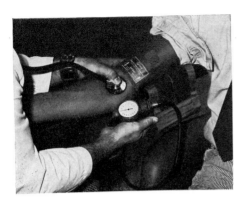

Fig. 5-2. Blood pressure recording. Cuff should be placed with the arrow over brachial artery. Stethoscope head should be positioned as shown. Exact procedure is described in text.

sure is the more significant and, if it is over 100 mm, the pressure should be retaken at a later time to assure the patient is not physiologically reacting to apprehension. If the diastolic pressure remains over 100 mm the patient should be referred to his physician for further evaluation. Ideally, the diastolic pressure should be about 80. The systolic pressure may vary considerably, but normally should be between 120 and 140, depending on age and physical stature. Thus, if a patient has a systolic pressure of over 150 mm, or a diastolic pressure of over 90, it would be wise to consider medical consultation if the pressure has been retaken several times to assure that it did not represent the results of anxiety or hyperactivity.

Laboratory Tests

A number of simple screening laboratory tests are available to the dentist today, which include techniques for taking and recording the bleeding and clotting time, lacrimal, salivary and blood glucose studies with test tape and microtechniques, and many other screening laboratory tests. These may be utilized if the medical history suggests a systemic ailment, or the patient may be referred to a clinical pathology laboratory. If there is a high degree of suspicion, however, it is more efficient to refer the patient

directly to a physician for a thorough physical examination.

Many other observations can be made by the astute examiner in considering the signs and symptoms suggestive of systemic disease. It is wise for the student and/or dentist to periodically review, by use of physical diagnosis texts, the methods for general physical diagnosis, and to employ those procedures, particularly the simpler ones, as part of the physical evaluation process. Again, the dentist is not expected to complete a thorough physical examination, but only to observe the general health of the patient for the more obvious signs and symptoms suggestive of systemic disease. This simple physical examination and health evaluation process provides a good basis for the determination of general health state of the patient and, included with a more detailed head and neck examination (covered later), provides the basis for a comprehensive plan of treatment for the patient.

BIBLIOGRAPHY

Arnold, M.: Psychological questionnaire design for oral diagnosis, J. Oral Med., *28,* 18, 1973.

Buckingham, W. B., Sparberg, M. and Brandfonbrener, M.: *A Primer of Clinical Diagnosis,* New York, Harper and Row, 1971.

Cheraskin, E.: Preventive medical case-finding opportunities and responsibilities of the dentist, Dent. Clin. North America, July, 1958.

Durocher, R. T. and Novak, A. J.: Iatrogenic disorders from the use of drugs, J. Dent. Med., *17,* 55, 1962.

Chue, P W. Y.: Interaction of drugs used in dentistry, Dent. Surv., p. 33, October, 1975.

Chue, P. W. Y.: Fundamental mechanisms of drug interaction, Dent. Surv., p. 37, September, 1975.

Hussar, D. A.: Interactions involving drugs used in dental practice. J. Amer. Dent. Ass., *87,* 349, 1973.

Gaffney, D. D.: Allergies in a dental practice, North-West Dent., *43,* 285, 1964.

Harrison, T. R., Adams, R. D., Bennett, I. L., Resnik, W. H., Thorn, G. W. and Wintrobe, M. M.: *Principles of Internal Medicine,* 5th Ed., New York, McGraw-Hill Book Co., 1966.

Kutscher, A. H., Zegarelli, E. V. and Hyman, G. A.: *Pharmacotherapeutics of Oral Disease,* New York, McGraw-Hill Book Co., 1964.

Land, M.: Management of emotional illness in dental practice, J. Amer. Dent. Ass., *73*, 631, 1966.

Liu, F. T. Y. and Lin, H. S.: Effect of some contraceptive steroids on growth and development of salivary glands and incidence of dental caries in female rats, J. Dent. Res., *48*, 477, 1969.

Macleod, J.: *Clinical Examination*, 2nd Ed., Edinburgh, E. and S. Livingstone Ltd., 1967.

McCarthy, F. M.: *Emergencies in Dental Practice*, Philadelphia, W. B. Saunders Co., 1967.

Merck Manual, 10th Ed., Rahway, New Jersey. Merck, Sharp and Dohme Research Laboratories, 1961.

Miller, A. S. and Pullon, P. A.: A system for electronic data retrieval and cross-tabulation in oral pathology, Oral Surg., *28*, 702, 1969.

Mitchell, D. F.: Undesirable side reactions to drugs, Dent. Clin. North America, March, 1968.

Morris, A. L.: The medical history in dental practice, J. Amer. Dent. Ass., *74*, 129, 1967.

Simmons, J. E.: *Psychiatric Examination of Children*, Philadelphia, Lea & Febiger, 1970.

Smith, J. W., Johnson, J. E. and Cluff, L. E.: Studies on the epidemiology of adverse drug reactions, II. An evaluation of penicillin allergy, New Eng. J. Med., *274*, 998, 1966.

Zegarelli, E. V. and Kutscher, A. H.: Oral moniliasis following intraoral topical corticosteroid therapy, J. Oral Ther. Pharm., *1*, 304, 1964.

Chapter 6

Common Diagnostic Techniques and Instruments

This chapter is designed to help you develop and perfect the skills of using common diagnostic techniques and instruments and to be able to evaluate the results of your findings. True learning of these skills can only come from applying these techniques.

INSPECTION

Effective positioning of the patient and adequate lighting are essential for proper inspection. Many techniques are used to "clear the field" for the examination. Fingers or instruments may be used as retractors. Irrigation, air and liquid sprays, suction and mouthwashes may be employed. A sponge may be wrapped around the tip of the tongue to move it about for more careful inspection. Sponges also are used to remove highlights by wiping surfaces dry, and to remove bacterial plaque, necrotic tissue or food debris. Wooden tongue blades serve as cheek retractors or tongue depressors. To depress the tongue so that the oropharynx may be examined, two blades are used together; to minimize gagging, the blade ends are placed slightly behind the mid-dorsum and pressure is exerted downward and forward. Special intraoral lighting equipment may be employed for direct visualization or transillumination. Filtered ultraviolet light used in a dark room will disclose certain fluorescent features or characteristics not apparent under incandescent light. Magnification is useful under some conditions.

PALPATION

Use of the sense of touch for investigation and as an aid to description is a highly developed art which too often has been neglected in dentistry. By touch, a surface may be found to be moist or dry, rough or smooth, or even of abnormal temperature, when these features are not necessarily apparent to the naked eye.

Experience reveals to the practitioner the normal consistency of a muscular organ such as the tongue or masticatory muscles; the consistency of the normal submaxillary salivary gland is important to recognize, as is that of a small submaxillary lymph node when it is rolled between the fingers of the examiner and the lower border of the mandible. The consistency of fat is readily apparent in contrast to a fluid-filled cavity within soft tissue. The induration of the tissues at the borders of a squamous cell carcinoma can be appreciated only by palpation.

Regular use of palpation during examinations will help one experience the range of normality to be expected. Then, when abnormality is encountered, the surface, consistency, size, compressibility, freedom of movement, and induction of pain or other sensations will reveal much of the nature of the abnormality (Figs. 2–5 and 2–8).

The examiner should use direct compression of tissues against underlying structures. Bidigital manipulation of tissues between the thumb and fingers of one hand is helpful. Bimanual manipulation should be used, as when an index finger of one hand explores the floor of the mouth while the opposing fingers of the other hand compress the tissues beneath. Every careful examination should refresh the mind of the examiner regarding the regional anatomy under inspection.

An orderly routine is important in the use of palpation as in any other phase of examination. One can begin by feeling the external ears and their lobes and the immediately surrounding tissue. Next, the fingers of both hands may be drawn down over the skin overlying the parotid glands. The normal parotid usually is not detectable, so if irregularity is encountered more careful inspection of this region is necessary.

Next, fingers may be placed in the preauricular region over the heads of the condyles, and the patient is asked to open and close and move his mandible from side to side. The condylar heads will be felt during these movements and any irregularity can be noted. The little fingers of each hand also may be placed in the external auditory canals and the condyle movement will be felt.

The masticatory musculature may be palpated during relaxation and contraction using bimanual external and intraoral palpation.

Finger pressure applied over the frontal and maxillary sinuses may induce discomfort from an infected sinus. Bidigital and bimanual palpation of the neck musculature, sites of regional lymph nodes, the trachea, thyroid and cricoid cartilages, and the hyoid bone should be routine. The pulsating carotid artery will be noted. Lateral displacement of the thyroid cartilage by the examiner will reveal the normal "thyroid crackle." One may palpate the neck structures while the patient holds his head erect or while he is relaxed. The head may be moved from side to side to facilitate this palpation.

Standing behind the patient, the examiner may use the fingers of his left hand to push the anterior neck structures toward the opposite side. With the patient's head dropped slightly forward, with muscles relaxed, the fingers of the opposite hand may be cupped and pushed medially; then these finger tips may be lifted slightly and drawn laterally to roll the compressed tissue under the inferior border of the mandible (Fig. 12–2). With practice one often will detect a submandibular node or two just as it slides between the fingers and the inferior notch of the mandible. If the consistency of the node is abnormal, or if undue pain is induced, further investigation is necessary.

The submental region may be explored bimanually. The texture of the lips and cheeks should be felt. The gingivae and hard palate should be palpated by a gently compressing finger. Palpating the alveolar process over the roots of teeth subjected to percussion may elicit pain if an acute infection is present. The searching finger may be used to compress the tongue to detect abnormality. The tonsils or the empty fossae may be felt with a deft finger which should also pass over the soft palate, a common site for mixed tumors of minor salivary glands. An overly elongated styloid process may sometimes be detected in the tonsillar fossa. The hamular process may be found above and behind the posterior tuberosity of the maxilla.

Prominent cortical surfaces of the jaws should be palpated extraorally and intraorally. After radiographic examination, palpation may help to localize any abnormal radiopacity or radiolucency. Detection of a thin compressible or absent cortex over a radiolucency may lead directly to the technique of aspiration. Contrarily, a radiopaque area that appears to be centrally located may actually be the result of a peripheral condition which may be palpable, such as a lingual torus or labial exostosis.

When abnormality is detected, the findings should be recorded. The size and consistency of a mass should be described and a notation made as to whether it is painful and whether it is fixed to neighboring tissues or freely movable.

Besides the fact that palpation should be done routinely to detect local abnormality, it should be employed for other reasons in special cases. For example, the elderly male with a chronic, ulcerated indurated lesion on the lower lip should be examined further to detect possible regional nodes involved suggesting metastasis from a possible carcinoma. Likewise, the patient with a history of tuberculosis, and an ulcer on the face, may have involved nodes nearby. Multiple and bilateral nodular enlargements should raise the possibility of the lymphomas and infectious mononucleosis.

With a fracture of the mandible, the two ends may be manipulated, revealing crepitation at the fracture site. The pressure of palpation may induce the flow of pus from an otherwise unobserved fistula or a natural tract such as the duct of a major salivary gland. Likewise, a small sialolith may be forced out through the normal orifice of a duct by a "milking" action.

DETERMINATION OF FUNCTION

This is an important part of the examination which the experienced practitioner does routinely and almost subconsciously.

Listen to speech and watch movements of the jaws and lips during the interrogation process. Speech aberrations of ankyloglossia, cleft palate and maxillary sinusitis are readily detectable.

While examining the buccal parietes run your fingers over the skin covering the parotid glands and observe clear saliva flowing from the orifice of Stensen's duct (Fig. 7–12). Likewise, observe the flow from Wharton's duct as you massage the submandibular and sublingual salivary glands. After drying the mucosa and observing the surface for a moment, you should be able to see tiny beads of secretions from the minor salivary glands. The absence of saliva under these conditions may reveal the cause of xerostomia. Pus or sialoliths expressed through the orifices will be discernible (Fig. 13–8).

Movements of the uvula and soft palate during phonation may reveal a hemiparalysis, and undue tremors of the tongue may be another sign of neurologic significance. Movements of the jaws during masticatory actions may reveal hypo- or hypermobility of jaws and teeth. The flow of thick mucus on the posterior wall of the oral pharynx (postnasal drip) may be indicative of sinusitis and nasopharyngeal inflammation.

AUSCULTATION

The simple act of listening during interrogation, palpation, and manipulation of tissues may reveal abnormal sounds. Clicking of the temporomandibular joint may be amplified by applying the stethoscope over the functioning joint. The ringing sound emitted from a tooth during percussion may denote ankylosis, or a dull sound may indicate looseness. Detection of a fracture line in a long bone such as the mandible may be aided by placing the stethoscope over a bony prominence on one side of the suspected line and percussing a bony prominence with a finger on the other side. Passage of the percussion sound through the stethoscope will be dulled if a fracture is present (Fig. 6–1). The stethoscope should not be

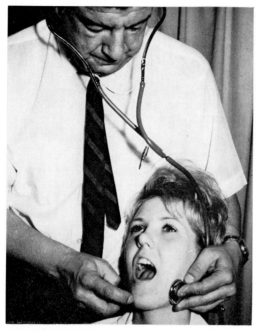

Fig. 6-1. Use of the stethoscope and percussion to locate fracture.

foreign to the dental office. It is used also with the sphygmomanometer to take the blood pressure. Heart sounds and respiratory noises can be evaluated by the experienced listener. Such experience would help one evaluate the status of an unconscious patient.

ASPIRATION

This refers to the withdrawal of fluids into a syringe from a body cavity for diag-

nostic purposes. Among dentists, the most widely recognized form of aspiration is performed prior to injecting a local anesthetic agent to assure that the needle is not located intravascularly.

Given a palpable lesion within soft tissue which appears to be full of fluid, or a radiolucent lesion within bone, the needle of the aspirating syringe usually can be placed within the suspected cavity and, when suction occurs, the fluid contents appear in the syringe. The rare nasolabial (nasoalveolar) cyst in the substance of the upper lip beneath the ala of the nose might yield a clear fluid as contained in many developmental cysts (Fig. 6–2D). The more common mucocele would yield a clear mucoid material. In the latter instance, the lesion may be evacuated, the syringe removed from the needle, and a corresponding amount of dilute tetracycline liquid placed in the barrel of the syringe and injected into the lesion. In the course of immediately subsequent surgery, after incision has exposed the lesion, the wound may be viewed under filtered ultraviolet light in a darkened room and the extent of the lesion will be marked by the yellow fluorescence of the tetracycline. The lesion then may easily be excised *in toto*.

A large circumscribed radiolucency is likely to be near the labial or buccal cortical plate, and palpation will reveal the loss of or thinness of the plate. The aspirating

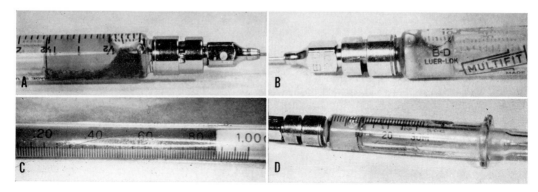

Fig. 6-2. Aspirating syringes filled with: *A,* straw-colored fluid tinged with blood from a large dentigerous cyst; *B,* pus from a chronic asymptomatic periapical abscess; *C,* blood drawn from a traumatic hemorrhagic bone cyst; *D,* clear, slightly grey solution drawn from a developmental nasoalveolar cyst.

needle usually can be placed within such a lesion through the missing or thin cortical plate with no more discomfort than is caused during injection of a local anesthetic. The most common intrabony cavity likely to contain cyst fluid is the periapical cyst and, secondly, the dentigerous cyst. Rather clear, straw-colored fluid may be obtained, or it may be blood tinged.

If pus is aspirated, it is obvious that an abscess is present whether primary or due to secondary infection of a cyst.

In the rather uncommon event that blood is aspirated, the lesion probably represents a traumatic hemorrhagic bone cyst, or the even less common central hemangioma of bone, or the rare aneurysmal bone cyst, which is least likely. Some central giant cell lesions may on occasion have sufficiently enlarged vascular spaces to yield blood during aspiration. If blood is obtained, caution is advocated. If a facial or intraoral hemangioma is present, the odds that the central bone lesion is also an hemangioma would increase.

The fact that nothing is obtained by this means may indicate that the operator has missed the central cavity; or that the contents of the cavity are semisolid, such as the caseous material seen in some developmental cysts; or that the radiolucent lesion is due to soft-tissue proliferation. Thus, even the negative finding is of some diagnostic importance.

Aspiration biopsy is another diagnostic technique, most often employed by the surgeon, wherein he uses a large bore needle with a special adapter that allows him to remove soft tissue as one does when using an apple corer. This technique is seldom recommended for the dentist or oral surgeon. It is more appropriate for use with a deep-seated node or liver biopsy.

PROBING

One of the most obvious examples of this technique is the use of the dental explorer for detecting dental caries. The tip of an explorer "sticks" in the soft carious material of an involved fissure, but not against the

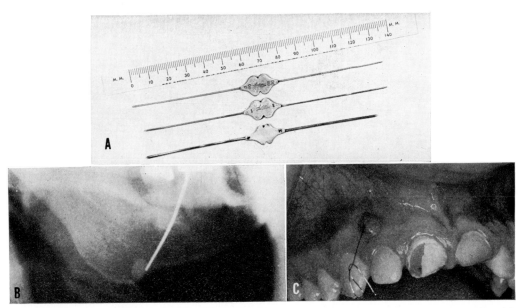

Fig. 6-3. Probes. *A,* Salivary gland duct probes. The #1 lacrimal probe also can be used for this purpose. *B,* Salivary gland probe contacting a small sialolith near the submaxillary salivary gland. (Mitchell, Year Book Medical Publishers, Inc., Practical Dental Monographs, Jan. 1965.) *C,* A fine orthodontic wire has been gently twirled to the depth of a fistula. An intraoral x-ray film would reveal which apex is involved.

hard enamel walls of a normal fissure. Another common instrument is the calibrated periodontal pocket probe. During its use, one may release the pus accumulated within a lateral periodontal abscess and thus establish the diagnosis and accomplish emergency treatment at the same time (Fig. 2–15). Part of an assessment of periodontal health includes recording sulcular and periodontal pocket depths.

The #1 lacrimal probe or a salivary duct probe (Fig. 6–3A and B) may be used to explore the patency of Stensen's or Wharton's ducts, or to explore the congenital lip pits in the midline of the lower lip, or at the lateral commissures. Fistulas or sinus tracts resulting from infection or intraoral openings may be explored similarly. Should the malleable, metallic probe prove cumbersome, a gutta percha point of the type used in endodontics may serve. "Twirling" an orthodontic tie wire and allowing it to follow the path of least resistance may also be helpful (Fig. 6–3C). In any event, once a probe of such nature is in place, selective radiographs should be taken to trace the tract.

TRANSILLUMINATION

Inspection of a lesion of soft or hard tissue may be enhanced by directing a strong light through it (Fig. 6–4). This technique is most commonly used by the otorhinolaryngologist in inspecting the sinuses. The dentist may

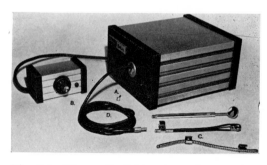

Fig. 6-4. Fiber optic light system: *A*, generator; *B*, rheostat; *C*, accessories; *D*, light guide. This instrument can be used to direct light of a controllable intensity to the bur of a handpiece, the dental mirror or through a transilluminator tip to improve visibility.

use this technique in a dark room by pointing an intense light source against the palate, directing the light through the maxillary sinuses and compressing the overlying soft tissue by drawing a thumb over the skin surface. Such technique allows one to compare the transmission of the light through one sinus as compared to the opposite side. A sinus filled with mucus, polyps, pus or a neoplasm will not transmit light onto the face as well as the clear sinus.

Transillumination was very popular prior to the extensive use of routine oral radiography. It was helpful in detecting periapical pathosis which failed to transmit the light and to detect interproximal caries in anterior teeth, as well as hidden restorations. It still is useful.

Transillumination also is valuable for inspecting tooth root surfaces for calculus after prophylaxis, or during gingivectomy. The gingivally impacted toothbrush bristle or other radiolucent foreign material may be revealed by transillumination and be unapparent in an x-ray film. As another example, a child was seen who had chewed paint from her bed and driven a square flake under the labial gingiva, which became inflamed. The flake was superimposed by the root of an incisor and not apparent in the radiograph. It was readily revealed by transillumination, and a dental explorer was inserted subgingivally and the thin flake of paint was removed. This child had been taken to many other dentists and physicians prior to this event, because of the square area of gingival erythema. This case illustrates the value of this diagnostic technique, and also illustrates the principle that if a lesion is angular or square a foreign body should be suspected.

FLUORESCENCE

The so-called Wood's lamp, black light or filtered ultraviolet light directed at tissues in the dark room, is an old technique used by physicians but relatively new in the hands of dentists (Fig. 6–5). Today it is widely used

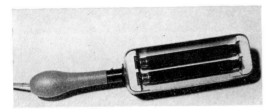

Fig. 6-5. An inexpensive source of filtered ultraviolet light to be used in a dark room to detect fluorescence.

to polymerize certain anterior restorative materials. Certain materials and tissues which appear normal or abnormal under incandescent light may glow vigorously under fluorescent light. One of the more common usages in the past has been to detect the presence of fluorescent parasites on the scalps of school children. Other medical uses have included investigation of skin diseases. Intravenous injections of fluorescein, a nontoxic, extremely fluorescent dye, have been made in patients suffering from diabetic gangrene, to delineate the region of adequate vascularization of a limb and to help determine the site of necessary amputation. Brain tumors have been shown to attract fluorescein thus injected, so that during an operation to remove a brain tumor the patient has been injected with the fluorescent dye; with the calvarium removed and the brain inspected under black light, the lesion then could be delineated for the surgeon.

The dentist may use filtered ultraviolet light to study skin and mucosal conditions. The normal skin of the nose of most patients reveals a concentration of orange fluorescent spots corresponding to the openings of sebaceous glands. This is due to a concentration of orange fluorescent bacteria. Burns *et al.* recorded many microorganisms with fluorescent qualities. Gross materia alba on teeth has revealed variations in fluorescence which may be related to variations in the microbial flora. Normal tongue coating is also rather orange in its fluorescence.

Many cases of intrinsic staining of teeth have occurred due to the administration of

the many different forms of tetracycline during tooth formation (p. 154). These drugs, like fluorescein, are vital dyes which are deposited in tissues that are calcifying. Thus periodic doses of tetracyclines in human beings will be found to be deposited in incremental lines of bone, dentin and cementum. The dental profession should be alert to the possibility that other medicaments of a fluorescent nature may act as vital dyes and thus stain developing teeth. Filtered ultraviolet light will reveal the yellow fluorescence of tetracycline in the dentin. It is a valuable tool for examining any questionable intrinsic stain of the teeth. The use of this instrument in forensic dentistry (Chap. 18) and in oral surgery has been noted elsewhere.

In the rare case of porphyria (porphyrinuria), developing teeth are dark stained, and are brilliantly fluorescent red.

As ultraviolet light becomes more popular as a diagnostic tool, other values will undoubtedly be identified.

THERAPEUTIC TRIAL

It is sometimes useful to treat a condition on the basis of a tentative diagnosis. The

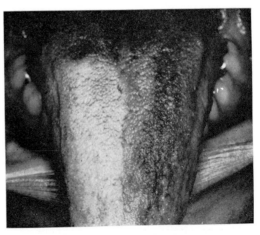

Fig. 6-6. Therapeutic trial. The tongue was covered completely with a dark brown coat, suspected to be due to medicine taken orally to reduce gastric acidity. Topical application of hydrogen peroxide to the right half of the tongue removed the bismuth stain and confirmed the tentative diagnosis.

result of treatment may lead to a more definitive diagnosis. For example, if pulpal pain may be arising from one of two or more teeth with open carious lesions, the application of eugenol to the prime suspect may relieve the pain, and a diagnosis made. Figure 6–6 shows this principle in demonstrating the origin of a dark stain on the dorsum of the tongue.

DENTAL TESTS

Percussion Test

This is the simplest test, hence the first used in diagnosing odontalgia. The end of the handle of a mouth mirror is tapped against the crown of the tooth. The force is exerted in the direction of the long axis of the tooth. If periodontal membrane fibers are the source of pain, whether they are periapical, lateral, or gingival, percussion will invoke a painful response. The proprioceptive fibers will help the patient and the operator locate the tooth. Tapping a "control" or sound tooth elsewhere in the mouth will clarify the degree of apprehension present. Tapping each cusp may reveal a fracture or "cracked tooth."

Contrary to the belief of many, most teeth with painful pulpitis are tender to percussion to some degree. The tooth subjected to a certain degree of orthodontic or other forceful tooth movement may be tender. A "high" restoration, gingivitis, periodontitis, a painful periodontal pocket or a lateral periodontal abscess may result in tenderness to percussion.

Percussion can be used to judge tooth mobility by palpating the tooth or alveolar gingivae over the root while it is being percussed. The ankylosed tooth will resound under percussion, whereas the sound of a normal or periodontally involved tooth will be more dull.

Instruments designed to assess tooth mobility for diagnostic purposes are promising, but not widely used at present.

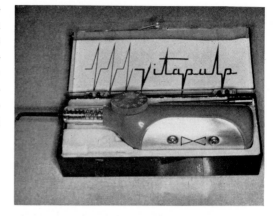

Fig. 6-7. A portable electrical pulp tester.

Electric Pulp Testing

The electrical pulp vitality test is used *only* to determine the presence or absence of vital nervous tissue within a pulp chamber. A painful response to the stimulus denotes vitality. The one advantage of the electrical test over the application of a hot metallic instrument or the dental bur is the fact that the controlled stimulus can be applied in a gradually increasing degree by means of the sensitive rheostats on the instruments, thus avoiding the induction of needlessly excessive pain. Used properly, the electrical test is a useful and reliable diagnostic aid (Fig. 6–7).

Reasons for Use

Before any tooth is restored, clasped or banded for movement the operator should know whether the pulp is vital; otherwise a necrotic pulp may be overlooked and at a later date pain may occur, resulting in embarrassment and revision of treatment. For example, if a tooth is non-vital and asymptomatic when banded, and subsequently becomes painful during orthodontic care, the patient and the orthodontist may feel that a cause-and-effect relationship has been demonstrated. Once orthodontic bands and archwires are in place, electrical test results have been shown to be confusing.

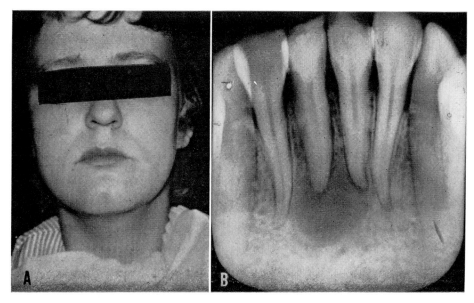

Fig. 6-8. *A,* The dimple on the chin has ulcerated and drained in the past and has been corrected by plastic surgery by a physician. Discomfort has recurred and the intraoral x-ray film in (*B*) demonstrates the source of the drainage.

Any tooth suspected to be non-vital should be tested. Discoloration, fracture, and deep carious lesions or restorations may indicate the need for testing. If an untreated non-vital tooth is detected, it is usually associated with a periapical granuloma, abscess, or cyst and of course such pathoses should be eradicated either by conservative endodontics, apical curettage or extraction. The dentist is obligated to treat such conditions whether or not they are symptomatic, because they may later become symptomatic or they may

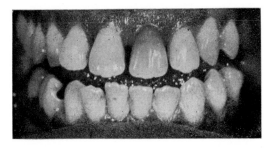

Fig. 6-9. The dark hue of the asymptomatic central incisor suggests the need for a pulp vitality test. (Mitchell in Healey, *Endodontics,* courtesy of the C. V. Mosby Co.)

serve as foci of infection (Figs. 6–8*A* and *B* and 6–9).

Electric pulp testing also is of value in the differential diagnosis of other conditions resembling the common lesions. Periapical radiolucency, especially in the lower incisor region of adults, initially may suggest a common periapical inflammatory reaction resulting from a non-vital pulp. However, if the pulp is found to be vital, and there are no other symptoms, a diagnosis of periapical cemental dysplasia (cementoma) is more likely and no treatment may be indicated.

If a lateral periodontal abscess has pointed or has formed a fistula, the condition may simulate a periapical abscess. If electrical pulp testing indicates that the pulp is vital, a periodontal approach to diagnosis and therapy would be indicated (Fig. 2–15).

Developmental abnormalities, neoplasms, and certain systemic diseases can cause radiolucent lesions which may be near the apical region only incidentally. If the associated teeth are not tested for vitality, one might make a tentative diagnosis of common periapical pathosis and overlook the possibility of such conditions as a developmental globulomaxillary cyst, a lateral periodontal cyst, an early ameloblastoma, a central giant cell lesion or hemangioma, a neurogenic neoplasm, eosinophilic granuloma, a lesion of multiple myeloma, malignant tumor metastasis or the so-called idiopathic (traumatic, hemorrhagic) bone cyst.

Instruments and Techniques

Unipolar high-frequency electrical testers are widely used. The Burton instrument* furnishes a high-frequency current controlled by means of a rheostat in one piece held in one hand. The applicator, to which the unipolar electrode is attached, is held in the other. The rheostat has three numerical zones: 1–7 "anteriors"; 7–11 "posteriors"; 11–14 "recheck zone." The responses to this instrument applied to normal anterior and posterior teeth in the mouth of a patient seldom vary more than 3 to 5 points over this scale of 14, making the "zones" rather meaningless.

If one moistens the tip of the tester (electrode) with water, toothpaste or other electrolyte and applies it to the thin skin on the back of the thumb, the stimulus usually will be felt between 10 and 14. When the stimulus is being delivered, the rheostat handpiece gives an auditory signal and a filament in the electrode portion glows with a faint orange neon light.

The Ritter instrument† has the rheostat and electrode incorporated into the single handpiece, and a revolving scale of 1 to 10 is used. Thus one hand can control the electrode and rheostat, while the other hand retracts. There is no auditory signal but a filament in the pole is seen to glow through the plastic coat. This instrument furnishes a stronger stimulus which can be felt readily through the skin, usually between 2 and 5,

and it becomes quite painful as the scale is increased to 8 or 10. Application to the heavily keratinized skin on the palmar surface of the hand may give no reaction. A low range of stimuli (1 to 4) usually invokes a response from normal anterior or posterior teeth.

The operator should determine whether the instrument is working by testing it on his skin before each use. The procedure should be briefly described to the patient and, if the patient is unfamiliar with it, the dentist should demonstrate, using the patient's thumb. This reduces apprehension and prepares the way for better cooperation. A "control" normal tooth should then be tested in a quadrant of the mouth other than that containing the "suspect" tooth. The tester point should be moistened and applied to sound enamel overlying sound dentin. With the anatomy of the pulp chamber in mind, the electrode should be pointed toward the pulp in the direction of the underlying dentinal tubules. The middle third of the labial or buccal surface of the crown usually is preferred, but any sound surface will suffice. Each cusp of a multirooted tooth should be tested. It seldom is necessary to isolate the tooth with cotton rolls and dry it before testing. The operator should avoid contact with a restoration in the tooth, or with the gingiva or other soft tissues. If the electrode touches denuded dentin, an early response results; similarly, a metallic restoration may serve as a better conductor. The patient should be asked to signal audibly or by the wave of a hand when the stimulus causes discomfort. His periocular musculature may be observed for wincing as a sign of pain. Numerical ratings for the test are recorded. The control test helps differentiate a true reaction to pain from an apprehensive response.

The examiner then proceeds to the suspected tooth and, if the pulp is non-vital, no response will be obtained. However, the stronger Ritter instrument sometimes may give confusing results in the numerical range

---

* Burton Manufacturing Corporation, Los Angeles, California.
† Ritter Manufacturing Corporation, Rochester, New York.

from 7 to 10, because occasionally a feedback through the retracted lips of the patient to the fingers of the operator occurs, and a false-positive reading may be given. Since most reactions to this instrument occur around 3, any reading of 7 or above may indicate abnormality. The pulp of a multi-rooted tooth may be only partially necrotic, so application of the tester point to cusps over the different roots may help explain varying results in some cases. The response must certainly vary with the extent of pulp necrosis (Fig. 10–7). A negative response should always be verified by retesting.

It has been said that an electrical pulp test may cause pain if the necrotic contents of the root canal are moist (pus) because the current may be carried to the vital periapical tissues. This seldom, if ever, is the case. If a periapical abscess exists, the tooth is often quite tender to percussion. If the pulp tester point is applied with any pressure, the patient may complain of pain induced by pressure rather than by the electrical stimulus; this is especially likely if he is overly apprehensive.

Patients with necrotic pulps were selected for study. Original electrical test results were negative. After endodontic cleansing and canal enlargement, the canals were filled with an electrolyte, and a sterile absorbent paper point was soaked in the same solution and inserted into the canals as far as possible. Another electrical test then was performed and no response was obtained.

Portable, battery-operated electrical testers are most practical and the least threatening to the patient. They operate almost identically to the "plug-in" type and they are inexpensive. The normal upper central incisors of several dentists responded to four different electrical pulp testers approximately as follows:

	Ritter	Burton	Pelton-Crane	Parkell
			Portable	
Average	1	4	3	4
Range	.5–3.5	2–7	2–7	2–7.5

Variation in response due to increasing age (thickness of dentin) or from tooth to tooth within the same mouth is not great. Diffuse pulpal calcifications and denticles are not associated with higher electrical test responses; however, large amounts of coronal secondary dentin are. Responses do not vary consistently with varying degrees of periodontal bone loss, nor do responses vary much from hour to hour or day to day in the same individual.

Responses occur earliest in the following order: lower incisors, upper incisors, cuspids, and premolars and molars, suggesting that tooth thickness probably is a factor in pulpal response to such tests.

The electric pulp test is a valuable, consistent, and accurate diagnostic test provided that the instrument is working properly, the patient is cooperative, and the operator is accurate in his technique and interpretation. If the results are questionable, it is good practice to use a simulated test at times in order to trick the patient and obtain true responses.

Thermal Pulp Testing

Thermal tests are used to help locate a tooth with painful pulpitis when the source of pain is not apparent. Fortunately, about 80 percent of teeth with painful pulpitis are at least somewhat sensitive to percussion, but the other 20 percent can cause extremely difficult diagnostic problems on occasion.

A piece of ice (Fig. 6–10) or a small pledget of cotton sprayed with ethyl chloride usually will suffice for the cold test. A heated cylindrical stick of temporary stopping (gutta percha) which softens at about 130° F furnishes a useful and reasonably consistent source of heat. When possible, these should be placed on sound enamel overlying sound dentin, as advocated for the electrical tests.

The sources of heat and cold should be applied to a "control" non-suspect tooth first to determine the patient's normal response

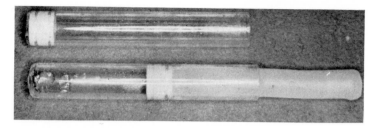

Fig. 6-10. Used anesthetic tubes filled with water and frozen are convenient for applying ice to the tooth surface. Five seconds is the optimal time.

or lack of response and to ascertain the degree of apprehension present. Then they are applied to a suspect tooth. The tooth with painful pulpitis nearly always will furnish an earlier, more severe, and prolonged painful response to one or both thermal tests. The patient should be asked if the pain induced feels like the toothache he had complained about.

An illustration of abnormal reaction to thermal stimuli occurs when one burns a finger superficially. The pain tends to persist if nothing is done. But if one touches the burned skin to something cool, the pain is relieved momentarily. Another example is the thumb struck with a hammer. Hot and cold water can relieve or stimulate pain depending on the degree of heat or cold. In neither instance is contraction or expansion of "gas" involved, as has been conjectured in relation to thermal stimuli. Gas-producing microorganisms have been demonstrated within infected pulps, but gas *per se* has not been demonstrated therein, nor is it a necessary consideration in evaluating the results of pulp tests.

Such tests must be judiciously used in addition to other observations of clinical or radiographic evidence of pulp exposure, careful evaluation of the periodontium through use of the periodontal pocket probe, and the percussion test.

With an understanding of the principles employed, ingenuity will help in some diffi-

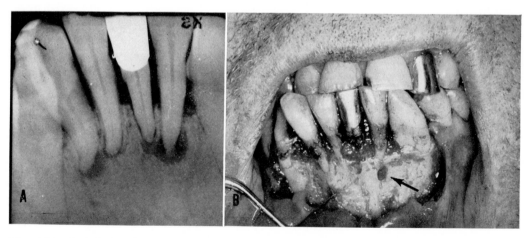

Fig. 6-11. *A*, Apical radiolucencies. *B*, The alveolar mucosa has been reflected to reveal the causes of the radiolucencies seen in the radiograph. A probe is inserted in an opening in the cortex. The arrow designates the other opening.

cult situations. For example, in the absence of an electrical tester a hot wax spatula can serve as an adequate vitality tester; however, if the pulp is vital, undue pain may result from this uncontrolled stimulus.

A tooth restored with a full crown presents a problem. If the usual methods to determine pulp vitality fail, the dental bur may be used. If pain is elicited when the dentin is reached, the hole may be filled with gold foil. If no pain occurs, one could proceed to the pulp in the first step of endodontic therapy.

Teeth with painless pulpitis are more common than those with painful pulpitis but, since there are no symptoms, they are not carefully inspected or tested and thus are overlooked according to Hasler and Mitchell. The dentist must have a high index of suspicion that such cases do exist; look for possible pulp exposure, and use percussion and thermal tests in an effort to detect and treat them before they become symptomatic.

No type of pulp test is adequate alone. The responses of children and mentally retarded patients frequently are confusing. Nevertheless, until diagnostic acumen has been much improved over that of the present day, every recognized test needs to be used on occasion if the best diagnostic efforts are to be made.

Figure 6–11*A* and *B* shows why transillumination, radiography and aspiration are practical for detecting periapical lesions.

BIBLIOGRAPHY

Baum, G., Greenwood, I., Slawski, S. and Smirnow, R.: Observation of internal structures of teeth by ultrasonography, Science, *139*, 495, 1963.

Bender, I. B. and Seltzer, S.: Oral fistula: Its diagnosis and treatment, Oral Surg., *14*, 1367, 1961.

Blozis, G. C.: Objective signs of disease, Dent. Clin. North America, March, 1968.

Burns, R. E., Greer, J. E., Mikhail, G. and Livingood, C. S.: The significance of coral-red fluorescence of the skin, Arch. Derm., *96*, 436, 1967.

Burrill, D. Y.: Pulp testing by determination of fusion frequency. J. Dent. Res., *41*, 437, 1962.

Christen, A. G. and Mitchell, D. F.: A fluorescent dye method for demonstrating leakage around dental restorations. J. Dent. Res., *45*, 1485, 1966.

Grossman, L. I., Lee, E. and Demp, E.: Isolation of gas-producing organisms from root canals, J. Dent. Res., *41*, 495, 1962.

Guthrie, T. J., McDonald, R. E. and Mitchell, D. F.: Dental pulp hemogram, J. Dent. Res., *44*, 678, 1965.

Hasler, J. F. and Mitchell, D. F.: Painless pulpitis, J. Amer. Dent. Ass., *81*, 671, 1970.

Halprin, K. M.: Diagnosis with Wood's light, J.A.M.A., *199*, 841, 1967.

Johnson, R. H.: The tetracyclines: A review of the literature—1948 through 1963, J. Oral Ther. Pharm., *1*, 190, 1964.

Johnson, R. H. and Mitchell, D. F.: The effects of tetracyclines on teeth and bones, J. Dent. Res., *45*, 86, 1966.

Kaplan, H.: The reagent-strip method for estimating blood glucose concentration. J. Amer. Dent. Ass., *74*, 1261, 1967.

Kutscher, A. H., Zegarelli, E. V., Fahn, B. S., Denning, C. R. and Douglas, R. N.: Tetracycline discoloration of teeth: Diagnosis by long-wave and short-wave ultraviolet light, Oral Surg., *23*, 91, 1967.

McDonald, R. E.: Diagnostic acids and vital pulp therapy for deciduous teeth, J. Amer. Dent. Ass., *53*, 14, 1956.

Mitchell, D. F. and Fahmy, H.: Test of seven agents for vital dye and intrinsic dental staining activity, J. Oral Ther. Pharm., *4*, 378, 1968.

Mumford, J. M. and Bjorn, H.: Problems in electric pulp-testing and dental algesimetry, Int. Dent. J., *12*, 161, 1962.

Pheulpin, J. L., Fiore-Donno, G. and Baume, L. J.: Les inflammations pulpaires: leurs diagnostics clinique et histopathologique, Rev. mens. suisse Odonto-stomatol., *77*, 701, 1967.

Phillips, L. J., Phillips, R. W. and Schnell, R. J.: Measurement of the electric conductivity of dental cement, J. Dent. Res., *34*, 839, 1955.

Ramadan, A. E. and Mitchell, D. F.: A roentgenographic study of experimental bone destruction, Oral Surg., *15*, 934, 1962.

Regan, J. E. and Mitchell, D. F.: An evaluation of periapical radiolucencies found in cadavers, J. Amer. Dent. Ass., *66*, 529, 1963.

Robinson, M.: Diagnosis of mandibular fractures by auscultation with percussion, Oral Surg., *12*, 173, 1959.

Rosenberg, E. W. and Fischer, R. W.: Improved method for intraoral patch testing, Arch. Derm., *87*, 115, 1963.

Rubach, W. C. and Mitchell, D. F.: Periodontal disease, age, and pulp status, Oral Surg., *19*, 482, 1965.

Seltzer, S., Bender, I. B. and Ziontz M.: The dy-
namics of pulp inflammation, Oral Surg., *16,*
846, 1963.
Shannon, I. L.: Physiologic baselines for total
protein in human parotid fluid collected without exogenous stimulation, J. Oral Med., *22,*
75, 1967.
Siekert, R. G. and Gibilisco, J. A.: Discoloration
of the teeth in alkaptonuria (ochronosis) and
parkinsonism, Oral Surg., *29,* 197, 1970.

Sorenson, F. M., Phatak, N. M. and Everett, F.
G.: Thermal pulp tester, J. Dent. Res., *41,*
961, 1962.
Taylor, R. C., Ware, W. H. and McDowell, J. A.:
Illumination of the oral cavity, J. Amer. Dent.
Ass., *74,* 1207, 1967.
Watt, D. M.: Recording the sounds of tooth
contact: A diagnostic technique for evalua-
tion of occlusal disturbances, Int. Dent. J.,
19, 221, 1969.

Chapter 7

Physical Examination by Anatomic Region

This chapter covers the topic of comprehensive physical examination on a regional basis. Utilizing the techniques of examination reviewed in Chapter 2, abnormalities of diagnostic importance which may be identified in each anatomic area are outlined. The information presented herein may be supplemented by reference to the more detailed descriptions of disease entities contained in succeeding sections.

The primary purpose of the physical examination is to collect, in an orderly and systematic fashion, clinical information about the individual patient. While the physical findings alone are frequently diagnostic, all pertinent data (health history, subjective symptoms, radiographic findings, indicated laboratory studies and/or consultations) must be used to establish a *clinical profile* of the patient and to arrive at the ultimate goal, a definitive diagnosis.

In this chapter, emphasis is placed on the observation and perception of abnormality. It will be apparent, however, that the clinical manifestations of disease constitute a spectrum of features ranging from subtle variations from normal to virtually pathognomonic clinical lesions. Thus, it is not possible to discuss or even list all of the variations of normality and departures from normalcy that may be seen by such simple observation. Rather, examples will be given not only to stimulate observational powers but also to encourage development of the vocabulary for recording purposes and for interprofessional communication.

GENERAL PHYSICAL APPEARANCE

From the time the patient appears until the completion of the interrogation, literally countless observations of his physical and mental well-being may be made. Body build, stature, posture, complexion, nutritional state and personal hygiene are among the first impressions the examiner obtains with the initial contact.

Personality traits as well as a variety of neural and neuromuscular disorders may be signified by often characteristic movements and gestures. The patient's "body language" will frequently telegraph his apprehension, call attention to nervous habits, or suggest other underlying problems. For example, unsightly teeth or severe malocclusion may explain why the patient holds a hand over the mouth while speaking, or even his introverted behavior.

Tremors of the hands, lips and tongue (often with bobbing and nodding of the head) are common in the elderly (senile tremor). In this regard, sudden onset of tremor and paralysis may be indicative of a recent "little stroke" or cerebrovascular accident. Other distinctive tremors are the intention tremor of multiple sclerosis, the coarse, pill-rolling, non-intention tremor of parkinsonism, and the fine, rapid, toxic tremors of thyrotoxicosis, uremia, alcoholism, etc. Tics, seen as transient involuntary contractions of the facial muscles or eyelids, often are related to stress. More severe spasms, or myoclonus, of the muscles of the face or oral cavity may indicate a central nervous system disorder. For example, *palatal myoclonus* is seen with lesions of the olivary body of the medulla.

An unusual gait may reflect a developmental deformity or neurologic disorder:

1. *Festinating gait*—characterized by short, dragging footsteps and body rigidity, seen in parkinsonism.
2. *Tabetic or ataxic gait*—an uncertain stamping or slapping of the foot with each step, noted with loss of proprioceptive sense in tabes dorsalis (tertiary syphilis).
3. *Waddling gait*—noted in patients with disorders involving the pelvic girdle musculature, such as progressive muscular dystrophy or Paget's disease with pelvic involvement.
4. *Scissors gait*—crisscrossing of the legs with the knees striking together with each step, as in spastic paraplegia or cerebral palsy.
5. *Staggering gait*—uncoordinated, stumbling gait, associated with drunkenness or paresis.

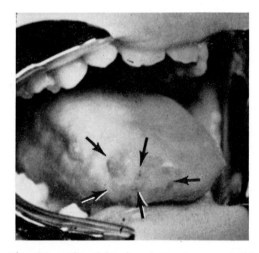

Fig. 7-1. The right tip of the tongue of this youngster has been ulcerated for several weeks. Biopsy of the lesion showed only chronic inflammation. The boy had a lurching gait as the result of chorea. It was finally established that he bit his tongue with each step. A plastic guard was made and the lesion disappeared.

6. *Choreic gait*—a lurching gait often associated with bobbing movements of the hands and head, noted in chorea (Fig. 7–1).
7. *Senile gait*—the feeble, calculated walk noted in elderly and often arthritic patients.

Functional disorders of nerve and muscle are discussed on pages 257–265. Other neuropathies and myopathies with associated pain are described on pages 291–295.

PHYSIOGNOMY

The facial features reflect the mood of the patient and his responsiveness to his surroundings. The physical examination should also note abnormalities of facial contour, function of the muscles of mastication (Fig. 7–2), and consistency and color of the facial tissues. Examination of the face should also include inspection of the eyes and their adnexa, the nose and ears (Fig. 7–3).

Congenital and hereditary disorders, disturbances in dental arch relationships, disease of the underlying soft tissues and bones, and general metabolic disturbances may

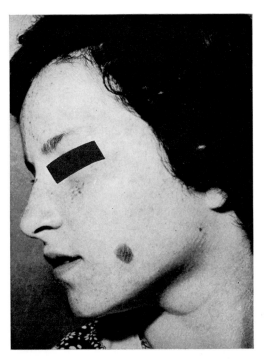

Fig. 7-3. A brown to black nevus is shown, and posterior to it a smaller one is just below the ear. Note the freckles.

manifest themselves as alterations in the physiognomy. Other examples include the obvious facial clefts, the notched upper lip commonly seen in the repaired cleft lip, the asymmetry of hemifacial hypertrophy and atrophy, the coarse facial features of acromegaly, the enlarged facial bones of Paget's disease, the bird-face of Pierre Robin syndrome, the round cherubic face of familial fibrous dysplasia, the adenoid facies of the adolescent, the myopathic facies of facioscapulohumeral muscular dystrophy, and the puffy facial features of mongolism.

Special attention to examination of the face, neck and salivary glands is given in Chapters 11, 12 and 13.

THE EYES, EARS AND NOSE

The eyes and their adnexa should be examined for any clinically obvious abnormalities. The horizontal position of the orbits, the size and shape of the orbital rims, the

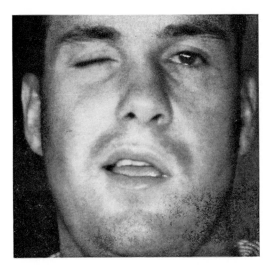

Fig. 7-2. Bell's palsy. The patient was asked to shut both eyes tightly and smile. Left facial paralysis is apparent.

prominence of the supraorbital ridges, and the interpupillary distances should be observed. The function of the eyelids, size and inclination in the palpebral fissures, tear secretion, color of the conjunctiva and iris, clearness of the sclera, and size and light responses of the pupils are noted.

Abnormalities of the orbits or their contents may be associated with several disorders of concern to the dentist. For example, developmental or growth disturbances affecting the cranial and facial bones may be manifest as hypo- or hypertelorism (Fig. 11–5A). A discrepancy in the horizontal plane or the orbits may suggest a previous orbital rim fracture or a tumor of the maxillary sinus. Exophthalmos is a well-known feature of Graves' disease. The blue sclera of osteogenesis imperfecta, yellow sclera of jaundice, the pinguecula of the bulbar conjunctiva in the aged, the coloboma and absence of eyelashes in Treacher Collins syndrome, the keratoconjunctivitis sicca of Sjögren's syndrome, the interstitial keratitis of congenital syphilis, the Bitot's spots of vitamin A deficiency, the iritis and conjunctivitis of Stevens-Johnson syndrome and Behcet's syndrome, the ptosis and miosis of Horner's syndrome, and the pinpoint pupils of drug addiction are other ocular disorders of concern.

The ears should be examined for symmetry, configuration, and position on the head.

Malformations of the ears (aural tags, preauricular pits and sinuses, low-set ears, etc.) often accompany other developmental defects involving the face or jaws (Figs. 1–2, 11–5). For example, congenital lip pits and fistulae have been associated with preauricular pits.

The configuration and symmetry of the nose should be noted. Nasal obstruction due to deviation of the septum, nasal polyps, or allergic rhinitis may be important considerations in the mouth breather. The saddle nose of congenital syphilis and achondroplasia may be easily recognized.

THE SKIN AND ITS APPENDAGES

The exposed skin of the face and neck as well as the extremities is readily observed in the physical examination. Its texture, elasticity and pigmentation (Figs. 7–3, 7–4) should be noted. The skin appendages (hair, nails, sweat glands, sebaceous glands) are of special interest since they have many features in common with the teeth.

Since most persons visit their dentist with greater frequency and regularity than their physician, the dentist has the opportunity to identify dermatologic changes of clinical significance. These include senile (solar) keratoses, basal cell carcinoma (Fig. 7–5), lichen planus, chronic discoid lupus erythematosus, pigmentary disorders, scars (Fig. 7–6), and others. In addition to those conditions of primary concern to the dermatologist, disorders of the skin or its appen-

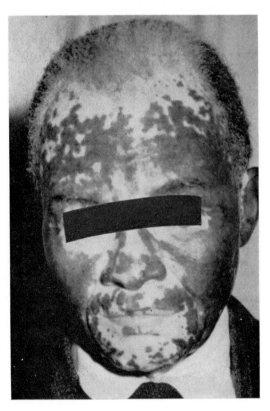

Fig. 7–4. Vitiligo. Gradual, symmetrical depigmentation.

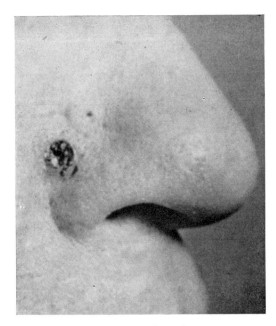

Fig. 7-5. An early basal cell carcinoma.

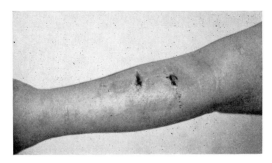

Fig. 7-6. Recent bite marks and older scars of the same origin on the forearm of a mentally retarded girl. The wounds were inflicted by an almost constant companion. (Courtesy of Louis Holmes.)

dages may be of value in arriving at the diagnosis of oral disease. The sparse hair, absence of sweat glands and partial anodontia of hereditary ectodermal dysplasia, the frequent concomitant skin and oral lesions of lichen planus, the plantar-palmar hyperkeratosis of juvenile periodontosis (Papillon-Lefevre syndrome), the associated basal cell nevi and odontogenic keratocysts, the koilonychia (spoon nails) and mucosal atrophy of Plummer-Vinson syndrome, and the dystrophic nails and kera-

totic oral lesions of pachyonychia congenita are examples. The skin additionally may present diagnostic "markers" of systemic disease: "target" lesions of erythema multiforme, cafe-au-lait spots of von Recklinghausen's disease, yellowing in hepatitis, bronzing in Addison's disease, acanthosis nigricans as a sign of internal malignancy, cyanosis of the fingernails in congestive heart failure, etc.

The dermatologic disorders are discussed in greater detail in Chapter 11.

THE EXTREMITIES

In the physical examination, the general muscular development and function of the limbs are noted. The hands in particular may reveal characteristics of the occupation of the patient; his temperament, as shown by nail biting (onychophagia); developmental defects such as adactyly, syndactyly, webbing and congenital amputations (Figs. 1–2, 11–4); arthritis (Fig. 7–7) (many rheumatoid arthritic patients have temporomandibular joint involvement); the simian crease of mongoloidism; clubbing of the fingers in cardiopulmonary disorders (Fig. 11–6), etc.

LIPS AND BUCCAL MUCOSA

Commence with visual and tactile examination of the lips to detect variations from

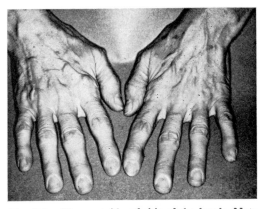

Fig. 7-7. Rheumatoid arthritis of the hands. Note the enlargement of the proximal phalanges. (Courtesy of William H. Binnie.)

Table 7-1. Common Lesions of the Lips and Buccal Mucosa

Lips

    Actinic (solar) keratosis
    Epidermoid carcinoma
    Mucocele
    Herpes labialis
    Lip pits
    Double lip
    Cleft lip

Buccal Mucosa

    Fordyce's granules
    Linea alba
    Lichen planus
    Hyperorthokeratosis
    Epidermoid carcinoma
    Fibroma
    Miscellaneous other benign tumors

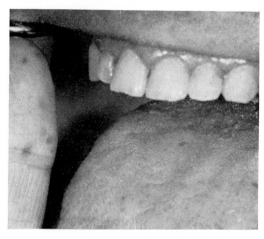

Fig. 7-8. Hereditary telangiectasia. The small red dots on the finger, tongue and elsewhere on the skin are characteristic.

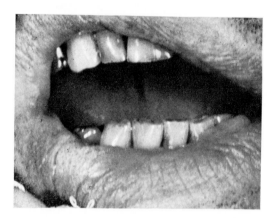

Fig. 7-9. Hyperkeratosis. An adherent white patch on the lower right lip of an aging male.

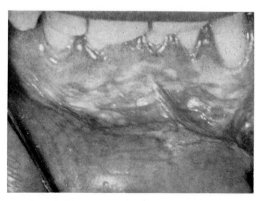

Fig. 7-10. Hyperkeratosis in the lower anterior labial sulcus associated with the use of snuff.

the normal in color, consistency, morphology and function (Fig. 7–8). The vermilion border and mucous membrane of the lips should be examined specifically for keratosis or ulceration (Table 7–1). *Actinic keratosis* (farmer's or sailor's lip) may be seen especially on the lower lip of elderly individuals or others exposed to much sun (Fig. 7–9). Since the lower lip in particular is a common location for *epidermoid carcinoma* (Fig. 1–17), especially in the aging male, ulceration, crusting or induration should be investigated thoroughly. Masses within the substance of the lips may not be visible when the lips are at rest. Bimanual or bidigital palpation of the skin and mucous membranes should extend to both the upper and lower mucobuccal folds.

The *mucocele* occurs with considerable frequency in the lower lip as a fluid-filled, palpable mass of recent origin (Fig. 1–5). In the aging, bluish varicosities are commonly seen on the inner surfaces of the lips, and deeper enlarged vessels are detectable by palpation. Tobacco-induced hyperkeratosis is common in snuff users who frequently

carry the quid in the lower anterior vestibule
(Fig. 7–10). The mucosa of the "snuff patch"
appears white and wrinkled, and the hyperkeratosis does not rub off. Accessory salivary
gland tumors are encountered on occasion
but almost invariably in the upper rather than
the lower lip. They usually are firm, well
circumscribed, and freely movable masses.
Higher in the mucobuccal fold near the base
of the ala of the nose, the rare *nasoalveolar*
(nasolabial) *cyst* may occur, and resemble
a deep-positioned mucocele.

Commissural lip pits (at the angles of the
mouth) are often overlooked since they may
be inadvertently hidden by the handle of the
mouth mirror during the routine examination. Such pits also occur on either side of
the midline of the lower lip. The *double lip*
involving the upper lip is an uncommon
defect (Fig. 7–11). Cleft lip, often associated with cleft alveolar process and palate,
is a developmental defect occurring in approximately 1 in 800 births.

Reflect the cheek mucosa one side at a
time and locate the orifice of Stensen's duct
on or beneath a soft papilla opposite the
upper first molar (Fig. 7–12). On occasion
it may be helpful to dry the mucosa with a
sponge. The buccal parietes are the most
common site for ectopic sebaceous glands
(*Fordyce's granules*) (Fig. 7–13) which
are also seen, less commonly, on the lips.
While these are of no clinical significance,
their occurrence should be noted during
the examination, since occasionally patients
become concerned if the granules are unexplained. A white line common on the

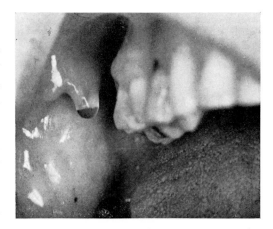

Fig. 7-12.   Parotid papilla in function.

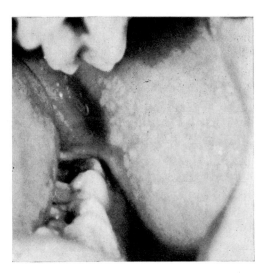

Fig. 7-13.   Fordyce's granules. These slightly
raised golden papules are characteristic.

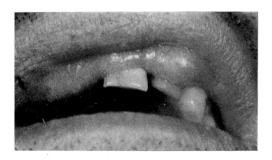

Fig. 7-11.   Double lip.

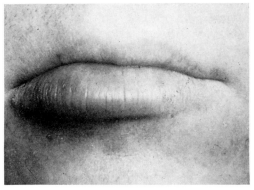

Fig. 7-14.   Angioneurotic edema of the lower lip.

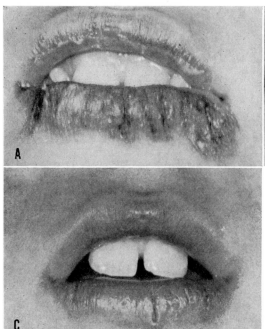

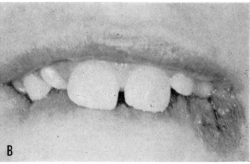

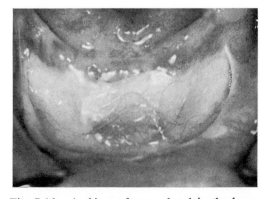

Fig. 7-15. Factitial injury. *A*, This 8-year-old girl apparently enjoyed several visits to physicians and dentists in the course of 7 months. Numerous medicaments had been prescribed. In an unguarded moment she was seen biting her lower lip, *B*. She and her mother were apprised of the fact. Orabase was prescribed for the lower lip 4 times daily. This was unpleasant when the patient indulged in her habit, and within 10 days the lip was healed to the extent seen in *C*. (Shafer, Hine and Levy, *Oral Pathology*, courtesy of the W. B. Saunders Co. and Ralph E. McDonald.)

buccal mucosa along the line of occlusion (*linea alba*) is related to trauma from the teeth or habitual negative intraoral pressure. Other white lesions of the buccal mucosa include *leukoedema* (Fig. 14–3), the lacy linear patterns of *lichen planus* (Figs. 1–24, 14–4), or the diffuse thickened mucosa of *hyperorthokeratosis* associated with smoking. Diffuse white lesions of congenital origin include the *white sponge nevus* and hereditary benign intraepithelial dyskeratosis (Fig. 4–19). *Epidermoid carcinoma* also may arise within leukoplakia on the buccal mucosa. Other lesions of the lips and buccal mucosa include the *hemangioma, papilloma, fibroma* (Fig. 2–5) and rarely the *granular cell myoblastoma. Angioneurotic edema* of the cheeks and lips (Fig. 7–14) is a diffuse enlargement due to allergy or hypersensitivity.

Factitial (self-induced) injury is commonly seen in the "cheek chewer" or, less commonly, the lip biter (Fig. 7–15). Intraoral skin grafts are occasionally used by plastic and oral surgeons (Fig. 7–16).

THE TONGUE AND FLOOR OF THE MOUTH

Both visual and manual examinations of the tongue and floor of the mouth are essential since these tissues may be the site of a variety of serious diseases (Table 7–2). Bimanual palpation of the floor of the mouth permits the identification of lesions arising in the major salivary glands, their ducts, and

Fig. 7-16. A skin graft was placed in the lower labial sulcular region many months before this photograph because of a gunshot wound. Hair can be seen growing on the skin surface.

Table 7-2. Common Tongue and Floor of Mouth Lesions

Tongue
- Traumatic ulcer
- Epidermoid carcinoma
- Lingual tonsil
- Lingual thyroid
- Fissured tongue
- Clefts of the tongue
- Median rhomboid glossitis
- Geographic tongue
- Glossitis
- Hairy tongue
- Miscellaneous benign neoplasms

Floor of Mouth
- Hyperkeratosis
- Epidermoid carcinoma
- Ranula
- Sialolithiasis
- Salivary gland neoplasms

the submaxillary lymph nodes as well as the covering and supporting tissues of these regions (Fig. 12–3).

The floor of the mouth is a common location for *hyperkeratotic lesions, epidermoid carcinoma, ranula, sialolithiasis* and, rarely, *neoplasms* of salivary gland origin.

A number of lesions of the tongue show some predilection for occurrence at certain anatomic sites such as the lateral border, dorsum, tip or ventral surface. In particular, the posterolateral border of the tongue is a common site for traumatic ulcer (Fig. 14–34), epidermoid carcinoma (Fig. 7–17) or specific granulomatous infections. The lingual tonsil (so-called foliate papillitis) appears as a red, elevated mass on the posterolateral portion of the tongue in the region of the foliate papillae and may be mistaken clinically for carcinoma (Fig. 7–19).

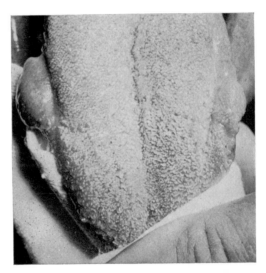

Fig. 7-18.   Tongue scars in an epileptic patient.

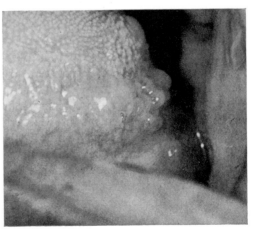

Fig. 7-19.   Red raised nodules of lingual tonsil on the lateral base of the tongue in the region of the foliate papillae.

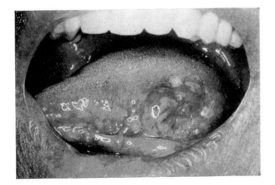

Fig. 7-17.   Squamous cell carcinoma. This indurated, tumefied, chronic, ulcerated lesion on the posterolateral surface of the tongue is typical of advanced carcinoma in an aging male.

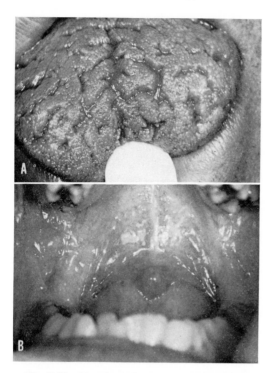

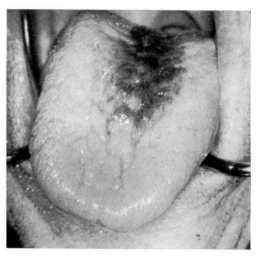

Fig. 7-21.   A brownish black hairy tongue.

Fig. 7-20.   Developmental abnormality. *A*, Fissured tongue. *B*, Hypermobility. The patient has placed the tongue in the nasopharynx.

Lesions of developmental origin commonly involve the dorsum of the tongue, *e.g.* fissured tongue (Fig. 7–20), cleft (bifid) tongue and median rhomboid glossitis which appears anterior to the circumvallate papillae in the midline (Fig. 7–23). Geographic tongue (glossitis migrans) manifests itself clinically as a serpiginous exfoliation of the filiform papillae over the dorsum, but occasionally extends onto the undersurface of the tongue (Figs. 7–24, 14–25). Other forms of glossitis typically involve the dorsum of the tongue and include Hunter's or Moeller's glossitis (pernicious anemia, sprue), the bald tongue of Sandwith (pellagra), "strawberry tongue" and "raspberry tongue" of scarlet fever and the atrophic tongue and mucosa of iron-deficiency anemia and Plummer-Vinson syndrome.

The common benign neoplasms of the tongue include papilloma (Figs. 1–15, 14–58), fibroma, hemangioma (Figs. 7–27, 14–

57) and, less commonly, the granular cell myoblastoma. The fibroma often occurs near the tip, while the papilloma involves papillae on the dorsum. The granular cell myoblastoma usually occurs on the dorsum (Fig. 14–63).

Carcinoma rarely occurs on the dorsum of the tongue except in those cases arising in a preexisting syphilitic glossitis. Hairy tongue sometimes results from oral medicaments (Figs. 7–21, 7–30). *Salivary gland tumors* and *lingual thyroid* may occur near the base of the tongue.

Traumatic ulcer, scar, thrombi, sialadenitis, mucocele and *fibroma* may occur on the anterior ventral surface or tip of the tongue.

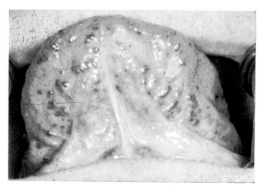

Fig. 7-22.   Varicosities characteristic of age on the under surface of the tongue.

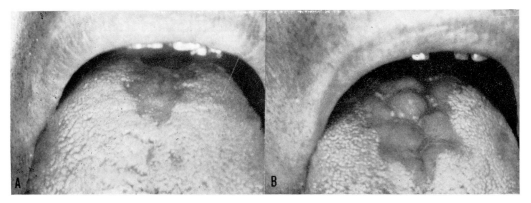

Fig. 7-23. Median rhomboid glossitis. A, Typical lesion neither rhomboid in shape nor inflamed. B, A more bizarre form. (Shafer, Hine and Levy, *Oral Pathology,* courtesy of W. B. Saunders Co.)

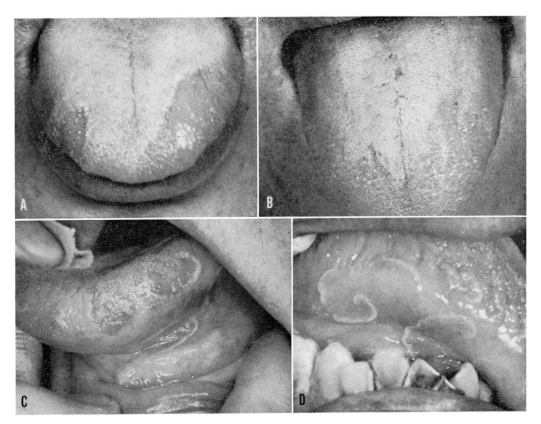

Fig. 7-24. Benign migratory glossitis (geographic tongue). *A,* The two lesions are red and devoid of filiform papillae although the fungiform papillae are apparent. The lesions are surrounded by a slightly raised white border. *B,* The same tongue 4 days later. *C,* Less commonly, the lesions are seen on the lateral border of the tongue and floor of the mouth. (Courtesy of N. H. Rowe.) *D,* A somewhat similar case.

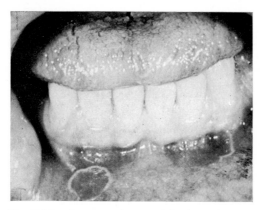

Fig. 7-25. An unusual case of benign migratory stomatitis on the lower lip of a medical student. Geographic tongue also was present. These lesions were observed periodically for nearly a year with little change except for their migratory characteristics.

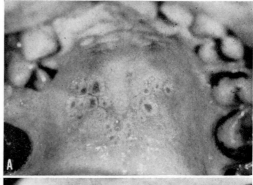

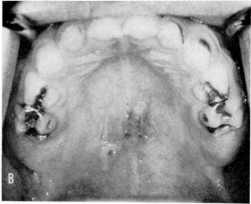

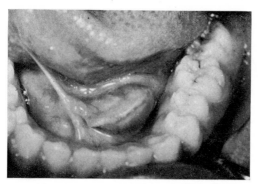

Fig. 7-26. Ranula. A small sialolith was present near the orifice of Wharton's duct, causing the swelling in the lower left floor of the mouth. (Shafer, Hine and Levy, *Oral Pathology,* courtesy of the W. B. Saunders Co.)

Fig. 7-28. Injuries. *A,* Nicotinic stomatitis of the palate. The orifices of the minor salivary glands are red, presumably protected by the functional flow of mucus, and the tissue around the orifices is adherent, raised hyperkeratosis. Note the tobacco staining of the teeth. *B,* Sucker-stick injury from a fall.

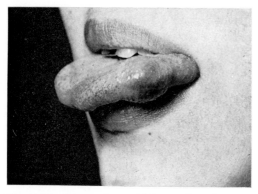

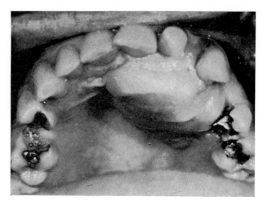

Fig. 7-27. Hemangioma. This purple lesion was present for as long as the patient could remember. It blanched on pressure.

Fig. 7-29. Lipoma. A very soft lesion of normal color in a patient with lipomatosis.

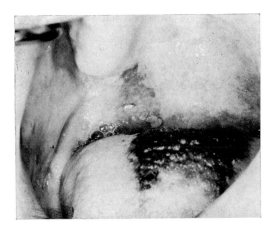

Fig. 7-30. Carcinoma-in-situ of the soft palate. A small biopsy had been made and pronounced negative. The patient was referred from otolaryngology to the dental clinic because of concern about the black hairy tongue. A cytological smear was positive, and subsequent larger biopsy of the erythematous lesion on the palate revealed the presence of preinvasive carcinoma. The interprofessional cooperation worked for the benefit of the patient.

PALATE AND OROPHARYNX

Observe and palpate the rugae, incisive papilla, palatal contour, the vibrating line and soft palate, the pterygoid hamulus and conceivably an elongated styloid process. Observe function of the movable parts during phonation. Note the uvula and palpate the pillars of the fauces and tonsils. With tongue depressed and during phonation, observe the posterior pharyngeal wall for the presence of small nodules of lymphatic tissue, injected vessels, erythema, postnasal drip and any lesions (Table 7–3). View the foliate papillae and lingual tonsils.

With the warm, inverted dental mirror or laryngeal mirror, and with the tongue depressed and extended, view the epiglottis. Look for signs of asymmetry, ulceration, color change, or departure from the normal consistency.

Question hoarseness which has persisted for more than 2 weeks. This is an important sign of laryngeal carcinoma, which is often associated with cigar smoking. Observe and question the patient regarding dysphagia or

Table 7-3. Common Palate and Pharynx Lesions

Palate
    Torus palatinus
    Clefts
    Denture injuries
    Stomatitis nicotina
    Salivary gland neoplasms
    Other neoplasms

Oropharynx
    Upper respiratory infections
    Exanthematous diseases
    Miscellaneous neoplasms

persistent sore throat. Newly occurring unilateral deafness, diplopia and tinnitus, or a postnasal hemorrhagic discharge may be indicative of malignancy in the nasopharynx. Constriction of the pupil (miosis), enophthalmos (the abnormal retraction of the eye into the socket), signs of paralysis or loss of sensation likewise are important.

The *torus palatinus* is present in approximately one-fifth of adult patients. Unerupted or impacted teeth, supernumerary teeth, dentigerous cysts and the several developmental cysts may be apparent upon palpation or with radiographic examination of the palate. Clefts of the palate and alveolar processes or surgically repaired clefts are not uncommon. Traumatic injuries occur in the child who falls on a sucker stick (Fig. 7–28B), pencil or toy. *Trophic ulcers* at sites of prior needle injections appear in the dense palatal mucosa. Denture injuries appear as diffuse erythema or *papillomatosis* in the vault of the hard palate. *Decubital ulcers* and *inflammatory fibrous hyperplasia* (epulis fissuratum) are seen in the mucosa adjacent to the denture borders.

A number of dermatologic and mucosal lesions frequently appear on the palate and oropharynx. *Stomatitis nicotina* (Fig. 7–28A), *leukoplakia,* and *carcinoma* are not rare. Extensions of disease from the teeth, maxillary sinus, or nasal cavity may be present clinically as inflammatory swelling, tissue enlargement or erythroplakia on the palate (Figs. 1–19, 7–30).

Petechiae, erythemas, ulcers, vesicles, and nodules are seen especially on the soft palate in a number of specific infections, exanthematous diseases and upper respiratory infections.

Lesions of diagnostic importance of the soft palate and oropharynx also include erythema (upper respiratory infections, exanthematous diseases), petechiae (infectious mononucleosis, leukemia), vesicles (herpangina), bullae (pemphigoid, pemphigus) and nodules (benign lymphonodular pharyngitis).

Papilloma (Fig. 7–46) and *adenoma* (Fig. 1–18) are among the more common benign neoplasms of the palate. *Squamous cell carcinoma* and *adenocarcinoma* (Fig. 7–32) are the most common forms of malignancy of

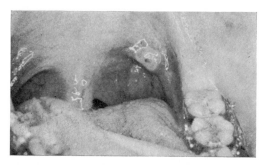

Fig. 7-33. An aphthous ulcer is seen on the anterior pillar of this young orthodontic patient. (See also Fig. 14-40 *A-D*.)

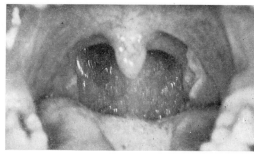

Fig. 7-34. The left tonsil is ulcerated and covered with a grey fibrinous membrane over the bleeding surface.

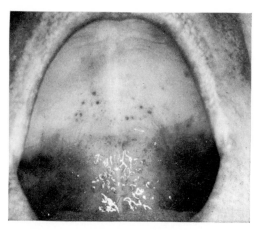

Fig. 7-31. Multiple small red petechiae are shown on the posterior hard palate. Thorough physical examination revealed no associated systemic disease. Nonetheless such lesions should be investigated thoroughly.

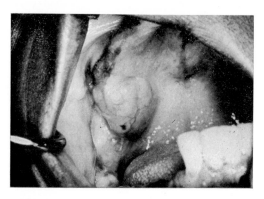

Fig. 7-32. An adenocarcinoma near the right posterior tuberosity.

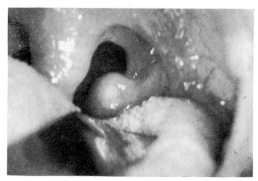

Fig. 7-35. A yellow circumscribed, peripheral lipoma of the tonsillar region.

this region. For the most part, squamous cell carcinoma generally occurs at the junction of the hard and soft palate or on the soft palate, whereas the pleomorphic adenoma and adenocarcinoma occur chiefly on the hard palate.

EXAMINATION OF THE JAWS

This examination includes direct observation, palpation, observations made during function, and thorough radiography. Recognize the differences in structure, size and radiodensity of the jaws of the child, the adult and the aged. Variations in stature of the patient, as in a frail, aged woman versus a large adult male, are to be considered along with the size of masticatory musculature, jaw bones, and the directly related radiodensity of the jaws. The many developmental abnormalities, inflammatory and infectious processes, neoplasms and signs of systemic diseases of the jaws are discussed in Chapter 15.

To examine the temporomandibular joints, observe the patient's face from the front while he opens and closes his mouth. Watch for deviation of the mandible to one side, limitation of movement, or hypermobility. The normal opening of the mouth is about 5 cm. Place the index fingers in the

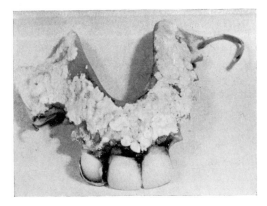

Fig. 7-36. A removable upper partial prosthesis which had not been removed from the mouth for 4 years. The patient thought it was a fixed device and sought dental care only because the teeth which had been clasped were badly decayed. Patient education is an important phase of treatment. (Mitchell, J. Indiana State Dent. Ass., Feb. 1958.)

external ear canals or just anterior to the tragus and feel the condyles move downward and forward as the patient opens. Listen and feel for any click or crepitus during movement. Palpate the masticatory muscles intra- and extraorally to detect undue tenderness. Apply the stethoscope to the side of the face over the condyle and listen to the joint sounds during mandibular movements.

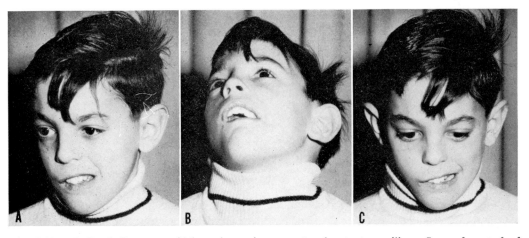

Fig. 7-37. *A, B, C,* Extrapyramidal syndrome in youngster due to tranquilizer. Loss of control of head and jaw-positioning musculature occurred. Child could not speak properly or close his mouth correctly. (Courtesy of David Dickey.)

Radiographs of both temporomandibular joints taken while the jaws are in the closed and opened positions are often used to rule out organic disease of the joints. Panoramic radiographs may also be useful. One must rule out the presence of primary and metastatic neoplasms of the condyle, fracture of the neck of the condyle or the fossa, ankylosis, dislocation, arthritis, condylar hyperplasia and other conditions. Rheumatoid, osteo-, infectious and traumatic arthritis are the most common forms of arthritis that involve these joints. Several other forms of arthritis seldom if ever do, so it is important to know the nature of any generalized arthritis the patient may have. Other conditions which have reportedly caused difficulty in the temporomandibular joints are scleroderma (Fig. 1–22), multiple myeloma (p. 291), and extensions of diseases of the ear, sinus, parotid gland and teeth.

Other conditions which have reportedly *simulated* temporomandibular joint involvement are brain tumor, hypertrophic coronoid processes and buccally erupting upper third molars impinging on masticatory muscles. Certain tranquilizers of the phenothiazine group have caused disturbances of mandibular positioning with resulting slurring of speech and anxiety in the extrapyramidal syndrome (Fig. 7–37).

EXAMINATION OF THE PERIODONTIUM

A common subjective complaint of patients with diseases of the periodontium is hemorrhage. The patient may have noticed blood on his pillow in the morning, or he may complain of excessive bleeding while brushing his teeth. Tenderness of the gingivae may result in the complaint of "sore gums." Halitosis and cacogeusia (bad taste) may be present. Occasionally, a complaint of "toothache" and/or swelling and trismus is made, especially in connection with pericoronitis or a lateral abscess involving a posterior tooth.

The medications the patient has used for the oral condition (aspirin, mouthwashes, antibiotics, ?) and any other therapeutic agents (Dilantin, tranquilizers, estrogens, the "pill") should be determined, since these may have a relationship to the oral findings.

A clear field for visualization, palpation and probing is essential for proper evaluation of the periodontium. Excessive amounts of food debris, materia alba or calculus may be removed with a spray or mouthwash, if necessary, or the gingivae and teeth may be wiped with gauze, or cleaned with compressed air. Rubbing the tissues with the finger may reveal desquamation. A double knot tied in dental floss which is then gently placed interdentally and drawn through the embrasures may displace foreign bodies or plaque. For example, the ubiquitous popcorn hull may be detected in this manner.

Palpation will reveal the consistency of diffuse inflammation, or the fluctuation of a lateral abscess. In addition, it may induce gingival crevicular hemorrhage, or pus may be expressed from periodontal pockets. Palpation of tooth crowns while asking the patient to grind his teeth will reveal excessive mobility, as will tapping the teeth. Percussion also may reveal abnormal sounds due to looseness or ankylosis, and tenderness. Diastemas and related "plunger cusps" which may cause food impaction should be recognized.

The periodontal pocket probe, calibrated in millimeters, should be inserted gently and pocket depth should be recorded (Fig. 2–15). The dental explorer may reveal overhanging restorations, calculus, foreign bodies and abnormalities of the dental root surfaces.

Alert use of the senses is imperative. One may see color changes, such as erythema, cyanosis, pigmentation, or the grey whiteness of ulceration. Changes in gingival morphology may be noted as in the case of a localized pyogenic granuloma or generalized gingival hyperplasia. Gingival recession should be noted and recorded whether or not an associated cause is apparent. A gingival

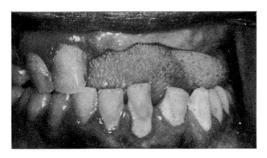

Fig. 7-38. Unilateral materia alba overlying calculus on the lower left side. This contrasts with the cleaner tooth surfaces on the patient's right due to self-cleansing action.

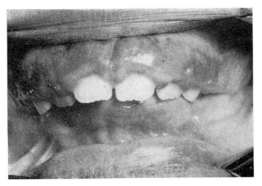

Fig. 7-39. Hereditary gingival fibromatosis, generalized. All of the teeth are present in the mouth of this teen-age Negro girl but most are completely hidden by the gingival overgrowth.

cleft associated with the pull of a labial frenum may be discerned. The presence of dentogingival plaque or calculus should be recorded. Disclosing solutions or tablets may reveal plaque that is otherwise not apparent. Supra- and subgingival calculus, especially common on the lingual of the lower anteriors and the buccal surfaces of the maxillary molars, should be detected.

The sense of smell may aid in detecting the acetone breath of the diabetic, the odor of the alcoholic or necrosis and bacterial overgrowth.

Radiographs, both periapical and bitewing types, reveal periodontal bone loss. One must recognize the limitations due to angulation and superimposition of teeth, tori or exostoses. Intracrevicular injection of radiopaque pastes to delineate the extent of periodontal pockets in radiographs, or the insertion of gutta percha points for the same reason, may be helpful.

The occlusion should be checked by visualization and palpation, and through the use of carbon marking paper inserted between the jaws during masticatory movements. The construction of study models may help one gain an insight into possible excessive pressures on individual teeth or soft tissues. The facets of wear on tooth surfaces may aid this evaluation.

Cytologic and bacterial smears, biopsy, and the therapeutic trial may be useful additional diagnostic measures on occasion.

Developmental Defects of the Periodontium

Developmental defects of the periodontium include clefts of the alveolar process (Figs. 4–15, 15–14), certain cysts (pp. 464–470) and dental anomalies (pp. 148–153). Knowledge of the embryonic and later developmental history of the region is basic to the diagnosis of such conditions. The generalized overgrowth of *hereditary gingival fibromatosis* is diagnosed by its appearance, intrafamilial occurrence, and the absence of other local or systemic predisposing factors (Fig. 7–39). Inflammation is not a prominent feature in this rare condition.

Atrophic and Hyperplastic Disorders

Atrophic and hyperplastic changes occur in the gingivae and other parts of the periodontium (Figs. 7–40, 7–41). Gingival recession associated with passive eruption, habit, aging, or with no obvious reason is an example of the former (Fig. 7–49). Generalized gingival hyperplasia may be pronounced in cases of Dilantin therapy (*Dilantin gingivitis*), *pregnancy gingivitis, leukemic gingivitis,* or simple *inflammatory hyperplasia* of the gingivae. The *pyogenic granuloma* (Figs. 1–8, 7–44*A,B,* 14–57, 14–64) is a common localized lesion which has many features in common with the *peripheral odontogenic*

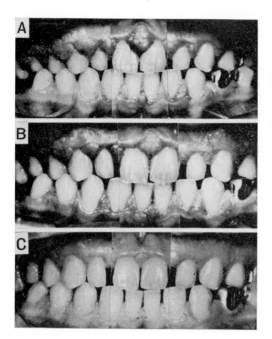

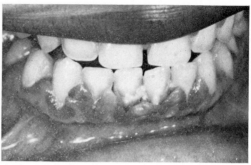

Fig. 7-41. Generalized chronic inflammatory gingival hyperplasia in association with subgingival plaque and calculus in the mouth of a young woman.

(*ossifying*) *fibroma and peripheral giant cell granuloma* (Fig. 14–65) of the gingiva.

Inflammatory and Infectious Diseases

Inflammation and infection underlie the most common diseases of the periodontium —non-specific gingivitis and periodontitis. These may be generalized or localized and they may result in ulceration, recession or gingival hyperplasia. Most commonly, plaque, calculus and other local factors such as food impaction, overhanging restorations

Fig. 7-40. Dilantin hyperplasia in a 30-year-old patient responding to toothbrushing and massage (Charters method). *A,* Before treatment; *B,* after prophylaxis and 3 months home care; *C,* one year. No alteration in Dilantin medication was made. (Eberle and Muhlemann, Schweiz. Monatsschrift für Zahnheilkunde, *70,* 395, 1960.)

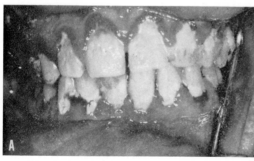

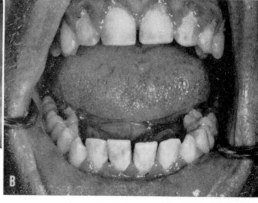

Fig. 7-42. Complete lack of oral hygiene in a young adult mentally retarded patient. *A,* The materia alba consists of masses of bacteria which are causing the red marginal gingivae and spontaneous hemorrhage at several sites. *B,* The same patient 4 days later after three topical applications of a topical antibiotic (vancomycin hydrochloride). No other therapy or home care was available. Notice the absence of spontaneous hemorrhage, the marked reduction in plaque and the reduction in the marginal gingivitis. Calculus is now apparent on the lower central incisors, whereas before it was completely covered with materia alba.

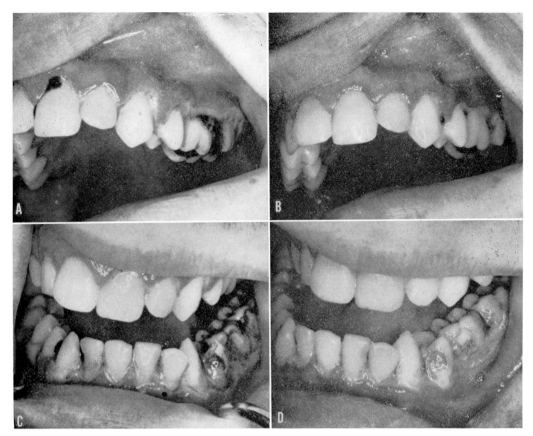

Fig. 7-43. Vincent's infection before (*A* and *C*) and 3 days after (*B* and *D*) one topical application of vancomycin hydrochloride. (Mitchell, Holmes, Martin, and Sakurai, J. Oral Ther. Pharm., *4*, 83, 1967.)

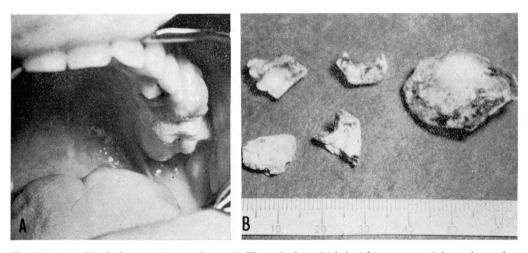

Fig. 7-44. *A*, Gingival pyogenic granuloma. *B*, The calculus which had been removed from the surface of the upper left quadrant. This middle-aged woman had noticed discomfort in this region several months before and avoided cleaning the region or chewing on that side. The calculus accumulated and the patient finally sought dental attention because she believed she had a "bony cancer." (Mitchell, J. Periodont., *27*, 273, 1956.)

and impingement of clasps are associated. Marginal gingival erythema and swelling, with or without malodor, discomfort, hemorrhage and pocket formation, are usually present.

Specific infections include *acute or chronic necrotizing ulcerative gingivitis* (NUG) or "Vincent's infection." This condition is recognized by the presence of gingival ulcers covered with a grey fibrin membrane and bacteria. This destruction most commonly involves the gingival papillae and interdental spaces. Finger pressure on the gingivae elicits hemorrhage from the ulcers. Poor oral hygiene, tenderness, malodor, fever and malaise may be associated. Stress appears to be an important predisposing factor. The diagnosis may be aided by a therapeutic trial. Cleaning the teeth usually results in improvement in a matter of hours or less. Systemic and/or topical antibiotic therapy will give similar results. Less commonly this infection involves a pericoronal operculum, the palatal and buccal mucosa, or the oropharynx (Vincent's angina).

Primary herpetic gingivostomatitis is a recognized entity seen most commonly in young children. The gingivae and other oral tissues are intensely inflamed. Ulcers subsequently form. Fever and lymphadenopathy accompany the oral lesions. Secondary or recurrent intraoral herpes simplex virus infection exhibits clusters of tiny vesicles on the hard palate, attached gingiva and edentulous alveolar ridge (Fig. 7–45). If gingival aphthae are present, the diagnosis of *aphthous gingivostomatitis* depends on the detection of typical aphthae elsewhere in the mouth, particularly on the movable mucous membranes (see pp. 394, 401). From a clinical standpoint, viruses and specific bacteria, using conventional office methods, seldom can be identified and unquestionably related to the clinical condition. Here again the therapeutic trial may be helpful. Duration of the condition with or without treatment is important, since such conditions tend to regress within a week or two. A history of periodic recurrence likewise aids the diagnosis.

Degenerative Disorders of the Periodontium

Periodontosis is a degenerative disease of the periodontium of unknown etiology. Fortunately it is rare, but when it occurs consternation is great (see below). All one can do is to treat associated local factors, and detect any possible systemic factors that may be involved. Genetic evaluation often is necessary (Chap. 4).

The young adult form of periodontosis is relatively common. It occurs more often

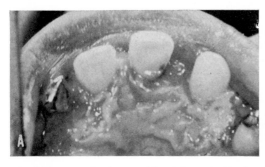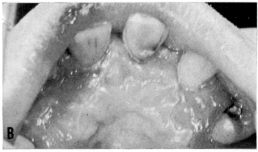

Fig. 7-45. *A,* Gingivopalatitis of 5 days' duration in a 40-year-old male. A physician had given him an injection of penicillin 2 days prior to this photograph. The condition remained unchanged. After examination here, he was advised to return in 3 days without any further treatment. *B,* At this time the lesions are healing, the ulcerated surfaces are erythematous but covered with epithelium. The final diagnosis was herpetic gingivostomatitis. Note the lesion on the upper lip in *B.* This is an example of "therapeutic trial" (penicillin) which, through failure, aided diagnosis.

among Negroids than among Caucasoids. No obvious local etiologic factors are present and the patient is often surprisingly free of both dental decay and calculus formation. The first permanent molars show severe vertical bone loss and subsequently the upper and lower incisors are involved (Fig. 7-48). The teeth loosen and tend to drift as pocket formation progresses and inflammation becomes superimposed. Any possible systemic factor such as diabetes, leukemia and genetic conditions must be ruled out, and local therapy is applied as in any form of periodontal disease. The necessity for home care is obvious. Splinting of teeth and judicious periodontal surgery may be employed in advanced cases.

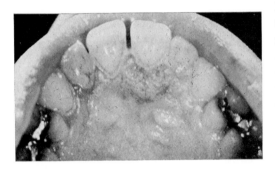

Fig. 7-46. A gingival papilloma lingual to the upper left central incisor. Three similar lesions were present elsewhere (papillomatosis).

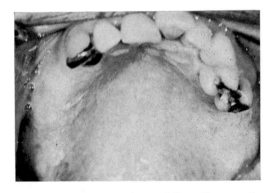

Fig. 7-47. Lichen planus bilaterally on the edentulous alveolar processes. In this location the typical lacy white lines of Wickham are less apparent and a rather hyperkeratotic diffuse plaque is seen instead.

Chronic desquamative gingivitis, etiology unknown, is most common among adult women. Desquamation is illustrated in Figure 2-14; another case is shown in Figure 14-21, and further discussion will be found on page 388.

Neoplasms of the Periodontium

Neoplasia may involve the periodontium. The most common neoplasms of the gingivae are papillomas (Fig. 7-46) and hemangiomas. Primary squamous cell carcinoma is the most common malignancy of the gingivae (Fig. 2-6). Adenocarcinoma does not arise primarily in the gingiva since glandular structures seldom occur there; it may however invade the periodontium from adjacent glandular tissue in the palate or maxillary sinus. Metastatic carcinoma and sarcoma involve the jaw bones on rare occasions. Spontaneous development of paresthesia and/or anesthesia of tissues innervated by the mandibular nerve may signify central malignancy, primary or metastatic, of the mandible. Any localized, severe osteolytic lesion without associated local factors should be considered suspect in relation to the latter. If a patient requests the removal of a loose tooth among otherwise healthy teeth with a healthy periodontium, the possibility of primary or metastatic malignancy should be considered, especially if the radiolucent lesion is ill defined and ragged and the tooth tests vital (Fig. 2-6). Biopsy in such a case is mandatory. The peripheral giant cell lesion of the gingiva is not uncommon (p. 427). Fibrous dysplasia of the jaws is not infrequent (p. 457).

Manifestations of Systemic Diseases

Diseases of other systems must be considered in the differential diagnosis of severe periodontal disease which appears not to be caused by local factors alone. Endocrine disturbances, blood dyscrasias, nutritional deficiency, dermatologic disorders, metabolic diseases, and certain genetic disorders are broad groups which must be investigated

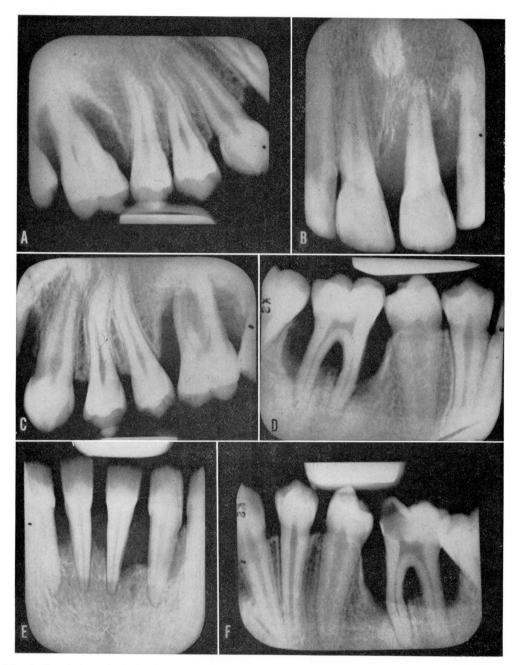

Fig. 7-48. *A* through *F*. Periodontosis in a young patient. Note the characteristic severe bone loss in the regions of the first permanent molars and the central incisors. Note the lack of apparent local factors. No systemic condition was revealed as contributory despite thorough physical examination.

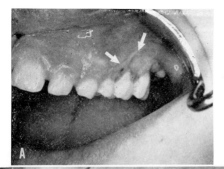

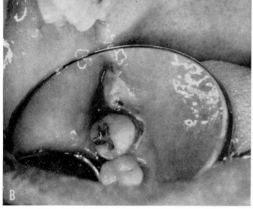

Fig. 7-49. Factitial gingival injuries. *A,* The alveolar bone on the buccal of the second deciduous and first permanent molars of this boy was exposed bilaterally. The youngster apparently had enjoyed several visits to dentists and physicians. Clinical laboratory studies including sternal marrow puncture had not revealed the cause. The boy finally admitted that he created these defects with his fingernails. (Hasler and Schultz, J. Periodont., *39,* 362, 1968.) *B,* Adult applied lemon extract to control toothache, causing ulceration.

according to the presenting signs and symptoms.

Diabetes mellitus (pp. 247–249, Figs. 9–17, 9–18), leukemic gingivitis (Fig. 1–20), histiocytosis X (pp. 488–489, Fig. 15–56) and scurvy in particular may simulate periodontal disease of local origin.

Certain dermatoses such as lichen planus (Fig. 7–47) or benign mucous membrane pemphigoid, erythema multiforme, lupus erythematosus, and pemphigus may involve the alveolar mucosa and gingiva (Chap. 14). Most often such gingival lesions will be associated with other more obvious lesions of

mucous membrane and skin. The periodontium also sometimes shows changes in the periodontal ligament space in scleroderma (Fig. 1–22).

Genetic conditions involving the periodontium to varying degrees include Papillon-Lefevre syndrome (Fig. 4–18), hypophosphatasia (Fig. 4–7 and p. 152), acatalasia, and Down's disease (mongolism, Fig. 4–13).

Certain drug effects, including idiosyncrasies, may cause periodontal changes—agranulocytosis (Fig. 14–50, p. 410), acrodynia (p. 362), and cortisonism.

EXAMINATION OF THE DENTITION

Invite the patient to comment regarding any problem involving the dentition. The mouth mirror, a sharp dental explorer, compressed air, a spoon excavator and dental floss may be needed. Using adequate illumination, retract the lips and cheeks and view the entire dentition in the opened and closed jaw positions to gain an overall impression of the problems that may exist. Record the jaw relationship according to Angle's classification I to III (p. 301). Palpate the labial or buccal surfaces of a few teeth while the patient grinds the teeth together to detect movement. Observe the jaws during opening, closing and chewing movements. Count the teeth and note those missing or possible supernumerary teeth present. Then, in an orderly manner, examine each individual tooth and tooth surface in the proper numerical order.

Use the senses to detect abnormality. Look for change in color, morphology, mobility and symmetry. Tap the individual teeth to detect unusual sounds due to looseness or ankylosis, and watch for reactions of the patient that reveal associated tenderness. Look for aesthetic factors which may be undesirable. Record developmental or acquired abnormality. Filtered ultraviolet light may aid in examining the teeth in a dark room for the detection of unusual fluorescence. If pain is present, additional diagnostic instruments and tests may be required (Chap. 6).

Developmental Defects of the Teeth

The teeth may exhibit a wide variety of developmental disturbances, ranging in severity from minor anomalies to extremely severe defects, some of which have serious implications. These developmental defects include abnormalities in number, size, shape or structure of the teeth. They may involve only a single tooth or affect all or most of the patient's teeth (Figs. 7–50, 7–51, 7–52).

Anodontia

Total anodontia, or complete absence of teeth, is extremely rare. Partial or total anodontia is seen in association with hereditary ectodermal dysplasia, in which there is also absence of sweat glands (anhidrosis),

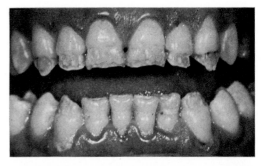

Fig. 7-52. Enamel hypoplasia (contemporaneous accretional dystrophy). It is apparent that some systemic upset occurred during the first year of the patient's life afflicting those portions of the teeth developing at that time.

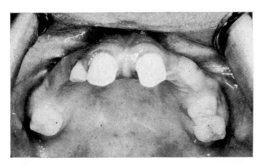

Fig. 7-50. Partial anodontia. No other ectodermal defects were detected. Note the parotid papillae of the functioning glands.

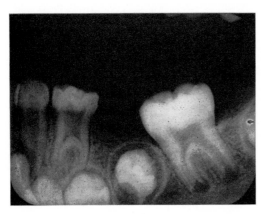

Fig. 7-51. Taurodontism in primary molar (Courtesy of Jose Garcia.)

salivary glands, nasopharyngeal mucous glands and sparse hair and eyebrows (Fig. 4–17). More commonly, partial anodontia is represented by congenitally missing third molars, maxillary lateral incisors or maxillary or mandibular second premolars (in descending order of frequency). Usually the condition is bilateral and an hereditary or familial pattern can sometimes be demonstrated (Fig. 7–50).

Indiscriminate irradiation of facial hemangiomas or other neoplasms in young children may cause inhibition of tooth formation in progress at the time. In this manner, *partial anodontia* results and radiation-sensitive tooth germs may be deformed or stunted, depending upon the age at the time the radiation therapy was given (Fig. 7–56).

Supernumerary Teeth

The mesiodens, seen in the midline of the anterior maxilla (Fig. 2–34), is the most common of the supernumerary teeth. It is followed in frequency by the maxillary fourth molar, maxillary paramolar, mandibular premolars and maxillary lateral incisors. Other supernumerary teeth are also seen on occasion (Fig. 2–12).

Multiple supernumerary teeth are characteristically found in *cleidocranial dysosto-*

sis (Fig. 11–8) and *Gardner's syndrome* (p. 482).

Dens in Dente (Dens Invaginatus)

The *dens in dente* is a developmental invagination of enamel in the crown of a tooth, most often the upper lateral incisor, but occasionally involving almost any tooth. Caries with the early development of pulp exposure may result in unexpected pulp pathosis (Fig. 7–57). For this reason, the minor dens in dente should be filled prophylactically as soon as it is recognized radiographically.

A comparable anomaly, *dens evaginatus*, is essentially the reverse of dens in dente. It appears as a cusp-like protuberance in the central fossa of the tooth crown. usually a premolar tooth. Another analogous defect is the *talon cusp* seen on the cingulum of the incisors. The protuberance of enamel and dentin (resembling an eagle talon) contains a pulp horn.

Gemination, Fusion, and Concrescence

Gemination, or "twinning," represents an aborted attempt of a single tooth bud to divide into two teeth. Often the division of the crown is complete, or nearly so, but there will be but a common pulp chamber and root.

Fusion represents two separate tooth buds which have united during an early stage of development. Thus, a single large tooth may form or, if the fusion occurred at a later stage, the crowns may be separate with confluent dentin in a common root (Fig. 7–58).

Concresence represents the fusion of two teeth by cementum only. Probably crowding together of the two separate teeth promotes the apposition and fusion of cementum.

Dilaceration

This condition represents a distinctive bend or curvature of the tooth root. Trauma or the presence of some intrabony lesion may account for the change. Dilaceration is of significance if extraction of the tooth should become necessary.

Microdontia, Macrodontia

Microdontia most commonly involves individual teeth, chiefly the maxillary lateral incisors (so-called peg lateral). Other than minor deviations from the average tooth size, microdontia is seldom generalized except in some cases of hypopituitarism arising in childhood (p. 252).

Macrodontia affecting all or several teeth is rarely seen except in some cases of pituitary giantism (p. 253) and in hemihypertrophy (p. 301). Single teeth with apparent macrodontia should be distinguished from gemination or fusion (see above).

Enamel Hypoplasia

Enamel hypoplasia, aplasia, and hypocalcification occur as a "contemporaneous accretional dystrophy" of the enamel surface which may take many forms. It is the most common defect of the teeth attributable to systemic diseases or disturbances. Several hereditary forms of enamel hypoplasia are also recognized. These have been differentiated according to the clinical types (pitting, vertical grooving, aplastic) and the mode of genetic transmission.

The most vulnerable time of the infant is the neonatal period and first year of life. The teeth most frequently affected are the permanent incisors and first permanent molars, the crowns of which are developing at this time. Any prolonged fever-inducing disease may cause enamel dystrophy. Childhood diseases, rickets, endocrine imbalances, nutritional deficiencies, ingestion of certain chemicals and other factors have been blamed.

Pits and grooves arranged horizontally and bilaterally are the most common defects (Fig. 7–52). Secondary (extrinsic) staining of the affected regions of the teeth is com-

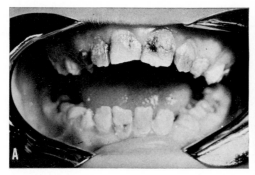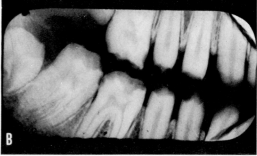

Fig. 7-53. Amelogenesis imperfecta of the hypocalcification type (hereditary brown teeth). The exposed dentin is brown and secondarily discolored due to extrinsic stains. Notice the absence of contact points and the sharp dentinal incisal edges. This teen-ager was an extreme introvert raised by an aunt who had suffered the same affliction, for which she had had all of her teeth extracted at an early age. After porcelain jacket crowns were constructed for the anterior teeth and full gold coverage for the posterior teeth, the patient underwent a noticeable, attractive personality change. *B,* A bite-wing film of another case showing normal pulp and dentin and an utter lack of enamel. (See also Fig. 4-10.)

mon. Such defects should not be confused with the developmental abnormalities of Hutchinsonian incisors and "mulberry molars" of congenital syphilis.

Amelogenesis Imperfecta (Hereditary Enamel Dysplasia, Hereditary Brown Enamel)

Amelogenesis imperfecta is a disturbance involving the enamel of all teeth of the deciduous and permanent dentitions. In the absence of enamel, the exposed dentin is brown, hence the term "hereditary brown teeth" (Fig. 7–53). The contour, color and lack of contact between the teeth are striking features (Fig. 4–10). Such patients are concerned with their appearance and there usually is no complaint of hypersensitivity to thermal changes because the patient has always lived with the problem and does not know the difference. The condition usually is transmitted as an autosomal dominant character. Chaudhry *et al.* reported the findings in 10 cases from 5 families with known pedigrees (Chap. 4). Management of these cases was discussed. Some of the patients were treated with temporary and later permanent crowns. Others more severely afflicted and with marked disturbances in occlusion received complete dentures after extraction of the teeth.

Dentinogenesis Imperfecta (Hereditary Opalescent Dentin)

In this disorder of the teeth, the hereditary factor responsible appears to be an autosomal dominant trait which is transmitted through affected subjects only (Table 4–2). Rare cases of *osteogenesis imperfecta* have been reported in association with dentinogenesis imperfecta, but the dental affliction occurs alone more often. Both the deciduous and the permanent dentitions are affected with the basic defect limited to dentin. The overlying enamel on incisal and occlusal surfaces may fracture off small bits at a time, presumably because of a defec-

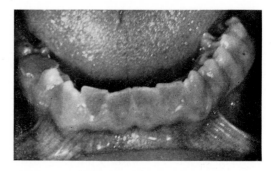

Fig. 7-54. Dentinogenesis imperfecta. The teeth are a translucent blue-grey. Note the extreme abrasion of the retained lower right deciduous molar. (Courtesy of Arden G. Christen.)

tive dentinoenamel junction. This may explain the severe, early attrition in some cases.

The color of the teeth is opalescent, ranging from a slightly golden brown to a bluish tinged color (Fig. 7–54). The morphology of the crowns of the teeth is within normal bounds. The roots are short and have a spiked appearance, and radiographically there is a tendency toward pulpal obliteration occurring at a young age (Fig. 4–16). No unusual tendency toward the development of periapical disease or dental caries was evident in this series. Management of such cases again depends to a degree on the problem of aesthetics. There apparently is no contraindication to the placement of full crowns or other restorations if adequate root support is present.

Dentinal Dysplasia ("Rootless Teeth")

Dentinal dysplasia is a rare defect of dentin which is inherited as an autosomal dominant trait. Except for some slight discoloration, the crowns of both the deciduous and permanent teeth appear normal. Radiographs, however, show short and pointed roots and absence of normal pulp chambers. Except for thin, threadlike canals in the teeth, the pulp chambers are filled with abnormal dentin which shows one or more peculiar crescent-shaped radiolucencies at right angles to the long axis of the root near the middle third of the tooth.

Taurodontism

This refers to a disturbance in the shape of the permanent and, occasionally, the de-

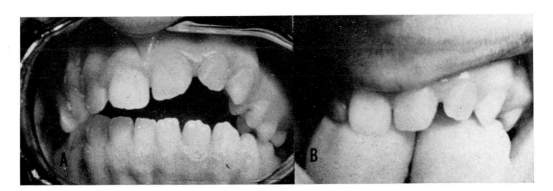

Fig. 7-55. *A*, Severe unilateral malocclusion associated with finger sucking, *B*.

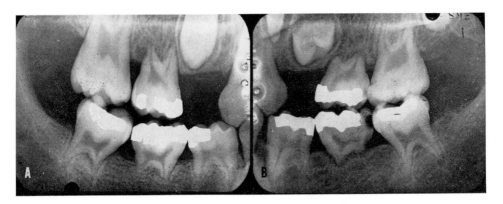

Fig. 7-56. Inhibition of root formation in a child treated with irradiation at an early age. (Shafer, Hine and Levy, *Oral Pathology*, courtesy of W. B. Saunders Co. and John Mink.)

ciduous molar teeth in which the teeth have some resemblance to those of the ungulates or cud-chewing animals such as the cow (taurus), as well as those of Neanderthal man. The crowns of affected molar teeth appear normal; however, radiographs show a marked elongation of the coronal pulp chamber in the coronal-apical dimension at the expense of the radicular pulp and roots. Because of this "stretched-out" appearance of the middle portion of the tooth, the bifurcation of the roots is located further apically than normal (Fig. 7–51).

Vitamin D Resistant Rickets (Familial Hypophosphatemia, Refractory Rickets, Phosphate Diabetes)

This familial disorder due to an inborn error of metabolism is thought to be a sex-linked dominant trait. The enamel is hypoplastic, the pulp chambers are large, and microscopic pulp exposures and their sequelae occur. Eruption may be delayed.

Hypophosphatasia (Hypophosphatasemia)

Hypophosphatasia is hereditary and transmitted as an autosomal recessive characteristic (Chap. 4). Alkaline phosphatase deficiency (hypophosphatasemia), rachitic-like bone changes, and early loosening of the teeth due to lack of or an inadequate type of cementum are characteristic (Fig. 4–7).

Regional Odontodysplasia ("Ghost Teeth," Odontogenic Dysplasia, Localized Arrested Tooth Development)

Recognition of this peculiar anomaly of the teeth is usually made radiographically. The affected teeth, which are most commonly the maxillary central and lateral incisors and canine on one side, show a marked reduction in density ("ghost teeth") with thin rims of dentin and enamel. The pulp chambers are correspondingly large. Attention is often directed to this area because of delay or failure of eruption of the involved teeth. Corresponding teeth on the opposite side of the arch are unaffected. The etiology is

unknown although "somatic mutation" or a latent viral infection involving the odontogenic apparatus of the anomalous teeth has been proposed. Since the teeth are poorly formed and unsightly, extraction is necessary.

Defects of Eruption and Exfoliation

Since the process of tooth eruption is intimately allied with growth of the individual, any factor which influences body growth may affect eruption (Table 7–4). Generalized delay in eruption has been noted in hypothyroidism and hypopituitarism (p. 245, Fig. 9–20). In the hereditary condition cleidocranial dysostosis, the jaws are overcrowded with retained unerupted teeth and sometimes with supernumerary teeth (Fig. 11–8). Other causes of generalized delay in tooth erup-

Table 7-4. Defects of Eruption and Exfoliation

Delayed Eruption (Generalized)
Hypothyroidism
Hypopituitarism
Cleidocranial dysostosis
Osteopetrosis
Fibromatosis gingivae
Chondroectodermal dysplasia
Gardner's syndrome
Mongolism
Infantile rickets
Achondroplastic dwarfism
Premature Exfoliation (Generalized)
Papillon-Lefevre syndrome
Acrodynia
Juvenile diabetes
Histiocytosis X
Cyclic neutropenia
Leukemia
Cherubism
Progeria
Hyperpituitarism
Dentinal dysplasia
Hypophosphatasia
Acatalasemia

tion include osteopetrosis, fibromatosis gingivae, chondroectodermal dysplasia (Ellis-van Creveld syndrome), Gardner's syndrome, mongolism, infantile rickets and achondroplastic dwarfism. Prolonged fever may cause moderate delay in tooth eruption.

Generalized premature loss of the deciduous teeth, and often of the permanent teeth as well, may be seen in children with Papillon-Lefevre syndrome (juvenile periodontosis), acrodynia, juvenile diabetes, histiocytosis X (Letterer-Siwe disease, Hand-Schüller-Christian disease), cyclic neutropenia, leukemia, familial fibrous dysplasia (cherubism), progeria, hyperpituitarism, dentinal dysplasia, hypophosphatasia and acatalasemia.

On the other hand, generalized premature eruption of the teeth is apparently a much less common occurrence. Individual teeth or pairs of teeth may be present at

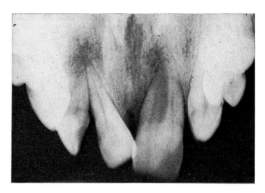

Fig. 7-58. Fusion apparently involving an upper central and lateral incisor. (Courtesy of Louis Holmes.)

birth (natal teeth) or erupt into the mouth during the first month (neonatal teeth). Often there is a familial history of natal or neonatal teeth. Some cases have been associated with chondroectodermal dysplasia, oculomandibular dyscephaly and pachyonychia congenita. Premature loss of a deciduous tooth will often permit the succeeding permanent tooth to erupt earlier than normal.

Cleidocranial dysostosis may predispose to *severe malposition and malocclusion*. Depending on the age of the patient at the onset of a pituitary or thyroid disturbance, jaw growth and tooth eruption may be affected with a variety of manifestations. Damaging or potentially injurious habits may affect tooth position (Fig. 7–55). Missing or supernumerary teeth, severe periodontal disease, trauma and neoplasia are some of the many factors that may contribute to tooth malposition.

Intrinsic Staining of Teeth

Intrinsic stains of the teeth are induced during the calcification of forming dentin by natural pigments of the body (hemoglobin, bile). Tooth color is also modified by high fluoride intake and tetracycline therapy during tooth development. While these latter agents are derived from outside the body, they are incorporated into the developing

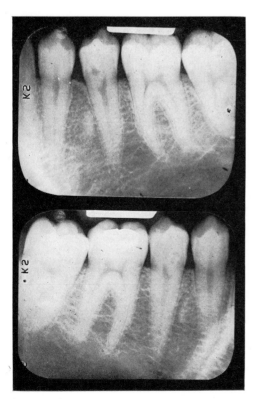

Fig. 7-57. Bilateral dens in dente of lower second premolars. (Courtesy of John McLaughlin.)

tooth structure and arbitrarily included with the intrinsic stains for convenience. The discoloration is apparent through the relatively unstained overlying enamel. The radicular dentin and cementum also are involved but, of course, such staining is seldom observed until after tooth exfoliation.

Jaundice, Erythroblastosis Fetalis

Any severe or prolonged *jaundice* occurring at a propitious time of tooth development may result in a greenish stain of calcifying tooth portions. The blue or green deciduous teeth of *erythroblastosis fetalis* have been seen as the result of the hemolytic jaundice occurring in surviving offspring incompatible with the mother as regards the Rh factor. Other conditions causing temporary episodes of hemolysis or metabolic insult, such as cerebral palsy or premature birth, may also induce intrinsic staining of developing teeth.

Porphyria

This hereditary disturbance of porphyrin metabolism causes intrinsic staining (Table 11–1, p. 232). Patients excrete reddish urine and the teeth are stained dark red; under the ultraviolet lamp, they fluoresce a brilliant crimson. Again, the dentin of the teeth developing at the time of birth is affected.

Dental Fluorosis ("Mottled Enamel")

This relatively common defect of developing teeth results from intake of excessive amounts of fluoride in the drinking water usually in excess of 1.5 parts per million (Fig. 1–23).

Although the enamel sometimes is hypoplastic in severe fluorosis, most commonly it is present in its entirety. Hypocalcification of developing zones causes it to appear chalky when erupted and extrinsic stains by foods and other materials later result in the characteristic brown mottling, a permanent affliction unless bleached or ground away. Accurate diagnosis of this condition is en-

hanced by fluoride analysis of the drinking water used by the patient at an early age. State departments of health can furnish the practitioner with charts designating high fluoride areas over the United States. The southwestern section of the United States and Colorado are common areas for the occurrence of fluorosis. The discovery and description of fluorosis by G. V. Black and Frederick F. McKay, in the region of Colorado Springs, and later work by H. Trendley Dean led to the discovery of the role of fluorides in inhibiting dental caries.

Tetracycline Staining

The tetracycline antibiotics, used widely since the latter 1950s, have resulted in many recent cases of intrinsic staining. The tetracycline* fluorophore is deposited in calcifying teeth and bone in a calcium complex of the inorganic portion of the tissues. The enamel incorporates comparatively little tetracycline except in extreme cases, when it also may exhibit hypoplasia (Fig. 7–59*A*). It may be difficult to ascertain whether the hypoplasia is due to tetracycline therapy or to the disease that was treated with the antibiotic. The dentin calcifying at the time exhibits incremental lines stained a faint dark brown when viewed in a ground section under incandescent light. When viewed through the fluorescent microscope (UV light), they are a brilliant yellow (Fig. 7–59*B*).

---

* Tetracycline. Achromycin (Lederle), Panmycin (Upjohn), Sumycin (Squibb), Tetracyn (Pfizer), and Tetrex (Bristol)
Chlortetracycline. Aureomycin (Lederle)
Demethylchlortetracycline. Declomycin (Lederle)
Oxytetracycline. Terramycin (Pfizer)
Rolitetracycline. Syntetrin (Bristol) and Velacycline (Squibb)
Methacycline. Rondomycin (Pfizer)
   The drug manufacturers have also combined the tetracyclines with other drugs. Examples of such preparations are as follows:
Achrostatin and Declostatin (Lederle)
Signemycin, Terra-cortril, Terrastatin and Tetrastatin (Pfizer)
Mysteclin-F (Squibb)
Comycin and Panalba (Upjohn)

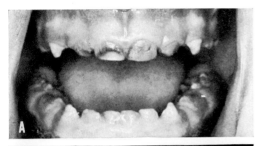

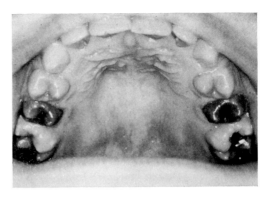

Fig. 7-60.   Tetracycline staining of the crowns of the upper second bicuspids. The upper second permanent molars also were stained. This denotes the chronological factor of dosage using these antibiotics. (Courtesy of Stanley Braun.)

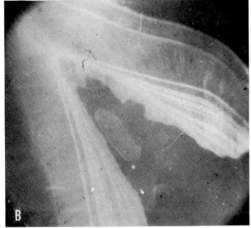

Fig. 7-59.   *A,* Tetracycline staining of the deciduous dentition. The cervical enamel of the upper centrals is slightly hypoplastic. The teeth are brown in color in incandescent light and fluoresce a brilliant yellow in a dark room under filtered ultraviolet light. *B,* Ground section of shed deciduous incisor of a child who had received eleven doses of tetracycline soon after birth (fluorescent photomicrograph).

Developing deciduous crowns of a fetus may be stained *in utero* during the last trimester of pregnancy when tetracyclines are administered to the mother.

Theoretically the crowns of anterior permanent teeth may be objectionably stained from birth up to the age of 7 or 8 years. Actually the likelihood of objectionable staining is greatest during the first 2 to 4 years, and the greater and more frequent the dosage the more intense the stain. The intensity of the stain has been shown in experimental rat teeth to be greatest with demethylchlor- and chlortetracycline, and less with the others (Johnson and Mitchell). Tetracyclines pass the placental "barrier" and also are ingested by the infant during breast feeding.

The teeth may appear grey to blue to deepening shades of brown (Fig. 7-60). When viewed under the filtered UV light in a dark room, they fluoresce yellow. The degree of fluorescence reportedly diminishes over the years, but the intrinsic stain visible in daylight remains. Reasonably effective correction of the aesthetic problem may be accomplished by bleaching the enamel surface.

Acquired Defects of the Teeth

The newly erupted tooth soon develops a pellicle consisting of bacteria and mucinous proteins and mucopolysaccharides from the saliva. This thin film, at first microscopic in nature, may serve as a basis for subsequently deposited extrinsic stains, disclosing solutions, salivary calculus and/or acidogenic and acidophilic bacteria which may, on protected tooth surfaces, be the basis for beginning dental caries activity. Thus, plaque is an infection at the very basis of dental caries and chronic periodontal disease. When the accumulation becomes thicker and apparent grossly, it is referred to as *materia alba.* Recent studies have shown that effective antibacterial agents will reduce this accumulation and prevent its recurrence, thus emphasizing its bacterial nature (Fig. 7–42).

Extrinsic Stains

Extrinsic stains deposited in the pellicle or thin plaque may come from foods, tobacco, chromogenic bacteria, medications and other colored materials placed within the mouth (Table 7–5). If the surface of the tooth is sound, such stains usually are readily removable by scaling and polishing. A thin cervical orange stain has been described on the teeth of patients with rheumatic fever. This probably is more related to prolonged antibiotic administration and its influence on oral flora than it is to the disease itself. Brown to black stains are common on the teeth of heavy smokers.

Brown is the most common colored stain among school children. Green, orange and black are less common in that order. A thin, brown line of stain near the cervix of the tooth in the mouths of patients with a low degree of susceptibility to dental caries has been described. This too would seem to be related to the unusual bacterial flora of such patients. The antibiotic vancomycin, when applied topically daily to the teeth of some patients for several days, causes a brown surface stain, especially in patients who smoke. Extrinsic stains and materia alba have been shown to fluoresce under UV light with different colors. The intimate interrelationships between pellicle, plaque, calculus, periodontal disease and dental caries make the variety of extrinsic stains a fertile field for further investigation.

Dental Caries

Dental caries, an infectious process, in all of its stages and its sequelae produces many changes in color and condition of the tooth structures. The detection of cavities is abetted by the knowledge of the teeth and surfaces most commonly involved. The occlusal pits and fissures of the posterior teeth usually are the first to be attacked, and subsequently the proximal surfaces. In contrast, the six lower anterior teeth usually are the last to be affected. Bite-wing radiographs are most valuable for detecting incipient proximal surface cavitation. All other tooth surfaces are best examined with direct light, a sharp explorer, and mouth mirror using reflected light. Transillumination and use of the UV light in a dark room will reveal otherwise undetectable alterations When dental floss is drawn between two teeth and it becomes frayed, this may indicate a sharp cavity or defective margin of a restoration. While viewing the occlusal surfaces, a suggestion of underlying proximal cavitation may be noted by the examiner when marginal ridges reveal a change in opacity as compared to the rest of the occlusal surface.

The patient's past experience with dental decay is obtained through the use of the DMF index—decayed, missing and filled teeth (pp. 57–59). These teeth are simply counted. The DMFS index is a more refined indication of caries experience. Evaluation of the degree of caries susceptibility of a patient can be aided by the use of "average" figures for children and young adults of different ages (Figs. 3–1 and 3–2).

A variety of caries susceptibility tests have been developed, the oldest of which is the *Lactobacillus acidophilus* count of collected, stimulated saliva. The Snyder test, a simple titration with color change resulting, has been useful as an indicator of bacterial acidogenesis. Such tests are useful in screen-

Table 7-5. Extrinsic Stains of the Teeth

Stained pellicle
Chromogenic bacteria
Tea, coffee, food
Tobacco
Iron
SnFl
Betel nut/pihu
 (nashumandi) berries
Chlorhexidine mouth washes

---

ing large groups of patients in experimental studies and epidemiologic surveys, but have not been found to be as effective for the individual patient. However, if a patient is obviously highly susceptible to decay, and if dietary restriction and other caries preventive techniques are employed, serial L.a. counts or Snyder tests may be helpful in determining the success of control measures and the degree of cooperation of the patient (see also p. 209).

Tooth Fracture

On occasion, a tooth will be traumatically *fractured* to the extent that a pulp exposure will occur. When only a crack occurs, it may be difficult to detect. A crack running buccolingually through the crown of a lower molar occasionally may be detectable in a radiograph. If the crack runs mesiodistally, obviously it will not be apparent in the conventional film. Persons with heavy masticatory musculature and evidence of clenching or grinding are prone to tooth fracture. A recent restoration left "high" may predispose to tooth fracture (Figs. 10–2, 10–3).

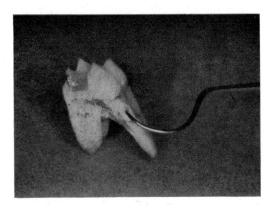

Fig. 7-61. An upper molar with symptoms of painful pulpitis; the cause was not apparent. After much clinical investigation and delay, the tooth was removed for sectioning. The tooth is shown after decalcification when a hole in the side of the root was observed. The explorer was readily inserted through the auxiliary lateral canal into the pulp chamber. The pulpitis had resulted from exposure due to gingival recession. (Courtesy of Robert E. Tarplee.)

Another cause for pulp exposure is the developmental *auxiliary lateral canal* opening onto the root surface which is exposed by gingival recession or periodontal disease (Figs. 7–61, 10–5). The pulp becomes infected and inflamed and the usual sequelae occur. Teeth with non-vital pulps change color toward grey to black if not treated endodontically soon after pulp death (Fig. 6–9). Even after endodontic therapy, especially if it is improper or incomplete, the crown may become darker with time. The tooth injured by a severe blow may immediately change color toward red to blue due to intrapulpal hemorrhage. Without endodontic treatment, the color may become darker as the pulp becomes necrotic. Should the pulp recover the discoloration may diminish.

Attrition

Occlusal and incisal *attrition* is a natural occurrence with advancing age. It is sometimes excessive in patients with bruxism or in those who use chewing tobacco in which there is a significant amount of abrasive soil (Fig. 2–28). Over the years, a certain amount of proximal surface wear becomes apparent, with the flattening of contact surfaces. This is a demonstration of the individuality of teeth and their movements during mastication. It is also an expression of "mesial drift" which is the tendency for teeth to move toward the midline due to their inclination, morphology, intercuspation and forces resulting from mastication.

Abrasion

Abnormal loss of tooth structure may be the result of habits of the individual. The carpenter who carries nails or the seamstress who habitually carries needles or pins between the teeth may develop incisal grooves. Bobby pins habitually opened by a patient (*e.g.* a beautician) using the incisal edge of a tooth may cause excessive wear, as will the habitual clenching on the stem of a pipe by a smoker. Unusual cervical wear of teeth has been noted in patients who use dental floss or the toothbrush overzealously causing grooves in the necks of the teeth.

Decalcification

Loss of tooth surfaces may result from the occupational or habitual exposure to acids. A common cause is the daily intake of lemon juice which patients take in different ways for various reasons. Professional singers or public speakers sometimes suck on lemons prior to a performance to clear their throats. Long distance runners who carry a section of lemon under their lips next to the labial surfaces of their anterior teeth to allay thirst may lose enamel in rather bizarre patterns. Patients with achlorhydria, for whom hydrochloric acid is prescribed daily or in more frequent dosages, may lose tooth substance if they do not shield their teeth from the acid. Patients with chronic vomiting or regurgitation may in time lose especially the lingual surface enamel of upper anterior teeth (Fig. 7–62).

Erosion

Dental erosion is a condition of unknown etiology in which enamel and dentin may be lost especially from labial and buccal sur-

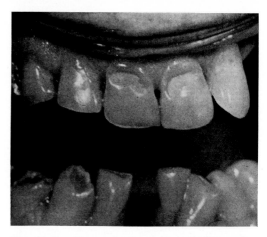

Fig. 7-63. The upper centrals of this patient developed erosion and were restored with silicate material. The lesions recurred. Note the eburnated, rounded gingival margins of the cavities. Attrition is apparent on the lower right cuspid and lateral.

faces leaving dished-out defects on the enamel and dentinal surfaces (Fig. 7–63). A similar defect sometimes results from overzealous toothbrush abrasion, but dental erosion is not due to this action alone. It has been observed in the teeth of handicapped patients who have never used a toothbrush. If the factor causing dental tissue loss can be found, it should be discontinued. Otherwise, management depends solely on restoration of the part in hopes of preventing further progression, pulp exposure or undesirable aesthetics.

Internal Resorption (Internal Granuloma, Pink Tooth of Mummery)

Internal resorption of a tooth is due to chronic inflammatory hyperplasia of the pulp either within the coronal portion or root canal. It sometimes is seen in teeth which have been traumatized by a single blow, or in teeth whose pulps have been exposed by any means including the dental bur. It is also seen on occasion in deciduous or permanent teeth which have been capped (unsuccessfully) with calcium hydroxide or other agents. Chronic inflamma-

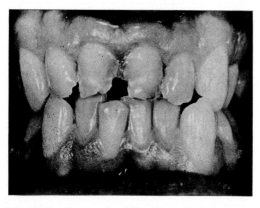

Fig. 7-62. Severe decalcification of the enamel and dentin of the upper incisors associated with a habit of regurgitation. Similar cases have been seen in patients for whom hydrochloric acid has been prescribed due to achlorhydria. Such patients should be advised to drink the solution through a straw and avoid contact with the teeth.

tory hyperplasia of the the confined pulp, with formation of multinucleated giant cells (odontoclasts), results in the resorption. This is comparable to the *pulp polyp* occasionally seen in the exposed deciduous or young permanent tooth; however, the polyp has room to expand outside the crown instead of within the pulp chamber. Internal resorption and/or pulp polyp formation should be treated endodontically before too much tooth destruction has occurred, or by extraction.

External Resorption

External resorption most commonly involves the tooth root, but on occasion the unerupted crown may be involved. This is usually due to periodontal (or pericoronal) disease, with chronic inflammatory hyperplasia of the connective tissue occurring and odontoclasia resulting. It is important to search for a likely cause in the past history of the tooth or in the condition of the pulp and periodontium. On occasion, eruption of a malposed neighboring tooth, a developing cyst or invading neoplasm may cause tooth resorption. Internal and external resorption are rarely "idiopathic."

Malposition

Malposition of teeth and malocclusion occasionally result from undesirable habits such as thumb or finger chewing (Fig. 7–55), abnormal posture during sleep and unusual effects from musical wind instruments or other objects frequently placed in the mouth. In periodontosis or advanced periodontitis, migration of the anterior teeth especially may call the attention of the patient to the periodontal problem.

Submerged Teeth

Some deciduous teeth undergo normal root resorption and shedding even in the absence of succedaneous teeth beneath them. Others in such situations may be maintained throughout most of adult life. There is no known explanation for this variation. Ab-

normally retained deciduous teeth may become ankylosed to bone. Sometimes they are "depressed" below the line of occlusion of neighboring normal teeth because of the ankylosis. This "submergence" is not due to pressure, but to ankylosis and lack of passive eruption. Tapping the ankylosed tooth results in an abnormal ringing sound as compared to a tooth with a normal "cushion" (periodontal membrane) (Fig. 2–19). Systemic causes of abnormal eruption and shedding of teeth are considered on page 152.

Hypercementosis

Increased cementum apposition on the tooth roots may follow a number of stimuli: chronic periapical inflammation, supraeruption of teeth following loss of an antagonist, secondary to trauma or fracture, and Paget's disease of bone.

Hypercementosis is readily identified radiographically as a bulbous thickening of the root contour. A distinct periodontal ligament space can be seen thus distinguishing it from true *tooth ankylosis*. However, if extraction of the tooth becomes necessary, difficulties may be experienced in either case.

Considerations of Occlusion

Recognition of any occlusal disharmony should precede treatment, especially for patients with periodontal disease. Loss or malposition of teeth may result in tipping of adjacent teeth with loss of continuity of the arch. Food impaction, impingement of opposing teeth on tissues due to overeruption or overbite, lack of self-cleansing tooth surfaces encouraging the accumulation of plaque and calculus, and excessive overloading of one or a few teeth in a quadrant all are examples of ill effects due to occlusal disturbances. Other local factors related to occlusion which can contribute to periodontal injury include the impingement on soft tissues by clasps, and the placement of a "high" recent restoration. When occlusal disturbances exist in a patient with habitual bruxism, the ill effects may be increased. Occlusal prematurities are also thought to induce bruxism.

In planning treatment all such factors should be considered for correction. Prior to extensive restorative therapy, a thorough evaluation of the occlusion should be undertaken. Often this is best done by use of diagnostic casts mounted on an articulator. The occlusal relationships can then be studied in detail, and reconstruction of the occlusal surfaces better planned.

The complexities of careful occlusal eval-

uation are such that textbooks have been written on this subject, to which the reader is referred for more information.

Equilibrating the occlusion of patients by selective grinding and placement of restorations has received much emphasis in dental education and practice in recent years. In spite of the fact that some of the advocates of this practice have the best of intentions, the rationale for performing it sometimes is questionable (Fig. 7–64).

The sensory mechanisms of the mouth cannot be overemphasized. The periodontal ligament contains many pain and proprioceptive nerve fibers which limit biting pressure and influence jaw position. Further, the mouth plays an important role in speech and expression of emotions, in sensual and sexual relationships, and in the use of teeth

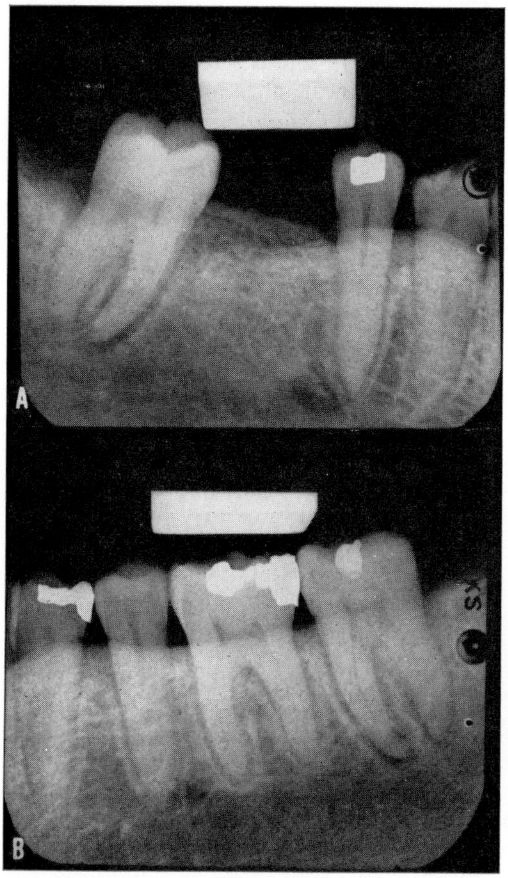

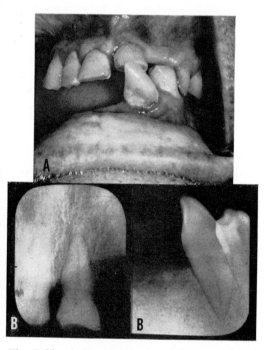

Fig. 7-64. Posterior roentgenograms of a patient suffering from iatrogenic traumatogenic occlusion. Increased periodontal membrane space resulting from a bite opening appliance worn for 18 months. Although the teeth were mobile, the height of the alveolar bone is essentially normal. (Swenson, J. Amer. Dent. Ass., 65, 345, 1962.)

Fig. 7-65. A, Traumatogenic occlusion is apparent in this patient with only the upper left central contacting the lower left canine for chewing purposes. The upper central is depressed approximately 2 mm when the patient closes. B, Radiographs of these two opposing teeth reveal surprisingly little periodontal destruction. The lower cuspid was quite firm.

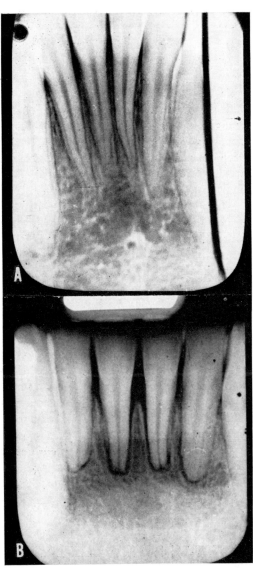

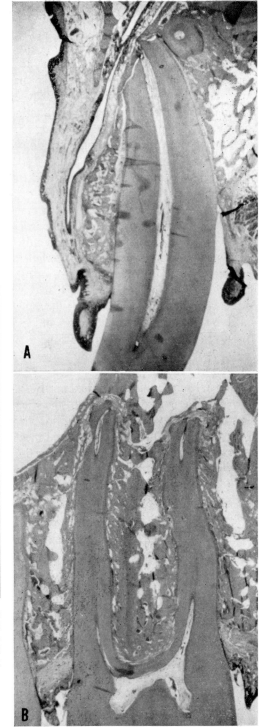

Fig. 7-66. Orthodontic root resorption. *A,* The lower incisors of a 12-year-old male before and *B,* 2½ years after orthodontic treatment. Cephalometric films had revealed that the crowns had been intruded as intended. This is not to say that judicious use of intrusive forces is harmful.

Fig. 7-67. Intrusive forces were used on the teeth of monkeys. *A,* Using injudicious force, the apex of the intruded upper central incisor was resorbed. Note the proximity of the nasopalatine canal. *B,* An intruded molar is shown. Note the apical resorption and that of the base of the crown in the interradicular region. Note the direction of the periodontal trabeculae indicative of the direction of tooth movement, and the proximity of the floor of the maxillary sinus. (Willian, Thesis, 1963.) A subsequent study demonstrated that the judicious use of intrusive forces could be accomplished with a minimum of root resorption. The pulps of these teeth, and those of other studies accomplished here, remained vital and unaffected by such remarkable occlusal "adjustment." (Dellinger, Amer. J. Orthod., *53,* 62, 1966.)

as tools. Thus, with disturbance of the emotions *or* the occlusion of an individual, tension, bruxism and clenching may result, sometimes contributing to the development of the temporomandibular pain dysfunction syndrome (Chap. 10) or increasing the severity of previously existing periodontal disease.

On the other hand, many minor occlusal interferences alone, such as "premature contacts" during lateral excursions of the mandible, have not been *proved* to be important in the *etiology* of: gingivitis, periodontitis, pulpitis, pulp necrosis, pulp stones, periapical cemental dysplasia, hypercementosis, or root resorption. Some practitioners have become so preoccupied with occlusion that they have failed to seek and eradicate the more obvious causative factors for most of these conditions (Figs. 7–65, 7–66, 7–67).

Consider these physiologic facts. The periodontal membrane is approximately 0.2 mm wide. The greater its function, the wider the membrane and the greater the mobility of the tooth. The thinnest periodontal membranes are found around unerupted or impacted teeth. Thus, the periodontal membrane is a plastic, dynamic connective tissue hammock which suspends the tooth from a plastic, viable bone. Kuhn demonstrated in a clinical experiment that the smallest measured force he used orthodontically resulted in tooth movement. This minimum force caused tooth movement of 1 mm within 1 week. Thus, if teeth are in "premature contact" and are struck repeatedly with significant force, they should move out of the way of this force and/or undergo attrition. During orthodontic tooth movement, teeth are often moved into "premature contact" and such minor imbalances do not result in detectable pathosis of the periodontium or pulp.

In the absence of clenching habits or bruxism, the teeth are in contact for only a few minutes per day. During mastication they seldom meet in occlusal or incisal contact, and then only at the end of a chewing cycle.

They are thus subjected to physiologic forces which do not cause the forms of pathosis listed previously. However, any immediate minor change in occlusion such as the placement of a high restoration is readily detectable by the proprioceptive system, and the patient tends to be overly aware of the change; this may result in unconscious clenching and bruxism. If it occurs during sleep, there may be tiring and soreness of the masticatory musculature and the periodontium on awakening.

Many animal experiments have demonstrated that gingivitis and periodontitis did not result from major imbalances of occlusion created by the placement of artificially "high" restorations. The microscopic findings showed that when teeth are placed in malposition and are subjected to malcontact they move if not locked in position. Resulting periodontitis has not been shown.

Clinical studies have been conducted in an effort to determine the influence of traumatogenic occlusion on the periodontium. By selective extraction of antagonists occlusal forces have been decreased on some teeth and increased on others. Radiographs, measurements of tooth mobility, radiotelemetry and indices of occlusal stress and oral hygiene have been used to assess this factor. Lovdal and co-workers stated that "The presumption that traumatic occlusion is an important etiological factor in periodontal disease is not substantiated by the present study."

Thus modification of the occlusion by such means as equilibration may be valuable in the treatment of some periodontal disease, or in the management of some cases of the temporomandibular pain dysfunction syndrome (myofascial pain–dysfunction syndrome). On the other hand, the matter must be kept in the proper perspective. It is not rational to attempt to prevent the occurrence of such problems by equilibrating the occlusion of all patients with healthy periodontiums, and with *no complaints* or objective signs of disease.

BIBLIOGRAPHY

Archard, H. O. and Witkop, C. J.: Hereditary hypophosphatemia (vitamin D-resistant rickets presenting dental manifestations), Oral Surg., *22*, 184, 1966.

Attstrom, R.: Presence of leukocytes in crevices of healthy and chronically inflamed gingivae, J. Periodont. Res., *5*, 42, 1970.

Attstrom, R. and Egleberg, J.: Emigration of blood neutrophils and monocytes into the gingival crevices, J. Periodont. Res., *5*, 48, 1970.

Baker, B. R.: Pits of the lip commissures in caucasoid males, Oral Surg., *21*, 56, 1966.

Balfs, D. J. and Hall, W.: Pain and the cracked tooth, J. Indiana Dent. Ass., *54*, 15, 1975.

Belding, J. H. and Anderson, W. R.: Treatment of desquamative gingivitis: report of cases, J. Amer. Dent. Ass., *77*, 612, 1968.

Berry, T. J.: *The Hand as a Mirror of Systemic Disease*, Philadelphia, F. A. Davis Co., 1963.

Beumer, J., Trowbridge, H. O., Silverman, S. and Eisenberg, E.: Childhood hypophosphatasia and the premature loss of teeth. A clinical and laboratory study of seven cases, Oral Surg., *35*, 631, 1973.

Bodenhoff, J. B. and Gorlin, R. J.: Natal and neonatal teeth, folklore and fact, Pediatrics, *32*, 1087, 1963.

Bowen, W. H.: The induction of rampant dental caries in monkeys (Macaca irus), Caries Res., *3*, 227, 1969.

Brookreson, K. R.: Dentinal dysplasia: report of a case, J. Amer. Dent. Ass., *77*, 608, 1968.

Brownstein, M. H. and Skolnik, P.: Papillon-Lefevre syndrome, Arch. Dermatol., *106*, 533, 1972.

Burch, M. S., Besley, K. W. and Samuels, H. S.: Regional odontodysplasia with associated midline mandibular cyst: report of case, J. Oral Surg., *31*, 44, 1973.

Casson, M. H.: Oral manifestations of primary hypophosphatasia, Brit. Dent. J., *127*, 561, 1969.

Castigliano, S. G.: Challenge to dentistry, Letters to the Editor, J. Amer. Dent. Ass., p. 321, February 1967.

Cohen, S. and Becker, G. L.: Origin, diagnosis and treatment of the dental manifestations of vitamin D-resistant rickets: review of the literature and report of case, J. Amer. Dent. Ass., *92*, 120, 1976.

Cohen, S. and Parkins, F. M.: Bleaching tetracycline-stained vital teeth, Oral Surg., *29*, 465, 1970.

Chusid, J. G. and McDonald, J. J.: *Correlative Neuroanatomy and Functional Neurology*, 12th Ed., Los Altos, Lange Medical Publications, 1964.

Fahmy, H., Rogers, W. E., Mitchell, D. F. and Brewer, H. E.: Effects of hypervitaminosis D on the periodontium of the hamster, J. Dent. Res., *40*, 870, 1961.

Formicola, A. J., Witte, E. T. and Curran, P. M.: A study of personality traits and acute necrotizing ulcerative gingivitis, J. Periodont., *41*, 36, 1970.

Fullimer, H. M., Gibson, W. A., Lazarus, G. S., Bladen, H. A. and Whedon, K. A.: The origin of collagenase in periodontal tissues of man, J. Dent. Res., *48*, 646, 1969.

Giansanti, J. S., Hrabak, R. P. and Waldron, C. A.: Palmar-plantar hyperkeratosis and concomitant periodontal destruction (Papillon-Lefèvre syndrome), Oral Surg., *36*, 40, 1973.

Greenfield, G. B., *et al.*: The hand as an indicator of generalized disease. Amer. J. Roentgen., *49*, 736, March, 1967.

Hooley, J. R.: The infant's mouth, J. Amer. Dent. Ass., *75*, 95, 1967.

Johnson, R. H. and Mitchell, D. F.: Effects of tetracyclines on teeth and bones, J. Dent. Res., *45*, 86, 1966.

Keyes, P. H.: The infectious and transmissible nature of experimental dental caries, Arch. Oral Biol., *1*, 304, 1960.

Keyes, P. H. and Jordan, H. V.: Periodontal lesions in the Syrian hamster, III. Findings related to an infectious and transmissible component, Arch. Oral Biol., *9*, 377, 1964.

Kirkman, D. B.: The location and incidence of accessory pulpal canals in periodontal pockets, J. Amer. Dent. Ass., *91*, 353, 1975.

Kisling, E. and Krebs, G.: Periodontal conditions in adult patients with mongolism (Down's syndrome), Acta Odont. Scand., *21*, 391, 1963.

Klein, H.: Dental fluorosis associated with hereditary diabetes insipidus, Oral Surg., *40*, 736, 1975.

Knapp, D. E.: Therapeutic control of apprehension and pain in adult dental patients, Dent. Clin. North America, March, 1968.

Kracke, R. R.: Delayed tooth eruption versus impaction, J. Dent. Child., *42*, 371, 1975.

Lynn, B. D.: "The pill" as an etiologic agent in hypertrophic gingivitis, Oral Surg., September, 1967.

Lysell, L.: Taurodontism: A case report and a survey of the literature, Odont. Rev., *13*, 158, 1962.

Mayhall, J. T.: Natal and neonatal teeth among the Tlinget Indians, J. Dent. Res., *46*, 748, 1967.

Miller, A. S., Brookreson, K. R. and Brody, B. A.: Lateral soft-palate fistula, Arch. Otolaryng., *91*, 198, 1970.

Mitchell, D. F.: Periodontal disease in the Syrian hamster, J. Amer. Dent. Ass., *49*, 177, 1954.

Mitchell, D. F. and Baker, B. R.: Topical antibiotic control of necrotizing gingivitis, J. Periodont., *39*, 21, 1968.

Mitchell, D. F. and Helman, E.: The role of periodontal foci of infection in systemic disease: An evaluation of the literature, J. Amer. Dent. Ass., *46*, 32, 1953.

Mitchell, D. F., Helman, E. and Chernausek, D. S.: Ammoniated dentifrices and hamster caries, Part III. Further studies on the effects of ingestion, Science, *116*, 537, 1952.

Mitchell, D. F. and Holmes, L. A.: Topical antibiotic control of dentogingival plaque, J. Periodont., *36*, 202, 1965.

Mitchell, D. F. and Johnson, M. J.: The nature of the gingival plaque in the hamster—production, prevention and removal, J. Dent. Res., *35*, 651, 1956.

Mitchell, D. F. and Shafer, W. G.: The effects of caries producing diets initiated at various stages of pre- and post-natal development of the hamster, J. Dent. Res., *28*, 424, 1949.

Panuska, H. J., Gorlin, R. J., Bearman, J. E. and Mitchell, D. F.: The effect of anticonvulsant drugs upon the gingiva—a series of analyses of 1048 patients, I. J. Periodont., *31*, 336, 1960, II. J. Periodont., *32*, 15, 1961.

Prescott, G. H., Mitchell, D. F. and Fahmy, H.: Procion dyes as matrix markers in growing bone and teeth, Amer. J. Phys. Anthrop., *29*, 219, 1968.

Ranney, R. R.: Specific antibody in gingiva and submandibular nodes of monkeys with allergic periodontal disease, J. Periodont. Res., *5*, 1, 1970.

Rizzo, A. A.: Absorption of bacterial endotoxin into rabbit gingival pocket tissue, Periodontics, *6*, 65, 1968.

Ross, W. L.: The dentist and cancer, Letters to the Editor, J. Amer. Dent. Ass., *74*, 1401, 1967.

Schiott, C. R. and Loe, H.: The origin and variation in number of leukocytes in the human saliva, J. Periodont. Res., *5*, 36, 1970.

Schneider, E. L.: Lip pits and congenital absence of second premolars: Varied expression of the lip pits syndrome, J. Med. Genetics, *10*, 346, 1973.

Selvig, K.: Attachment of plaque and calculus to the tooth surfaces, J. Periodont. Res., *5*, 8, 1970.

Shafer, W. G., Hine, M. K. and Levy, B. M.: *A Textbook of Oral Pathology,* 3rd Ed., Philadelphia, W. B. Saunders Co., 1974.

Shifman, A. and Buchner, A.: Taurodontism. Report of sixteen cases in Israel, Oral Surg., *41*, 400, 1976.

Siekert, R. G., and Gibilisco, J. A.: Discoloration of the teeth in alkaptonuria (ochronosis) and parkinsonism, Oral Surg., *29*, 197, 1970.

Skouggard, M. R., Bay, I. and Klinkhamer, J. M.: Correlations between gingivitis and orogranulocytic migratory rate, J. Dent. Res., *48*, 716, 1969.

Sutcliffe, P.: Extrinsic tooth stains in children, Dent. Pract., *17*, 175, 1967.

Terz, J. J. and Farr, H. W.: Carcinoma of the tonsillar fossa, Surg. Gynec. Obstet., *125*, 581, 1967.

Trodahl, J. N., *et al.*: The pigmentation of dental tissues in erythropoietic (congenital) porphyria, J. Oral Path., *1*, 159, 1971.

Vogel, R. I.: Intrinsic and extrinsic discoloration of the dentition (a literature review), J. Oral Med., *30*, 99, 1975.

Wesley, R. K., Wysocki, G. P., Mintz, S. M. and Jackson, J.: Dentin dysplasia type I, Oral Surg., *41*, 516, 1976.

Yamane, G. M., El-Mostehy, M. R. and Panuska, H. J.: Dental signs of systemic disturbances, Dent. Clin. North America, March, 1968.

Occlusion

Bhaskar, S. N. and Frisch, J.: Occlusion and periodontal disease, Int. Dent. J., *17*, 251, 1967.

Burstone, C. J.: Biomechanics of Tooth Movement in *Vistas in Orthodontics* (Kraus, B. S. and Riedel, R. A., eds.), Philadelphia, Lea & Febiger, pp. 197–213, 1962.

Kuhn, R. J.: Force values and rate of distal movement of the mandibular first permanent molar. Thesis, Indiana University School of Dentistry, 1959.

Lovdal, A., Schei, O., Waerhaug, J. and Arno, A.: Tooth mobility and alveolar bone resorption as a function of occlusal stress and oral hygiene, Acta Odont. Scand., *17*, 61, 1959.

Pameijer, Jan H. N., Glickman, I. and Roeber, F. W.: Intraoral occlusal telemetry III. Tooth contacts in chewing, swallowing and bruxism, J. Periodont., *40*, 5, 253, 1969.

Ramfjord, S. P. and Ash, M. M., Jr.: *Occlusion,* Philadelphia, W. B. Saunders Co., 1966.

Ramfjord, S. P. and Kohler, C. A.: Periodontal reaction to functional occlusal stress, J. Periodont., *29*, 3095, 1959.

Richardson, E. R.: Comparative thickness of the human periodontal membrane of functioning versus non-functioning teeth, J. Oral Med., *22*, 120, 1967

Victor, M. and Adams, R. D.: Vertigo and disorders of equilibrium and gait, in *Principles of Internal Medicine,* 5th Ed. (Harrison, T. R. *et al.*, eds.), New York, McGraw-Hill Book Co., pp. 213–218, 1966.

Waerhaug, J.: Current basis for prevention of periodontal disease, Int. Dent. J., *17*, 267, 1967.

World Workshop in Periodontics, Ann Arbor, Mich., June 1966. Ramfjord, S. P., Kerr, D. A. and Ash, M. M., eds., Copyright, University of Michigan, pp. 458.

Chapter 8

Radiographic Examination

In 1895, Professor Wilhelm Konrad Roentgen of Wurzburg, Bavaria, discovered the x ray, which has since come to bear his name. He found that when electrons from a cathode tube encountered dense matter, a new ray was produced which was capable of penetrating objects opaque to ordinary light. These roentgen rays could be registered on a photographic emulsion and, when the emulsion was properly developed, an image resulted which was quite different from an ordinary light exposure. Within a year after this discovery, an American dentist, Dr. C. Edmund Kells, had made the first dental roentgenograph. In 1909, Dr. Howard R. Raper of Indiana was instrumental in having the first dental x-ray machine installed in a dental school. Since that time, the field of oral roentgenography has expanded until it is now indispensable in the practice of dentistry. It is so basic to oral diagnosis that Sarner states that it is a dentist's "duty" to take roentgenographs as part of the oral examination.

Roentgenography is essentially photography using the roentgen ray rather than the light ray to activate the film emulsion. *Roentgenology* may be defined as: the study of the art of making and interpreting roentgenographs. *Radiology* is often used as a synonym and, although it does not specify the type of radiant energy used, it is a less cumbersome word. In practice, however, roentgenology and radiology are often used interchangeably, as are roentgenograph and roentgenogram and radiograph and radiogram. Even more loosely used is the term *x ray,* which properly refers to the roentgen ray but is often used to represent the whole field of roentgenography, or to refer specifically to the film before or after development.

BASIC THEORY OF RADIOGRAPHIC EXAMINATION AND FILM DEVELOPMENT

The roentgen ray is generated in an x-ray machine by the bombardment of electrons from a cathode onto a heavy metal anode target. The anode target then emits these short wavelength electromagnetic vibrations in all directions. Only a small number of these emissions are useful, the rest being absorbed by the shield around the tube head. Roentgen rays, like light rays, have wavelength, amplitude, and power, and these may be adjusted by changing the kilovoltage peak (*kvp*) or milliamperage (*ma*) settings on the machine. High *kv* settings result in rays which are very penetrating, while low settings result in rays which are termed "soft" and are not as penetrating. The *useful beam* (primary beam) is the more penetrating one, so the "soft" rays are often filtered out by use of aluminum filters (later described). This beam, once it leaves the machine, may be deflected by any object it strikes, resulting in "stray radiation," or it may cause that object to emit "secondary radiation." Roentgen rays travel in a straight line. When these rays strike an object, that object may emit these "softer" rays of its own. All rays other than the primary beam constitute a hazard to the operator and patient and should be controlled as much as possible.

Body tissues tend to filter roentgen rays to a greater or lesser extent, depending upon their density. Those tissues which are very dense such as teeth and bone are relatively *radiopaque,* while soft tissues are relatively *radiolucent.* The degree of opacity or lucency revealed on the exposed film also depends upon the strength of the primary beam, hence the use of these terms should be qualified in this respect.

Some dental x-ray units operate at a fixed *kvp* or *ma,* while most can be regulated within a range of 10 to 20 *ma* and 65 to 100 *kvp.* The average operating range usually is 70 *kvp* and 15 *ma.* Optimum penetration with a minimum health hazard is obtained at 100 *kvp* and 15 *ma.* Selection of the exposure time must take into account the settings as well as the sensitivity of the film used and the density of the structure to be examined.

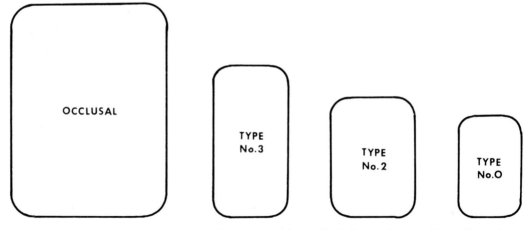

Fig. 8-1. Diagram of comparative sizes of the commonly available intraoral x-ray films. The occlusal film may also be used for extraoral radiography. (Reduced approximately one third.)

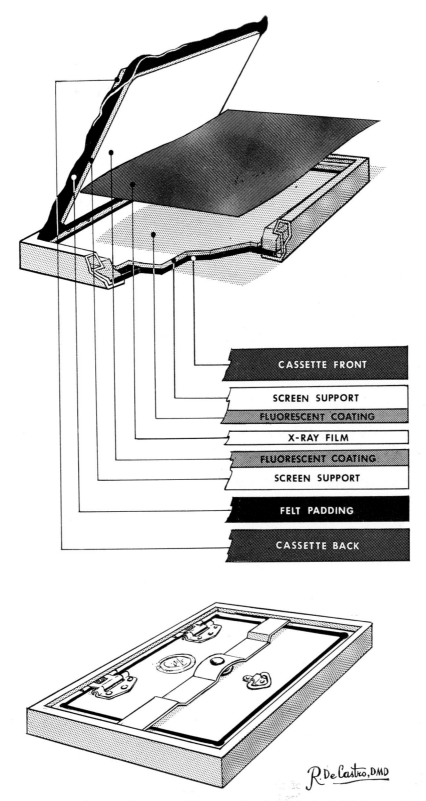

CASSETTE FRONT

SCREEN SUPPORT

FLUORESCENT COATING

X-RAY FILM

FLUORESCENT COATING

SCREEN SUPPORT

FELT PADDING

CASSETTE BACK

R. DeCastro, DMD

Fig. 8-2. Cross section of extraoral cassette. The x-ray film should be loaded in the cassette as shown, in the darkroom. The intensifying screen serves to convert the roentgen rays to light rays and allows for a lower exposure time.

Intraoral x-ray films are available in several different sizes (Fig. 8–1), including the occlusal type, and use about five different speeds. Selection of the size and speed of the film depends upon the needs of the examiner. These films are enclosed in light-proof packets with lead backings to absorb secondary radiation.

Extraoral x-ray film comes in several sizes and may be prepackaged, but usually must be loaded into a special holder called a cassette. This must be done in the darkroom. Some cassettes have screens next to the film which fluoresce when irradiated (intensifying screens) and create a more positive image with less exposure (Fig. 8–2). Grids are sometimes built into cassettes to filter out non-parallel rays before they strike the film.

An x-ray film consists of a flexible cellulose acetate base which is coated on one or both sides with a gelatin emulsion containing a silver halide (Fig. 8–3). The speed or sensitivity of the film depends upon the thickness of the emulsion and size of the silver halide crystals. Thicker emulsions and larger crystals result in faster, more sensitive films, but the larger crystals result in poorer detail and contrast, hence film speed, exposure time, *kvp* and *ma* settings must be balanced to get the detail and contrast desired with a minimum of hazard to the patient.

When the roentgen rays strike the emulsion, they render it developable by activation of the silver halide salts. The latent image thus created is developed and made permanent by immersing the film in a series of solutions in the darkroom. The time necessary for complete development and fixation depends upon the type of solution used, the exposure time, and the temperature of the solution. Thus it can be seen that many variables must be controlled in order to produce good diagnostic radiographs.

RADIATION SAFETY

The fact that roentgen rays are dangerous must never be forgotten. Overexposure can cause erythema, alopecia, surface burns, changes in the red and white cell count, osteoradionecrosis, sterility and cancer. Some of these changes do not become evident for many years, so the operator may be lulled into a false sense of security and may become careless in the use of x-ray equipment. The exact nature of the cellular damage due to such radiation is not clearly understood, nor is the minimal acceptable dose well defined. Nevertheless, radiographs taken with a minimum of exposure furnish diagnostic benefits which far outweigh the risk of potential damage.

The tissues which are most vulnerable to severe damage are the more primitive ones such as the gonads, and this principle is followed therapeutically in treating primitive cell (anaplastic) neoplasms with roentgen rays. The gonadal radiation received from a full mouth intraoral survey is very slight, however, and the total body radiation received is minimal when compared to natural radiation received from ground and cosmic sources during a lifetime.

In considering radiation hazards, one must always keep in mind the differences between total and local body radiation as well as acute versus chronic exposures. Many laymen have become fearful of diagnostic radiation because of a poor understanding of these differences. The patient should be reassured that the danger from the diagnostic use of radiation is minimal if proper precautions are taken.

Many states have "Radiation Control Acts" which require registration of all

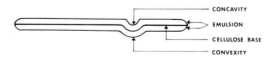

CONCAVITY
EMULSION
CELLULOSE BASE
CONVEXITY

Fig. 8-3. Cross section of double emulsion film. Most intraoral films today are of this type with emulsion on both sides. This makes the film more sensitive and allows for a reduction in exposure time.

sources of radiation, including dental x-ray machines. Information on radiation hazards and registration of machines can be obtained from state boards of health or from the American Dental Association, as well as from several excellent textbooks on oral radiology.

From a practical standpoint, several principles should be followed to reduce unnecessary exposure to the operator, auxiliary personnel and the patient.

1. Choose good x-ray equipment; make sure that there are no leaks in the shielding around the tube head and that the primary beam is properly filtered.
2. Use a timer cord more than 5 feet long, so the operator can stand away from the tube head during exposure, or behind a lead shield. Remember that roentgen rays pass readily through ordinary walls. This fact should be considered when the machine is installed in an office and lead or concrete shielding in the walls should be used when indicated.
3. Make sure that the primary beam is well collimated (focused) to a zone about 3 inches in diameter at the cone end.
4. The long cone technique reduces local body exposure.
5. Fast film requires less radiation to activate the emulsion.
6. Proper techniques reduce the need for retakes.
7. Lead aprons, especially for women during the first 6 months of pregnancy, are desirable.
8. The machine should be monitored at periodic intervals.
9. Adequate filtration of the primary beam should be accomplished with use of an aluminum filter 1.5 to 2 mm thick or its equivalent.
10. High kilovoltage should be used whenever possible.
11. All personnel in the dental office should at least occasionally wear film badges or other monitoring devices and have them checked periodically.
12. Above all, resist temptation to take shortcuts, such as holding the film in the patient's mouth, or steadying the tube head with your hand.

INDICATIONS FOR RADIOGRAPHIC EXAMINATION

Radiographic examination has become a routine part of any thorough oral examination; however, it is not a substitute for a good clinical examination. After the initial examination, the regions in question should then be examined radiographically. The usual routine involves a 14-film intraoral survey of the teeth and jaws, plus 2 or 4 bite-wing films.

Before the films are exposed, the patient should be questioned regarding any contraindications to the use of diagnostic radiation. Generally, it is wise to limit the amount of radiation given to a patient with a history of previous radiation therapy for cancer or other reasons, but this should not interfere with the thoroughness of an examination. The same is true for the pregnant patient. Another reason for questioning a patient before taking radiographs is to detect the presence of possible contagious diseases. Likewise a history of jaw fracture or previous surgery for tumors or cysts of the jaws should prompt the examiner to take special films as a follow-up to examine the previous operation site for evidence of possible recurrence or other complications.

In examining the completed radiographs, it must be remembered that a film records in only two dimensions and a third dimension should not be "read into" the radiogram. *Anything* between the ray source and the film which is opaque to roentgen rays will register on the film. The frequent occurrence of artifacts (p. 38) such as foreshortening, elongation, malprocessing, film scratches, and the almost innumerable other "outside" factors can complicate or mar the diagnostic qualities of a film. Once all facets of radiography are understood, however, these things become less of a problem.

THE ROUTINE INTRAORAL RADIOGRAPHIC EXAMINATION

The frequency of taking radiographic surveys should be determined on an individual patient basis (age, caries, and periodontal health), rather than on a preset regular interval.

It is not intended here to discuss the technical details of taking individual radiographs, since this is well covered in textbooks on the subject. There are many excellent though different methods of obtaining good intraoral radiographs. All should be based on the premise of obtaining good films efficiently and with a minimum of exposure to the patient and a minimum of distortion of the image. Often "starting angles" are quoted and since every mouth differs these are useful only as a "start." The principle of bisecting the angle between the long axis of the object (tooth) and the film, and directing the rays at right angles to this line, is still basic and is necessary to limit distortion to a minimum in the maxilla and some positions in the mandible. If this principle is completely understood, it should be possible to take a good set of films with the patient seated in any position.

Film holders are also available from commercial firms. These holders attach to the cone of the x-ray machine and help reduce mistakes such as foreshortening and elongation.

When examining radiographs, it is important to understand certain principles.

Orientation

The film should first be oriented with respect to the region being examined. For example, in viewing an intraoral periapical film it should be determined whether it is of the maxilla or mandible. The anatomic portion of the arch and the side involved should be determined. If an intraoral film is examined with the depression toward the examiner, it is as though the examiner were standing on the tongue of the patient and looking out. Often films are mounted with the convexity toward the viewer and the film

is read as if the examiner were looking at the patient. (This is true for all illustrations in this text.)

Tooth Count

In examining a complete intraoral series of films, the viewer should account for each tooth; this will prevent overlooking impactions, missing and supernumerary teeth.

Normal Anatomy and Age

The technique used and the anatomic structures which may create an image on the film should be fully understood. Otherwise normal structures may be mistaken for pathoses.

The patient's age should be considered and it must be remembered that many changes take place within the jaws of younger individuals. A rarefaction at the apex of a tooth, for example, could represent incomplete development of the root apex in a 12 year old or a periapical granuloma in a 30 year old.

Radiopacity and Radiolucency

Dense structures (with high atomic numbers) block passage of roentgen rays and result in lightened areas on the film (radiopacity). Sinus cavities, intrabony canals, and foramina are seen as radiolucent areas on the film. These terms are relative and depend also on exposure, development and other variables.

Examples

The following are illustrations of individual films used in a complete intraoral radiographic survey. The first 9 films (Figs. 8–4 to 8–12) represent one-half of a complete survey with minor pathoses or none. The next 7 films (Figs. 8–13 to 8–19) represent the other half with evidence suggestive of more severe disease. Obviously these are selected films from different patients.

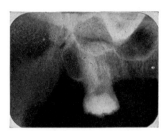

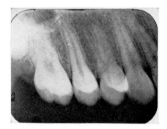

Figure 8–4. Maxillary right molar exposure. Region included: tuberosity, third and second molars. Anatomic structures often visible: (1) coronoid process; (2) pterygoid hamulus; (3) maxillary sinus; (4) zygomatic arch and process; (5) dentin and pulp chambers of teeth; (6) periodontal ligament space; (7) lamina dura (cribriform plate); (8) crest of alveolar bone, and (9) trabeculation of the alveolar bone.

Normally the second and first molars are also shown in this exposure. The third molar present appears normal in this two-dimensional plane with no evidence of a break in the continuity of the enamel or other irregularities. The roots are straight. The pulp chamber is normal in size for this middle-aged adult and the lamina dura and periodontal ligament space are rather indistinct. The trabecular bone pattern is typical for this age group. The maxillary sinus is radiolucent as it should be normally; however, it is wise to compare it with the film on the opposite side. The radiopaque wall of the sinus and crest of the alveolar bone are also normal.

Figure 8–5. Maxillary right premolar exposure. Region included: first molar through cuspid. Anatomic structures often visible: (1) anterior part of the maxillary sinus; (2) U-shaped radiopaque zygomatic process of the maxilla (not shown).

The rather large pulp chamber and canal of the cuspid tooth in this view as well as the pulp chambers and canals of the other teeth suggest that this patient is in his early middle age. The crestal bone height is essentially normal and there is no suggestion of periodontal disease. Both roots of the first bicuspid are available. The lamina dura and periodontal ligament spaces are easily seen around the root of the second bicuspid. Distal to the apex of the first molar is a radiopaque mass which is suggestive of an impacted second molar. An additional film would be necessary in order to demonstrate the impaction.

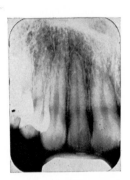

Figure 8–6. Maxillary right cuspid exposure. Region included: first premolar through right central incisor. Anatomic structures often visible: (1) right nasal fossa; (2) incisive foramen (not visible). Occasionally a dark line is seen in the upper right-hand corner of a film that has been exposed in this area due to the film bending necessary to place the film properly in this portion of the arch.

The radiolucent area in the upper right-hand corner of the film represents the right side of the nasal fossa. The radiopaque area in the lower border of the film is due to the *bite block* which was used to hold the film in place. The trabecular pattern of the bone is normal. The relative radiolucency around the apices of the central, lateral and cuspid teeth represents the cuspid fossa or depression.

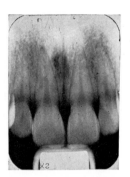

Figure 8–7. Maxillary central incisor exposure. Region included: the right through the left maxillary lateral incisors. Anatomic structures often visible: (1) median anterior maxillary suture; (2) incisive foramen and part of incisive canal; (3) nasal fossae (not present); (4) median nasal septum or cartilage (not present); (5) outline of soft tissue of nose (not present).

The very large pulp chambers and canals as well as the rounded proximoincisal angles indicates that this patient is in the early teens. The radiolucency between the central incisor roots represents the incisive foramen. Again, the bite block is visible.

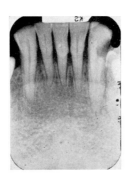

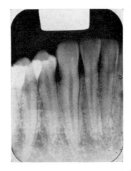

Figure 8–8. Mandibular central incisor exposure. Region included: mandibular right cuspid through mandibular left cuspid. Anatomic structures often visible: (1) genial spine and lingual foramen; (2) mental prominence (radiopaque).

The very small thread-like pulp chambers and canals of these teeth as well as the sharp proximal angles indicate that this patient is older, probably in his sixties. The opaque collars around the mandibular left central and lateral incisors represent calculus and there is evidence of advanced bone loss. On the mandibular left cuspid, there is a radiolucency on the distal which represents a carious lesion. The depth of this lesion is difficult to determine from this film because of the angulation. Note: Mandibular right cuspid is missing.

Figure 8–9. Mandibular right cuspid exposure. Region included: second premolar through right central incisor. Anatomic structures often visible: (1) mental foramen (not shown); (2) alveolar bone.

The mental foramen may be present as a radiolucency near the apex of either premolar or between them. Occasionally it must be differentiated from periapical pathosis by pulp testing the associated tooth. The horizontal angulation is such that there is overlapping of the incisors and premolars. The tooth of primary interest in this view is the cuspid. Note that the roots of the teeth are straight.

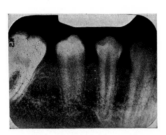

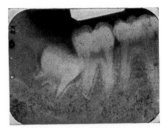

Figure 8–10. Mandibular right premolar exposure. Region included: second molar through lower right cuspid. Anatomic structures often visible: (1) mental foramen (not present); (2) alveolar bone; (3) mandibular tori (not present).

This film allows a good examination of the roots of the premolars and first molar teeth as well as the surrounding trabecular bone pattern. At the apex of the teeth there may often be seen the radiolucent inferior alveolar canal; however, it is not present in this particular exposure. The first molar is missing and the second molar is tilted mesially. The apparently enlarged pulp chamber and canal of the second bicuspid are due to rotation of the tooth—the canal is being viewed from what would ordinarily be the proximal side. It is suggested that this patient is between 10 and 12 years of age because the apex of the second premolar has not yet been completed.

Figure 8–11. Mandibular right molar exposure. Region included: third molar through mandibular right first molar. Anatomic structures often visible: (1) anterior border of the ramus and external oblique line; (2) mylohyoid line (not visible); (3) inferior alveolar canal; (4) impacted third molar.

This exposure is also valuable to examine for root curvatures before surgery or other irregularities in the roots of the molar teeth. In this exposure there is a mesioangular impaction of the third molar with a follicular space around the crown. The inferior alveolar canal can be seen apical to the third molar. An occlusal projection should be taken prior to removing this tooth in order to locate it buccolingually with respect to the second molar. There is suggestion of caries on the mesial of the first molar.

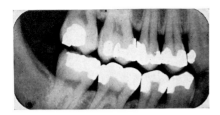

Figure 8–12. Right bite-wing film. This is a post-treatment film made to check for contour and overhangs and residual caries. No decay is shown. The maxillary second premolar and first molar have overhangs on the distal and mesial respectively at the gingival line angle. Most restorations in this film are quite deep; however, the contour is good in the lower molars and premolars. Restorations in the lower arch represent inlays which have been cemented to place while the upper teeth are restored with amalgam. Calcific metamorphosis can be noted in the coronal portion of the pulp in the maxillary right second molar adjacent to the deep restoration. The crestal bone level is quite good for this patient in early middle age. A pulp stone is present in the maxillary first molar. There are no other significant pathoses visible.

EXAMINATION OF COMMON FINDINGS SUGGESTIVE OF PATHOSES

During the examination of a complete intraoral radiographic series of films, any variations from normal should be studied thoroughly and attempts should be made to explain these variations. Additional films and other diagnostic procedures are often necessary to establish a diagnosis. For example, if the examiner sees a radiolucency at the apex of a tooth, he should note whether it is round or irregular and whether its border is sharp or fuzzy, opaque or lucent. A well-circumscribed, round radiolucency with a radiopaque border usually indicates that the lesion is slow growing or arrested, while an irregular, poorly demarcated area without an opaque lining suggests more rapid growth of an osteolytic lesion. The radiolo-gist should be able to "see osteoblasts and osteoclasts at work," in his mind's eye when he is interpreting a film, in much the same way that he understands the anatomy and physiology of structures he is examining when he palpates tissues clinically.

Caries

Detection of interproximal caries is one of the chief reasons for taking radiographs. The caries process may involve only the enamel, but it may include the dentin and even the pulp. It should be understood that a carious lesion is usually deeper than it appears on the radiograph. Dentin sclerosis can sometimes be seen deep in the carious lesion. This represents an attempt at repair, as does the "dentin bridge" of reparative dentin seen on the pulpal side of a successful pulp-capping treatment. Although occlusal caries is best detected clinically, it may often be seen radiographically. This is likewise true of facial and lingual carious lesions. It should again be stressed that it is not possible to tell facial from lingual on the film.

Periodontal Disease

Another important facet of radiographic examination is to detect evidence of advanced periodontal diseases. These are often manifested early by loss of crestal bone and later by further loss of alveolar bone either locally or generally and in a horizontal or a vertical direction. Often calculus, overhanging restorations, or other causes may be seen which give suggestions as to the etiology. Clinical demonstration of pocket formation is usual, however, except in early cases of periodontosis. The radiograph may be used to follow the progress of the disease after treatment, but it may be stressed that changes in exposure time can often mislead the examiner into thinking that the bone level has improved. Usually this is due to a decreased exposure time, resulting in better visualization of crestal bone, rather than to true bone regrowth.

Impacted, Supernumerary, and Congenitally Missing Teeth

Impactions occur in a descending order of frequency as follows: mandibular third molars, maxillary cuspids, maxillary third molars, mandibular first premolars and maxillary first premolars.

Supernumerary teeth are most often seen in the maxillary third molar region (disto- and paramolars), between the maxillary central incisors (mesiodens), and in the mandibular premolar regions. These findings are seldom demonstrable except by use of radiographs.

The following teeth are most commonly congenitally missing: third molars, maxillary lateral incisors, and mandibular and maxillary premolars. When there are missing, supernumerary, or impacted teeth, an effort should be made to explain these findings. There may be multiple unerupted teeth because deficient mandibular or maxillary growth on an hereditary basis has limited the arch space, or because a hypofunction of the thyroid or anterior pituitary gland has resulted in an insufficient growth potential. Multiple supernumerary teeth may be part of an overall systemic syndrome (cleidocranial dysostosis) or may merely represent an hereditary predisposition. Multiple missing teeth (anodontia) may also be explained on an hereditary basis as part of a systemic condition such as ectodermal dysplasia.

Anatomic Changes of the Teeth

Numbers and shapes of tooth roots can be determined radiographically. This is most important to the dentist contemplating tooth removal or endodontic therapy. Teeth with poorly formed roots may make poor abutments for prostheses.

Retained Roots

Due to the morphology of the roots of the deciduous lower molars, their root tips are sometimes not resorbed during eruption of the lower bicuspids, and remnants may be detectable radiographically throughout life.

Retained roots, broken during extraction, often are asymptomatic and are found in routine radiographic examination. There may be evidence of a PDL space and lamina dura around the root. A history of difficult tooth extraction is most helpful in completing this diagnosis.

Examples

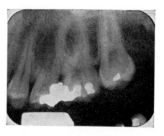

Figure 8–13. Maxillary left molar exposure. If the morphology of the teeth is carefully studied, it will be noted that there is a retained deciduous second molar and an absent permanent second bicuspid. The maxillary third molar is not present. The radiopacity near the apex of the first molar represents part of the zygomatic process of the maxilla. The roots of the maxillary first molar are curved and those of the deciduous molar are barely discernible, suggesting that they have been partially resorbed. This film should have been placed higher so that the second molar apices would be visible.

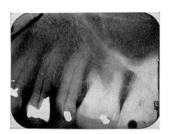

Figure 8–14. Maxillary left premolar exposure. The radiolucency apical to the distal-occlusal restoration on the first bicuspid represents a carious lesion, as does the mesial darkness on the second premolar. The radiolucency above the molars is due to the maxillary sinus. The reason the buccal roots on the first molar appear short with respect to the palatal root is that the vertical angulation of the roentgen-ray cone is increased above normal, shortening the closest roots and elongating the farthest.

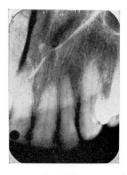

Figure 8–15. Maxillary cuspid exposure. An ill-defined radiolucency can be noted at the apex of the lateral incisor. This tooth also has mesial caries. Pulp tests revealed that this tooth was non-vital; therefore, a diagnosis of granuloma, cyst, or chronic periapical abscess was made. This tooth is treatable endodontically because the root canal is straight. Decay is present on the distal and mesial of the left central and on the mesial of the right central incisor. There may be caries on the distal of the cuspid; however, superimposition of the first bicuspid makes this interpretation difficult. The dark line in the upper left corner of the film represents film bending, which could have been eliminated with another technique. The radiolucent area adjacent to it is the nasal fossa, and in the right upper region is the anterior portion of the maxillary sinus. The roots of all teeth present in this film are straight. The relatively sharp proximal incisal angle indicates attrition. The patient is in late middle age and the small pulp canals confirm this.

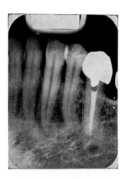

Figure 8–16. Mandibular left cuspid exposure. This film reveals attrition suggestive of bruxism and/or a heavy anterior occlusion because of the sharp proximal incisal angles. The patient is middle aged as suggested by the relatively small pulp chambers and canals. The second premolar has been treated by root canal therapy and the filling material is well condensed. There is a modified post and core crown on this tooth; however, the post is shorter than is usually acceptable. There is a void between the end of the post and the beginning of the root canal material which is filled with radiolucent cement. The radiolucency below the apex of the second premolar represents the mental foramen and it can be differentiated from periapical pathosis because of its distance from the apex of this tooth. At the apex of the cuspid tooth there appears to be a small radiolucency surrounded by diffuse radiopacity, suggesting the need for a pulp vitality test. The relative radiolucency surrounding the middle and apical thirds of all the teeth represents the depression on the facial surface of the mandible rather than pathologic change. The trabecular pattern is normal.

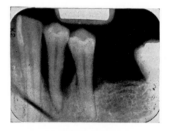

Figure 8–17. Mandibular left premolar exposure. Around the premolars excessive loss of bone indicative of severe periodontal disease is seen. The radiolucency on the distal of the root of the first premolar represents external resorption from the granulomatous tissue present in the periodontal area. These teeth were quite mobile and ultimately will be extracted. The mandibular left first molar is missing and there is no evidence of the socket present so it has been missing for a long time. Again, evidence of film bending is present and is associated with the exposure technique used.

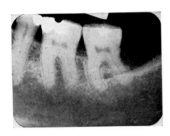

Figure 8–18. Mandibular left molar exposure. The small pulp chambers and indistinct pulp canals suggest that this patient is in his later years. The flat occlusal plane suggests that the patient either clenches or grinds his teeth or chews tobacco (the latter being the case). There is some hypercementosis on the distal root of the second molar and some physiologic decrease in the amount of bone apical to the roots of the teeth. The third molar is not present. Restorations are present in all teeth shown. There is slight adumbration on the distal of the second premolar and the mesial of the first molar near the alveolar crest. The crestal bone height is quite good.

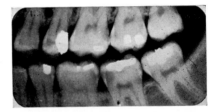

Figure 8–19. Bite-wing left side. This view is particularly useful in the detection of proximal surface caries and judging the depth of this destruction. It is also valuable for examining the dentin and pulps. Restorations may be checked for depth, the presence of base materials, and overhanging or shy margins. This is also an excellent exposure to examine crestal bone height for periodontal disease. Often these films are used after treatment to detect faulty restorative technique. Periodic use of the bite-wing film may be justified for the patient who is especially susceptible to dental caries.

Mesial caries in the lower second molar, distal caries in the first molar, mesial caries of the upper second bicuspid and distal decay of the first bicuspid are seen. There is distal caries on the mandibular second bicuspid, first molar and mesial and distal caries on the mandibular second molar. The opaque areas represent metallic restorations, probably amalgam. There is some calcific metamorphosis in all six molars present.

OTHER RADIOGRAPHIC TECHNIQUES

Edentulous Survey

The need for an edentulous survey has been demonstrated by the fact that about one-fifth of edentulous patients have undesirable conditions revealed by such radiographs.

There are several ways in which the clinically edentulous maxillary and mandibular ridges can be examined radiographically. One method is to take a 10-film intraoral survey. This resembles the 14-film survey previously described, but fewer films are necessary due to the reduced complexity of the anatomy of edentulous jaws.

Another such survey involves the use of four long bite-wing films positioned as periapical films from the cuspid through the third molar regions. Two occlusal films for the anterior maxilla and mandible may be used. Only 6 exposures are necessary.

Two extraoral lateral oblique projections are sometimes used to examine the ridges of the maxilla and mandible on either side. Then two occlusal films of the anterior maxilla and mandible suffice for these areas. This technique requires only 4 exposures.

If available, the simplest method of surveying the edentulous ridges is the panographic survey, which can then be supplemented, if necessary, with individual intraoral films.

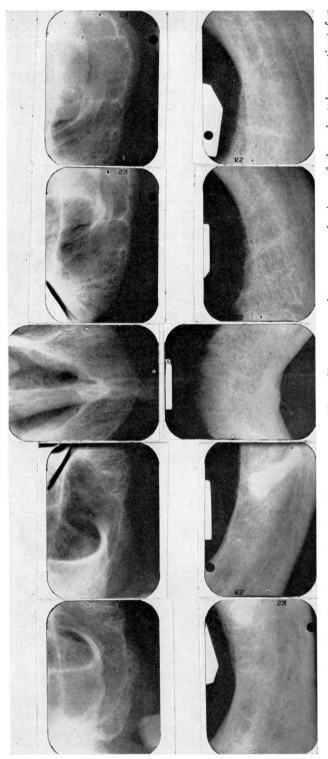

Figure 8–20. Ten-film intraoral edentulous survey. These films are used to survey the jaws of the edentulous patient for evidences of root tips or other pathologic or anatomic abnormalities, prior to making upper and lower dentures. There is an impacted premolar in the right mandibular region. No other gross abnormalities are found except for the enlarged maxillary sinuses. These enlarged or pneumatized sinuses are often seen in patients of advanced age.

Pedodontic Survey

As in the edentulous survey there are several methods of examining the jaws of the dentulous child. These methods may be varied according to the sizes of the ridges and the space available.

One method in the older child is to take an ordinary intraoral 14-film survey, plus bite-wings (Fig. 8–21).

Another method is to take an intraoral survey covering the areas where teeth are present using a fewer number of films and including bite-wings.

In the younger child (mixed dentition) sometimes it is valuable to use a combined intra-extraoral survey because of the problems associated with controlling a patient of this age. This can be done by taking an anterior maxillary and mandibular occlusal projection, and then using adult periapical film in a flat plane in the region of the deciduous and permanent molars, making the projection much as one would make an occlusal projection. This can be done in all four quadrants making the complete survey with a total of six exposures.

Any of these methods is adequate to survey the jaws of a child provided that all areas are covered in the survey and provided that bite-wing films are included in order to detect interproximal caries.

Occlusal Film Radiography

The occlusal film, which is a larger film than the periapical, is often used in intra- and extraoral radiography. This film is most often used to examine the anterior maxilla or mandible, but it may be used extraorally

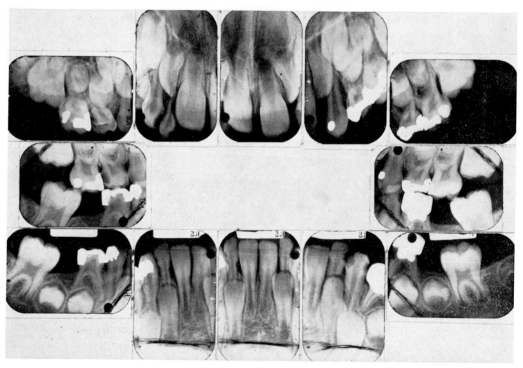

Figure 8–21. Pedodontic survey. This is a 10-film survey of a patient between 6 and 7 years of age. Bite-wing films are also included. Note that the mandibular first (6 year) molars have erupted, whereas the maxillary first molars are in the process of erupting. The permanent central incisors, maxillary and mandibular, have erupted and permanent teeth in many areas are still unerupted. The patient has multiple carious lesions.

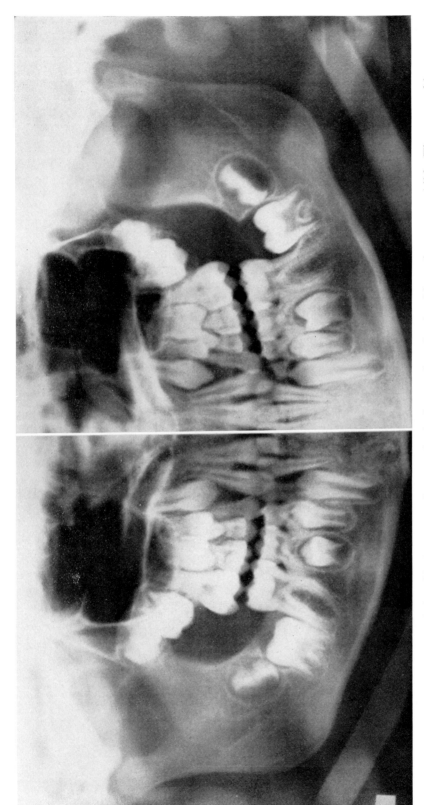

Figure 8–22. Panorex of child. This is an excellent method of surveying the dentition of a young child. The coronoid processes, the condyles in their fossae, and the inferior border of the mandible are easily noted. The maxillary sinuses are visible, as are all the erupted and unerupted teeth. This type of film, however, is not useful for the detection of small carious lesions, and bite-wing films (anterior and posterior) are often used to supplement the panoramic view for this reason.

to examine such areas as the angle and body of the mandible, soft tissues in the neck, or even the hand or other parts of the body. When taking an occlusal film of the anterior maxilla, or one side of the maxilla, it should be remembered that the x-ray beam *must be directed* perpendicular to the line bisecting the plane of the film and the object to be examined. Failure to do so results in distortion. The same is true when examining the mandible in the incisal region or in edentulous regions, or the floor of the mouth for signs of sialoliths or foreign bodies.

When an impacted third molar is present, an occlusal film may be used for a lateral oblique projection, especially if the impaction is located so that it is difficult to demonstrate on an intraoral periapical film. This provides a good view for the location of the tooth in a vertical plane. A film placed along the occlusal plane may then be used to locate the tooth buccolingually. The occlusal film may also be used in special types of crossfire projections to examine the zygomatic arch, the incisive canal region, or even the parotid and submaxillary glands.

SPECIAL INTRAORAL TECHNIQUES

Location of Foreign Body

Since as previously mentioned an individual film can only record in two dimensions it is difficult to locate a foreign body. It is often possible by using several serial radiographs to locate the foreign body in three dimensions. If, for example, a foreign body is located opposite a molar tooth, several serial films can be taken from the posterior toward the anterior. When these are examined, if the foreign body is located lingual to the teeth it will appear to move anteriorly as the more anteriorly placed films are viewed. If, however, the foreign body is located buccal to the teeth, it will appear to move posteriorly as the anteriorly placed films are examined (Fig. 8–23*A* and *B*). An occlusal plane projection often helps locate the foreign bodies in a mediolateral position. This same principle can be applied in a vertical direction. Should a broken needle be lost in the soft tissues it is sometimes possible to locate this needle by inserting another needle to a known depth and then taking radiographs in different planes. The unknown foreign body can then be located with reference to the latter.

It must again be stressed that occasionally a foreign body will appear to be located centrally in the maxilla or mandible when actually it is in the lip, the palatal mucosa or elsewhere.

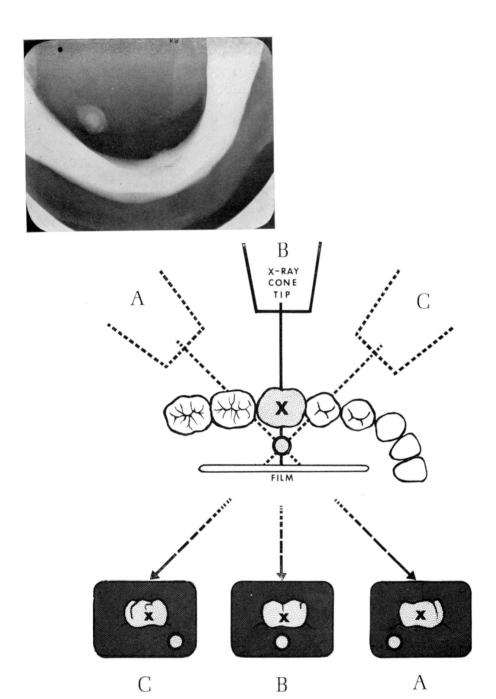

Figure 8–23. *Above,* Occlusal film of edentulous anterior mandible. In this projection no teeth are present in the anterior part of the mandible. The outline of the lip and of the tongue can be seen readily. The mass in the lower right floor of the mouth represents a sialolith which may or may not be palpable clinically. *Below,* Location of a foreign body buccolingually with respect to a given tooth (*A*). Since a radiograph only records in two dimensions, a foreign body cannot be located in depth unless several films are taken. If a foreign body is noted as in film (*B*), an additional film such as (*A*) might be taken with the cone and x-ray beam directed at a different horizontal angle. If the foreign body is located lingual to the tooth (*x*) in question, the object will move distally on the second film (*A*). The reverse is true if the foreign body is located buccal to the tooth.

Tracing a Fistulous Tract

If a fistulous tract is present, but the origin is not known, a radiograph can be taken with an orthodontic wire threaded in the tract to its depth. Radiopaque media likewise can be injected into these fistulae before taking radiographs and the tooth or object causing the problem can often be identified.

Examination for Intrabony Pockets

When an intrabony pocket is suspected, a gutta percha point similar to those used in endodontic therapy may be placed to the depth of the gingival pocket and periapical or bite-wing films then are exposed. The opaque point will reveal the depth of the pocket as compared to the crest of the alveolar bone. This is a good method of surveying the extent of periodontal disease both prior to treatment and during treatment to ascertain progress of the therapy.

Delineation of Cystic Spaces

Occasionally in the maxilla there are cystic areas adjacent to the maxillary sinus and it becomes difficult to determine whether they communicate with the sinus. A large 18-gauge needle on a Luer Lok syringe can be used to inject a radiopaque media into these cystic spaces. Radiographs then will reveal whether there is a direct communication between these areas and the sinus proper.

Other Uses

There is an almost inconceivable variation in the possible uses of intraoral films to examine certain areas and structures. As mentioned before, most routine films are taken at routine angles in routine locations; however, the good oral radiologist can vary any of these techniques to locate and discern areas or lesions within any of the soft or hard tissues in the region of the face. The uses depend upon the knowledge and ingenuity of the examining dentist.

EXTRAORAL TECHNIQUES, USES, AND INTERPRETATION

Most of these extraoral films other than the occlusal type are made using a 5 by 7 or 10 by 12 inch x-ray film in a cassette.

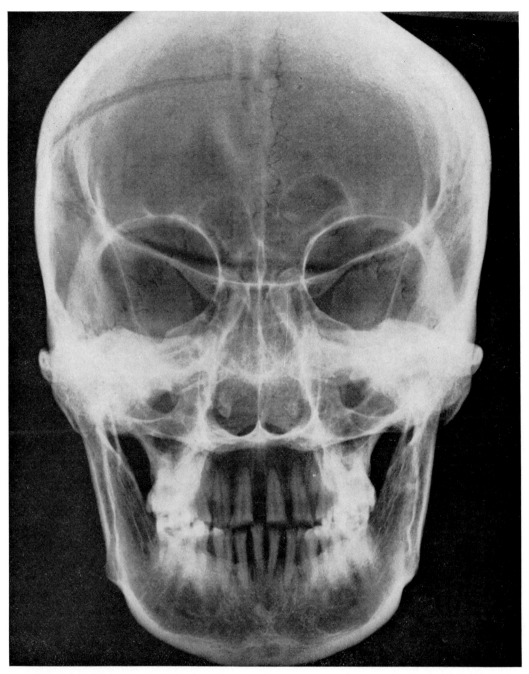

Figure 8–24. Posteroanterior versus anteroposterior. This posteroanterior (PA) radiograph is taken by placing the patient's nose and forehead against the film and directing the beam through the head perpendicular to the film. It is useful for the examination of the middle third of the face in the horizontal plane, and the mandible. It is preferred to the anteroposterior (AP) projection, because of the principle that the object located nearest to the film shows best. Hence, if we are interested in the middle third of the face, the PA projection should be used. The examination of the anterior mandible, maxilla, middle third of the face, orbits and ramus for fractures and other signs of disease is best accomplished by this projection. The coronoid processes, heads of the condyles and the symphysis of the mandible are usually obliterated by the superimposition of other structures.

This film is taken of a dry skull so the detail is much better. Films taken of the living head with soft tissue present will not show this detail. It is quite useful to have a dry skull available when viewing head plates to help determine anatomic landmarks.

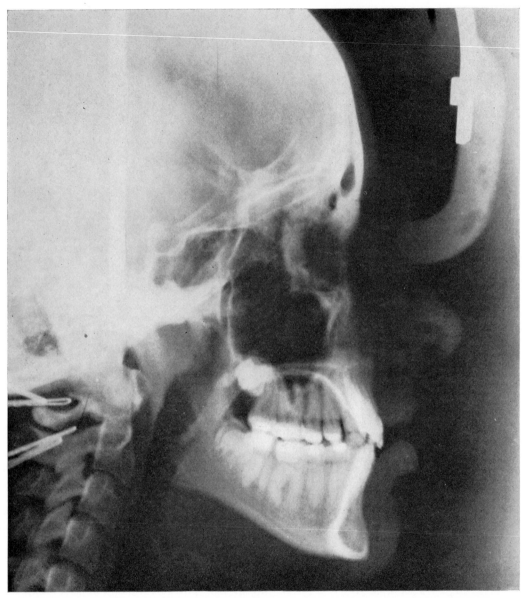

Figure 8–25. Lateral head plate. This film is particularly useful for the examination of the skull in a sagittal plane. The orthodontist uses this in cephalometric techniques for measuring growth and development of the maxillae and mandible in this plane. Because there is much superimposition, the use of this projection is limited. Examination of such structures as the mandible and the maxillary sinuses is difficult because they are superimposed upon each other, although in this film it appears as if they can be seen quite clearly. Note the clarity of the soft tissues of the face, and the hairpins below the ear region.

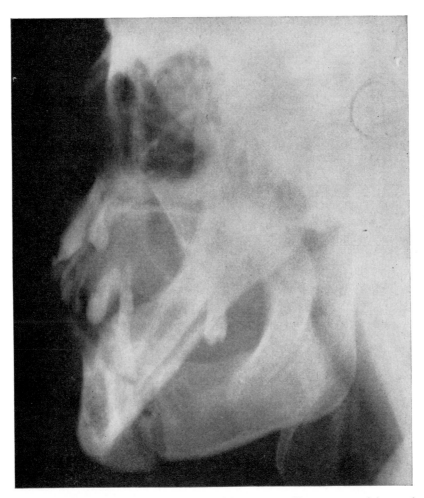

Figure 8–26.   Lateral oblique of the mandible. These films are used in preference to the lateral head plate for the examination of the ramus and body of one side of the mandible. The lateral oblique eliminates superimposition. Fractures, impacted teeth, and other lesions are readily visible. As a general rule, it is wise to examine similar films of both sides for comparison. Pathologic conditions are usually not bilateral, while developmental defects often are present on either side.

This particular projection shows the outline of part of the hyoid bone just below the angle of the mandible. It also shows a comminuted fracture in the mental foramen region, with slight displacement of the fragments.

EXAMINATION OF SPECIAL ANATOMIC AREAS

Sialography

The salivary glands are not normally visible on ordinary radiographs. Calcifications such as sialoliths quite frequently will show on ordinary films. However, if there are symptoms in the submaxillary, sublingual or parotid gland regions it may be necessary to examine these glands and their ductal and acinar patterns more carefully. This can be done by forcing a radiopaque media through the orifice of the ducts (Wharton's and Stensen's) into the glands and then, keeping this media in place, taking radiographs. For the submandibular or sublingual gland, a modified lateral oblique is the best type of projection. For the parotid gland, a modified PA of the injected side is useful. This is done by having the patient puff his cheek

out, forcing the parotid gland away from the lateral border of the mandible and then taking a posteroanterior exposure with the x-ray beam parallel to the lateral surface of the ramus. Lateral head plates also are useful occasionally to examine the parotid gland that has been injected with this media. Close examination of the films often reveals strictures or stenosis of the ducts which indicate that some trauma or infection is or has been present. If the infection has been long standing, the ducts may resemble a string of sausages (sialodochitis). If there has been chronic obstruction, the gland itself may be filled with the media which has become confluent or puddled. Should a tumor be present, the ductal pattern may be interrupted in that area, or if a cyst is present it may be filled with the media. This technique has another advantage in that the media used has some therapeutic value and in a chronic sialadenitis it promotes drainage.

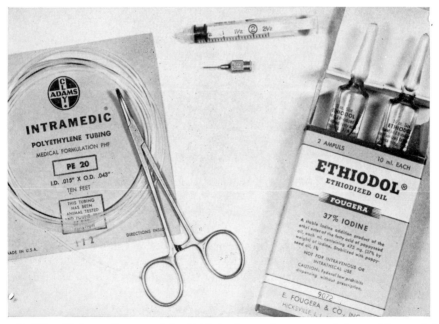

Figure 8–27.   Sialography materials. This is the equipment used for making a sialograph of the submaxillary, sublingual and parotid glands. It consists of a radiopaque media, a small polyethylene tube which is threaded into the orifice of the salivary gland duct, and a syringe to carry the media through the tube into the gland. (Fast and Forest, Dent. Clin. North America, March, 1968.)

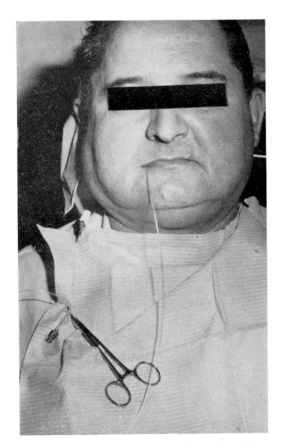

Figure 8–28. Tube in place for sialograph. The polyethylene tube has been placed
in Stensen's duct. Note the enlargement of
the parotid gland due to the filling with the
radiopaque media. Considerable pressure
may be required to fill the gland. This should
be applied slowly to avoid discomfort.

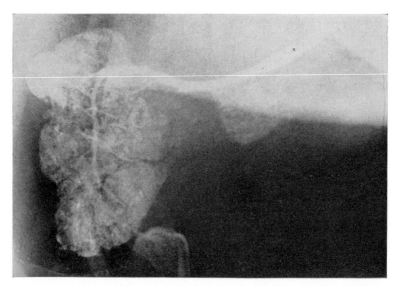

Figure 8–29.   Modified lateral oblique sialograph. This shows the normal submaxillary and sublingual glands filled with the radiopaque media. Note the branching of the ducts within the gland and the complete filling. The hyoid bone is barely discernible over the well-displayed thyroid cartilage.

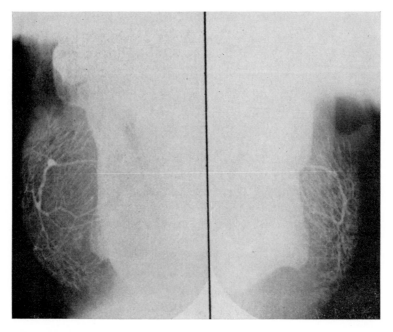

Figure 8–30.   Parotid gland sialographs, modified PA projections of the right and left parotid glands produced after filling the glands with the radiopaque media. While the patient puffs his cheeks out, the beam is directed parallel to the lateral border of the ramus of the mandible. Note the fine ductal pattern of these glands.

Temporomandibular Joint Radiography

One of the most difficult areas of the body to examine radiographically is the temporomandibular joint. This is because of the anatomic interference on the radiograph by the petrous portion of the temporal bone superomedially, the mastoid process posteriorly, and the zygoma superoanteriorly. These structures make necessary special techniques to view the joints from their different aspects. There are three basic types of TMJ radiographs: *transcranial projection* (lateral or oblique); *anteroposterior* (including transorbital projection); *infracranial* projection (submentovertex, or basal projection). Other types used are panoramic, tomograms and laminagrams.

Transcranial Projection (A Modified Lateral Head Plate)

Burnout Technique. This is a method of examining the right or left joint using the principle that the object closest to the film shows most readily on the film. This gives a very good view in a sagittal plane.

The Modified Oblique Transcranial Projection (using the 15° angle board). By this method the patient's head is in a fixed position and the rays are directed to the skull through the temporomandibular joint in question. Since all of these things are controlled, the joint can be examined at frequent intervals and the films compared (Fig. 8–31).

Anteroposterior

Transorbital Projection or Modified Mayer Projection. In this method the rays are directed through the orbit and then through the temporomandibular joint onto the film which is placed behind the head. This gives a good view of the head of the condyle in the frontal plane (Fig. 8–32).

Anteroposterior or Posteroanterior Projection. This view can be used to examine the

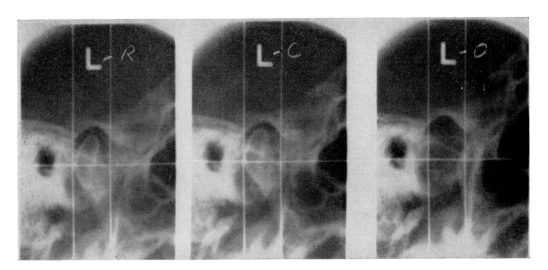

Figure 8–31. TMJ radiograph (transcranial projection). This film demonstrates the relationship of the head of the condyle to the glenoid fossa in resting, closed and opened position. Note the normal space between the depth of the glenoid fossa and the head of the condyle. Note, in the open position, the condyle's relationship to the anterior articular eminence. In order to orient oneself when reading these films, one should first locate the external auditory canal. This film demonstrates an essentially normal temporomandibular joint.

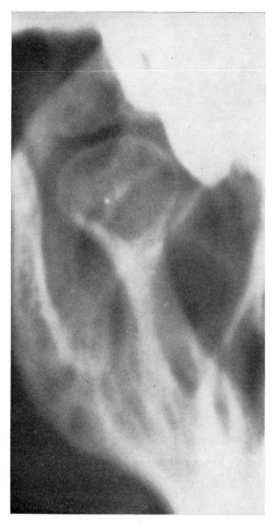

Figure 8–32.   TMJ radiograph (transorbital projection). This projection is taken in an AP direction through the orbit. It is useful for examination of the head and neck of the condyle in this plane. This radiograph demonstrates an essentially normal condyle and condylar neck.

neck and occasionally the head of the condyle in a frontal plane. The ramus is also readily visible in this plane. A modification of the AP view which gives a better delineation of the neck of the condyle is the Townes projection or reverse Townes projection which is a modified PA. These projections, because of the difference in angulation, result in elongation of both rami and condylar necks.

Infracranial Projection (Submentovertex or Basal Projection)

This is a method for viewing the neck and head of the condyles from the inferior aspect. The film is placed above the skull; the direction of the beam is parallel to the posterior of the ramus and enters from the midline beneath the mandible and floor of the mouth. This projection is also valuable for examining the inferior border of the mandible and other structures at the base of the skull as well as the zygomatic arches.

Other Methods of Examining the Temporomandibular Joint

Tomograms (planagrams, laminagrams, panoramic) are methods of examining the temporomandibular joint which require special equipment. The Panorex has been previously discussed. The laminagram is taken by having the source of radiation and the film itself rotate around the patient; the resultant film then gives a blurred image except for the structure of interest.

Stereoradiography, polytomography and arthrography have also been suggested as means of examining the temporomandibular joint; however, information regarding the success of these techniques is at this time incomplete, A more recent method involves a cineradiographic circle unit, in which the film and radiation source rotate around the patient and this is coupled with electromyographic recordings of the muscle of mastication. Because of the superimposition of normal anatomic structures and the variations in individuals, it becomes very difficult to select as best any single technique for examining the temporomandibular joint. One should not be easily frustrated because of failure with any particular technique but should strive to try different methods of examining the joint until good views are obtained.

Although most temporomandibular joint radiographs may be negative for any signs of pathoses, they still should be taken when there are any symptoms or signs of disease in the area. Such things as fractures, spurs or erosions of the head of the condyle suggestive of previous trauma or arthritis are easy to see.

Many authors consider the size of the interarticular space important when examining temporomandibular joint films. This is risky because technical difficulties in exposing these are often misleading. It is, however, important when there are clinical signs.

of ankylosis and no joint space is visible. The transcranial projection is valuable for examining the glenoid fossae and the relationship of the head of the condyle in function. If, in the open position, the condyle is far anterior to the anterior articular eminence, the patient can be considered to have hypermobility of that joint; to the contrary, if, in the open position, the head of the condyle has not moved out of the glenoid fossa, the patient can be considered to have hypomobility. Conditions such as these can be present on either or both sides and films of both joints should always be taken for comparison.

Submentovertical Projection

This projection is used primarily to examine the outline of the zygomatic arches and base of the skull. It is also valuable for viewing the ramus, neck, and head of the condyles for changes in morphology in the transverse plane, and for fractures.

Waters' Sinus Film

The Waters' sinus film is a modified PA used to examine the sinuses and the bones of the middle third of the face in this plane. It is often used for evaluation of expected fractures of the middle third of the face and for suspected sinusitis and tumors. The sinuses normally are radiolucent.

Lateral Neck Plates

These films are taken with a decreased exposure time in order to show any calcification such as phleboliths, sialoliths, calcified lymph nodes, or opaque foreign bodies in the soft tissue of the neck. These can be taken either in a PA or lateral-medial plane.

Panographic Examination

An innovation in extraoral facial radiography is the panoramic view which involves a rather complicated machine capable of taking a continuous type of laminagram. This method is quite useful for examining the jaws for fractures and gross bony lesions or for examining areas such as the submandibular glands, the maxillary area including the orbits and the mandibular ramus. Since detail is poor, slight changes may not be visible.

RADIOGRAPHY AND TRAUMA

In some hospitals there are standard radiographic series used to examine patients with facial trauma for fractures. Trauma to the right mandible might suggest a fracture series including temporomandibular joint films, right and left lateral obliques of the mandible. Trauma to the mental region of the mandible likewise suggests to the radiologist a series including a PA, submental vertical and temporomandibular joint films, as well as intraoral occlusal of the mandible, to rule out fractures of the condyle and symphysis regions.

The radiograph is important to the oral surgeon not only to detect fractures but also to study the alignment after reduction and to follow the healing process. Radiographs have definite and important medicolegal ramifications.

BIBLIOGRAPHY

Berkman, M.D.: Pedodontic radiographic interpretation, Dent. Radiogr. Photogr., *44,* 27, 1971.

Castigliano, S. G.: Sialography of the submaxillary salivary gland: A new technique, Amer. J. Roentgen., *87,* 385, 1962.

Chiles, J. L. and Gores, R. J.: *Anatomic Interpretation of the Orthopantomogram,* Oral Surg., *35,* 564, 1973.

Coin, C. G.: Tomography of the temporomandibular joint, Dent. Radiogr. Photogr., *47,* 23, 1974.

Dachi, S. F. and Howell, F. V.: A survey of 3,874 routine full-mouth radiographs, II. A study of impacted teeth, Oral Surg., *14,* 1165, 1961.

Ennis, L. M., Berry, H. M. and Phillips, J. E.: *Dental Roentgenology,* 6th Ed., Philadelphia, Lea & Febiger, 1967.

Garusi, G. F.: *Salivary Glands in Radiographic Diagnosis,* New York, S. Karger, 1964.

Hettwer, K. J.: Simplified duct cannulation in sialography, Oral Surg., *28,* 649, 1969.

Mandel, L. and Baurmash, H.: The role of sialography in extraparotid disease, Oral Surg., *31,* 164, 1971.

Morris, C. R., Marano, P. D., Swimley, D. C. and Runco, J. G.: Abnormalities noted on panoramic radiographs, Oral Surg., *28,* 772, 1969.

Ollerenshaw, R. and Rose, S.: Sialography—a valuable diagnostic method, Dent. Radiogr. Photogr., *29,* 37, 1956.

O'Shaughnessy, P. E. and Mitchell, D. F.: Effect of altering physical roentgenographic factors on patient radiation dose levels, J. Amer. Dent. Ass., *69,* 335, 1964.

Regan, J. E. and Mitchell, D. F.: Roentgenographic and dissection measurements of alveolar crest height, J. Amer. Dent. Ass., *66,* 356, 1963.

Sicher, H.: *Oral Anatomy,* 4th Ed., St. Louis, C. V. Mosby Co., 1965.

Wainwright, W. W.: *Dental Radiology,* New York, McGraw-Hill Book Co., 1965.

Yale, Seymour H.: Dent. Clin. North America, Symposium on Oral Roentgenology, July, 1961.

Chapter 9

Laboratory Diagnosis: Use of the Oral and Clinical Pathology Laboratories

Myotonic Dystrophy
Congenital Myotonia
Paramyotonia Congenita
Hypotonia
Myasthenia Gravis
Multiple Sclerosis
Parkinson's Syndrome
"Motor System Disease"
Poliomyelitis
Cerebral Palsy
Epilepsy

Properly utilized, the laboratory examination yields important and often essential information necessary for the diagnosis of oral and systemic diseases. Although most dentists recognize the tissue biopsy and cytologic smear as useful diagnostic procedures, many are unfamiliar with or are reluctant to use other laboratory tests that may be indicated. Knowledge of the indications for certain of the more commonly used tests of importance in dentistry as well as their interpretation and clinical significance is essential to the thorough examination.

The laboratory examination is used to supplement the findings of the physical examination rather than as a shortcut to instant diagnosis. Although unsuspected diseases are sometimes discovered with the routine tests given hospitalized patients, the vast majority of cases identified by laboratory methods are first suspected on the basis of a thorough history and physical examination. Thus, specific tests ordinarily are requested when necessary to confirm or rule out possible diagnoses established from the clinical findings. In some instances, it may be necessary to repeat a test if the results are inconsistent with the clinical features or symptoms of the case. It is equally important to avoid selecting tests that are unlikely to provide meaningful information in a given case, since many of the tests are time consuming and expensive.

As with nearly all special examination procedures, the results of a given test taken alone are of little diagnostic significance and must be correlated with other clinical and laboratory findings to be useful.

The selection of a laboratory test presupposes a knowledge of what information the test will provide and the clinical significance of the results obtained. Generally, the simpler tests are employed first, with orderly progression to more elaborate tests that may be necessary.

The dentist should know the normal range of values for the more commonly used tests and understand the significance of abnormal results. Suitable references should be kept at hand which furnish the normal values for less frequently used tests (Appendix Table 1).

"Normal" values for laboratory tests are defined as the mean ± 2 standard deviations. Thus, 5 percent of the laboratory values obtained from normal patients would be expected to be borderline or outside the normal range. Inasmuch as the techniques used in performing even standard tests may vary, normal values acceptable to the particular laboratory being used should be obtained.

TISSUE BIOPSY

Biopsy refers to the removal, usually by surgical means, of living tissues for the purpose of microscopic examination. Because of the relative ease with which small samples of tissues can be removed from the oral cavity, biopsy is one of the most commonly used and reliable tests available to the dentist. The procedures are simple and can be performed by the dentist with a minimum of time and effort and with little inconvenience to the patient. In most instances, obtaining a satisfactory tissue sample for microscopic diagnosis is considerably less difficult than extracting a tooth or performing a gingivectomy.

Indications for the Tissue Biopsy

The best known indication for performing a biopsy is to establish a diagnosis in cases of suspected neoplastic disease. Thus, biopsy may be performed in cases of suspected benign or malignant neoplasms or, in the event cancer is obvious, to determine the specific type of neoplasm and the degree of differentiation.

Some lesions are biopsied because they present few or no diagnostic signs or symptoms suggestive of the diagnosis. For example, the chronic non-specific ulcer may represent epidermoid carcinoma, a specific granulomatous infection, or traumatic (inflammatory) ulcer, lesions which cannot be differentiated on a clinical basis alone.

Biopsy of some lesions may be performed to confirm a clinical diagnosis which seems to be obvious. For this reason, it is the practice of some to submit all tissue removed during treatment for microscopic examination. Examples include periapical lesions, gingivectomy tissue and denture injury hyperplasia. Such practice serves to improve the dentist's clinical judgment and diagnostic skill and provides better insight into the condition under treatment. In addition, it inspires the confidence of the patient in the dentist's thoroughness and interest in his welfare. On occasion, the clinical diagnosis may prove to be in error upon microscopic examination.

Because the oral tissues are easily accessible, biopsy may be performed as an adjunctive diagnostic procedure in a variety of suspected metabolic diseases. It has been utilized with some success to show diabetic arteriopathy, amyloidosis, connective tissue diseases (including Sjögren's syndrome), cystic fibrosis and sarcoidosis.

Biopsy may be performed as a form of therapy for the patient with cancerphobia. This fear may be expressed openly by the patient who may relate accounts of friends or relatives who died of cancer. In some instances, the patient may seek consultation on some other pretext but question the dentist at length about one or more innocuous lesions in the mouth, finally asking the dentist if he thinks the lesion is cancer. If there is any doubt about the clinical diagnosis, or the patient still suspects cancer, biopsy is completely justified. The patient may be shown the written report "proving" that no tumor is present.

Contraindications for Biopsy

There are some contraindications for a tissue biopsy. Obviously, sound clinical judgment must be used as for any surgical procedure. Thus, extreme debilitation, cardiac disease, acute infection, undue bleeding tendency, or other conditions contraindicating minor surgery also apply to biopsy.

In most instances, biopsy should not be performed in cases of clinically obvious cancer. Such patients should be referred directly to the individual or center who will carry out the definitive treatment. Biopsy of the lesion simply results in unnecessary delay and, conceivably, could induce local spread or metastasis. Of primary importance, however, is the need to establish a definitive diagnosis and commence therapy with the least possible delay.

Selection of the Biopsy Site

If only a small portion of the lesion is to be removed for histologic examination, care should be used to obtain tissue which is representative of the active lesion under study. The central portions of the specimen may exhibit areas of necrosis which will be of little value to the pathologist in interpretation of the histologic findings. Often, the extreme edges of a lesion may show reactive tissue not characteristic of the main lesion. Although most oral surgeons attempt to obtain adjacent normal tissue as well as the diseased tissue within the same specimen, this is of less importance than being certain the sample is representative of the lesion proper. A common error is to fail to remove sufficient depth of tissue, particularly in the epithelial dysplasias where there may be marked thickening of the keratin or spinous layers of the epithelium (Fig. 14–2). If the lesion overlies bone as on the hard palate, the incision should be made down to bone.

In cases of multiple or diffuse lesions, several smaller specimens properly identified will ordinarily be of greater diagnostic value than one larger biopsy. Since certain portions of the diffuse lesions may simply be reactive, the additional samples materially increase the chances for a definitive microscopic diagnosis.

The *toluidine blue test* has been utilized to help identify the best site for biopsy of suspected cancer and to outline the lateral extent of the lesional tissue. The technique entails painting the lesion with 2 percent toluidine blue followed by thorough irrigation with saline or water to remove excess dye. Those areas retaining the royal blue stain are considered most appropriate for biopsy. This test is based on the affinity of the dye for cells actively synthesizing nucleic acid. Unfortunately, regenerating epithelium in the healing ulcer as well as dysplastic epithelial cells and mucus bind the dye, thereby making interpretation difficult. Conversely, keratotic lesions (some of which may be cancer) do not retain the dye. For these reasons, some authorities have questioned the value of this test.

Types of Biopsies

Incisional Biopsy

The *incisional biopsy* refers to the removal of a small portion of the lesion, usually a wedge-shaped or elliptical specimen (Fig. 9–1). This type of biopsy is used for large or diffuse lesions in which the diagnosis is the primary concern of the dentist. For this reason, a second procedure is generally necessary to remove or treat the remainder of the clinical lesion.

Excisional Biopsy

This refers to the removal of the entire lesion (Fig. 9–2). All small lesions and certain large lesions which can be removed without extensive surgery should be excised in their entirety. In addition, suspected pigmented nevi and vascular malformations should be excised rather than incised. If cancer can reasonably be expected but is not clinically certain, generous lateral and deep margins of normal tissue should be obtained to avoid transection of neoplastic cells if present.

The most satisfactory biopsy specimens therefore are obtained by surgical excision of all or part of the clinical lesion. The use of electrocautery is not indicated, especially with small specimens; coagulation of the cells with resulting distortion and difficulty of interpretation may occur. Although electrocautery offers excellent control of hemorrhage, postoperative healing may be delayed somewhat as well. If for special reasons electrocautery is desired, its use should be restricted to large specimens and the method of removal should be indicated on the history sheet.

Punch Biopsy

The *punch biopsy* utilizes a specially designed instrument for the removal of a small segment of tissue. The instrument may be forceps-like with cup-shaped cutting edges or cylindrically shaped, much like a corkborer. While it is convenient to use in some situations, the small size of the specimen obtained and the likelihood of crushing the tissue limit its usefulness in the oral cavity.

Needle or Aspiration Biopsy

This refers to the removal of small bits of tissue or fluids from deep structures by means of a large gauge needle (Vim-Silverman needle) and stylet. It is sometimes used for deep-seated and relatively inaccessible soft tissue lesions (*e.g.* suspected tumors of major salivary glands). Tissues obtained in this manner are quite small and difficult to orient for tissue sectioning. However, aspiration of suspected cyst-like lesions in bone is often diagnostic and may, in the case of a central hemangioma, avert serious bleeding complications. Aspirated material may be submitted to a laboratory where it can be treated as a cytologic smear or centrifuged and the sediment handled as a tissue biopsy.

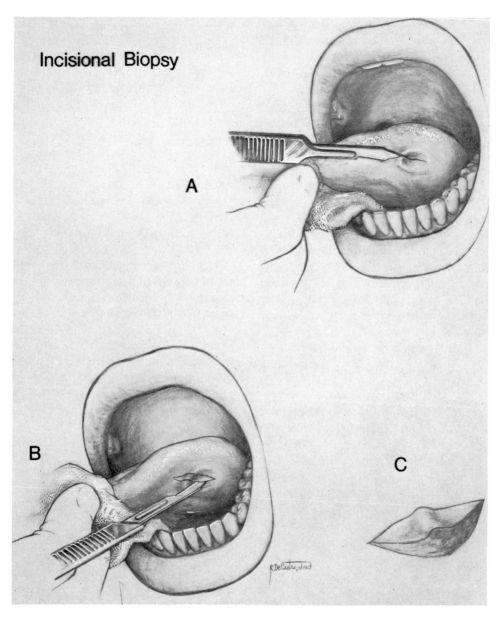

Fig. 9-1.   Incisional biopsy.

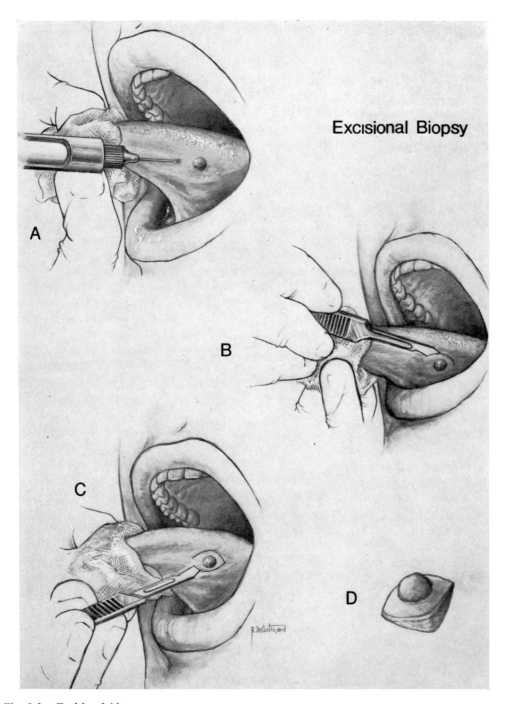

Fig. 9-2. Excisional biopsy.

Exploratory Biopsy

Tissue obtained during surgical exploration of a lesion such as that which might be encountered centrally within bone is sometimes called an exploratory biopsy. Frequently biopsy may not be anticipated prior to the surgical exploration but tissue is found which grossly indicates the need for histologic examination. Biopsies of this type are sometimes referred to as unplanned biopsies.

Care of the Biopsy Specimen

Proper handling of the specimen removed for histologic examination will greatly facilitate the preparation of the histologic sections and interpretation by the pathologist. Common artifacts caused by improper handling of the biopsy specimen include crushing, drying, improper fixation and freezing. It is often helpful to include a small sketch of the lesion *in situ* so that important anatomic landmarks may be identified by the pathologist. The placement of a suture in one end of the specimen will serve to orient it for the pathologist and may be of some significance in the event that tumor cells may have been transected on one or more borders.

Care should be used not to crush the tissue with hemostats or other instruments used for immobilizing the tissues during surgical removal. The tissue to be removed should be grasped at the extreme edge with a tissue forceps or immobilized by holding with a suture or a dental explorer placed through one margin.

Excessive drying of the specimen will significantly alter cytologic detail and occasionally prevent a definite microscopic diagnosis. To avoid drying or even possible loss of the tissue, the biopsy should be placed immediately in previously prepared bottles of fixative upon its removal from the mouth.

In order to preserve histologic detail, chemical fixation of the tissue is necessary. The most commonly used and reliable fixative is 10 percent formalin which is readily available at nearly all pharmacies. A volume of approximately 10 times that of the specimen is adequate. With extremely bulky masses of tissue, inadequate penetration of the fixative in the central portions may result unless the mass is carefully cut into smaller segments. If pulp tissue is to be studied, the root apex should be cut or fractured off, or the tooth ground down under water on one or more surfaces.

Since cases requiring biopsy are often found unexpectedly, a supply of fixative should be kept on hand at all times. Specially prepared mailing containers complete with biopsy history sheets and specimen bottles containing fixative are available from oral pathology laboratories. In the event formalin is not available, reasonably satisfactory fixation may be obtained with ethyl alcohol or even alcohol-containing beverages.

Freezing artifacts may inadvertently occur if the specimen remains in a corner mailbox overnight in the winter months. Because of the large ice crystals which form in the specimen, marked distortion of the cells and tissue occurs and diagnosis is difficult or even impossible. The severity of these artifacts is increased if repeated freezing and thawing occur.

Preparation of the Biopsy History Sheet

A written clinical history and description of the lesion to be examined should accompany the specimen to the laboratory. History sheet forms are available from most oral pathology laboratories. However, the history may be submitted in the form of a letter or other note describing the pertinent features.

The same principles apply to preparing the biopsy history sheet as they do to the dental examination in general. The age, sex and occupation of the patient should be included since these may materially affect the final microscopic diagnosis. Since a variety of systemic diseases may be manifest in the oral cavity, information about the patient's medical history or evidence of systemic disease should be described. Because of the occasional metastasis of a variety of malignant neoplasms to the oral cavity, a history of neoplastic disease in any part of the body should be indicated. In like manner, the past dental history may have an important bearing on the case. The presence of infected teeth, periodontal disease, previous extractions in the region or other factors may be of importance to the oral pathologist.

The lesion should be fully described, including measurements of size and descriptions of color and consistency of the lesion. A common error is to omit the location of the lesion, even though an otherwise detailed history has been provided. Frequently, a small sketch of the defect will be helpful. Symptoms such as pain or tenderness as well as their duration and relationship to any previous incident in the patient's dental or medical history may be of diagnostic importance. Appropriate radiographs, clinical photographs, results of laboratory tests and other pertinent material should also accompany the specimen to the laboratory.

Interpretation of the Biopsy Report

The written biopsy report returned to the dentist consists of a microscopic description of the specimen submitted and a microscopic diagnosis which is based in part on the clinical history and description. For example, granulation tissue seen microscopically would be diagnosed as periapical granuloma provided the clinical history indicated that the tissue had been removed from the apical region of a non-vital tooth.

The most important portion of the biopsy report is the microscopic description which outlines in detail those features on which the diagnosis is based. Careful study of the description will often provide the dentist with additional insight into the character of the lesion which may not be immediately apparent from the diagnostic terms given. Some knowledge of basic pathologic processes then is useful to obtain the greatest benefit from the biopsy report.

It should be emphasized that a negative biopsy report does not necessarily rule out the possibility of cancer or some other serious disease. Obviously, if the microscopic diagnosis is inconsistent with the clinical features presented by the patient, further evaluation of the case by both the pathologist and the dentist is required. Review of the case by direct personal contact with the pathologist will resolve a number of these problems or suggest other possible approaches to diagnosis. In certain cases, it must be concluded that the specimen submitted is not representative of the disease and the biopsy must be repeated.

ORAL EXFOLIATIVE CYTOLOGY

Exfoliative cytology refers to the removal of surface cells for cytologic examination. Although the study of exfoliated cells for the diagnosis of cancer was first described well over 100 years ago, it was not until Papanicolaou established a technique for the study of cervical smears that it became a recognized diagnostic procedure. Cytology is a useful procedure for sites such as the uterine cervix, or for the examination of expectorated cells from the lung; however, direct observation and surgical biopsy are readily accomplished in the mouth. For this and other reasons, oral exfoliative cytology had not been utilized to any great degree in dentistry until recently. A number of studies have been undertaken in the past several years to demonstrate the usefulness and reliability of the oral cytologic smear. At present the cytologic smear technique is being used both for diagnostic purposes and for routine screening of patients with oral lesions of various types. If this method is to be used, its indications and limitations should be fully understood.

Indications for Oral Exfoliative Cytology

Oral exfoliative cytology is used most frequently in cases of suspected epidermoid carcinoma. Because of the seriousness of this disease, biopsy is the diagnostic procedure of choice in highly suspicious lesions. However, cytology may be useful for patients who refuse biopsy or are poor surgical risks.

If biopsy is not immediately feasible, a cytologic smear may be obtained quickly and without inconvenience to the patient. Since carcinoma of the oral cavity in its early stages may be remarkably innocuous appearing, its nature may not be suspected. Thus, exfoliative cytology is indicated for those cases in which biopsy is not planned and for those erythematous lesions which appear to be relatively harmless.

Contraindications for Oral Cytology

Exfoliative cytology is not indicated in cases of obvious cancer. Such patients should be referred immediately for histologic diagnosis and treatment. There is no justification in delaying this referral for the period of time necessary to obtain the cytologic report. A histologic diagnosis will be required in any event since definitive treatment cannot be based on a cytologic smear.

Smears of obviously keratotic lesions of the oral cavity are not indicated since these specimens almost invariably are composed only of superficial keratinizing cells of no diagnostic value.

Obviously, cytologic smears scraped from the mucosal surface are of no value for those deep-seated lesions or masses which do not communicate with the surface.

Advantages of Oral Cytology

The main advantages of oral cytologic techniques are the ease with which the sample can be obtained, the minimum equipment required, the convenience and lack of pain to the patient, and the ease of preparation of the specimens.

Disadvantages of Oral Cytology

The disadvantages of the exfoliative cytologic smear technique are mainly those related to the interpretation of the specimen. Further, a definitive diagnosis is not obtained with this procedure; rather, only the presence or absence of malignant cells is established. A positive diagnosis necessitates a second procedure for biopsy to confirm that a malignant neoplasm is present, and its type and degree of differentiation. The method is of no value in hyperkeratotic lesions. If a negative smear is obtained, a false sense of security may prevent adequate follow-up of a given lesion. Re-observation and repetition of the smear often are indicated.

Oral Cytology Technique

The lesion to be smeared should be cleansed of debris and mucin with a moist sponge. Two or more 1×3 inch glass slides and the fixative should be at hand. Cells are obtained by scraping the surface of the lesion several times with a moistened tongue blade, metal cement spatula or other instrument. Scrapings are spread evenly over the central portion of the slide and the cells are fixed immediately with ethylene glycol, alcohol, or other cytologic fixatives available commercially. It is important to write the patient's name in ordinary lead pencil on the frosted end of the slide so the technician can determine on which surface of the glass the cells were smeared. To assure representative cells from the lesion, at least two smears should be prepared for each lesion to be examined. After the fixative has dried, the slides should be submitted to the laboratory along with an appropriate history describing the features of the lesion as described for biopsy above.

Interpretation of the Cytology Report

The cytology report describes, often in tabular form, the relative numbers of cell types representing the various layers of the epithelium and their degree of differentiation. An indication of the types and numbers of inflammatory cells, histiocytes, fibroblasts, microorganisms and other cells may be similarly tabulated. In some instances a brief description of any unusual cytologic features is presented. Generally, the smears are graded according to one of several cytologic classifications to indicate if the smear is negative, suspicious or positive for malignant cells (Fig. 9–3). The classification used by

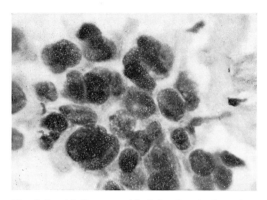

Fig. 9-3.   Malignant epithelial cells obtained from an area of erythroplasia on the anterior fauces in a 47-year-old male. The epithelial cells show nuclear hyperchromatism, pleomorphism and an increased nuclear cytoplasmic ratio. A diagnosis of epidermoid carcinoma was established by biopsy.

the laboratory is usually given on the report form and often states in a general way the clinical significance of the findings described. A commonly used classification is given in Table 9-1.

It should again be emphasized that a negative cytology report is not proof that neoplastic disease does not exist. If a lesion persists, biopsy should be done in the ab-

sence of any other positive diagnostic features.

Other Uses for Exfoliative Cytology

Cytologic smears have been utilized in the diagnosis of a variety of oral conditions. They have been of some value in identification of certain specific infections of the oral mucosa such as candidiasis and fusospirochetal infections, and in the identification of epithelial dysplasias of the oral mucosa such as hereditary benign intraepithelial dyskeratosis (Witkop) and the white sponge nevus (p. 378, Fig. 4–19). Certain vesicular diseases, chiefly those showing acantholysis, may exhibit suggestive or even pathognomonic cytologic features. For example, the so-called fried-egg cells are considered strongly suggestive of pemphigus (Fig. 14–23). Certain viral infections such as primary herpes simplex (Fig. 7–45) and herpes zoster may exhibit characteristic multinucleated cells if material is obtained fresh from an intact vesicle. Patients receiving radiation therapy, chemotherapy and those suspected of having megaloblastic anemia are reported to show characteristic cytologic

Table 9-1. Cytologic Diagnosis.

	Cytology Report	Interpretation
Class I	Normal cells.	All cells normal, cancer unlikely.
Class II	Atypical cytology; no evidence of malignancy.	Morphologic alteration of cells; probable inflammatory reaction rather than malignant transformation.
Class III	Cytology suggestive of but not conclusive for malignancy.	Morphologic changes indeterminate for carcinoma; biopsy indicated.
Class IV	Cytology strongly suggestive of malignancy.	Morphologic features mostly typical of cancer; biopsy mandatory.
Class V	Cytology conclusive for malignancy.	Biopsy mandatory.

changes. Sex-chromatin studies of exfoliated buccal epithelial cells are useful procedures in Klinefelter's syndrome and sex identification (p. 525). Whitten has reviewed a large number of benign oral lesions and outlined the cytologic features that appear consistently in many of them.

Fluids aspirated or expressed from underlying "cystic" defects will sometimes yield cells of diagnostic value especially if the aspirate is centrifuged at the laboratory before spreading it on the slide (Fig. 6–2).

EXAMINATION OF THE SALIVA

The application of standard laboratory procedures to the analysis of saliva has only recently been utilized for diagnostic purposes. Although most clinical laboratories are not presently prepared to conduct elaborate salivary analyses, these services will probably become available as additional applications are devised. Studies have already established the usefulness of salivary analyses in the diagnosis of cystic fibrosis of the pancreas (mucoviscidosis) and the monitoring of heavy metal intoxication in industrial workers, digitalis levels in arrhythmias and cardiac failure, and urea levels in hemodialysis. Considerable experimental and clinical evidence supports the concept of a dental caries-salivary gland-endocrine gland axis and salivary analyses may prove useful in these areas. Blood group antigens present in the saliva also provide important data, particularly in genetic studies and forensic investigations of bite marks in criminal assault cases (p. 526).

Salivary flow, viscosity, pH and composition may reflect disorders of the salivary glands proper, their neural and humoral regulators and other parameters of body metabolism.

Salivary Flow and Volume

The clinical examination should routinely include some gross estimation of the quantity of the saliva since the presence of xerostomia and sialorrhea often provides important clues

in diagnosis (p. 359). The salivary flow ranges from 1000 to 1500 ml in 24 hours. The submaxillary gland contributes approximately 70 percent of the total volume while the parotid and sublingual glands contribute about 25 percent and 5 percent respectively. Thus, secretory activity of the salivary glands occurs at the rate of about 1 ml per minute but may drop to 0.25 ml per minute during periods of inactivity or sleep. Salivary flow is increased following administration of sympathomimetic (epinephrine, norepinephrine) and parasympathomimetic (acetylcholine, methancholine, pilocarpine) drugs. Sympatholytic drugs (ergot, dibenamine) and parasympatholytic drugs (atropine, scopolamine) reduce salivary secretion. Similar effects are induced by a number of other common drugs, including the ganglionic blocking agents used for the treatment of hypertension.

Salivary Viscosity

Parotid saliva is of low viscosity and contains more amylase than the submaxillary secretion, which is of high viscosity and is high in mucoprotein. Salivary proteins account for the physical characteristics of saliva. Saliva is hypotonic to plasma and has a specific gravity ranging from 1.002 to 1.012.

Salivary pH

Salivary pH depends chiefly on the concentration of salivary CO_2 and, in turn, upon the blood CO_2. It ranges from 5.75 to 7.05 with most cases falling within the 6.35 to 6.85 range. Bicarbonates and phosphates of the saliva act as buffers and for this reason salivary pH is relatively constant. With loss of CO_2, the saliva becomes more alkaline. As for the blood, salivary pH may be elevated in hyperventilation or lowered in case of bicarbonate ingestion.

Salivary Electrolytes

Many physiologic and pathologic processes are reflected in the chemical composition of the saliva, chiefly the salivary electrolytes. Systemic diseases (asthma, hypertension, cystic fibrosis), drug therapy (aspirin, cortisone, digitalis), hormonal changes (pregnancy, menstruation, Addison's disease, Cushing's syndrome) and stress alter salivary electrolytes. The potassium concentration of saliva is relatively high (30.0 mEq/L), exceeding that of the plasma. Desoxycortisone administration causes an increase in salivary potassium and a fall in salivary chloride and sodium. Stress, such as that following surgical procedures, causes elevation of salivary potassium and calcium. Determinations of salivary sodium/potassium ratios have been shown to vary inversely with the level of adrenocortical salt-retaining activity in essential hypertension and primary aldosteronism. The sodium/potassium ratio is high in Addison's disease and low in Cushing's syndrome and salt deprivation. Free 17-hydroxycorticosteroid levels in the parotid saliva parallel those of the serum in Cushing's syndrome and adrenal hyporesponsiveness to ACTH.

Elevated salivary calcium and phosphorus levels are found in children with cystic fibrosis and asthma. While these values alone cannot differentiate the two diseases in a child with pulmonary signs, biopsy of the accessory (labial) salivary glands shows characteristic changes in cystic fibrosis.

Salivary Enzymes

The saliva contains upwards of 30 different enzymes, of which amylase is the best known. The salivary enzymes (which may be derived from glands, microorganisms or salivary leukocytes) are grouped as carbohydrases (*e.g.* amylase, lysozyme, beta glucuronidase, hyaluronidase, mucinase), esterases (*e.g.* acid and alkaline phosphatase, lipase, acetylcholinesterase), transferring enzymes (*e.g.* catalase, peroxidase, succinic dehydrogenase), proteolytic enzymes (proteinase, peptidase, urease) and others (carbonic anhydrase, aldolase, etc.). Parotid saliva contains approximately 4 times as much amylase as submaxillary and sublingual saliva, and is unrelated to the salivary flow rate. Salivary lysozyme is found in concentrations up to 8 times that of serum. It is of interest that parotid saliva acid phosphatase activity has been found to be significantly elevated in patients with both metastatic and nonmetastatic carcinoma of the prostate.

The submaxillary saliva in patients with cystic fibrosis shows increased levels of calcium, total protein, urea, uric acid, hexose, fucose and amylase, acid and alkaline ribonuclease, and lysosome activity. Immunodiffusion of submaxillary saliva and serum from patients with cystic fibrosis also shows significant elevations of immunoglobulin (IgA). Grossly the submaxillary saliva is cloudy or turbid.

CARIES ACTIVITY TESTS

Various tests have been devised to measure the caries activity of the individual. Much controversy has surrounded this subject. The tests have been based upon such parameters as salivary microorganisms, salivary buffering capacity and other chemical characteristics of saliva. For the most part, the tests indicate the individual's potential to develop caries in the future rather than the actual activity at the present time. For example, persons who are obviously caries immune may exhibit features seen in caries-active individuals such as high *Lactobacillus acidophilus* counts (L.a.), poor buffering capacity or high viscosity of the saliva. Although such methods do not clearly distinguish between those individuals who are caries free and those who are caries immune, they may provide certain guidelines for the institution of caries preventive measures such as dietary control, fluoride treatment or other preventive measures. Likewise, periodic tests may aid in assessing the degree of cooperation a patient may be furnishing in following dietary restrictions.

The caries activity tests include: (*a*) wafer test, (*b*) glucose clearance test, (*c*) modified Wach test, (*d*) Snyder test, (*e*) L.a. count, (*f*) Green test, (*g*) salivary flow test and (*h*) salivary viscosity test.

The Snyder test and the lactobacillus count have been the most popular caries activity tests. Judiciously used, they provide reasonable criteria on which to base recommendations to the patient. In addition, they may provide a quantitative means by which to impress on the patient the importance of dietary control, good toothbrushing habits, plaque control measures, and other methods to suppress caries. Such tests also have been used in assessing and predicting the general caries activity of groups of individuals serving as subjects in epidemiologic or experimental studies of dental caries.

HEMATOLOGY

A variety of diseases may reflect changes of diagnostic importance in one or more of the several components of the blood. The hematologic examination is conducted routinely for all hospitalized patients, for those with suspected hemorrhagic problems, and for the diagnosis of several oral and systemic diseases characterized by changes in the peripheral blood.

The hematology examination includes evaluation of the formed elements (erythrocytes, leukocytes, platelets) of the blood and bone marrow as well as a vast array of tests of hemostasis (*e.g.* bleeding and clotting factors). Although certain of these tests require a minimal amount of equipment and experience and may be performed in the dental office, the majority require the facilities of a clinical pathology laboratory to ensure accuracy.

The "routine hemogram" or complete blood count (CBC) usually includes a total

Table 9-2. The Hematology Report Form.

NAME _____ Room No. _____ Hosp. No. _____

Physician _____

Procedure	Normal	Patient	Procedure	Normal	Patient
RBC	4-6,000,000		Segs	50 to 70%	
Hemoglobin	12-16 gm.		Bands	2-6%	
WBC	5,000-10,000		Juveniles	0 to 1%	
Bleed-Time	2 to 3 min.		Myelocytes	0%	
Coag. Time	3 to 8 min.		Eosinophils	1 to 3%	
Platelet	200-300,000		Basophils	0 to 1%	
Reticulocyte	.2-1.5%		Lymphocytes	20 to 40%	
Sed. Rate	10 to 25 mm		Lymphoblasts	0%	
Hematocrit	37 to 50%		Monocytes	2 to 8%	
			Monoblasts	0%	
			Remarks		

Technician _____ Director of Laboratories _____

Date _____ Date Rec'd: _____

HEMATOLOGY

red blood cell count, a hematocrit, or total and differential white blood cell count, hemoglobin determination and a smear for morphology (Table 9–2).

The Red Blood Cells

Examination of the red blood cells entails determinations of numbers, size, shape and quality of the cells. Indications for erythrocyte determinations in the outpatient usually are based on generalized and often vague symptoms of fatigue, shortness of breath, headache, dizziness, pallor or glossitis. These symptoms may be suggestive of anemia, most commonly iron deficiency anemia (Fig. 14–47).

Blood Smears

Blood smears are useful for evaluation of red blood cell size, shape, maturity and staining properties (Fig. 9–4). Some of these morphologic or tinctorial changes and their significance are described below.

Anisocytosis. Abnormal size of the erythrocyte indicates defective maturation and is seen in iron deficiency (hypochromic-microcytic) anemia and pernicious (hyperchromic-macrocytic) anemia.

Poikilocytosis. Abnormal shapes of the red blood cells are seen in most anemias, particularly pernicious anemia.

Polychromatophilia. Basophilic stippling or a bluish tinge to portions of the red blood cell indicates young red blood cells in the peripheral blood. These changes together with circulating reticulocytes (nucleated red blood cells) occur in several blood dyscrasias.

Howell-Jolly Bodies, Cabot's Rings. These structures represent residual fragments of the red blood cell nucleus and are seen in Banti's syndrome and other forms of "splenic anemia" and following splenectomy.

Sickle Cells. Moon or sickle-shaped red blood cells are characteristic of the sickle cell trait and sickle cell anemia (p. 409). Because of the abnormal hemoglobins present, sickling occurs in special preparations using low oxygen tension (Fig. 9–5). The character of the abnormal hemoglobin (hemoglobin S) can be demonstrated by electrophoretic methods.

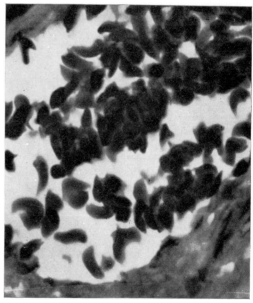

Fig. 9-5. Sickle cell anemia. "Sickling" of erythrocytes in a blood vessel is shown similar to that produced in the laboratory under lowered oxygen tension. Sickling of erythrocytes is not necessarily seen in routine tissue sections in either sickle cell anemia or sickle cell trait (p. 409). Rather, local conditions of vascular stasis or delayed fixation may result in lowered oxygen tension and sickling. (Courtesy of W. G. Sprague.)

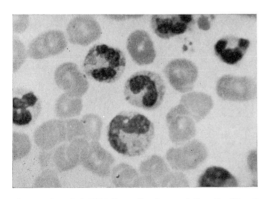

Fig. 9-4. A Wright-stained peripheral blood smear showing polymorphonuclear leukocytes (neutrophils) and erythrocytes. The clear areas within the erythrocytes correspond to the central concavity characteristic of these cells.

Target Cells. A small dot of basophilic material resembling the bullseye of a target is seen in Mediterranean anemia (thalassemia), sickle cell anemia and certain hypochromic anemias.

Erythrocyte Count

The total erythrocyte count provides a reasonable estimate of the number of circulating red blood cells which may vary according to the age and sex of the individual (see Appendix, Table 1, p. 405). The adult erythrocyte count may range greatly from 4 to 5.4 million cells per mm³, and figures for the adult female are usually less.

Hematocrit

Because of the rather considerable error in red blood cell counts, the hematocrit (packed cell volume after centrifugation) has proven to be a more informative test. The volume of packed red blood cells in a given sample of peripheral blood is a quantitative measure of the percentage of the total blood made up by red blood cells. The normal adult female exhibits hematocrit values of 38 to 46 percent, while the adult male will show normal values of 41 to 50 percent red blood cells.

Hemoglobin

Normal hemoglobin values range from 12 to 16 gm per 100 ml (grams percent) of blood in normal adult females; males show a range of 14 to 18 gm percent.

Lesser values obtained with these tests are suggestive of anemia, but more elaborate tests are required to identify the particular type. Remembering that anemias may be classified according to their basic etiology, defects in the circulating red blood cells may be due to decreased production, defective maturation or increased destruction. Thus, anemia may be manifest as too few cells, abnormal cells in size or shape, and cells deficient in hemoglobin.

Red Blood Cell Indices

Utilizing the information gained from the total erythrocyte count (rbc per mm³), hemoglobin (Hgb) determination and the hematocrit cell volume (percent cell volume, PCV), it is possible to calculate several *red blood cell indices*: mean corpuscular volume (MCV), mean corpuscular hemoglobin (MCH) and mean corpuscular hemoglobin concentration (MCHC).

The values obtained correlate cell numbers, cell volume and hemoglobin concentrations. The *mean corpuscular volume* (volume of a red blood cell) would obviously be increased in macrocytic anemia and reduced in microcytic anemia. The *mean corpuscular hemoglobin* value represents the amount of hemoglobin per red blood cell and would be reduced in hypochromic microcytic anemia. It would be increased, on the other hand, in macrocytic anemia since the larger cell would ordinarily contain more hemoglobin than the normal red blood cell. The *mean corpuscular hemoglobin concentration* represents the amount of hemoglobin expressed as a percentage of the volume of a red blood cell. Thus this value would be essentially normal for all the several anemias except hypochromic-microcytic anemia.

Erythrocyte Sedimentation Rate (ESR)

This measurement of the rate at which erythrocytes settle out in oxalated blood is used as a general screening test. While it is highly sensitive to variations in erythrocyte size and shape, cell volume and serum protein concentration and type, it has little specificity. An accelerated ESR generally indicates changes in the plasma proteins and may be seen in acute and chronic inflammatory reactions, destructive tumors and the lymphomas. Decreased values are found in polycythemia, hypochromic-microcytic anemia, hypofibrinogenemia and the hemoglobinopathies. Normal values for the adult male are 0 to 19 mm/hr and for the female 0 to 15 mm/hr. ESR values increase with increasing age of the patient.

The White Blood Cells

The normal number of circulating leukocytes may vary over a considerable range depending upon the age, sex and physiologic status of the patient. The white blood cell count in children is ordinarily higher than for adults (see Appendix, Table 1). In most laboratories, the normal range of white blood cells in the adult patient is 5 to 10,000 per mm^3 (Table 9–2). Physiologic increases in circulating white blood cells may be seen following extreme muscular activity, meals, exposure to extremes of temperature, administration of epinephrine, and during pregnancy and labor.

The differential leukocyte counts may be expressed either as the relative number of each type of white blood cells or the absolute number per volume of blood for each cell type. Depending upon the laboratory, normal values for the differential white blood cell count are as follows:

	Percent
Band neutrophils	2–6
Segmented neutrophils	50–70
Lymphocytes	20–40
Monocytes	2–8
Eosinophils	1–3
Basophils	0–1

Leukocytosis

An increase in the total white blood cells is referred to as leukocytosis. This is seen in a variety of infectious diseases most of which show a marked relative increase in the percentage of neutrophils in the circulating blood.

Except for physiologic leukocytosis, an increase in the total white cell count usually indicates the presence of infection. It should be noted, however, that certain other conditions are necessary for leukocytosis to occur.

The microorganism must be of a type capable of calling forth leukocytes; the infection must not be overwhelming; and the bone marrow must be capable of producing leukocytes. Leukocytosis also may occur in protein shock, allergy, intestinal obstruction and after severe hemorrhage.

Specific types of leukocytosis may suggest a specific diagnosis. A *neutrophilic leukocytosis* is seen in most acute infections, after severe hemorrhage, in myelogenous leukemia and, at times, in association with rapidly growing malignant tumors. *Eosinophilia* is typically found in allergic conditions, parasitic infestations, some endocrine disorders (*e.g.* Addison's disease and ovarian dysfunction), and following x-ray therapy.

Lymphocytosis usually occurs in lymphatic leukemia, infectious mononucleosis, whooping cough, following irradiation and during convalescence from infection. *Monocytosis* may occur in subacute bacterial endocarditis, Hodgkin's disease, malaria and tuberculosis.

Leukopenia

Certain infections such as measles, mumps, typhoid fever, influenza and infectious mononucleosis may depress the number of circulating white blood cells. This also occurs in pernicious anemia, aplastic anemia, and aleukemic leukemia. A variety of drugs or other toxic agents and radiation may de-

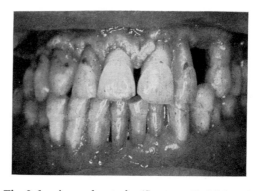

Fig. 9-6. Agranulocytosis. (Swenson, Reddish and Manne, J. Periodont., *36*, 466, 1965.)

press the bone marrow to such an extent that leukopenia results.

Reduction in the number of granulocytes (neutrophils, for all practical purposes) is referred to as *agranulocytosis* or granulocytopenia and is seen most commonly as a result of drug sensitivity or toxicity (Fig. 9–6). *Cyclic neutropenia* is a disease in which there is a precipitous drop in the number of circulating neutrophils at regular intervals, usually a 21-day period.

The Differential (Shilling) Count

The differential white blood cell count also may reflect the severity of an infection (and the response of the host) by demonstrating a change in the ratio between the number of young and adult leukocytes. An increase in young forms of neutrophils with a few lobes or "bands" is called a "shift to the left." Thus, a high neutrophil count occurs with an increase in young cells as a result of a rapid outpouring from the bone marrow in response to an acute need, before cellular growth and differentiation are complete. In depression of bone marrow function there is an increase in the number of immature forms but with a decreased total neutrophil count. This latter reaction has been termed "degenerative shift to the left." Prolongation of this response indicates a poor prognosis. On the other hand, if the total leukocyte count decreases but the neutrophils show more mature forms, it indicates the host is overcoming the infection. Further, reappearance of eosinophils, monocytes, and lymphocytes indicates reduction of the acute stage of infection and likely recovery.

Pernicious anemia is one of the few diseases in which the appearance of a larger number of very mature neutrophils or "shift to the right" is of diagnostic importance. Thus, the presence of large, hypersegmented neutrophils is indicative of folic acid or vitamin B_{12} deficiency.

The appearance of early developmental forms of leukocytes in the blood usually indicates serious illness and, if the immature cells are abnormal, the patient may have leukemia (Figs. 1–20 and 14–45). However, in aleukemic leukemia, it may be necessary to supplement the absolute and differential counts with bone marrow smears. Infectious mononucleosis may also produce atypical lymphocytes in the circulating blood, and a positive sheep cell agglutination (Paul Bunnell) test is confirmatory (pp. 234, 339).

It is apparent that the response of the bone marrow determines the character and number of leukocytes in the peripheral blood. Conversely, the nature of the circulating cells may give a clue as to whether the defense mechanism is adequately responding to the infectious agent or other etiologic factor.

LE Test

The LE test determines the presence of LE factor, an antinuclear autoantibody, in plasma of patients with systemic lupus erythematosus (p. 330). Damaged nuclear material from leukocytes is released and other leukocytes form a characteristic clump or rosette about these LE bodies to phagocytize the structure. A positive LE test is found in approximately 80 percent of the patients with systemic lupus erythematosus and on occasion in patients with rheumatoid arthritis, chronic discoid lupus erythematosus (p. 329), lupoid hepatitis and certain drug reactions.

Platelets

Platelets are derived from fragments of megakaryocytes of the bone marrow and subsequently appear in the peripheral blood as small bodies 2 to 4 microns in diameter. They contain several biochemical substances including serotonin (5-hydroxytryptamine), histamine and thromboplastin. Their chief function is in blood clotting and clot retraction.

Depending upon the laboratory method used, normal values of platelets may range from 200,000 to 400,000 per mm^3. Since methods for the determination of platelets vary among laboratories, it is important to obtain the normal values of the particular laboratory (Table 9–2). Some physiologic variation in numbers of platelets occurs. Like erythrocytes, blood platelets tend to increase in individuals living in high altitudes. Further, the numbers of platelets tend to increase somewhat during the winter months.

Defects of the platelets may be either numerical, functional or both. Increases in numbers of platelets may be physiologic or occur concurrently with certain other diseases, chiefly those which are associated with bone marrow activity of normal hematopoietic tissue such as posthemorrhagic states. Decreases in the number of platelets occur physiologically and when there is destruction, replacement, atrophy or degeneration of the normal hematopoietic tissue, e.g. myelophthisic anemia, most leukemias, infections, drug intoxication, allergy, and other bone marrow diseases. This condition is referred to as secondary thrombocytopenia. In addition, decreased platelets without known or obvious cause are seen in primary (idiopathic) thrombocytopenic purpura. In some instances (thrombocytopathic purpura, thrombocythemia), the platelet count is normal or even increased but the platelets are structurally or functionally abnormal.

Further references to these conditions are made in a following section and on page 411 et seq.

Bone Marrow Examination

Examination of the bone marrow is used to supplement studies of the peripheral blood in the refractory anemias and hemoglobinopathies, thrombocytopenias, leukemias, myeloproliferative disorders, lipid and non-lipid reticuloendothelioses and other hematologic disorders. This procedure should not be carried out if one of the coagulopathies is suspected. Bone marrow samples are obtained by aspiration or open biopsy, usually from the sternum but occasionally from the iliac crest or lateral process of a vertebra. The myelogram is analogous to the differential cell count in that the relative numbers and maturity of the developing blood cells are tabulated. Additionally, the presence of tumor cells in metastatic disease, myeloma, Gaucher's disease, the lymphomas, etc. as well as certain parasitic diseases (malaria, histoplasmosis, etc.) may be identified.

BLOOD COAGULATION AND HEMORRHAGIC DISORDERS

Potential hemorrhagic problems in the dental patient must be recognized prior to clinical treatment (p. 405). Signs and symptoms of some significance include a history of frequent nosebleeds, gingival bleeding of unexplained nature, or a tendency to develop petechiae or bruises of the skin following minor injury. The history of postoperative bleeding following minor wounds or tooth extraction should be considered of some consequence. In particular, oozing of blood from the wound followed by bleeding some hours later are signs indicating further tests. The history should establish whether or not the patient is receiving anticoagulant therapy which could be responsible for the bleeding tendency.

Hemostasis

The recognition and diagnosis of the disorders of the hemostatic mechanism are predicated on a clear understanding of the pathophysiology of bleeding, coagulation and clot lysis.

Primary Hemostasis

Both platelets (thrombocytes) and blood vessels play a significant role in the control of hemorrhage. With disruption of the blood vessel wall, the vessels reflexly constrict and retract, and platelets adhere to the exposed collagen. Once exposed to collagen, the platelets release several active factors (serotonin, adenosine diphosphate or ADP, platelet factor III, etc.) which account for vasoconstriction, aggregation of more platelets and the formation of a loose platelet plug.

In this manner, bleeding is controlled within a few minutes.

Primary hemostasis is therefore dependent upon an adequate number of circulating platelets of good quality and, additionally, of responsive blood vessels with viable endothelium and perivascular connective tissue.

The factors which have been identified as being involved in the clotting mechanism are:

I   Fibrinogen
II   Prothrombin
III   Thromboplastin
IV   Calcium
V   Proaccelerin
VI   No factor assigned
VII   Proconvertin
VIII Antihemophiliac factor (AHF)
IX   Plasma thromboplastin component (PTC)
X   Stuart factor
XI   Plasma thromboplastin antecedent (PTA)
XII   Hageman factor
XIII Fibrin stabilizing factor (FSF)

Coagulation

Secondary hemostasis is initiated by exposure of blood to injured tissue and the release of tissue thromboplastin via the so-called extrinsic pathway. Simultaneously, Hageman factor (XII), upon exposure to collagen, is activated (XIIa) and a series of reactions termed the intrinsic pathway is triggered. The extrinsic and intrinsic systems combine to activate factor X and the common pathway in which prothrombin is converted to thrombin and fibrinogen is converted to fibrin (Fig. 9–7). In this manner, fibrin is deposited in the loose hemostatic plug and, as the fibrin is further polymerized by the action of fibrin stabilizing factor (XIII), a definitive clot is formed which controls further loss of blood.

Fibrinolysis

In the normal circulation, small fragments of fibrin are continuously being deposited on the inner surface of the vessel wall just as circulating platelets function to plug small leaks which constantly appear in the capillaries. This unwanted fibrin is cleared through the activation of plasminogen by an activator enzyme probably produced in the liver. The dissolution of the blood clot at the termination of the healing process occurs by essentially the same mechanism.

Endogenous plasminogen activators are present in trace amounts in endothelium and all body fluids, including saliva, and the lysosomal granules of leukocytes. Conditions of stress with the release of vasoactive amines, fever, shock, infection, lung surgery and metastatic carcinoma of the prostate have been associated with the release of excessive plasminogen activators.

Exogenous plasminogen activators include aspirin and those produced by microorganisms (*e.g.* streptokinase). The "kinases" are sometimes used therapeutically to reduce postoperative edema.

Circulating inhibitors of plasminogen activation (antiplasmin) are probably alpha globulins, produced in the liver. Abnormal fibrinolysis may be inhibited therapeutically by the administration of epsilon aminocaproic acid. This agent has also been used preoperatively in the hemophilia C patient since factors V, VIII and IX appear to be susceptible to the enzymatic action of plasminogen.

Tests for Bleeding and Coagulation Disorders

The diagnosis of hemorrhagic disorders must establish that a possible disturbance exists on the basis of the clinical history and examination; then appropriate screening tests to confirm or rule out the existence of a bleeding problem must be selected.

Tourniquet (Rumpel-Leede) Test

This test is mainly used as a simple screening method to determine vascular integrity. A blood pressure cuff is inflated to the midpoint between systolic and diastolic pressure and held for 5 minutes. The blood pressure

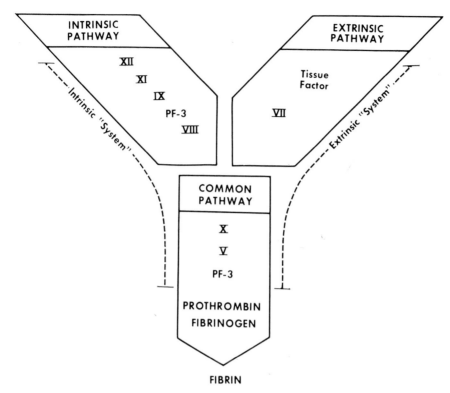

Fig. 9-7. Blood coagulation. The cascade or waterfall hypothesis of blood coagulation (adapted in part from Wintrobe and others) demonstrates the interaction of the 12 plasma clotting factors resulting in the ultimate conversion of fibrinogen into a fibrin clot. The extrinsic system is activated by contact of blood with tissue, releasing tissue thromboplastin which combines with factor VII; the intrinsic system is initiated by Hageman factor contact with exposed collagen in the injured vessel wall and subsequent transformations of factors XI, IX, and VIII. In the common pathway, factor X is activated and combines with factor V, PF3 (platelet factor 3, a phospholipid), and calcium to form prothrombinase, which in turn splits prothrombin into the proteolytic enzyme thrombin. Thrombin converts fibrinogen into soluble fibrin monomer. FSF (XIII) polymerizes the monomer into a stabile, cross-linked fibrin polymer. (From Wintrobe, *Clinical Hematology,* 7th Ed., Philadelphia, Lea & Febiger, 1974.)

cuff is removed and the petechiae are counted after a 5-minute waiting period. Less than 10 petechiae in a 2.5-cm circle on the flexor surface of the forearm is considered normal. This test provides some estimate of capillary fragility and, indirectly, platelet function.

Bleeding Time

Following a standard skin wound made with a special lancet, sterile filter paper is used at 10-second intervals to blot the drops of blood until bleeding stops. Normally, this requires 2 to 6 minutes. This test also provides some measure of vascular integrity and the physical ability of platelets to plug the severed capillaries, but does not differentiate the two conditions. It correlates well with blood prothrombin levels.

Disturbances in the vascular integrity which typically show alterations of these test results include non-thrombocytopenic purpura, severe infectious diseases, drug sensitivity and vitamin C deficiency.

Platelet Counts

Platelets provide an important source of thromboplastin. In addition, they physically plug the severed capillaries and regulate bleeding time. (It should be noted that fibrin clots are necessary to block the bleeding from larger blood vessels.)

Disturbances in platelets, the most common cause of bleeding disorders, may be due to deficiencies in numbers of platelets (thrombocytopenia) or quality of the platelets (thrombasthenia). The most common diseases in this category are primary and secondary thrombocytopenic purpura (p. 412). The frequent association of disturbance in platelet numbers or quality with increased capillary fragility is poorly understood but may be related to the function of platelets to plug small, otherwise insignificant, defects in the capillary wall.

Clot Retraction Time

This test provides an estimate of platelet activity. Blood placed in a test tube will clot and subsequently retract from the serum of the blood beginning within 2 hours. Retraction will be complete within 24 hours. Failure of the blood clot to retract indicates a decreased number of platelets or a failure of the platelets to disintegrate and release thromboplastin.

Partial Thromboplastin Time

This test is especially useful as a screening test for factor VIII and IX deficiencies or circulating anticoagulants. Prolonged test values will be found in relatively severe deficiencies of any of the other coagulation factors of the intrinsic and common pathways (Fig. 9–7). A calcium deficiency (factor IV) of sufficient magnitude to interfere with blood coagulation is highly unlikely.

The normal range of partial thromboplastin time is 35 to 50 sec, with 10-sec increases above normal considered significant. If abnormal values are obtained for this test, additional procedures are required to identify the specific factor that might be involved (p. 216). In addition to deficient or defective platelets, hereditary deficiencies of clotting factors (*e.g.* hemophilia, Christ-

mas disease) must be considered. AHG is the most likely defect to be expected.

Prothrombin Time

This test is designed to evaluate the function of the extrinsic and common pathways (Fig. 9–7). Thus, prothrombin values will be prolonged with deficiencies of factors I, II, V, VII and X as well as in the presence of circulating anticoagulants. Since this test does not reflect disorders involving factors VIII, IX, XI and XII, the partial thromboplastin test should be run concurrently with prothrombin time.

If a clot does not form or appears to be physically defective in this test, fibrinogen deficiency should be suspected.

If prothrombin time is prolonged, procedures may be modified to help identify the specific disorder such as a circulating anticoagulant or heparin, factor V deficiency or factor VII deficiency (Stypven time test).

Whole Blood Clotting Time

This test provides an estimate of all three phases of coagulation but chiefly stage I of the blood clotting mechanism. Normal values (Lee-White, glass tubes) range from 3 to 8 minutes. While not a highly sensitive test, the whole blood clotting time is of value since it is prolonged in severe factor deficiencies other than thrombocytopenia, factor VII and factor XIII defects.

Hemorrhagic diseases of significance to the dentist are listed in Table 9–3. Laboratory findings useful in their diagnosis are given.

Euglobulin Lysis Time

The laboratory evaluation of fibrinolysis is made by determination of the euglobulin lysis time (normal, 2 to 4 hr). A modification of this method has also been used for the estimation of fibrinolytic activity in saliva.

Table 9-3. Hemorrhagic Diatheses

	TT	PC	BT	PTT	PT
Defects of:					
Vascular integrity					
Hereditary hemorrhagic telangiectasia	O				
Vitamin C deficiency	O				
Platelet number					
Thrombocytopenia	●	●	●		
Thrombocythemia	O	●	●		
Platelet function					
Thrombocytopathia	●		●		
Thrombocytasthenia	●		●		
Coagulation factors (hereditary)					
Intrinsic pathway					
VIII (AHF) – Hemophilia A				●	
VIII – Von Willebrand's disease	O		●	O	
IX (PTC) – Hemophilia B				●	
XI (PTA) – Hemophilia C				O	
XII – Hageman factor deficiency				●	
Common pathway					
II – Prothrombin deficiency				●	●
I – Afibrinogenemia			O	●	●
V – Factor V deficiency				●	●
X – Factor X deficiency				O	●
XIII – Factor XIII deficiency				●	●
Extrinsic pathway					
III – No defect recognized					
VII – Factor VII deficiency				●	●
Coagulation factors (acquired)					
Liver disease			O	●	●
Vitamin K deficiency				●	●
Anticoagulant therapy reaction				●	●
Disseminated intravascular coagulopathy				●	●
Fibrinolysis				●	●

TT = Tourniquet test
PC = Platelet count
BT = Bleeding time
PTT = Partial thromboplastin time
PT = Prothrombin time

● Abnormal test O variable test

Disorders of Hemostasis

The hemorrhagic diatheses encompass a broad spectrum of disease entities and clinical conditions of diverse etiology and pathogenesis. These may be acquired or hereditary in origin and grouped according to the particular phase of hemostasis affected: *i.e.* primary hemostasis, blood coagulation or fibrinolysis.

Disorders of primary hemostasis reflect defects of capillary integrity, the supporting connective tissue and/or platelet number and quality.

Blood coagulation disorders are those in which there is an hereditary or acquired defect involving one of the blood clotting factors.

The fibrinolytic disorders are largely acquired although a factor XIII deficiency may result in an unstable, poorly polymerized fibrin clot which is susceptible to fibrinolytic action. Aspirin medications not only interfere with platelet aggregation and the plugging of capillary leaks but activate the fibrinolytic system. Liver disease is often associated with clotting factor abnormalities and reduced antiplasmin levels.

Disturbances in Primary Hemostasis

Thrombocytopenic purpura
Non-thrombocytopenic purpura
Aldrich's syndrome
Thrombocytasthenia
Thrombocytopathia
Thrombocythemia
Vitamin C deficiency
Hereditary hemorrhagic telangiectasia

Disturbances in Blood Coagulation

Hemophilia A
Von Willebrand's disease
Hemophilia B
Hemophilia C
Acquired coagulation defects

Disturbances in Fibrinolysis

Anticoagulant medication reaction
Disseminated intravascular coagulation
Factor XIII deficiency
Liver disease
Circulating endogenous anticoagulants

SERUM CHEMISTRY

The fluid portion (plasma) of the blood contains a remarkable number of substances carried in transport to various parts of the body. If whole blood is allowed to clot, the remaining fluid is called serum. Plasma and serum are almost identical in composition except that in the latter certain of the clotting factors and fibrinogen have been removed with the clot.

The Biochemical Profile

Automation of many of the routine laboratory determinations has become a practicality in many clinical laboratories through advanced instrumentation. With sophisticated instruments such as the Auto-Analyzer or Sequential Multiple Analyzer (SMA 12/60, Technicon Corp.), multiple analyses may be carried out on small samples of various body fluids. For example, approximately 2 ml of serum introduced into the system is split into 12 portions and automatically subjected to the appropriate biochemical reaction, and the results are recorded on a strip-chart recorder. A single sample can be processed in approximately 8 minutes. While automation has permitted obvious savings in time and laboratory personnel, it has also made possible more comprehensive screening of hospital patients on admission and earlier diagnosis of unsuspected disease processes.

The results of the automated analysis are recorded as red pen tracings on a graph (Fig. 9–8*A*–*C*). Shaded areas on the graph illustrate the normal value ranges for each of the 12 parameters usually tested: calcium, inorganic phosphorus, glucose, blood urea nitrogen (BUN), uric acid, cholesterol, total protein, albumin, bilirubin, alkaline phosphatase, lactic dehydrogenase (LDH) and serum glutamic oxaloacetic transaminase (SGOT). In this manner, a biochemical profile is obtained with those findings which deviate from the normal range readily apparent. Further, specific patterns (profiles) of disease, not apparent with single labora-

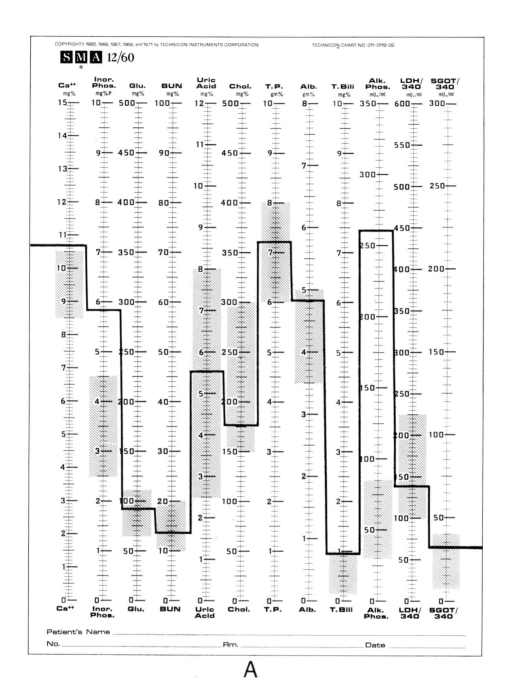

A

Fig. 9-8*A*. The normal pattern of a 12-year-old child. The increased alkaline phosphatase and inorganic phosphorus are due to bone growth. The alkaline phosphatase is heat labile, and therefore bone in origin.

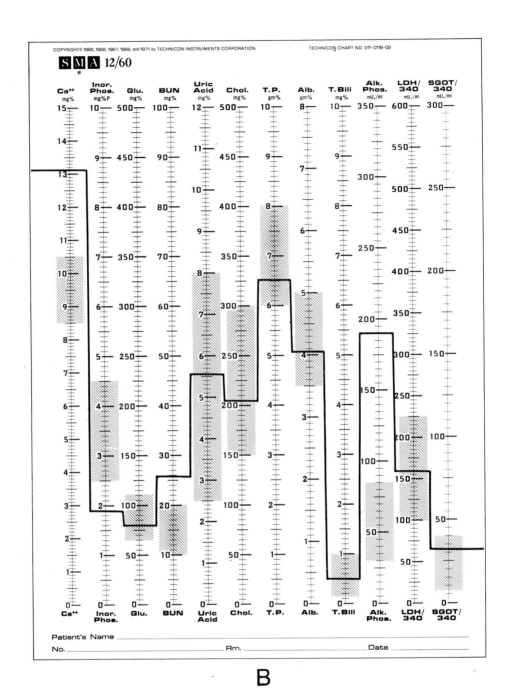

B

Fig. 9-8B. Pattern of primary hyperparathyroidism. The elevated calcium, decreased phosphorus, and elevated alkaline phosphatase are hallmarks of this disease. The alkaline phosphatase is heat labile, and therefore bone in origin. The slight elevation in BUN is due to renal calcinosis.

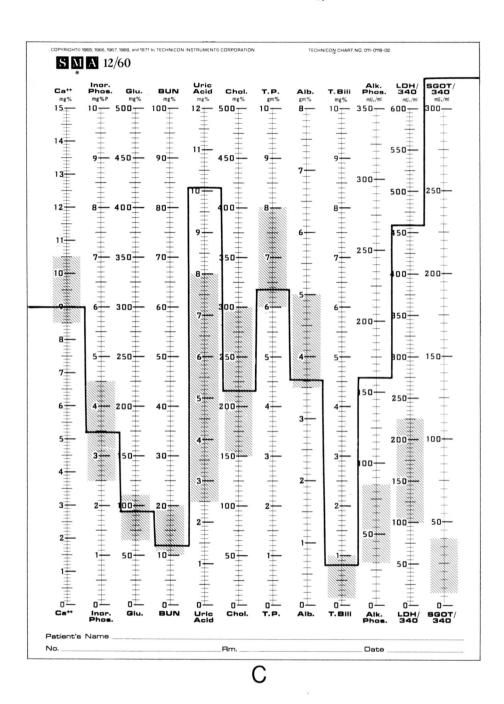

C

Fig. 9-8C. Pattern frequently seen in infectious mononucleosis with anicteric hepatitis. The elevated liver enzymes with a normal bilirubin are characteristic. The elevated uric acid is due to white cell proliferation. (Fig. 9-8 from Preston, J. A. and Troxel, D. B., *Biochemical Profiling in Diagnostic Medicine,* copyright 1971 by Technicon Instrument Corporation, Tarrytown, New York.)

tory tests, can be recognized. For example, the influence of bone growth on profiles obtained in normal children is reflected in the markedly elevated alkaline phosphatase and inorganic phosphate levels. Other characteristic patterns are found in the elderly, during pregnancy and associated with specific disease states.

Plasma Proteins

The chief plasma proteins, albumin, globulin and fibrinogen, serve a number of specific functions. These include maintenance of osmotic pressure, buffering, the transport of hormones such as thyroxin, insulin and steroids, the transport of antibodies, and blood clotting. Thus, a number of congenital, inflammatory, infectious, neoplastic, and metabolic disease processes will show associated changes in the quantity and/or quality of the plasma proteins.

Normal Serum Protein Values

Normal values for total serum proteins are 6 to 8 gm per 100 ml. Normal values for the individual proteins are: albumin 4.0 to 5.0 gm per 100 ml; globulin 2.0 to 3.0 gm per 100 ml; albumin/globulin ratio 1.5 to 2.5:1.

The globulin fraction may be further separated by electrophoresis into alpha 1, alpha 2, beta 1, beta 2 and gamma globulins. The gamma globulin levels reflect antibody formation.

Disturbances in the quantity of the serum proteins are called *dysproteinemias* while those characterized by chemically abnormal proteins are referred to as *paraproteinemias*.

The Dysproteinemias

Quantitative defects in the serum proteins are most commonly seen secondarily to another basic disease process. Rarely, primary

Table 9-4. Blood Chemistry Report Form.

NAME			Room No.	Hosp. No.	
Physician					
Procedure	Normal	Patient	Procedure	Normal	Patient
Total Protein	6.0-8.0 gm%		Glucose	80-120 mg%	
Albumin	3.5-5.5 gm%		Amylase	80-150 Units	
Globulin	1.3-3.3 gm%		Lipase	0.2-1.5 Units	
Fibrinogen	.2 to .6 gm %		Uric Acid	2-5.6 mg%	
A—G Ratio	1.5-2.5 to 1		NPN	25-40 mg%	
Total Bilirubin	0.2-1.0 mg%		BUN	8-18 mg%	
VanDenBergh direct	0.0-0.2 mg%		Calcium	9-11 mg%	
VanDenBergh indirect	0.2-0.8 mg%		PBI	4-8 mcg	
Cholesterol	150-250 mg%		CO$_2$ Combining Power	55-75 vol.%	
Esters	70-80%		Creatinine	1.0-2.0 mg%	
Alk. Phos.	2.2-8.6 S.G.R. Units		Transaminase	4-40 Units-SGOT	
Acid Phos.	0.0-2.0 S.G.R. Units			5-35 Units-SGPT	
Prothrombin	90-100%		Sodium	135-150 meg/1	
Icterus Index	4 to 6 Units		Potassium	4.0-5.5 meg1/	
BSP	0-6%		Bicarbonite	55-65 mg%	
Thymol	2-4 Units		Gamma Glob.	.5 to .7 mg%	
Ceph. Floc. 24 Hours	neg.		Chlorides	570-620 mg%	
Ceph. Floc. 48 Hours	1 plus		PSP 1 hour	40-50%	
Phosphorus	Adults - 3-4.5		PSP 2 hour	30-40% ret'd	
Phosphorus	Children - 5-6.5				
Technician		Director of Laboratories			
Date Collected:		Date Rec'd:			

CHEMISTRY

types representing congenital deficiencies (agammaglobulinemia, afibrinogenemia) of these proteins are encountered.

Disturbances in the total serum proteins occur because of inadequate protein intake, inadequate absorption from the gastrointestinal tract, inadequate protein synthesis in the liver, or excessive excretion of protein in the urine. It follows that reductions in the total serum proteins and hypoalbuminemia are seen in starvation, intestinal diseases (sprue), liver diseases (cirrhosis), and kidney disease (nephrotic syndrome). Marked edema due to decreased osmotic pressure characterizes these conditions.

Elevated levels of albumin are not seen except in cases of dehydration or the hemoconcentration of shock.

Hyperglobulinemia

Changes in the serum globulins usually are manifest as increases in one or more of the fractions. While these alterations will not ordinarily provide a definitive diagnosis, they do provide important information relative to the general body response to a given disease process and often suggest the basic pathologic process present.

Increases in the alpha globulins are often associated with acute febrile processes and wasting diseases (*e.g.* tuberculosis, carcinoma). Increased alpha globulins associated with hypoalbuminemia occur in nephrosis, acute rheumatic fever and other acute infections.

Increases in the beta globulins are seen in cases of increased serum lipids such as hepatitis, cirrhosis and probably arteriosclerosis.

The gamma globulins show an elevated response to the antigenic stimuli of most infectious agents. Conditions showing elevated gamma globulin include cirrhosis, hepatitis, lupus erythematosus, rheumatoid arthritis, multiple myeloma, sarcoidosis, myelogenous leukemia, monocytic leukemia and Hodgkin's disease.

Agammaglobulinemia

This is an hereditary deficiency of gamma globulin. Since these patients are unable to form antibodies they are particularly susceptible to infectious agents.

The Paraproteinemias

Qualitative disturbances in the serum proteins are referred to as paraproteinemias. They are identified by their characteristic electrophoretic patterns and other tests.

Bence Jones Protein

The best known of the paraproteins is Bence Jones protein which occurs almost exclusively in multiple myeloma (Fig. 15–53) and macroglobulinemia. This protein, which is similar to gamma globulin, is of relatively low molecular weight and thus readily spills over into the urine. It is easily identified in the urine since the protein coagulates at 40 to 60° C and then disappears upon boiling.

Cryoglobulins

The cryoglobulins are abnormal serum proteins which gel below 30° C and are generally found in association with multiple myeloma and hyperglobulinemia.

Macroglobulinemia of Waldenström

This condition is characterized by abnormally large globulin molecules in the blood found in association with several diseases such as myeloma and other dysproteinemias.

Myoglobulinemia

This refers to the presence of muscle proteins in the blood. These proteins are most easily identified in the urine. Since the molecules are relatively large, kidney blockage and failure develop in many instances. Myoglobulinemias may occur following severe muscle injury (rhabdomyolysis, p. 292) and in a rare hereditary condition called *hereditary idiopathic nocturnal hemoglobinuria*.

C-Reactive Protein

An abnormal beta globulin fraction called C-reactive protein may be identified in the serum in cases of inflammatory or infectious processes. It is an especially sensitive indicator of the progress of rheumatic fever. Recent studies have shown C-reactive protein to be elevated in periodontal disease. Using commercially available C-reactive protein antiserum mixed with an equal amount of the patient's serum in a test tube, a precipitate is formed in positive cases. The size of the flocculus in the test tube is reported as 1+ to 4+ and is used as a measure of the presence or absence of inflammation.

Serum Calcium

Calcium is present in the blood serum in a protein-bound form and a diffusible (ionizable) form. The latter is highly labile, entering in equilibrium with the extravascular compartments and bone. Values for serum calcium measure chiefly the protein-bound component and range from 9 to 11 mg per 100 ml.

Parathyroid hormone mobilizes calcium from the bones when the serum calcium level falls. Reciprocal changes in serum phosphorus occur through the direct effect of parathormone on tubular reabsorption of phosphates. Conversely, calcium spills over into the urine when serum calcium values rise above the normal threshold levels.

Examples of disturbances in serum calcium values are found in the following conditions:

Hypercalcemia

1° hyperparathyroidism
2° hyperparathyroidism
1°, 2° malignant bone tumors
Vitamin D intoxication
Milk-alkali syndrome
Immobilization
Polycythemia vera
Sarcoidosis
Idiopathic hypercalcemia

Hypocalcemia

Idiopathic hypoparathyroidism
2° hypoparathyroidism
   (2° to surgery or irradiation)
Rickets
Renal rickets (osteomalacia)
Steatorrhea, celiac disease

Serum Phosphorus

Inorganic phosphate is present in the serum as a reciprocal of the serum calcium (Ca/P ratio) and is regulated in part by the phosphaturic effect of parathyroid hormone on the kidney tubules, *i.e.* the hormone inhibits renal tubular reabsorption of phosphate. Thus, disturbances in serum phosphate levels occur in renal disease (nephritis, de Fanconi syndrome, secondary hyperparathyroidism), parathyroid disease and other conditions in which there are defects in calcium balance. Serum phosphate is decreased in primary hyperparathyroidism, rickets, osteomalacia, and vitamin D-resistant rickets ("phosphate diabetes," hypophosphatemia). Elevated values are found in hypoparathyroidism, renal insufficiency and hypervitaminosis D.

Serum Alkaline Phosphatase

Metabolic bone activity, such as active growth, causes elevation in serum alkaline phosphatase. For this reason, normal values will be considerably higher in children than in adults and higher in generalized bone disease than in disease involving only a single bone. Elevated values for serum alkaline phosphatase are found in hyperparathyroidism, Paget's disease of bone, osteomalacia, rickets, osteosarcoma and tumors metastatic to bone. Decreased values are found in hypophosphatasia (hypophosphatasemia), chronic anemia, scurvy, and hypothyroidism.

Serum Acid Phosphatase

Abnormally elevated values of serum acid phosphatase are diagnostic of metastatic carcinoma of the prostate. Elevated serum acid phosphatase is also seen in the adult form of Gaucher's disease.

Serum Amylase

Determinations of serum amylase are of value in the diagnosis of mumps (epidemic parotitis), acute pancreatitis and cystic fibrosis of the pancreas.

It is of interest that the saliva normally contains high levels of amylase and that inflammation of the salivary glands may be accompanied by significant elevation of amylase in the serum. Electrophoretic studies have confirmed that the increased serum amylase in such cases is derived from the salivary enzyme. Sialolithiasis, which is accompanied by sialadenitis of the blocked gland, may also show some elevation of serum amylase.

Marked elevations of serum amylase are seen following therapeutic or accidental irradiation of the salivary glands and it has been suggested that this laboratory test may be useful as a screening test and biologic indicator in radiation exposure of these tissues. Elevated serum amylase values may also occur in intestinal obstruction, postoperatively in laparotomy patients, and following the administration of certain of the opiates.

Blood Urea Nitrogen (BUN)

By-products of protein metabolism appear in the circulating blood in increased amounts in advanced renal disease. The BUN test is preferred to the non-protein nitrogen test. The normal BUN value is 9 to 19 mg per 100 ml.

Carbon Dioxide Combining Power

This test is useul in suspected disturbances in acid-base balance. The range of normal values for carbon dioxide combining power is 21 to 28 mEq/L or 50 to 65 vol percent. Lowered values are seen in metabolic acidosis, diabetic acidosis, diarrhea, Addison's disease, hyperventilation (respiratory alkalosis) or other conditions in which there is excess loss of carbon dioxide from the lungs or accumulation of acidic products in the circulation. Elevated carbon dioxide values suggestive of acidosis are found in severe respiratory diseases such as emphysema.

Serum Electrolytes

Values for serum chlorides, serum sodium and serum potassium should be determined when there is reason to suspect a disturbance in electrolyte balance (Table 9–5). Normal values for each of these are given in the Appendix. Examples of specific conditions in which disturbances in these electrolytes may be expected include: elevated serum chloride in kidney disease and dehydration; decreased serum chloride due to vomiting and diarrhea. Elevated serum sodium occurs in dehydration and as the result of corticoid administration. Sodium deficiency may result from excessive perspiration, kidney disease and Addison's disease (Figs. 11–18 and 14–13). Elevated serum potassium occurs with adrenal cortical insufficiency and renal failure, whereas potassium deficiency results from diarrhea and diabetic acidosis.

EXAMINATION OF LIVER FUNCTION

Tests of Liver Function

A large variety of laboratory tests reflect, directly or indirectly, the complexities of liver function. Serum chemistry and enzymology for serum proteins, transaminases, alkaline phosphatase, uric acid and BUN; blood clotting tests for fibrinogen, prothrombin and antiplasmin; and certain tests of endocrine function may all be modified by the state of liver function or disease. The more common tests of liver function are listed below, with their normal laboratory values and clinical significance.

Icterus Index

This test measures the approximate concentration of bilirubin in the serum and is used principally to follow patient progress in

Table 9-5. Electrolyte Balance Report Form.

NAME			Room No.		Hosp. No.	

Physician

Meq./L	Normal Electrolytes	Patient Electrolytes	Meq./L
200			200
175			175
155	Cation Anion	Cation Anion	155
125	Na 142 HCO₃ 27		125
100			100
75			75
50	Cl. 103		50
25	Ca 5.0 Sulfate Phos.		25
0	K 5.0 Mg 3.0 Prot'n 20 Organic Acid 10		0

Technician   Director of Laboratories

Date   (SEE OTHER SIDE)

ELECTROLYTE BALANCE

Normal Electrolytes			Patient Electrolytes		
CATIONS	MG%	MEQ/L	CATIONS	MG%	MEQ/L
Sodium	315-350	135-150	Sodium		
Potassium	16-22	4.0-5.5	Potassium		
Calcium	9-12	4.5-5.8	Calcium		
Magnesium	1.6-2.9	1.4-2.4	Magnesium		
Total	358 mg %	155 |mEq/L	Total		
Anions	mg %	mEq/L	Anions	mg %	mEq/L
Bicarbonate	55-65	25-29	Bicarbonate		
Chlorides	570-620	98-106	Chlorides		
Phosphates	3.0-4.5	1.7-2.6	Phosphates		
Sulfates	.3-2.0	.2-1.3	Sulfates		
Organic Acid	14-28	4-8	Organic Acid		
Proteinate	6-8,000	14.6-19.4	Proteinate		
TOTAL	6,948 mg %	155 mEq/L	TOTAL		

Table 9-6. Serology Report Form.

NAME		Room No.	Hosp. No.
Physician			
Procedure	**Report**	**Procedure**	**Report**
Kline		Heterophile	
VDRL		Guinea Pig	
Mazzini		Coombs Direct	
Wassermann		Coombs Indirect	
Kahn (Qual)		Antistreptolysin	
Kahn (Quant)		Cold Agglutins	
Kolmer		A-Z Pregnancy	
VDRL (Quant)			
Technician		Director of Laboratories	
Date Collected:			
Date Rec'd:			

SEROLOGY

cases of jaundice. Normal values range from 4 to 6 icterus units.

Serum Bilirubin (Direct and Indirect van den Bergh)

The direct van den Bergh reaction measures the serum concentration of bilirubin glucuronides which are elevated in obstructive jaundice. The indirect van den Bergh reaction measures unconjugated bilirubin which is elevated in hemolytic and neonatal jaundice, the latter principally because of Rh, ABO or other blood group incompatibility. In hepatitis, both conjugated and unconjugated bilirubin levels are elevated. Normal values of total serum bilirubin in adults range from 0.1 to 0.8 mg/100 ml Malloy-Evelyn units. Direct values are normally 0.1 to 0.2 mg/100 ml and the indirect values are 0.1 to 0.6 mg/100 ml. Normal neonate values are several times higher, especially in the first week after birth.

Urinary Urobilinogen

Measurement of urinary urobilinogen, the end-product of bilirubin metabolism, is useful in the detection of early hepatitis. Since the injured liver cells are unable to remove urobilinogen from the portal blood, it is excreted by the kidneys in increasing amounts as the hepatitis progresses. In obstructive jaundice, few or no bile pigments are carried to the intestine and thus fecal urobilinogen is decreased, thereby accounting for the typical clay-colored stools of obstructive jaundice. Normal values are 0.1 to 1.0 Ehrlich units/2 hr.

Cephalin-Cholesterol Flocculation

Now rarely used, this test is an indication of increased globulin and decreased albumin in the serum. Thus, a positive test may indicate hepatitis, cirrhosis or hepatic necrosis. Normal values are expressed as negative or 1+ reactions.

Thymol Turbidity

The thymol turbidity test is an indicator of hepatitis much like the cephalin-cholesterol flocculation test, but additionally it is reactive to the elevated serum lipoproteins associated with nephrosis. Normal values are expressed as 0 to 5 Shank-Hoagland units. In most laboratories, the thymol turbidity test and cephalin-cholesterol flocculation have been largely superseded by other methods.

Bromsulphalein (BSP) Test

This test measures the excretory function of the liver following injection of BSP dye. Normal values show less than 6 percent retention of the dye in the serum after 45 minutes. In cirrhosis, up to 45 percent retention of the dye may occur.

Liver Function Disorders

It is recognized that hepatic disease may have related oral manifestations: disorders of blood coagulation and fibrinolysis complicating oral surgical procedures; pigmentations of the skin, mucous membranes and teeth; transmission of serum hepatitis (p. 54); and even a possible relationship to oral cancer. Such oral conditions have been associated with hepatic cirrhosis, obstructive jaundice, hemolytic jaundice, vitamin K deficiency, hemosiderosis and hemochromatosis. In addition, disorders of the reticuloendothelial system and other metabolic disturbances may exhibit hepatomegaly or hepatosplenomegaly with oral involvement.

Signs and symptoms of disease of the liver or biliary tract include jaundice, clay-colored stools, abdominal pain or "colic," bleeding diatheses, spider angiomas of sun-exposed skin, esophageal varices, hemorrhoids, caput medusae or collateral veins around the umbilicus, and hepatomegaly.

The oral examination will sometimes reveal jaundice or icterus, most evident in sclera of the eyes and ventral surface of the tongue, spontaneous gingival bleeding or postoperative hemorrhage.

Hepatic Cirrhosis

Replacement of liver parenchymal cells by scar tissue (cirrhosis) may follow toxic liver damage (from alcoholism, carbon tetrachloride exposure, anesthesia, hypersensitivity to drugs, etc.), specific infections (hepatitis, syphilis, schistosomiasis), cardiovascular disease and metabolic disturbances. Types of cirrhosis include portal (Laennec's) cirrhosis, postnecrotic cirrhosis, biliary cirrhosis and cardiac cirrhosis.

With progressive loss of functional liver cells in cirrhosis, biosynthesis of blood coagulation factors is impaired (p. 414).

Vitamin K Deficiency

The role of this vitamin in the biosynthesis of the vitamin K dependent coagulation factors in the liver is discussed on page 414. Normal bile production and excretion are required for normal absorption of the fat-soluble vitamins A, D and K.

Obstructive Jaundice

Obstruction of the hepatic or common bile ducts by gallstones or tumor causes pain or biliary colic, vomiting, nausea and other gastrointestinal symptoms. Jaundice, resulting from absorption of bilirubin and bile salts into the circulating blood, may follow according to the degree of occlusion and the functional capacity of the gallbladder.

Hemolytic Jaundice

Abnormal destruction of red blood cells (hemolytic anemia, p. 410) may produce mild jaundice; however, if there is additionally primary hepatic disease jaundice may be severe. The hemolytic disorders include the hereditary hemoglobinopathies (sickle cell anemia, thalassemia, p. 409), immune disorders (autoimmune hemolytic disease, erythroblastosis fetalis, p. 154), and hemolysis associated with physical and chemical agents (lead poisoning, burns, antimalarial drugs, etc.).

Hemosiderosis

In systemic hemosiderosis, generalized accumulations of hemosiderin pigment are found in various tissues, including those of the oral cavity. The condition is caused by increased absorption of iron (seen with high dietary intake, alcoholism or cirrhosis) or by increased red blood cell destruction (as in the hemolytic anemias or transfusion reactions).

Hemochromatosis

Like hemosiderosis, hemochromatosis is an iron storage disorder; however, the disease produces extensive damage in various organs and pigmentation of the skin. The combination of hepatomegaly, pancreas involvement with diabetes mellitus and skin pigmentation is termed "bronze diabetes" (p. 321).

Hepatosplenomegaly

Enlargements of the liver and/or spleen may accompany several systemic and metabolic diseases of concern to the dentist. Hepatomegaly is caused by (1) alterations in the flow of blood or bile, (2) infiltration of metabolic substances, or (3) reticuloendo-

thelial cell disorders. Enlargements of the spleen commonly occur in conjunction with liver disorders, numerous infections, blood dyscrasias and the reticuloendothelioses.

EXAMINATION OF THE URINE

The routine urinalysis provides information of a qualitative and semiquantitative nature (Table 9–8). Volume, color, pH, specific gravity, protein content, presence of ketone bodies, sediment and urinary glucose determinations are useful as screening tests for a wide spectrum of diseases. Abnormal findings in regard to any of these factors should be confirmed by repeating the urinalysis. The cause and significance of abnormalities are then established by additional, more specific diagnostic procedures. A wide variety of qualitative and quantitative tests are available for the demonstration of specific substances in the urine.

Rapid Tests

So-called dip-and-read tests for the rapid screening of the various body fluids are available commercially. Most utilize urine, although serum, plasma, whole blood or stools may also be examined with these reagent systems. Appropriate reagents are incorporated into small tapes which are dipped into the fluid being examined and then compared with color charts for the laboratory value (Fig. 9–16). Tapes are available for

Hepatomegaly	*Splenomegaly*
Congestive heart failure	Histoplasmosis
Obstructive jaundice	Malaria
Amyloidosis	Tuberculosis
Glycogen storage disease	Infectious mononucleosis
Lymphomas and leukemia	Hepatic cirrhosis
Gaucher's disease	Hemolytic anemias
Histoplasmosis	Pernicious anemia
Letterer-Siwe disease	Iron deficiency anemia
Hepatitis	Thrombocytopenic purpura
Infectious mononucleosis	Niemann-Pick disease
Hemochromatosis	Gaucher's disease
	Histiocytosis X
	Lupus erythematosus
	Amyloidosis
	Polycythemia vera

Table 9-8. Urinalysis Report Form.

NAME				
Physician		Room No.	Hosp. No.	
Color		Microscopic:		
Character		White Cells		
Reaction		Red Cells		
Sp. Gravity		Epith Cells		
Albumin		Casts		
Sugar		Bacteria		
Acetone		Mucous		
Diacetic Acid		Crystals		
Bile				
Urob. Titer				
Technician		Director of Laboratories		
Date Collected:		Date Rec'd:		

URINALYSIS

single tests (*e.g.* Tes-Tape for urinary glucose, Eli Lilly) or for multiple tests (*e.g.* Bili-Labstix for urinary pH, protein, glucose, ketone bodies, bilirubin and occult blood, Ames Co.). Other rapid dip-and-read or tablet tests are used for phenylketonuria, salicylate intoxication, blood urea nitrogen (BUN), etc.

Urinary Volume

Normal urinary output of an adult male ranges from 1,200 to 1,500 ml per 24 hours. Decreased volume (oliguria, < 500 ml) occurs in acute glomerulonephritis, impaired renal function, congestive heart failure, severe burns, diarrhea and other conditions characterized by dehydration. Increased urinary output (polyuria, > 2,000 ml) is seen in diabetes mellitus, diabetes insipidus, with diuretic therapy, and in certain stages of chronic glomerulonephritis.

Color of the Urine

The normal color of the urine is a light amber. It may be modified by the degree of concentration and by the presence of hemoglobin, bile pigments, pus or fat.

The urine will appear red if significant numbers of red blood cells, hemoglobin or porphyrins are present. Intact red blood cells generally indicate hemorrhage somewhere in the urinary tract, whereas hemoglobinuria suggests hemolysis of red cells in the circulating blood or possibly in the kidney. Porphyrins in the urine (porphyrinuria) give it a bright red color which fluoresces in ultraviolet light. Acquired porphyria has been reported following ingestion of certain fungicides and chemical agents. Congenital porphyria is characterized by red urine, photodermatitis and erythrodontia (p. 154).

Bilirubin in the urine may appear as various shades of yellow-brown to dark brown or black depending on its concentration. It may be present because of hepatitis, obstructive biliary diseases and hemolysis. A faint fluorescence is seen in ultraviolet light.

In diabetes mellitus, the urine may be a pale green. Black urine may indicate malignant melanoma. In addition, a variety of drugs as well as vitamin C spill over into the urine, giving it a characteristic color.

Urinary pH

The pH of the urine is slightly acid. Increased pH occurs in renal insufficiency, potassium deficiency, and systemic alkalosis (p. 227). An acid pH of the urine is found in acidosis (diabetic coma) and prolonged fevers.

Urine Specific Gravity

The normal specific gravity of urine ranges from 1.003 to 1.030. Specific gravity determinations reflect the concentration of substances dissolved in urine. This is increased in simple dehydration. Increased concentrations of glucose and proteins seen in diabetes mellitus and nephrosis, respectively, cause an elevated specific gravity. The specific gravity of urine is decreased in diabetes insipidus and acute nephritis in which there is reduced concentration of urine.

Urinary Sediments

Various cells, crystals, and casts in the urinary sediment may suggest the presence of disease, usually in the kidney or urinary tract. Normally, desquamated epithelial cells, a few leukocytes and bacteria, and oxalate, phosphate and urate crystals are found in the sediment.

Pus cells, red blood cells, cystine or tyrosine crystals and casts are considered abnormal and require additional studies. Red blood cells are seen in the sediment in urinary tract bleeding and in glomerulonephritis. Red cell casts, leukocyte casts, and fatty, waxy, hyaline or granular casts may be of significance in certain renal diseases.

Urinary Protein

Proteinuria in significant quantities may indicate increased glomerular permeability to serum proteins and is seen in several renal diseases and other disease states such as multiple myeloma. Albumin, of smaller molecular weight than globulin, filters through the glomerulus more readily than globulin. Thus, proteinuria is often called albuminuria since only about one-tenth of the protein is globulin. Bence Jones protein may be demonstrated in the urine in most cases of multiple myeloma and macroglobulinemia (p. 225). Protein may appear in the urine in congestive heart failure or following a large meal.

Urinary Glucose

See Tests for Pancreatic Function (p. 245).

IMMUNOLOGY AND SEROLOGY

Immunologic and serologic laboratory procedures based on the presence of immune substances in various body fluids and tissues are utilized for the detection and measurement of antibodies in infectious diseases, autoimmune diseases, immunologic disorders, and hypersensitivity states. These methods may be employed directly in the identification of microorganisms or, in cases such as syphilis and viral infections where the organism is not readily isolated, the effects of the agent on the host (antibody production) can be measured indirectly. Additionally, several skin tests also utilize the principle of antigen-antibody response in tests for allergy, hypersensitivity and immunity.

Examples of immunologic and serologic tests of diagnostic importance are given below, with their clinical applications.

Agglutination Tests

Tests of this type are employed as a rapid means of detecting serum antibodies or specific microorganisms or their products. In essence, slide agglutination tests are based on antigen-antibody reactions in which the patient's serum, thought to contain a specific antibody, is mixed with a suspension containing a known antigen. Tests of this general type are used in blood typing, syphilis (VDRL) testing and identification of certain bacteria.

Latex Agglutination Test

Rheumatoid factor can be demonstrated in the blood, joint fluids and tissues of most patients with rheumatoid arthritis with the latex agglutination test. Latex particles coated with human or rabbit IgG agglutinate with the antigamma globulin antibodies (antiantibodies) or rheumatoid factor of the test material.

Complement-Fixation Tests

These tests are based upon the use of serum known to contain specific antibodies which may be mixed with a suspension of the material thought to contain the pathogenic agent (antigen). The resulting antigen-antibody complex binds and inactivates (fixes) the complement present in the serum. This method is also used to determine the presence of antibodies in the patient's serum against known antigens. These tests are especially useful in the identification of viral infections and syphilis.

Heterophil Agglutination Test (Paul Bunnell Test)

In this diagnostic test for infectious mononucleosis, agglutinins (heterophil antibodies) against sheep red blood cells are demonstrated in the patient's serum. Titers up to 1:28 are found normally in serum, whereas in infectious mononucleosis titers of 1:224 or higher are considered positive if the clinical findings are consistent with the diagnosis.

Monospot Slide Test

A commercially available kit is available as a rapid screening test for infectious mon-

onucleosis. Horse instead of sheep erythrocytes are used.

Immunoelectrophoresis Tests

In this method, the serum to be analyzed is separated by electrophoresis (see p. 224) and various antisera are applied. Precipitin lines are formed as antigens and antibodies diffuse toward each other.

Immunofluorescence (Fluorescent Antibody) Tests

Antibodies which are coupled by covalent bonds to fluorescein, a fluorescent dye, react with their specific antigens and can be demonstrated with fluorescent microscopy. Thus, this method can be used to demonstrate antigens in or outside of cells—bacteria, rickettsia, viruses, protozoa, tissue antigens, hormones and enzymes.

Fluorescent antibody tests are also valuable diagnostic tools to supplement the clinical examination and tissue biopsy for the differential diagnosis of several vesiculobullous and connective tissue diseases. These tests are diagnostic for pemphigus (p. 390), bullous pemphigoid, benign mucous membrane (cicatricial) pemphigoid and dermatitis herpetiformis (p. 386). While less specific for chronic discoid and systemic lupus erythematosus (p. 330), bullous and erosive lichen planus (p. 389), and porphyria, the tests are nevertheless helpful in the total evaluation of these difficult diagnostic problems. Because the specimens require special handling (e.g. quick-freezing), the procedures are best managed by the dermatologist or immunologist.

The indirect fluorescence test is used for the detection of unknown antibody including autoantibodies and isoantibodies in the serum (immunofluorescent serology). The direct fluorescence test is used to demonstrate bound immunoglobulins and complement by its interaction with labeled antihuman immunoglobulin and complement conjugates in the tissue biopsy (immunohistology).

The most reliable diagnostic test for the infectious stages of syphilis (chancre, mucous patch) is the demonstration of *Treponema pallidum* by dark-field examination. In the absence of primary or secondary lesions, syphilis can be diagnosed only by the use of one of several serologic tests. Most of these tests rely on the demonstration of syphilis reagin, an antibody-like substance formed in response to the microorganism. The serologic tests for syphilis are unlikely to be positive during the incubation period of the disease.

Common serologic tests for the diagnosis of syphilis are the Wassermann (complement-fixation test) and the Kline, Kahn, Eagle, Hinton, Mazzini and VDRL (Venereal Disease Research Laboratory) tests. These latter are precipitation (flocculation) tests. An additional test of value is the *Treponema pallidum* immobilization test which may be used when a suspected false-positive result has been obtained with the routine tests. A number of diseases (severe febrile diseases, upper respiratory infections, measles, chickenpox, infectious hepatitis, infectious mononucleosis, disseminated lupus erythematosus and narcotic addiction) may give false-positive results. If the biologic false-positive serology persists over an extended period of time, sarcoidosis, malignant lymphoma or collagen disease should be ruled out (see also pp. 327, 338 and 340).

Miscellaneous Diagnostic Skin Tests

Skin tests are occasionally useful for the dentist or his consultants. Performed in the office of the appropriate physician (allergist, dermatologist), skin tests are usually requested when a specific diagnosis is to be confirmed or ruled out.

Most skin tests will involve intracutaneous injection, transcutaneous administration or patch tests. In the intracutaneous injection, the appropriate fluid is introduced under the epithelium but not into the subcutis.

With the transcutaneous type of test, small scratches are made in the epidermis and the test fluid (usually an allergen) is applied to the scratch. For patch tests, the test substance is applied directly to the intact skin.

Most positive skin test reactions represent one of the following:

1. *Toxin-antitoxin neutralization*—Erythema develops within 12 to 72 hours unless the injected toxin is neutralized by circulating antibodies. Examples are the Schick test for susceptibility for diphtheria and the Dick test for susceptibility to scarlet fever.
2. *Immediate reaction (anaphylactic reaction)*—Reactions occur within 5 to 20 minutes as an erythema or wheal and then disappear, usually within 1 hour. Immediate reactions, associated with circulating antibodies, are characteristically seen in various allergies and horse serum sensitivity.
3. *Delayed hypersensitivity (tuberculin reaction)*—Signs of induration and erythema appear in 24 to 48 hours and occasionally last for several days. Indicative of cell-mediated hypersensitivity, the tuberculin reaction is utilized in the diagnosis of several infectious diseases of bacterial, viral, mycotic, protozoan and metazoan origin. The test material is ordinarily an extract or a filtrate of the cultured organism or tissue obtained from a patient known to have the disease.

Mantoux Test

The classical model for delayed hypersensitivity, this test involves the intradermal injection of PPD (purified protein derivative). An area of induration 0.5 cm in diameter after 48 hours is considered positive, *i.e.* the patient has had experience with *Mycobacterium tuberculosis* but does not necessarily have active tuberculosis.

Kveim Test

This test for sarcoidosis involves the intracutaneous injection of a saline suspension prepared from lymph nodes of patients with known sarcoidosis (p. 338).

Histoplasmin Test

Used for the diagnosis of histoplasmosis (p. 241), the test material is derived from a culture filtrate of *Histoplasma capsulatum*.

Cat-Scratch Antigen Test

In suspected cat-scratch disease (benign lymphoreticulosis, p. 239), antigen is prepared from heat-treated suppurative material obtained from a known case of the disease. A positive reaction occurs in most cases within 48 hours.

Patch Tests

Test materials may be placed in direct contact with the skin in cases of suspected contact dermatitis (dermatitis venenata) or contact stomatitis (stomatitis venenata, p. 392). It should be noted that the suspected agent (1) may simply act as an irritant or (2) act as an antigen or hapten and induce a cell-mediated reaction after repeated exposure or prolonged contact. Examples of common contact allergens are nickel, *Rhus* antigen (poison-ivy), lipstick and other cosmetics, and medicaments such as local anesthetic solutions, antihistamines and other topical agents.

Reactions to Dental Materials

Although rarely proven, hypersensitivity to denture or filling materials is occasionally suspected. Most cases are probably actually due to physical or microbial irritation of the mucous membrane in contact with the material in question. Nevertheless, the patient may insist that an allergy exists or, on occasion, the patient's physician may refer the patient to the dentist with that clinical diagnosis. In such cases, a patch test may be performed. The test material is placed in direct contact with skin of the inner surface of the forearm, covered with a layer of gauze or cellophane, and held with adhesive tape. After 24 to 48 hours the skin is examined for evidence of erythema or other reaction.

Care should be taken to avoid misinterpretation of local irritation because of the physical nature of the material being tested. In cases of suspected acrylic allergy, the actual denture or scrapings from the denture may be used for testing. If the reaction is considered to be positive, the test should be repeated and additional material of another brand of recently cured acrylic should also be examined with a view toward choosing a restorative material to which the patient is not sensitive.

On occasion, the dental patient will give a history of being "allergic" to local anesthetics. In most instances, careful questioning will show that syncope occurred following injection of the local anesthetic but that no other untoward effects developed. Such findings suggest that the syncope was secondary to apprehension rather than a direct effect of the anesthetic agent. Nevertheless, the dentist should proceed with caution and be prepared to handle any side reactions should they develop (see Chap. 19). In addition to carrying out the precautions necessary to rule out an actual hypersensitivity or idiosyncrasy in the patient, the dentist can minimize the chances of syncope by good "chairside manner," careful technique, and premedication. Too-rapid injection of the anesthetic, inadvertent intravenous administration, and lack of a vasoconstrictor in the anesthetic may also induce syncope or even toxic reactions. Overdose of a local anesthetic is not likely in routine dental procedures although it should be noted that in cases of severe liver disease detoxification of the anesthetic is delayed.

Signs of toxicity to the anesthetic agent should be recognized promptly. Restlessness, tremor, and central nervous system stimulation, followed by depression and shock, are ominous signs requiring specific emergency measures.

A history of allergic response (hypersensitivity) to an anesthetic agent requires that a safe local anesthetic be selected or that general anesthesia be employed for dental operations. Since cross-sensitivity of the different groups of available local anesthetics is not likely, a safe local anesthetic can usually be selected.

The occurrence of angioneurotic edema, bronchospasm, skin rash or anaphylaxis following previous local anesthetic administration suggests the need for hypersensitivity tests. Skin tests, while not necessarily predictive of an actual allergic response should the offending agent be administered, are useful as screening procedures. Further, dermal tests are not reliable for identification of delayed responses such as urticaria. The conjunctiva and the sublingual oral mucosa are often more effective in establishing allergy to local anesthetics. Dermal, conjunctival and sublingual tests are best performed by or under the supervision of an allergist and require careful monitoring of the patient's blood pressure and other vital signs.

MICROBIOLOGICAL EXAMINATIONS

Because of the considerable reliance on antibiotics, bacterial smears and cultures are infrequently used in dental practice. The mixed population of microorganisms of the oral cavity complicates the isolation and culture of organisms suspected of causing a specific oral infection. With the development of more specific skin tests, fluorescent antibody methods, antibody titer and other laboratory procedures, diagnosis of certain specific infections is often accomplished more quickly than possible with bacterial smears and cultures.

In years past, routine oral smears for the demonstration of Vincent's organisms were required for food handlers. However, it has been clearly established that Vincent's infection cannot be diagnosed with any accuracy by this method inasmuch as these organisms are common inhabitants of the normal oral cavity. Although in Vincent's infection and candidiasis the causative organisms are predominant in routine smears, such findings can only be suggestive and must be corre-

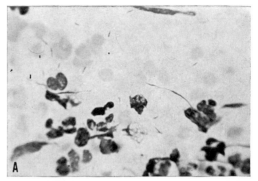
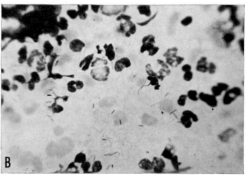

Fig. 9-9. *A* and *B*, Giemsa stained smear of suspected Vincent's ulcer of the lower lip showing numerous dark staining leukocytes and histiocytes, pale erythrocytes, fusiform bacilli and delicate thread-like *Borrelia vincentii*. "Punched-out" gingival papillae with pseudomembrane formation supported the diagnosis of Vincent's ulcer.

lated with the clinical features of the respective diseases (Fig. 9–9; pp. 144, 376). A clinical trial of a specific therapeutic agent sometimes serves as a diagnostic measure.

If bacterial specimens are collected to aid in diagnosis, a careful technique must be employed to avoid contamination from adjacent uninvolved regions of the oral cavity. Material for routine smears must be handled as carefully as material collected for biologic cultures. Special collection procedures may be required depending upon what methods of identification are to be used by the laboratory. The laboratory concerned should be contacted prior to obtaining the specimen for specific instructions on these points. Some general rules regarding smears and cultures are as follows:

1. The specimen should be collected prior to the use of antiseptics or antibiotics applied either topically or systemically.
2. All material should be managed carefully to avoid infection of the operator and the spread of infection in the patient.
3. If the amount of material available is scanty, sterile cotton swabs or absorbent paper points may be used to obtain the specimen.
4. Aspirated solutions should be placed in a sterile test tube for subsequent centrifugation and smearing at the laboratory.
5. The specimen should be labeled clearly and submitted promptly.

Bacterial Smears

Routine smears are spread over the slide and flamed for fixation. Gram's stain is commonly used to determine morphology and whether the organisms are gram-positive or gram-negative. If possible, several smears should be submitted for examination since the laboratory may wish to use differential staining methods.

Routine Cultures

Ordinarily, it is best to send the swab used to obtain the specimen directly to the laboratory in a sterile test tube (Fig. 9–10). In this way the laboratory may then select the appropriate media on which to commence culture, basing the choice on the history and differential diagnosis submitted. If the laboratory supplies agar plates (usually

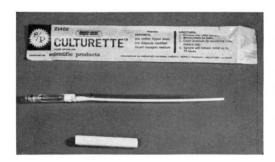

Fig. 9-10. Culturette for bacterial cultures. The Culturette (Scientific Products) contains a sterile swab and a storage tube with Stuart transport medium. Samples will remain moist up to 72 hours to permit transportation to the laboratory.

blood agar or thioglycollate media), routine streaking of the plate may be performed in the dental office provided sterile methods are used. Thioglycollate broth may also be used by stabbing the medium with the swab or other instrument used in collecting the specimen. If a swab is used, this is usually left in the culture broth and sent to the laboratory with the tube.

Antibiotic Sensitivity Tests

Although the majority of the common oral infections are controlled by the body's own defenses once localization and drainage have occurred, antibiotic therapy is indicated in some instances. Most oral infections respond readily to penicillin or erythromycin, either of which is effective against streptococci and other gram-positive organisms. Severe infections, particularly those that fail to respond to the usual therapy, or those in patients with a known allergy to penicillin, require the use of the antibiotic sensitivity test to permit the selection of appropriate agents for control of the predominating organisms. Erythromycin is the most likely substitute for penicillin.

The collection of the material must be done carefully. If the infection is deep seated, it may be necessary to incise and drain the lesion in order to obtain representative material from the most active site. With surface infections, care should be taken to avoid contamination from adjacent unaffected areas. The specimen may be placed directly into a sterile culture tube or, if several hours will be required to deliver the material to the laboratory, it may be inoculated into thioglycollate broth or streaked on an agar plate.

On receipt, laboratory personnel will place wafer discs permeated with various antibiotics on the culture plate on which the organism is growing and, following overnight incubation, zones of growth inhibition will be noted (Fig. 9–11). Usually the sensitivity of the organisms to the antibiotics can be determined within 48 hours and the ther-

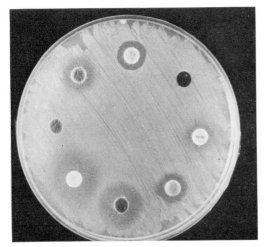

Fig. 9-11. Antibiotic sensitivity test using standard staphylococci test organisms. Sharply outlined area around disc of vancomycin at 12:00 o'clock indicates bactericidal activity. Bacteriostatic activity is shown as a diffuse ring of inhibition around other antibiotic pellets. A control pellet with no activity is located at approximately 2:00 o'clock. (Courtesy of Howard R. Kuder.)

apy already begun may be altered or continued as indicated (Table 9-9).

Bacterial Infections

Most bacterial infections of the oral cavity are of pulpal or periodontal origin and consist predominately of microorganisms native to the flora of the mouth. Thus, both pure and mixed cultures obtained from the usual dental infection might demonstrate *Strep. viridans, Staph. epidermidis, Staph. aureus, Strep. micros, Actinomyces, Ps. aeruginosa, Lactobacillus sp.,* and others. Ordinarily, however, smears or cultures are not required unless there are unusual presenting signs or therapy proves ineffective, making it necessary to identify the specific causative organism.

In addition to the common dental infections, certain other specific bacterial infections may be encountered. These include

Table 9-9. Antibiotic Sensitivity Report Form.

Name	RM	HOSPITAL NO.
PHYSICIAN		
Source of Material		
Direct Smear Reveals		
Culture Reveals (A) Predominant Organism		
(B) Other Organism (s)		

ANTIBIOTICS	A	B	S-ensitive	A	B	R-esistant	A	B
1. Aureomycin			12. Novobiocin			23. Tetracycline		
2. Bacitracin			13. Nystatin			24. Vancocin		
3. Chloromycetin			14. Oleandomycin			SULFAS		
4. Coly-mycin			15. Prostaphlin			1. Kynex		
5. Declomycin			16. Penicillin			2. Elkosin		
6. Erythromycin			17. PolymxinB			3. Gantrisin		
7. Furacin			18. Seromycin			4. Thiosulfa		
8. Furadantin			19. Spontin			5. Triple Sulfa		
9. Furoxone			20. Streptomycin			6. Sulfadiazine		
10. Kanamycin			21. Staphcillin			7. Sulfamerazine		
11. Neomycin			22. Terramycin					

Technician	Director of Laboratories
Date Collected:	Date Rec'd.
(see other side)	**ANTIBIOTIC SENSITIVITY**

tuberculosis (pp. 55, 338, 399), syphilis (pp. 53, 235, 377, 400), noma (p. 402), pyostomatitis vegetans (p. 394), acute ulceromembranous gingivitis (p. 400), gonorrhea (pp. 54, 402), tetanus and rheumatic fever and rheumatic heart disease (p. 50).

Mycotic Infections

The pathogenic fungi are relatively inert organisms which must exist on a host as parasites or saprophytes. They do not produce exotoxin or endotoxin but act chiefly as foreign bodies and thereby often induce an exuberant granulomatous response, especially the deep mycoses. Several are endemic in certain geographic locations such as the midwest (histoplasmosis), Kentucky and surrounding areas (N.A. blastomycosis), South America (S.A. blastomycosis) and the southwest and far west (coccidioidomycosis or San Joaquin Valley fever).

Closely related to bacteria (*e.g.* the *Actinomyces,* which are considered higher bacteria with features of branching), the fungi show dimorphism or growth in different forms under different conditions. Both segmented and non-segmented filaments or hyphae, round bodies (spores) and collections of rounded bodies (endospores) are common growth forms in tissue. Because many of the fungi have thick capsules they are effectively protected from phagocytosis and resist specific therapy. Some may even parasitize histiocytes (*e.g.* histoplasmosis, cryptococcosis). Further, the capsule is antigenic, capable of inducing immune bodies which serve as the basis for complement-fixation tests for diagnosis.

As "opportunists" and natural residents of the oral cavity and bowel, some of the mycotic organisms such as *Actinomyces* and *Candida* produce disease when local conditions are optimal for growth. Secondary mycotic infections must therefore be considered in debilitated patients with pre-existing malignancies, especially malignant lymphoma and leukemia. Certain therapeutic regimens which may modify the normal

bacterial flora (*e.g.* broad-spectrum antibiotics), depress the immune mechanism (*e.g.* irradiation, chemotherapy or steroid therapy in the cancer patient or transplant patient), or modify tissue metabolism (*e.g.* the patient with diabetes) may also predispose to mycotic infections. In refractory cases of candidosis it is essential that concomitant diabetes or other endocrine disease such as hypoparathyroidism be ruled out. Likewise, mucormycosis involving antral and oral mucosa is a frequent complication of diabetic acidosis, leukemia, terminal malignancy, etc.

Candidosis

In suspected candidosis (moniliasis) the superficial white plaques ("thrush") are scraped from the surface of the oral mucosa and smeared on a slide (Fig. 14–9*A–D*). Treatment of the smear with a drop of sodium hydroxide will permit better identification of *Candida albicans,* which will be seen microscopically as a tangled mass of mycelia and yeast-like cells (Fig. 9–12). Culture is carried out on corn-meal agar or Sabouraud's medium (Figs. 9–12 and 9–13).

Actinomycosis

The suppurative material from lesions of actinomycosis frequently will exhibit yellow sulfur granules representing colonies of the organism *Actinomyces israelii,* more accurately classified as a higher bacterium. Such material may be spread over a slide for

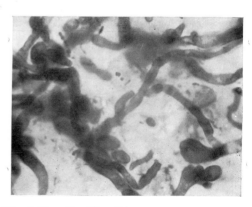

Fig. 9-12. *Candida albicans.*

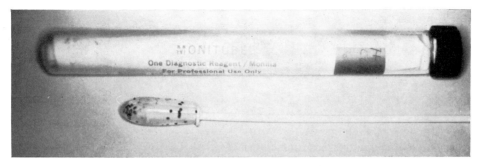

Fig. 9-13. Diagnostic media swabs. Minitubes (Laboratory Diagnostic Co.) used in suspected monilial infections. Positive cultures develop dark brown to black colonies in 24 to 36 hours at room temperature.

microscopic examination of the unstained specimen. The sulfur granules, ranging up to 3 mm in diameter, are hard and may be crushed under a coverslip. With Gram's stain, the central mass stains a deep blue, whereas the radiating clubs around the periphery stain red. A similar staining reaction is seen in tissue biopsies. This anaerobe may be grown on veal infusion broth or thioglycollate medium. It must be differentiated on occasion from the aerobic actinomycete *Nocardia asteroides* by special methods.

Blastomycosis

This disease which often resembles tuberculosis also occurs as a cutaneous granulomatous infection. Since it is pus producing, it may simulate actinomycosis clinically. The budding, double-contoured organisms (*Blastomyces dermatitidis*) may be demonstrated

in wet preparations from the pus as well as in biopsy material (Fig. 9–14). Culture is carried out on Sabouraud's medium. In cases of systemic infection, complement-fixing antibodies may be demonstrated in the serum of the patient.

Histoplasmosis

The causative organism *Histoplasma capsulatum* may be cultured on blood agar. In superficial granulomatous lesions in the oral cavity biopsy is used to demonstrate the organisms within histiocytes (Fig. 9–15). Since histoplasmosis is endemic in certain areas of the United States (such as the south central and Great Lakes regions), a positive histoplasmin skin test indicates evidence of past or present infection. With the skin test, cross reactions with other mycotic infections may also be present. A complement-fixation

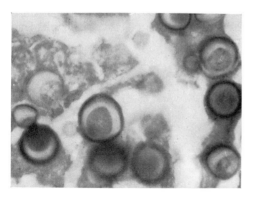

Fig. 9-14. *Blastomyces dermatitidis.*

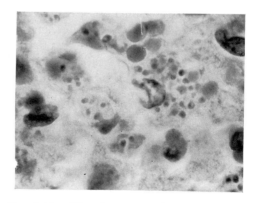

Fig. 9-15. *Histoplasma capsulatum.*

test indicates the presence of antibodies which are of low titer in primary stages of the infection but tend to increase with progression of the disease.

Mucormycosis (Phycomycosis)

The *Phycomycetes* are a group of large, ubiquitous, non-septate fungi of low virulence which may cause superficial infections of the skin, ears, nose, and sinuses. These infections often appear as complications of other debilitating conditions (see above), sometimes with a fulminating course and wide dissemination. Infection of the maxillary antrum may extend into the oral cavity where it may simulate an antro-oral polyp or even carcinoma. The organisms are most readily identified in histologic sections where they often show only a minimal inflammatory response.

Viral Infections

The diagnosis of viral diseases is ordinarily made on the basis of typical clinical manifestations and predictable clinical course. Fortunately, most common viral diseases such as measles, mumps, varicella, influenza, herpes and upper respiratory infections present characteristic clinical patterns and are identified without elaborate tests (p. 324). In other instances, viral "inclusion bodies" may be seen in biopsy specimens of the diseased tissue. These structures may be either intranuclear or intracytoplasmic and represent colonies or clumps of viruses. For example, certain skin warts, molluscum contagiosum (p. 313), primary herpes simplex (p. 207) and herpes zoster (p. 326) typically exhibit inclusion bodies. These features together with the clinical findings are sufficient to make the diagnosis.

Viral infections of more obscure nature present greater difficulties in diagnosis. Unfortunately, viruses cannot be cultured on artificial media but require living tissues such as embryonated chicken egg, or living cells grown in tissue culture. Identification of suspected virus material by these methods is extremely difficult and time consuming. In most cases, serologic methods such as the complement-fixation test, hemagglutination-inhibition test, precipitation tests, neutralization tests and fluorescent antibody tests are employed (pp. 233–235).

Weathers and Griffin have successfully employed the fluorescent antibody technique for identification of herpetic infections of the oral cavity. Briefly, the method involves the use of fluorescein isothiocyanate labeled herpes simplex antibody which binds to the organisms. The resulting complex exhibits a characteristic fluorescence when examined with a fluorescent microscope. It seems certain that the method will eventually be useful in the diagnosis of other specific infections of the oral cavity.

Parasitic Infections

The protozoal and helminth infections are rarely seen in the oral and paraoral tissues, as the few case reports in the literature would suggest. It is entirely possible, however, that certain of these parasitic diseases, once considered as "rare tropical diseases," will increase in frequency because of the surge in international travel and the scattered brushfire wars in remote parts of the world.

Among the protozoal infections, leishmaniasis, trichomoniasis, trypanosomiasis (Chagas' disease) and toxoplasmosis are reported to exhibit oral involvement on occasion. Toxoplasmosis is important in the differential diagnosis of cervical lymphadenopathy (p. 333).

Helminth infections also have been reported in the oral tissues, most notably trichinosis (p. 292), but cysticerosis, ascariasis, strongyloidiasis, myiasis, schistomoniasis (*Bilharzia*), *Echinococcus* (hydatid) disease and hookworm disease (cutaneous larva migrans) as well.

Laboratory diagnosis is made chiefly through biopsy of oral lesions, lymph node biopsy and/or stool cultures.

EXAMINATION OF THE ENDOCRINE SYSTEM

Certain functional disturbances of the endocrine glands manifest changes of diagnostic importance in the oral tissues. Frequently, these signs and symptoms appear relatively early in the disease, often before generalized symptoms become of sufficient magnitude to cause the patient to seek medical attention. The alert dentist will recognize the clinical significance of acetone breath (diabetes mellitus), the recent appearance of gingival pigmentation (Addison's disease), diffuse enlargement of the tongue, coarsening of facial features, and gradual enlargement of the mandible (acromegaly), the significance of certain central giant cell lesions of the jawbones (hyperparathyroidism), retention of deciduous teeth associated with failure of somatic growth (hypopituitarism), and similar features suggestive of endocrine disease.

It should be emphasized that disturbances in endocrine function often manifest fairly specific clinical signs and symptoms which are of diagnostic importance to the dentist. The patient manifesting such signs should be referred for further medical evaluation since the definitive diagnosis of many of the endocrine disturbances is a complex process. The consultation will be most productive if the dentist is not only familiar with the clinical manifestations of the suspected endocrine dysfunction but understands the diagnostic significance of the endocrine tests employed as well.

Tests of Thyroid Function

Disturbances in thyroid function typically present generalized symptoms and physical changes of greater diagnostic importance than the more subtle oral changes. The clinical manifestations depend upon the age of onset and the functional state of the gland, *i.e.* whether the patient is hyperthyroid, hypothyroid or euthyroid (Fig. 12–6).

Diffuse or nodular enlargements of the thyroid and their clinical significance are discussed on pages 341 to 343. Medical evaluation of all thyroid enlargements should be requested inasmuch as neoplastic changes as well as functional disturbances may develop.

Other signs of thyroid dysfunction may be correlated with the recognized functions of the thyroid gland. The chief thyroid hormone, thyroxin (T_4), is an iodine-containing amino acid which regulates cell metabolism. T_3, a more active form of thyroxin, is secreted in small amounts by the gland. At the cellular level, T_3 is derived from T_4 by deiodination. Thyroxin causes increased oxygen consumption at the cellular level and is of importance in lipid and carbohydrate metabolism. Its influence on growth and maturation is chiefly manifest in children. Thyroid function is controlled by the thyroid-stimulating hormone (TSH) of the anterior pituitary through a feedback mechanism induced by the level of circulating thyroid hormone.

The metabolically active thyroid hormones (T_4, T_3) in the circulating blood are loosely bound to carrier proteins as thyroxin-binding globulin (TBG), thyroxin-binding prealbumin (TBPA) and serum albumin. A relatively minute amount of free thyroxin (FT_4) is released as required and enters target cells where it is physiologically active.

Tests of thyroid function are designed to measure the parameters of hormone activity described above. As for almost any laboratory test, the various tests taken individually cannot be considered diagnostic but must be correlated with the results of other tests as well as with the clinical features. Certain drugs, especially those containing iodine, invalidate some of the tests.

The principal tests of thyroid function and their significance are described in the following paragraphs.

Basal Metabolic Rate (BMR)

This old, infrequently used test measures oxygen consumption in the resting and fasting state and is most useful in monitoring changes in an individual during therapy. Oxygen consumption in a healthy, young adult male is approximately 40 cal/sqM/hr and in a female, 35 cal/sqM/hr. Since the BMR varies with the age, sex and body build of the individual, the value is expressed in the laboratory report as a percentage of normal. A variation of ±15 percent of the normal is acceptable.

Protein-Bound Iodine (PBI)

PBI has been used for many years for estimating thyroid function but, with the development of more definitive thyroid function tests, is now considered largely outmoded. Approximately 95 percent of the protein-bound iodine in the circulating blood is in "thyroxin" with the remainder found in monoiodotyrosine, thyroglobulin and other forms of the thyroid hormone. Normal values for PBI show a range of 4 to 8 μg per 100 ml.

Butanol-Extractable Iodine (BEI)

This test measures the iodine level of thyroxin but not the iodine of other forms of thyroid hormone. The normal range of BEI is 3 to 7 μg per 100 ml. The BEI test is routinely used by some laboratories.

Triiodothyronine Uptake Test

An *in vitro* test, the triiodothyronine (RBC—T_3) uptake test, gives normal values of 11.5 to 19 percent (male) and 11 to 17 percent (female).

Serum Thyroxin Test

Determinations of serum thyroxin may be made in cases of prior treatment with non-hormonal iodine. Normal values show a rather wide range of 4 to 11 μg per 100 ml.

Thyroxin-Binding Globulin (TBG), Thyroxin-Binding Pre-Albumin (TBPA)

Determination of proteins which bind thyroxin are made by TBG and TBPA tests. Less commonly used, these tests must be correlated with PBI and serum thyroxin values.

Radioactive Iodine Uptake

Radioactive iodine (^{131}I) administered orally concentrates mainly in the thyroid gland and can be measured with a scintillation (gamma ray) counter placed over the neck. Gammagrams are prepared from readings taken at intervals up to 48 hours. The percent of the ^{131}I dose in the normal thyroid gland at 2 hours is approximately 20 percent with progressive increases seen up to 50 percent by 24 and 48 hours. Iodine^{131} uptake studies are useful for evaluation of thyroid enlargements for possible neoplasms and identification of metastatic thyroid tumor. In therapeutic doses, ^{131}I may be used to treat some functional neoplasms and hyperplasias of the thyroid.

Thyroid-Stimulating Hormone (TSH) Administration

Thyroid function is controlled by TSH secreted by the anterior pituitary. Apparent thyroid dysfunction may actually be caused by an anterior pituitary disturbance in TSH secretion. TSH administration would cause a normal thyroxin response (PBI, ^{131}I uptake) if the defect is primarily in the TSH secretory mechanism (pituitary myxedema).

Desiccated Thyroid Administration

This "test" is usually carried out as a clinical trial. If symptoms thought to be due to hypothyroidism are relieved, more definitive diagnostic tests may be indicated.

Interpretation of Thyroid Function Tests

The several available tests of thyroid function measure corresponding parameters of the gland physiology. It follows that no single test will be universally diagnostic. Rather, the results of the clinical findings must be correlated with the values obtained with appropriate thyroid function tests. Some laboratory and associated clinical findings in several thyroid disturbances are outlined below.

Disturbances of Thyroid Function

Cretinism

Hypothyroidism present in children from birth results in cretinism. Without treatment these children become increasingly retarded and show a characteristic facies. The skin becomes rough and scaly with a yellowish tint and the facial features become thickened. The tongue may enlarge and protrude from the mouth as early as the second or third month and the eyes are widely spaced. The nose is wide and flat and the lips are thickened. These children develop pot bellies and exhibit fat pads on the back of the shoulders and the buttocks. Body growth is retarded and the eruption of the teeth is delayed.

Myxedema

Hypothyroidism occurring in adults is characterized by subcutaneous edema, dry skin, coarse or sparse hair, husky voice, slow speech and mental dullness. The BMR is well below normal. The level of PBI may be reduced to below 2 μg per 100 ml, and the ^{131}I uptake is low.

Juvenile myxedema refers to the development of hypothyroidism in a previously normal child, i.e. there was normal growth and development prior to the onset of the endocrine symptoms. Treatment must be initiated early in both cretinism and juvenile myxedema if permanent damage is to be avoided.

Hyperthyroidism (Thyrotoxicosis)

Hyperfunction of the thyroid gland is characterized by loss of weight, constant fatigue, intolerance to heat, tremor, nervousness and increased irritability. The skin is generally warm and moist. The patient is anxious and exhibits fine tremor of the fingers. Exophthalmos and goiter may be present.

The laboratory examination is essential for the diagnosis of hyperthyroidism. The BMR is elevated in cases of moderate severity to a range from +30 to +60. The PBI is elevated

and the ^{131}I uptake value shows a sharp rise within the first 2 hours of administration, approaching 70 percent of the ^{131}I dose administered.

Thyroid crisis or storm, an acute exacerbation of the symptoms of hyperthyroidism, may follow severe infection or other illness in untreated or inadequately treated hyperthyroid patients. While these often serious complications of thyrotoxicosis can be averted by adequate thyroid treatment, they are of special significance to the dentist in patient management. The hyperthyroid should not be subjected to undue stress and is extremely hypersensitive to vasoconstrictors even in the small amounts contained in local anesthetics.

Tests of Pancreatic Endocrine Function

The islets of Langerhans of the pancreas secrete the hormones insulin and glucagon. These hormones regulate intermediary metabolism, chiefly carbohydrate metabolism. Insulin is secreted by the beta cells and glucagon by the alpha cells of the islets. The basic effect of insulin activity is to lower blood glucose and promote its transport across cell membranes. Glucagon, on the other hand, acts largely as an anti-insulin hormone, providing a check and balance to the action of insulin. By stimulation of liver glycogenolysis, glucagon elevates blood glucose. While complex interrelationships among the several endocrine glands serve to regulate pancreatic activity and carbohydrate metabolism the chief disease of concern to the dentist is diabetes mellitus.

The principal laboratory tests of value in the diagnosis of diabetes mellitus are determination of serum glucose, glucose tolerance test and urinary glucose test (Table 9–10).

Serum Glucose Test

The normal fasting blood sugar is 60 to 100 mg per 100 ml. A high carbohydrate meal will normally cause a rise of the blood sugar to approximately 150 mg per 100 ml within 30 minutes to 1 hour. With normal

9

Table 9-10. Glucose Tolerance Test Report Form.

MG%	HOURS ½ 1 2 3 4 5 6		Name			
600			Room		Hosp. No.	
560						
520			Physician			
480			Spec.	Blood	Urine Acet.	Urine Sugar
440						
400	Severe Diabetes		Fast			
360			½ Hour			
320						
280	Mild Diabetes		1 Hour			
240	Liver Disease		2 Hour			
200	Hyperthyroidism		3 Hour			
160	Normal					
120			4 Hour			
80	Addisons		5 Hour			
40	Hyperinsulinism, Hypothyroidism		6 Hour			

Technician	Director of Laboratories
Date	
Date Rec.	
GLUCOSE TOLERANCE	

insulin function, the blood sugar values return to the normal fasting level within 2 hours. Values above 170 mg per 100 ml are considered diagnostic of diabetes mellitus. At this level, the excess serum glucose will spill over the renal threshold into the urine.

A number of rapid screening methods for determination of blood or urinary glucose are available. These may be employed as a routine procedure in the office by the dentist. One method involves the use of a commercial preparation called Dextrostix for estimating blood glucose values (Fig. 9–16). In addition to their diagnostic value and as screening tests, such methods are of considerable value in cases of suspected diabetic coma or insulin shock.

Glucose Tolerance Test

This more complicated test provides an accurate measure of the response of the pancreas to measured oral or intravenous doses of glucose. Under controlled conditions measured carbohydrate preparatory diets are fed for 3 days orally. Specific amounts of glucose are then given orally or intravenously and the blood glucose is measured at frequent intervals up to 3 hours. With normal function, the 1-hour blood glucose determination should show less than 160 mg glucose per 100 ml. At 2 hours the normal values would be less than 120 mg per 100 ml. In the diabetic, the 1-hour specimen of serum glucose will be in excess of 180 mg per 100 ml.

Urinary Glucose

The demonstration of glucose in the urine in diabetes is the simplest test used for the identification of the diabetic. Obviously it is not the most effective test since it reflects

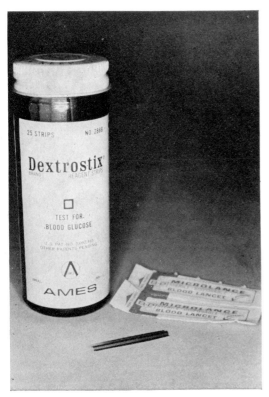

Fig. 9-16. Commercially available reagent strips such as Dextrostix are useful in screening patients for elevated blood glucose.

Disturbances of Pancreatic Endocrine Function

Diabetes Mellitus

The clinical signs of diabetes may be detected by the alert dentist who will recognize abrupt changes in the health of the periodontium, failure of the periodontal tissues to respond to routine therapy, or acetone (fruity) breath odor (Figs. 9–17, 9–18*A* and *B*). While these signs and symptoms are not in themselves diagnostic, they may suggest the need for medical consultation.

The onset of diabetes mellitus may be quite abrupt in children and young adults, whereas in older individuals gradual onset is the rule. Unrecognized cases may exhibit progressive periodontal bone loss more severe than might be expected from local factors.

Patients with diabetes commonly exhibit polyuria with daily outputs often in excess of 3 liters. Polydipsia, polyphagia, drowsiness and loss of weight and strength are common features. Uncontrolled diabetics fail to heal properly and may develop atrophic ulcers of the feet and legs as circulation becomes progressively impaired. The labora-

the spilling over of glucose into the urine in cases of hyperglycemia. This test is often used in conjunction with the glucose tolerance test, and also as a screening procedure.

Ketosis and Acidosis

Associated with disturbances of carbohydrate metabolism, disturbances in protein and fat metabolism also occur. Accumulation of the products of fat metabolism results in acidosis. Acetone, acetoacetic acid and beta hydroxybutyric acid are toxic and eventually may aid in the production of diabetic coma. Serum ketone bodies can be measured qualitatively to assess the severity of ketosis. Ketone acids and acetone may be detected in the urine of uncontrolled diabetics, often up to 60 gm per day.

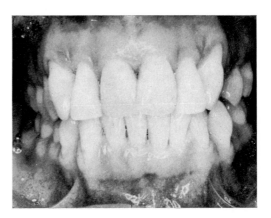

Fig. 9-17. Clinical appearance of gingiva of patient with unsuspected diabetes mellitus. The health of the gingiva in this case was maintained, largely because of excellent hygiene. However, there were deep periodontal pocket formation and severe alveolar bone loss, all of which occurred within a period of 1 year. (Courtesy of Marshall S. Manne.)

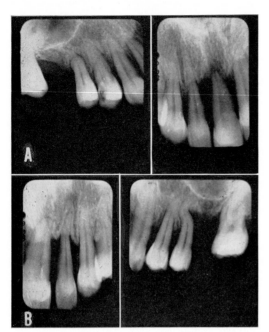

Fig. 9-18. *A* and *B,* Intraoral radiographs of adult with poorly controlled diabetes mellitus. The extensive periodontal bone loss necessitated full mouth extractions.

tory values which are of significance in diagnosis are as follows: (*a*) urinary glucose, (*b*) high specific gravity of the urine, (*c*) ketone bodies in the urine, (*d*) proteinuria, (*e*) urinary casts, and (*f*) elevated blood sugar.

Complications of diabetes mellitus include acidosis, diabetic coma and insulin shock. Patients with severe diabetes may show unusual susceptibility to infections and frequently exhibit poor healing. Thus, infection and gangrene particularly of the feet and ankles are common complications and result from secondary disturbances in circulation. Retinitis, hypertension associated with vascular changes, cataracts, and motor and sensory changes associated with peripheral neuropathy complicate the disease. These patients frequently develop boils (furuncles, carbuncles), a feature which in itself should suggest the need for serum or urinary glucose determinations. Diabetics will sometimes exhibit secondary mycotic infections such as candidiasis and mucormycosis (p. 242).

Early Recognition of Diabetes

In addition to those clinical features described above that are characteristic of active diabetes, a number of clinical signs and symptoms suggestive of early, mild diabetes may be recognized. While these are not specific for diabetes, they are of sufficient importance to warrant screening tests to rule out such a diagnosis.

Inasmuch as the inherent "resistance" of the diabetic is reduced, he is subject to a variety of infections, especially staphylococcal, manifested as furuncles and carbuncles, not ordinarily seen in the healthy individual. Most particularly oral or vulvovaginal candidiasis is common in mild diabetes (p. 240). Yellow pigmentation of the skin resembling jaundice or carotenemia but without involvement of the sclera may be present in the early diabetic. As the diabetic state becomes established, small erythematous papules or yellow, depressed plaques appear on the skin with some frequency. In addition, brown pigmented, ovoid patches are sometimes seen on the ankles or the pretibial regions.

The simplicity of some screening tests (*e.g.* urine sugar) justify their use when any of the above signs are recognized during examination.

Hypoglycemia

Hypoglycemia may result from the secretion of excess insulin. Other causes are excessive injection of insulin, missing a meal, and strenuous physical activity. Signs and symptoms of hypoglycemia include hunger, tachycardia, pallor, sweating, chills and syncope.

The diagnosis of hypoglycemia is made on the basis of blood sugar determinations similar to those used for diabetes. Care should be taken to establish proper control situations to ensure that a normal transient hypoglycemia is not present. It is particularly important to determine the underlying cause inasmuch as a wide variety of diseases, both those primary in the pancreas and those related to other tissues, may be responsible. Hyperinsulinism may occur in hypertrophy and hyperplasia or benign and malignant neoplasia of the pancreatic islet cell tissue. Certain disturbances of the pituitary, adrenal (p. 254) and thyroid glands also may modify the secretion and activity of insulin. Postnatal hypoglycemia is seen in *Beckwith's hypoglycemic syndrome* (p. 431).

The administration of readily available carbohydrates such as sugar water, orange juice or even milk will generally relieve the immediate symptoms of hypoglycemia and raise the blood sugar to a normal level.

Tests of Parathyroid Function

The parathyroid hormone regulates calcium and phosphorus metabolism chiefly by inhibiting phosphate reabsorption and possibly by enhancing reabsorption of calcium in the renal tubules. In addition, parathormone mobilizes calcium from the bones. Thus parathyroid gland secretion increases serum calcium, increases urinary phosphate and lowers serum phosphate. Hormone production in the parathyroid gland is stimulated when the serum calcium level falls or the serum phosphate level rises. Conversely, parathormone secretion is inhibited by hypercalcemia or by hypophosphatemia.

Disturbances in calcium and phosphorus metabolism may be associated directly with the functional activity of the parathyroid gland, secondarily with renal tubular disease and indirectly with vitamin D absorption or metabolism.

Serum and Urinary Chemistry

Laboratory examinations useful in determining these data are: serum calcium, phosphorus and alkaline phosphatase (p. 226), urinary calcium and phosphate and other renal function tests (pp. 231–233). The rationale for use and clinical significance of these tests are described here insofar as they are applicable to the specific disturbances of parathyroid function described in following sections.

Radiographic Skeletal Survey

The "brown tumors" of hyperparathyroidism (von Recklinghausen's disease of bone) are sometimes discovered in routine intraoral radiographs (Fig. 9–19). They are radiolucent defects without cortication and may vary considerably in size and shape (p. 451). In addition to these defects (osteitis fibrosa cystica), a "ground-glass" appearance of the trabecular pattern and loss of lamina dura have been described. Once the nature of the radiolucent defect has been determined by appropriate tests, a skeletal radiographic survey should be performed to determine the size and location of other "brown tumors." Periodic radiographic examination of the radiolucent lesions may be helpful in evalu-

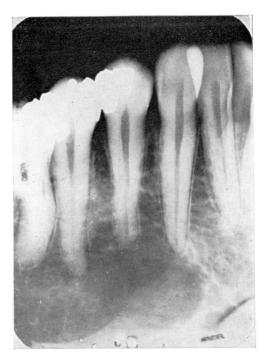

Fig. 9-19. Radiolucency discovered on routine periapical radiographs. The teeth in the area tested vital. Biopsy revealed a giant cell lesion shown to be a "brown tumor" of hyperparathyroidism by appropriate tests. (Courtesy of A. P. Chaudhry.)

ating therapy since they heal once the parathyroid hyperfunction is corrected.

Bone Biopsy

Microscopic examination of the "cystic" bone lesions in hyperparathyroidism reveals a central giant cell lesion of bone. Inasmuch as the central giant cell granuloma of bone and the "brown tumor" of hyperparathyroidism are histologically identical, additional workup is required to confirm or rule out the latter condition.

Disturbances of Parathyroid Function

Hypoparathyroidism

Hypofunction of the parathyroid gland occurs most commonly following accidental removal of the parathyroid gland at thyroidectomy. In rare instances, hypoparathyroidism may follow acute systemic infection or may be due to congenital absence of the gland. An autoimmune mechanism may be operative in some "idiopathic" forms.

Tetany induced by the hypocalcemia of hypoparathyroidism is characterized by tonic muscle contractions, gastric pain, nausea and convulsions. *Chvostek's sign* (twitching of facial muscles following tapping of the skin overlying the facial nerve) is usually positive. Spasm of muscles of the arm causing flexion of the wrist and thumb with extension of the fingers (*Trousseau's sign*) can often be induced, even in mild tetany, by applying a blood pressure cuff for a few minutes. If the disease is active during tooth development the teeth may be malformed. Administration of calcium salts and large doses of vitamin D relieves the condition.

Pseudohypoparathyroidism

A rare hereditary sex-linked dominant disturbance in which there is a failure of end-organ (kidney tubules, bone) response to parathormone, pseudohypoparathyroidism causes enamel hypoplasia, short and tapering roots of the teeth, mandibular exostoses and coarse bone trabeculations. Other signs

and symptoms related to the hypocalcemia are similar to those found in postsurgical or idiopathic hypoparathyroidism.

Another rare condition which exhibits similar physical findings has been called *pseudopseudohypoparathyroidism.*

Primary Hyperparathyroidism

Hyperfunction of the parathyroid glands as a result of gland hyperplasia or neoplasia is referred to as primary hyperparathyroidism. The principal signs and symptoms are related to hypercalcemia, hypercalciuria and bone lesions. Physical changes in the glands seldom occur.

The ionizable (diffusible) component of the serum calcium accounts for nearly all of the increased serum calcium in hyperparathyroidism (p. 226). Further, parathyroid hyperplasia generally results in higher serum calcium values than parathyroid adenoma.

Hypercalcemia produces generalized symptoms of irritability, anorexia, nausea and dysphagia. Weakness, reduced muscle tone and laxity of ligaments may be present. Eye lesions ("band keratopathy" and conjunctival calcification), gastric and duodenal ulcers and acute pancreatitis are associated findings believed to be caused by the elevated serum calcium.

Hypercalciuria is chiefly responsible for the nephrolithiasis that may occur. These stones, composed of calcium oxalate or calcium phosphate, may precede other physical findings in the disease. In severe cases, nephrocalcinosis, severe renal disease or renal failure may develop.

The bone lesions of hyperparathyroidism are described as "cysts" or "brown tumors" and appear as multiple radiolucent defects (osteitis fibrosa cystica generalisata). Bone tenderness or pain often causes the patient to seek professional advice. Pathologic fractures may occur. Biopsy reveals the "cysts" to be composed of giant cell lesions histologically identical to the central giant cell granuloma (see p. 463). Although bone lesions are not demonstrable in all cases of hyperparathyroidism, their occurrence in the jaws offers the dentist both the opportunity and the responsibility to establish the diagnosis.

Secondary Hyperparathyroidism

Hyperplasia with increased functional activity of the parathyroid glands may occur secondarily to renal diseases (chronic interstitial nephritis, cystinosis or Lignac-Fanconi disease, polycystic kidney). The resulting retention of phosphate induces parathyroid hyperfunction (functional hyperplasia) and mobilization of calcium salts from the bones. Since excess phosphates may be excreted by way of the intestinal tract, the formation of insoluble calcium phosphates in the intestine prevents adequate calcium absorption.

Secondary hyperparathyroidism of long standing in adults is evident clinically as osteitis fibrosa cystica. In children, these disturbances in calcium and phosphorus metabolism occurring secondarily to renal disease result in marked skeletal deformity, stunting of growth, and other developmental defects referred to as renal rickets.

Tertiary Hyperparathyroidism

With the advent of kidney transplants and routine kidney dialysis, a new disorder, tertiary hyperparathyroidism, is occasionally seen. Chronic renal acidosis with lowering of serum calcium stimulates parathyroid activity (secondary hyperparathyroidism). In some cases, however, the gland becomes autonomous and fails to respond to the feedback mechanism of increased serum calcium (tertiary hyperparathyroidism). Metastatic calcifications form in the already damaged kidneys and, additionally, these patients experience severe bone pain. Calcium is likewise deposited in a transplanted kidney, thereby compromising its success. For this reason, partial parathyroidectomy is sometimes done prior to kidney transplant.

Tests of Pituitary Function

The several hormones secreted by the anterior and posterior lobes of the pituitary gland function chiefly to regulate somatic growth and functional activity of other endocrine glands, influence water balance, fat and nitrogen metabolism, and stimulate parturition (Table 9–11). Regulation of pituitary

Table 9-11. Pituitary Hormones.

Hormone	Chief Activity
Anterior pituitary	
Growth hormone (STH)	Stimulates body growth
Thyroid-stimulating hormone (TSH)	Stimulates secretion of thyroxin
Adrenocorticotrophic hormone (ACTH)	Stimulates secretion of cortisone
Follicle-stimulating hormone (FSH)	Stimulates ovarian follicle and spermatogenesis
Luteinizing hormone (LH)	Stimulates luteinization of ovarian follicle, and testosterone secretion
Luteotrophic hormone (LTH)	Maintains corpus luteum of pregnancy, stimulates lactation
Pars intermedia	
Melanocyte-stimulating hormone (MSH)	Stimulates melanocytes
Posterior pituitary	
Vasopressin, antidiuretic hormone (ADH)	Promotes renal water retention
Oxytocin	Stimulates uterine contractions

activity is mediated by way of the hypothalamus through a complex feedback mechanism involving circulating hormones from other endocrine glands and direct neural pathways from higher centers. It follows that disturbances in pituitary function may be due to hypothalamic lesions; hyperplastic, neoplastic, atrophic or destructive disease in the pituitary gland; or, secondarily, to functional (feedback) disturbances in other endocrine glands. Overproduction of the trophic hormones of the pituitary gland will induce hyperactivity of the specific target gland, whereas underproduction of these hormones by the pituitary is evident as a hypofunction of the target gland. The chief example of this interrelationship is between the pituitary gland and the adrenal cortex. Adrenocorticotrophic hormone (ACTH) regulates the secretory activity of the adrenal cortex which in turn provides a check and balance for pituitary secretion of this hormone (p. 256). A similar relationship is seen between the pituitary gland and the thyroid through secretory activity of thyrotrophic hormone (p. 243). Other trophic hormones of the pituitary control activity of the gonads, the somatic tissues (STH), the mammary glands (lactogenic hormone) and the uterus (oxytocin).

Although some of the hormones of the pituitary as well as other endocrine glands may be identified directly in body fluids such as the serum or urine, others undergo considerable metabolic change and cannot be recovered in their original state. In many instances the activity of these hormones must be identified by their physiologic action (bioassay) or by a number of indirect methods.

Direct demonstration of most specific pituitary hormones requires elaborate chemical procedures and/or assay in animals. Because of the association of adrenal cortex activity and pituitary function many of the tests of adrenal function reflect the condition of the pituitary. Certain of these tests will be described in the following section on adrenal glands.

Lateral head plates showing the size and shape of the sella turcica are occasionally useful in the diagnosis of lesions of the pituitary. The pituitary ameloblastoma typically exhibits calcified structures suggesting the diagnosis. Slow-growing benign neoplasms of the pituitary or pituitary hyperplasia may occasionally show enlargement or erosion of the sella turcica.

Radiographic examination of the epiphyseal plates of the long bones and the growth centers of the hands are often useful for bone age determinations in evaluation of growth disturbances of pituitary origin.

Disturbances of Pituitary Function

The pituitary dysfunctions of interest to the dentist are those related to the secretion of somatotropic growth hormone (STH) and adrenocorticotropic hormone (ACTH). Such dysfunctions include pituitary dwarfism (Figs. 9–20, 9–21), pituitary giantism, acromegaly (Fig. 1–21) and the alarm (stress) reaction of Selye. Other pituitary disturbances of special concern to the dentist include the craniopharyngioma (pituitary ameloblastoma), and diabetes insipidus occurring in association with part of the triad of Hand-Schüller-Christian disease (p. 488, Fig. 15–56).

Hypofunction of the pituitary gland secondary to extensive neoplastic disease, cyst,

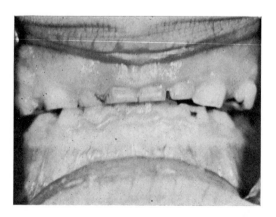

Fig. 9-20. Hypopituitarism in a 24-year-old female. The retained deciduous teeth show marked attrition. The patient was of normal intelligence and of small but well-proportioned stature.

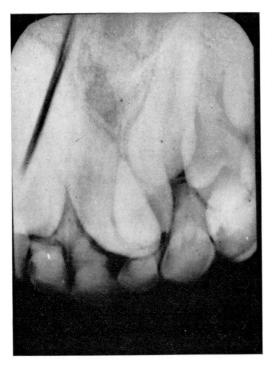

Fig. 9-21. Intraoral radiographs showing retained deciduous teeth and unerupted permanent teeth in the pituitary dwarf shown in Figure 9-20. Because of the small size of the jaws, the permanent teeth are in malposition.

metastatic tumor or infarction results in diminution of all the trophic hormones of the pituitary with secondary effects in target organs and tissues. Hypothyroidism may also develop secondarily because of the reduced thyrotrophic hormone. *Diabetes insipidus* occasionally follows diminished antidiuretic hormone production. Cases occurring before puberty will exhibit very low blood sugar and *pituitary dwarfism* because of absence of growth hormones (Figs. 9–20, 9–21). Such dwarfs are generally of normal intelligence (in contrast to the cretin) and are well proportioned (in contrast to the achondroplastic dwarf). Gonadotropic hormone deficiency may also be present causing amenorrhea or azoospermia and loss of libido and pubic hair.

Other possible causes of pituitary destruction may occur postpartum (Sheehan's syndrome) or as septic infarction due to puerperal infection. In addition to signs and symptoms related to specific hormone deficit, the patient with *panhypopituitarism* typically develops a fawn color with increased wrinkling of skin of the face about the eyes and around the mouth.

Giantism

Excess production of growth hormone prior to epiphyseal closure results in remarkable growth. Individuals may reach heights of 8 feet or more and show corresponding enlargement of the jaws.

Acromegaly

Overproduction of pituitary growth hormones in an adult after epiphyseal closure results in an increase in the size of the hands, feet and mandible and a coarsening of soft tissues, particularly of the face (Fig. 1–21). The tongue may be markedly enlarged and produce separation of the teeth with diastema formation (p. 431). Condylar growth causes marked prognathism.

Tests of Adrenal Function

The adrenal gland consists of two parts, the medulla and the cortex. The adrenal medulla, primarily under control of the sympathetic nervous system, elaborates the catecholamines (epinephrine, norepinephrine, dopamine) which cause vasoconstriction, acceleration of the heart rate, relaxation of bronchial and intestinal musculature, and promote the breakdown of glycogen.

Evidence indicates that the separate zones of the adrenal cortex secrete different adrenal cortical hormones (Race *et al.*). These are as follows: zona glomerulosa, aldosterone (11-desoxycorticosterone); zona fasciculata, 11- and 11-17-hydroxycorticoids (glucocorticoid); zona reticularis, androgens (17-ketosteroids, some testosterone or estrogens). Further, disturbances in adrenal function may involve each of these zones selectively or all of them concurrently. Thus, the range of clinical manifestations of adrenal cortical disturbances will vary according to the specific zones involved as well as the respective target organs and tissues affected. The cortical hormones exert widespread metabolic effects in the body.

The mineralocorticoids (*e.g.* aldosterone) promote the retention of sodium and the urinary excretion of potassium. Thus altered mineralocorticoid secretions may cause serious electrolyte disturbances.

The glucocorticoids (*e.g.* cortisone) influence anabolic and catabolic processes generally and cellular metabolism specifically. It is therefore of significance that these hormones not only exert an effect upon metabolism of protein, fat and carbohydrates, but also influence cellular activity of fibroblasts, the formation of ground substance and collagen fibers, and the process of inflammation.

The androgenic hormones exert an influence on secondary sex characteristics.

It is apparent therefore that disturbances in either the pituitary or the adrenal gland may produce complex metabolic disturbances manifest not only in the glands proper but in their respective target organs and tissues. Selection of specific tests to identify the nature of the defects should be under the direction of a physician. Accordingly, detailed descriptions of specific tests to evaluate either pituitary or adrenal gland function would be of little value here. Only the general nature of certain of the more frequently used tests and their rationale for use will be mentioned.

Laboratory tests useful in the diagnosis of adrenal cortical dysfunction are directed toward demonstration of the degradation products of the hormones in the blood or urine, or are functional tests to demonstrate their physiologic activity. The most important of the tests using blood serum measure corticoids and serum electrolytes.

Vanillylmandelic Acid (VMA)

Vanillylmandelic acid is a metabolite common to all three catecholamines produced by the adrenal medulla. VMA serves as the basis for laboratory tests useful in the diagnosis of neoplasms of the adrenal medulla and other neurocristopathies sometimes found in the oral regions.

ACTH Stimulation Test

In this functional test, a single intramuscular injection of α^{1-24}-corticotropin is administered and the plasma cortisol level is measured after 30 minutes. A normal response of the adrenal cortex is shown by a threefold rise in plasma cortisol over the preinjection level. Absence of a cortical response to ACTH is characteristic of Addison's disease.

Metyrapone Test

This test is utilized to determine pituitary (ACTH) reserve. It is of value in suspected pituitary tumors, hypopituitarism and to establish the responsiveness of the ACTH secreting mechanism of patients who have received long-term steroid therapy. Metyrapone given orally every 4 hours for 6 doses causes a twofold increase in total urinary 17-hydroxycorticosteroids or a tenfold increase in plasma 11-deoxycortisol. Failure to respond to the metyrapone test with a normal response to the ACTH stimulation test indicates intact adrenal glands but a lack of pituitary reserve.

Dexamethasone Suppression Test

Another screening test for hypercortisolism, this test normally causes plasma cortisol to fall to less than 5 mg/100 ml in 24 hours, thereby excluding Cushing's syndrome from the differential diagnosis. In cases of abnormal response to this test, the diagnosis of Cushing's syndrome can be confirmed by urinary free cortisol determinations which are elevated in virtually all cases.

Water Diuresis Test

The stimulating effect of cortisol on glomerular filtration is measured by the water diuresis test. The patient with Addison's disease excretes a lesser volume of urine.

Urinary 17-Hydroxycorticosteroids

A more specific test of adrenal cortical function measures urinary 17-hydroxycorticoids following ACTH administration. A marked increase in urinary 17-hydroxycorticoids with further increases as the test is continued is considered normal. Again, patients with Addison's disease or other cortical hypofunction would not exhibit this response. This test is useful in ruling out the possibility of pituitary dysfunction producing secondary changes in adrenal cortical activity.

Disturbances of Adrenal Function

Conditions involving the cortex of the adrenal gland primarily or by way of the pituitary include the adrenal crisis, Addison's disease, Cushing's syndrome, the adrenogenital syndrome and stress.

Adrenal Crisis (Acute Adrenocortical Insufficiency)

The adrenal crisis may follow rapid, severe destruction of the adrenal cortex by infection or thrombosis of major vessels. Acute stress in patients following surgery, particularly those who have already been subject to stress by disease or previous ACTH or cortisone therapy, may precipitate adrenal crisis. Because of the effects of cortisone on circulating eosinophils of the blood, the direct eosinophil count is of value in the diagnosis of adrenal crisis.

Addison's Disease

Primary adrenocortical insufficiency may follow destruction of the adrenal cortex. Overwork or autoimmune mechanisms have been suggested for a number of cases of this disease. A significant number of cases are due to tuberculosis or other miscellaneous infections, hemorrhage or thrombosis of the gland (Fig. 11–18).

The initial findings of Addison's disease are mainly non-specific and related to generalized weakness and fatigue. It is of con-

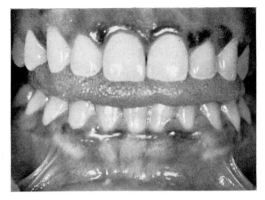

Fig. 9-22. Melanin pigmentation of gingiva in Addison's disease. The recent appearance of the pigmentation of the gingiva and skin as well as other signs and symptoms would rule out the differential diagnosis of physiologic pigmentation.

siderable diagnostic significance that prolonged recovery periods from uncomplicated infectious processes such as those occurring about the teeth or jaws may be present. These features would suggest Addison's disease, particularly if there has been recent development of typical melanin pigmentation of the mucous membranes, loss of weight, emaciation, muscular weakness, feeble heart action, lowered blood pressure and anemia. Pigmentation of the skin is a highly reliable sign in primary adrenal insufficiency (p. 321). (Insufficiency occurring secondarily to reduced pituitary ACTH production rarely induces melanin pigmentation.) The patient may undergo crises of hypoglycemia (p. 248). Marked depression may also accompany the disease. Glucocorticoid and mineralocorticoid substitution therapy is used to maintain patients with this condition.

Cushing's Syndrome

Cushing's syndrome refers to the condition of increased glucocorticoid activity for whatever reason, whereas *Cushing's disease* is due to an abnormal regulation of ACTH secretion. Inasmuch as both conditions cause nearly identical symptoms, they will be considered together.

The most common cause of Cushing's syndrome is the therapeutic use of adrenal corticosteroids. Since the diagnosis is readily obvious from the clinical history, laboratory work is generally unnecessary except to determine pituitary reserve in cases of long-term therapy.

The *basophil adenoma* of the pituitary generally secretes abnormal amounts of ACTH with resultant hyperadrenocorticism and increased 17-hydroxycorticoids in the plasma and the urine. Other comparable hormones may also be increased. The *chromophobe adenoma* may also be a functional tumor, producing great amounts of ACTH. In some cases, erosion of the sella turcica or disturbances in vision due to pressure on the optic chiasm are presenting signs.

Functional tumors of the adrenal cortex or cortical hyperplasia secondary to ACTH production may result in increased amounts of the major hormones of this gland. These patients typically exhibit a moon face, increased collections of fat over the fat pads of the shoulder (buffalo hump), truncal obesity, and purple striae of the abdomen. Hypertension, glycosuria (not controlled by insulin therapy) and albuminuria characterize this disease. Osteoporosis occurs in most cases, and, in children, reduction in growth activity. Compression fractures of the vertebrae may complicate the condition.

Adrenogenital Syndromes

Androgenic (masculinizing) hormones are normally secreted by the adrenal cortex in sufficient quantities to influence sex characteristics. The 17-ketosteroids and testosterone particularly produce bizarre clinical changes when secreted in excess. Since the adrenal androgens promote protein synthesis as well as enhance male sex characteristics and inhibit female sex characteristics, adrenal androgen excess results in increased muscle strength and bone development as well as in masculinization.

The clinical manifestations of the adreno-genital syndromes differs considerably depending upon the sex of the individual and the age of onset. In the female, hirsutism, deepening of the voice, amenorrhea, enlargement of the clitoris, development of a male escutcheon and other masculine features characterize the condition. In the male prior to puberty, the clinical manifestations are somewhat similar to those seen in precocious puberty.

The diagnosis of the adrenogenital syndromes is based upon evaluation of the clinical features together with elevation of urinary 17-ketosteroids. Such features without elevated 17-ketosteroids indicate the presence of an ovarian tumor (arrhenoblastoma) or testicular tumor.

Pheochromocytoma (Functional Paraganglioma)

The pheochromocytoma of the adrenal medulla occurs chiefly in the adult patient 30 to 50 years of age. However, the tumor may occur at extra-adrenal sites and some cases have been reported in children. Although benign pheochromocytomas are most common, malignant forms with distant metastasis are seen in about 10 percent of cases. Since the tumor releases substantial amounts of catecholamines, predominately norepinephrine, hypertension is the chief presenting symptom. Additionally, sweating, tachycardia and postural hypotension occur. The hypertension thus differs from essential hypertension. The diagnosis is based on the identification of a tumor mass, usually by aortography and presacral air insufflation, and the demonstration of free catecholamines and vanillylmandelic acid (VMA) in the urine.

The pheochromocytoma is of special significance since it may occur as one manifestation of the *familial multiple endocrine adenomatosis syndrome* (*Wermer's syndrome*). With this condition, a variety of endocrine hyperplasias or neoplasias may occur simultaneously and in various combinations. These may involve the parathyroids, islets of Langerhans, anterior pituitary, adrenal and/or thyroid glands.

Pheochromocytoma has been reported to occur in association with: (1) neurofibromatosis (p. 429), (2) Von Hippel-Lindau disease, (3) neurofibromatosis–hyperparathyroidism–Zollinger-Ellison syndrome (islet cell tumor–gastric hypersecretion–gastric ulcers), (4) neurofibromatosis–medullary carcinoma of thyroid–parathyroid adenoma, (5) medullary carcinoma of thyroid–mucosal neuromas (multiple mucosal neuroma syndrome, Sipple's syndrome).

Neuroblastoma–Ganglioneuroma

One of the most common forms of cancer in young children, neuroblastomas arise most commonly in the adrenal gland. They may also occur in the paravertebral sympathetic chain, abdominal viscera, retina of the eye (retinoblastoma), jaw, nose, bladder and other sites. Catecholamines and their metabolite vanillylmandelic acid (VMA) appear in the urine. Metastasis may be widespread, involving chiefly the liver, lungs, and bones, including the jaws. While these tumors are highly malignant, a few cases undergo spontaneous maturation to less aggressive forms, ganglioneuroblastoma and ganglioneuroma. The latter is completely benign. This transition is more likely to occur if the neuroblastoma is present at birth or in the first year of life.

Neuropolyendocrine Syndrome (Sipple's Syndrome)

This apparently autosomal dominant syndrome is characterized by familial occurrence, multiple mucosal neuromas, medullary carcinoma of the thyroid, and pheochromocytoma. The mucosal neuromas appear as numerous elevated nodules on the lips and tongue soon after birth (p. 421). The medullary carcinoma of the thyroid and the pheochromocytoma of the adrenal medulla may not be clinically apparent until the late teens or adulthood. As noted in a previous section, catecholamines secreted by the pheochromocytoma may cause hypertension, postural hypotension, sweating, headache, nausea, and other symptoms. Elevated urinary VMA is characteristic. The most serious aspect of Sipple's syndrome is the thyroid medullary carcinoma which frequently metastasizes to cause death (p. 343).

NERVE AND MUSCLE FUNCTION DISORDERS

The evaluation and diagnosis of nerve and muscle function disorders of the oral regions are predicated on (1) an understanding of functional neuroanatomy to aid in identifying the *anatomic site* of the disease process, and (2) the correlation of the clinical findings with recognized disease entities. While elaborate neurologic tests and laboratory examinations may be required in problem cases, careful observation, detailed interrogation and a few simple functional tests will usually suggest the component of the neural or neuromuscular apparatus which is primarily affected.

Disturbances of Motor Function

Motor function disturbances are most readily recognized by observation of the patient's body movements, facial expression, speech, jaw movements, and swallowing functions. A "frozen" expression, difficulty in enunciating certain sounds or the inability to smile, whistle, suck liquids through a straw or blow up a balloon will indicate weakness or paralysis of the muscles of facial expression. "Jaw drop" or the inability to close forcibly or execute lateral excursions of the jaws points to disturbances involving the muscles of mastication. Disorders of the pharyngeal, palatal, tongue, and/or cheek musculature will often produce dysphagia, dysarthria, nasal speech, regurgitation of food and/or trapping of food in the buccal vestibule. Palpation of the involved muscle may elicit pain (myositis) or demonstrate increased warmth, trismus, enlargement, spasticity, fasciculation, atonia or atrophy. Percussion of normal muscle will produce a brief reflex contraction; certain neuromuscular disorders, on the other hand, will show prolonged, spasmodic contraction (percussion myotonia) by tapping the tongue or other muscles with a dull instrument.

Weakness or paralysis of the oral and facial muscles may develop secondary to lesions located in the central nervous system, the motor nerve trunk, the myoneural junction or the muscle proper. In some instances paralysis is sudden, as in Bell's palsy. In other instances the onset of motor function loss is gradual, involving a few fascicles of the muscle and gradually extending to affect an entire muscle or group of muscles. Weakness of muscle after a period of exercise, following by a prolonged recovery period, is characteristic of the myasthenias.

Functional disturbances of the neuromuscular apparatus secondary to lesions in the central nervous system can exhibit a variety of clinical features reflected in the function of the muscle supplied. Muscle coordination is generally impaired, with the involvement of single muscles or groups of muscles depending upon the extent and character of the disease process involved. The affected muscles may show tremor, fasciculation, hypotonia, myotonia, paralysis or atrophy. In some cases, associated sensory disturbances are present as well (e.g. epilepsy). Diseases of importance within this group include cerebral palsy, multiple sclerosis, poliomyelitis, the "motor system" diseases and Parkinson's disease.

Disturbances of Sensory Function

Disorders of the sensory nerves (or their receptors) may affect one or several of the recognized senses (sight, hearing, smell, touch, pressure, temperature, kinesthesia, proprioception, taste, pain), depending upon the type and number of sensory units involved. For the most part, the several forms of neuritis and neuralgia (p. 293) are characterized by lowered sensory thresholds (hyperesthesia), most particularly for pain. Loss of sensory perception is an equally significant symptom and is most commonly manifest in the oral cavity as paresthesia or anesthesia.

Paresthesia, Anesthesia

The loss of general sensory perception of the cranial nerves may be gradual or abrupt. It should be noted that new denture wearers will often complain for a time of some loss of taste and reduced touch and temperature sensation over the mucosal surfaces covered by the denture. In addition, there may be temporary sialorrhea which may further modify sensory function.

Paresthesia or anesthesia of the lower lip and corner of the mouth is of much greater clinical significance, since this may be the first indication of primary or metastatic tumor in the mandible. Because the onset is usually gradual, the patient may not be aware of the change until it is somewhat advanced. For the most part, the patient describes the sensation as a tingling (paresthesia) or numbness (anesthesia) similar to that experienced during block anesthesia of the mandibular nerve.

Loss of Taste

Disturbances in taste sensation are more difficult to establish since taste not only is dependent upon normally functioning receptors and sensory nerves but is modified by visual, olfactory and psychogenic stimuli and salivary flow. The chorda tympani branch of the facial nerve (VII) supplies taste receptors for the anterior two-thirds of the tongue. The posterior one-third of the tongue is supplied by the glossopharyngeal nerve (IX) while the vagus nerve (X) supplies the pharyngeal aspect of the tongue, the soft palate and the epiglottis. General sensory perception is supplied to the anterior two-thirds of the tongue by the trigeminal nerve (V_3) and to the posterior one-third by IX.

Disturbances of Autonomic Function

Autonomic nervous system control of internal homeostasis may be modified by psychic stimuli (fight or flight), vegetative requirements, and certain drugs and hormones. Sympathetic innervation of the skin of the face and scalp is from the superior cervical ganglion by way of plexuses distributed along branches of the external carotid artery. Both sympathetic and parasympathetic nerves supply the salivary glands, intrinsic muscles of the eye and mucous membranes through the cranial autonomic ganglia (ciliary, sphenopalatine, otic, submaxillary). Flushing or blanching of the face, hyperhidrosis or anhidrosis, ptosis, miosis or dilatation of the pupils, nasal congestion, lacrimation and alterations in the quantity and/or character of saliva are suggestive of autonomic dysfunction. Since the autonomic system is anatomically and functionally integrated with other parts of the nervous system, signs and symptoms frequently overlap.

Autonomic signs are commonly seen in conjunction with the atypical neuralgias, Horner's syndrome, auriculotemporal syndrome, crocodile-tears syndrome, Raynaud's disease (p. 261) and familial dysautonomia (p. 362).

Tests of Nerve and Muscle Function

The simpler tests of nerve and muscle function are designed to demonstrate sensory perception, response to autonomic stimulation and neuromotor activity. These may be supplemented by microscopic tissue examination and clinical laboratory studies.

General Sensory Perception Tests

Touch, temperature, and pressure sensations may be simply tested by stimulating the skin or mucosa with a needle, wisps of cotton, electric pulp tester, or hot and cold glass tubes. By charting the changes from normal, the involved nerve(s) can usually be identified. Two-point discrimination, the ability to perceive two simultaneous stimuli applied in close approximation, is most highly developed on the fingertips, lips, and tip of the tongue. Normal values will be less than 0.3 cm.

Taste Perception Tests

The primary taste sensations are sweet, salty, sour and bitter. Secondary taste sensations represent combinations of the primary tastes modified or enhanced by texture (touch), temperature, and odor of the substance being tasted. Primary taste function is tested by applying solutions of salt, sugar water, vinegar or quinine to different portions of the tongue and recording the physiologic response. The fungiform papillae may contain all four types of receptors, whereas the circumvallate papillae contain only bitter receptors. Inasmuch as these endorgans of taste are quite specific, failure of the patient to recognize one or more of the test substances at given points on the tongue is not abnormal.

Reflex Testing

The reflex arc involves a receptor, the afferent (sensory) neuron, central nervous system synapses, the efferent (motor) neuron and the effector (muscle, gland). Interruption of the arc at any point abolishes the typical response.

The *superficial reflexes* of the mucous membranes include the corneal (conjunctival) reflex, nasal (sneeze) reflex, uvular reflex, and pharyngeal (gag) reflex.

Deep reflexes are typified by the well-known patellar (knee-jerk) reflex. The maxillary (jaw-jerk) reflex follows tapping on an instrument placed on the lower anterior teeth or hitting the point of the chin with the jaws slightly open. With a normal response, the jaw is forced open slightly and closes reflexly, just short of the teeth coming into direct contact. Deep reflexes, normally inhibited by higher centers in the brain, are exaggerated in cases of lesions of the motor cortex. Absence of superficial reflexes combined with exaggerated deep reflexes generally indicates upper motor neuron disease.

Visceral reflexes of interest include the several pupillary reflexes, the carotid sinus reflex, the oculocardiac reflex and the ciliospinal reflex. In the carotid sinus reflex, pressure over the carotid sinus normally causes a fall of blood pressure and slowing of the heart. Fainting (carotid sinus syncope) occurs with prolonged pressure over this area. Absence of the carotid sinus reflex indicates involvement of cranial nerves IX or X. The oculocardiac reflex, induced by pressure over the eyeballs, induces slowing of the heart if nerves V and X are normal. The ciliospinal reflex, induced by painful skin stimulation such as pinching the neck, causes dilatation of the pupil and indicates normal function of the cervical sympathetics. In Horner's syndrome, this reflex is abolished.

Autonomic Drug Tests

A number of drugs specifically stimulate or inhibit autonomic nerve impulses. For example, sympathomimetic (epinephrine, amphetamines) and parasympathomimetic (acetylcholine, pilocarpine) drugs stimulate salivary flow while parasympatholytic (atropine) drugs inhibit the flow, producing a more viscid secretion. The vasodilators and vasoconstrictors may be used to test autonomic response.

Sweat Test of Minor

Disturbances of the sympathetic system may be tested by thermoregulatory sweating. Aspirin (0.5 gm) is administered one-half hour prior to the test. An iodine solution is painted over the skin area to be tested and allowed to dry. The area is then dusted with starch powder and sweating is induced by giving the patient hot liquids and covering him with electric blankets. Sweating facilitates a reaction between the iodine and starch, giving a blue-black coloration. Skin resistance to the passage of small electric currents is also used to test sweat gland function.

Nerve Conduction Test

This test utilizes the application of galvanic shock directly to the nerve trunk or the muscle and is useful in localizing the given lesion either proximal or distal to the point of application. Thus, if direct application of galvanic stimulus to the muscle elicits a contraction, but to the motor nerve trunk does not, the defect may be assumed to be within the nerve.

Electromyography

The recording of bioelectric activity in muscle is a useful procedure which has had increased application to dental problems in recent years. Distinctive variations in wave forms and sounds are often pathognomonic of the basic disease process involved. Electromyography has been used to study normal functional patterns of the muscles of mastication and has permitted the identification and correction of occlusal abnormalities associated with bruxism. The results obtained with electromyography are objective and, in the hands of a trained individual, are reliable tools particularly in the diagnosis and prognosis of functional disturbances involving the central nervous system or motor neurons, of peripheral nerve injury and disease, of disturbances of the myoneural junction and of primary myopathies.

Muscle Biopsy

Biopsy of muscle may be useful in the diagnosis of muscle disease in some instances, although many of the primary myopathies frequently present a similar histologic appearance. The muscle biopsy does provide confirming evidence, in conjunction with other clinical and laboratory findings, in the diagnosis of such primary muscle diseases as muscular dystrophy and polymyositis. The presence of nematodes (*e.g.* trichinosis, p. 292) and certain other specific infectious agents may occasionally be identified in muscle sections. Such diseases as myasthenia gravis, reported to be characterized by "lymphorrhages," usually show non-specific changes in the muscle biopsy.

Creatine and Creatinine

Creatine and creatinine of the blood and urine reflect muscle catabolism and are of some diagnostic importance in such diseases as the muscular dystrophies. Creatinine, which is normally present in the blood and urine, shows a distinct fall in value with progressive muscle breakdown and loss of muscle function in the muscular dystrophies. On the other hand, creatine, which is normally converted to creatinine before excretion in the urine, shows a corresponding increase as muscle function is lost.

Serum Creatine Phosphokinase (CPK)

CPK has been a particularly useful test in the identification of active progressive muscular dystrophy and of those individuals believed to be suspected carriers of the gene or who do not yet exhibit clinical signs of the disease. CPK is also elevated in myocardial infarction but is normal in neuromuscular atrophies.

Aldolase is a fairly specific but less sensitive test for patients with suspected muscular dystrophy or other primary myopathies.

Serum Glutamic Oxaloacetic Transaminase (SGOT)

This test also reflects degree of muscle breakdown and has been particularly valuable in evaluation of patients with myocardial infarction. Because of the muscle breakdown products elaborated, values of SGOT are also increased in muscular dystrophy.

Lactic Dehydrogenase (LDH)

Like CPK and SGOT, this enzyme is liberated in the bloodstream in cases of muscle breakdown. Thus, elevated values are seen in myocardial infarction and other myopathies (*e.g.* myositis, rhabdomyolysis, muscular dystrophy, etc.). If a biochemical profile (p. 220) is done, concurrent elevations of all three of the above enzymes may be seen in the chronic myopathies. In myocardial infarction, the peak elevations of CPK, SGOT and LDH will vary according to age of the infarct. Isolated elevation of LDH may indicate the presence of renal carcinoma or other visceral cancer.

Specific Functional Neuropathies and Myopathies

Several functional disorders of the sensory-motor system manifest in the oral regions are described in the following sections. Those which are characterized by pain, including functional myositis, neuritis and neuralgia, are discussed on pages 292–295.

Auriculotemporal Nerve Syndrome (Gustatory Sweating, Frey's Syndrome)

In this bizarre condition, flushing and sweating of the face on the affected side occur with eating or taste stimulation. The condition follows injury or surgery to the auriculotemporal nerve in which the salivary parasympathetics reinnervate the facial sweat glands. Some individuals exhibit gustatory sweating following the ingestion of highly spiced foods, chocolate, or certain cheeses. Gustatory sweating may also be present in *diabetic autonomic neuropathy.*

Gustatory rhinorrhea has been reported in a rare case following radical parotidectomy.

Horner's Syndrome (Sympathetic Ophthalmoplegia)

This disorder of the autonomic nervous system follows damage or pressure on the cervical sympathetic ganglia which causes unilateral ptosis, miosis, enophthalmos, anhidrosis and flushing of the face.

Raynaud's Phenomenon

Paroxysmal vasoconstriction of the arteries and arterioles of the fingers (Raynaud's disease), when seen in conjunction with certain of the collagen diseases, chiefly scleroderma, is referred to as Raynaud's phenomenon. The fingers become pale or cyanotic upon exposure to cold or emotional upset; reactive hyperemia follows.

Bell's Palsy

Sudden unilateral (facial nerve) paralysis of the muscles of facial expression may arise following exposure to cold, surgery or trauma, infections, or for no obvious reason. There is drooping of the corner of the mouth with drooling of saliva and inability to whistle, wrinkle the forehead, wink or close the eye (Fig. 7–2). With attempts to close the eyes, the eyeball on the involved side turns upward (Bell's phenomenon). Additional signs and symptoms are present if the lesion is located more proximally along the facial nerve or its branches. For example, lesions proximal to the stylomastoid foramen in the facial canal cause loss of taste to the anterior two-thirds of the tongue and reduced salivation (chorda tympani involvement). Hyperacusis (stapedius muscle involvement) occurs in lesions higher in the canal and VIIIth nerve deafness may be present when the lesion affects the internal auditory meatus.

Melkersson-Rosenthal Syndrome

Recurring Bell's palsy, cheilitis granulomatosa (p. 430), fissured or scrotal tongue and facial edema characterize this unusual condition. The recurring facial edema must be differentiated from angioneurotic edema (Fig. 7–14).

Ramsey Hunt Syndrome

In this condition, Bell's palsy is associated with herpes zoster (p. 326) of the geniculate ganglion and tympanic membrane.

Marcus Gunn (Jaw-Winking) Phenomenon

With congenital ptosis, movement of the mandible to the contralateral side causes elevation of the ptotic eyelid.

Inverted Marcus Gunn (Marin-Amat) Syndrome

Sometimes seen during the recovery period in Bell's palsy, this condition exhibits closure of the eyes upon forceful opening of the mouth.

Crocodile-Tears Syndrome

Eating (or taste stimulation) causes lacrimation in this unusual condition. The syndrome is due to atypical nerve regeneration following VIIth nerve injury. It is therefore analogous to the "gustatory sweating" of Frey's syndrome (p. 261).

Bilateral Facial Palsy

Bulbar disease should be suspected in cases of bilateral VIIth nerve paralysis of recent onset if uveoparotitis or other etiologic factors can be ruled out. Facial diplegia has been reported in association with infectious mononucleosis.

Uveoparotid Fever (Heerfordt's Syndrome)

Seventh nerve paralysis, and other cranial nerve involvement, may be seen in up to half of the patients with uveoparotitis (p. 358).

Congenital Facial Diplegia (Moebius Syndrome)

Congenital nuclear aplasia and/or congenital facial muscle aplasia is the most likely basis for the bilateral facial paralysis characteristic of this syndrome.

Orofacial Dyskinesia (Facial Spasm, Paroxysmal Hyperkinesia of Facial Muscles, Neck-Face Syndrome, Extrapyramidal Syndrome, etc.)

Characterized by involuntary twitching of the facial muscles, various forms of this spectrum of conditions have been associated with extrapyramidal disorders, phenothiazine therapy and disorders of dental proprioception. The signs range from severe muscle spasms to purposeless, uncoordinated lip-smacking, grimacing and pouting movements. Vermicular tongue movements may precede tardive dyskinesia and the full syndrome may be aborted if the use of antipsychotic drugs can be stopped.

Meniere's Disease (Paroxysmal Vertigo)

This disturbance of endolymphatic fluid pressures in the labyrinth of the middle ear and the cochlear division of the VIIIth nerve is characterized by tinnitus, vertigo, deafness and nausea. The condition occurs chiefly in the middle-aged or elderly and should be differentiated clinically from vascular disorders which may produce similar symptoms.

Unilateral Vagal Paralysis

Soft palate paralysis, anesthesia of the pharynx and larynx, hoarseness, nasal speech and dysphagia on the affected side are seen in Xth nerve disturbances. The particular combination of signs and symptoms will vary according to the site of the causative lesion.

Hypoglossal Nerve Disturbances

Lesions involving the XIth nerve are suggested by paralysis of the tongue with fasciculation and atrophy. Tremors and atrophy of the tongue are also seen in "motor system" disease (*progressive bulbar palsy, progressive muscular atrophy and amyotrophic lateral sclerosis*).

Progressive Muscular Dystrophy (Generalized Familial Muscular Dystrophy, Pseudohypertrophic Muscular Dystrophy of Duchenne)

This disease occurs in boys as a sex-linked recessive trait. It arises prior to 5 years of age with progressive involvement of striated muscles, beginning in the proximal girdles first and extending to the distal muscles as the disease progresses. Initially, these patients exhibit Gower's maneuver, an attempt to arise from the floor by walking up the legs with the hands. The calves of the legs show gross enlargement (pseudohypertrophy). En-

largement of the tongue and speech difficulty follow in the late stages. Flaring and diastema formation of the anterior teeth, due to oral and facial muscle imbalance, are common. Few affected children live to maturity.

Facioscapulohumeral Muscular Dystrophy (Mild Restricted Muscular Dystrophy of Landouzy and Dejerine)

This form of muscular dystrophy differs from the progressive familial type in that it may arise at any age, usually the second decade, and may affect either males or females. It has a slow, prolonged course but is rarely fatal. The disease does not exhibit pseudohypertrophy but rather shows progressive atrophy and degeneration involving mainly the shoulder girdle and facial muscles. Because of involvement of the facial muscles, the face has a mask-like appearance. The patient is unable to pucker the lips or whistle and difficulty in speech is encountered.

Oculopharyngeal Muscular Dystrophy

A late-onset form of muscular dystrophy inherited as a dominant trait, oculopharyngeal muscular dystrophy affects chiefly the facial, oral and pharyngeal musculature.

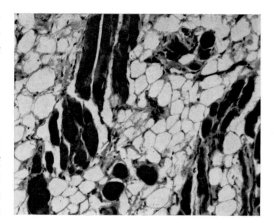

Fig. 9-23. Oculopharyngeal muscular dystrophy. Photomicrograph of tongue muscle showing scattered residual striated muscle fibers and surrounding fat tissue. Fat replacement of striated muscle of the tongue. Only scattered intact muscle fibers remain. (Courtesy of Stanley Weitzner.)

There is a characteristic "myopathic facies" with weakness, flaccid paralysis and atrophy. The muscle fibers show progressive replacement by fat (Fig. 9–23).

Myotonic Dystrophy

This progressive familial disease is characterized by myotonia (failure of relaxation after muscle contraction), followed by marked weakness and atrophy of muscles. Percussion of the muscle ("percussion myotonia") causes contraction of the muscle with slow relaxation. For example, tapping of the tongue with an instrument causes prolonged contraction of the intrinsic muscles. The disease is slowly progressive over many years and eventually causes the death of the patient.

Congenital Myotonia

This disease of childhood is characterized by a true hypertrophy of the muscle so that the individual appears as a small Hercules. Eventually, the enlarged muscles weaken and atrophy. Percussion myotonia is marked and generally the patient has considerable difficulty in initiation of speech. Death does not occur as a direct result of the disease.

Paramyotonia Congenita

This rare muscle disease is characterized by myotonia only upon exposure to cold. However, in common with the other forms of myotonia, percussion myotonia is elicited in the intrinsic muscle of the tongue.

Hypotonia

Reduced or absent tonus in the striated muscles is characteristic of a variety of diseases of infancy (floppy infant syndrome) and includes such primary muscle diseases as infantile muscular dystrophy, polymyositis, central core disease and other neural or neuromuscular conditions.

Myasthenia Gravis

Abnormal fatigue and weakness of muscle following exercise, with a long recovery period, characterize the myasthenias. In general these represent disturbances of muscle excitation and contractility often referable to defects of transmission at the myoneural junction. The most important of these to dentists is *myasthenia gravis,* a disorder characterized by ready fatigue of muscle following mild exercise and a long recovery period. It occurs most commonly in the 20- to 50-year age group and shows some predilection for females. The initial manifestation of myasthenia gravis is often in the external ocular muscles, with resulting ptosis and diplopia. This is followed shortly by involvement of facial, neck and limb muscles. Quite often the patient exhibits dysarthria and dysphagia. Because of weakness and fatigue in the temporal and masseter muscles, the mouth of the patient will hang open as fatigue develops. Ergograph (grip) tracings exhibit the quantitative loss of strength, which is restored promptly by anticholinesterase drugs. Muscle biopsies are not in themselves diagnostic; rather, the diagnosis is made on the basis of clinical findings and the ability of cholinesterase inhibitors to restore muscle strength and function. Considerable evidence has accumulated to suggest that myasthenia gravis represents an autoimmune disease in which the patient reacts to his own muscle proteins or, more specifically, to those tissues of the myoneural junction.

Multiple Sclerosis

This "demyelinating disease" of the central nervous system commonly arises in young adults from 20 to 40 years of age. While the initial expression of the disease varies with the location and severity of the white matter involvement, typical features are weakness of the extremities and an ataxic gait (p. 126), visual disturbances (diplopia), skin paresthesia, mood changes and autonomic system involvement with loss of bladder control. The classical Charcot's triad includes intention tremor, nystagmus and "scanning" or "staccato" speech. Facial and masticatory muscle weakness may be early signs. The disease runs a progressive, down-hill course which may range from a few months to many years.

Parkinson's Syndrome (Paralysis Agitans)

This neuromuscular disorder is character-ized by resting or non-intention tremors and a propulsion or festination gait (p. 126). The disease has an insidious onset in individuals in their 50s or 60s, with increasing rigidity and tremors. "Pill-rolling" tremors of the fingers and bobbing head movements as well as dysphagia and dysarthria are typical fea-tures. As the patient's disability progresses, often over several years, emotional problems sometimes arise; however, mental faculties are not affected.

"Motor System Disease"

This broad term includes at least three clinical states: progressive muscular atrophy, progressive bulbar palsy and amyotrophic lateral sclerosis. These are characterized by corticospinal and anterior horn cell degener-ation and either bulbar or limb muscle in-volvement. In the bulbar forms (progressive bulbar palsy, amyotrophic lateral sclerosis), the tongue, pharyngeal and laryngeal mus-cles are affected, with resultant dysphagia, dysarthria and hyperactive jaw-jerk reflex (p. 259). Interestingly the tongue may be involved early, with fasciculation and tremor followed by extreme atrophy. The motor system diseases affect adults, usually in the third to fifth decades, with death occurring within five years of onset.

Poliomyelitis (Infantile Paralysis)

With the widespread use of live oral vac-cines, the incidence of poliomyelitis has de-clined remarkably in recent years. The onset of the paralytic form of the disease is sud-den, with fever, sore throat, headache and stiff neck followed by flaccid paralysis. In bulbar poliomyelitis, the motor neurons of the cranial nerves are affected, often with resultant unilateral or bilateral paralysis of the facial or masticatory muscles.

Cerebral Palsy (Little's Disease)

Non-progressive disorders of motor func-tion present since infancy or early childhood and characterized by involuntary muscle con-tractions, rigidity, atonia or tremors are broadly referred to as cerebral palsy. Clini-cal forms of this heterogeneous group of conditions include spastic, athetoid, ataxic, rigid and tremorous types. Up to half of the cases exhibit associated mental retardation. Dental management of the cerebral palsy patient poses special problems with behav-ior, dietary and oral hygiene control and operative procedures.

Epilepsy

Epilepsy is characterized by sudden, tran-sient seizures affecting chiefly the motor sys-tem, although sensory, autonomic and psy-chic components may be involved as well. In the *grand mal* form, the patient loses consciousness and will fall to the floor. Con-vulsions follow, often with gnashing of the teeth and biting injuries to the tongue. Sub-sequently, there is a period of sleep and stupor of up to 4 hours with the victim un-able to recall little if anything of the attack. Described by laymen as "fits," the patient recognizes only the loss of consciousness and may claim or admit only to "fainting spells."

With *petit mal* seizures, there may be momentary loss of consciousness with a blank expression or myoclonic jerks, after which the individual resumes his normal ac-tivities. Commonly, the eyes of the patient roll upward and all voluntary actions are stopped for a few moments.

Diagnosis is based chiefly on the clinical history of typical seizures and electroenceph-alography. Anticonvulsant drugs, particularly diphenylhydantoin (Dilantin sodium) or phenobarbital, are generally effective in con-trolling the seizures. An undesirable side effect of Dilantin therapy is marked gingival hyperplasia (Fig. 7–40) which may require gingivectomy and, if possible, substitution of another drug such as phenobarbital.

BIBLIOGRAPHY

Tissue Biopsy

Bhaskar, S. N.: Oral pathology in the dental office: Survey of 20,575 biopsy specimens, J. Amer. Dent. Ass., 76, 761, 1968.

Cooke, B. E. D.: The diagnosis of bullous lesions affecting the oral mucosa, Brit. Dent. J., 109, 83, 1960.

Friedlander, A. H.: Use of a needle biopsy in oral and maxillofacial surgery, Oral Surg., 41, 411, 1976.

Keene, J. J. Jr.: Arteriosclerotic changes within the diabetic oral vasculature, J. Dent. Res., 54, 77, 1975.

Schwartz, H. C. and Olson, D. J.: Amyloidosis: A rational approach to diagnosis by intraoral biopsy, Oral Surg., 39, 837, 1975.

Strong, M. S., Vaughn, C. W. and Incze, J.: Toluidine blue in diagnosis of cancer of the larynx, Arch. Otolaryngol., 91, 515, 1970.

Weisman, M. I.: The importance of biopsy in endodontics, Oral Surg., 40, 153, 1975.

Zajicek, J., Eneroth, E-M. and Jakobssen, P.: Aspiration biopsy of salivary gland tumors. VI. Morphologic studies on smears and histologic sections from mucoepidermoid carcinoma, Acta Cytol., 20, 35, 1976.

Oral Exfoliative Cytology

Alling, C. C. and Secord, R. T.: A technique for oral exfoliative cytology, Oral Surg., 17, 668, 1964.

Goldsby, J. W. and Staats, O. J.: Nuclear changes of intraoral exfoliated cells in six patients with sickle-cell disease, Oral Surg., 16, 1042, 1963.

Hayes, R. L., Berg, G. W. and Ross, W. L.: Oral cytology: its value and its limitations, J. Amer. Dent. Ass., 79, 649, 1969.

Medak, H., Burlakow, P., Cohen, L., McGrew, E. and Tiecke, R.: Correlation of cytology and clinical findings in pemphigus vulgaris, J. Oral Med., 28, 4, 1973.

Shapiro, B. L. and Gorlin, R. J.: An analysis of oral cytodiagnosis, Cancer, 17, 1477, 1964.

Shedd, D. P., Hukill, P. B., Bahn, S. and Ferraro, R. H.: Further appraisal of in vivo staining properties of oral cancer, Arch. Surg., 95, 16, 1967.

Whitten, J. B. Jr.: Diagnostic cytology of the oral mucous membranes. Thesis, Master of Science in Dentistry, Indiana University School of Dentistry, 1966.

Whitten, J. B. Jr.: Cytologic examination of aspirated material from cysts or cyst-like lesions, Oral Surg., 25, 710, 1968.

Examination of the Saliva

Abelson, D. C., Wotman, S., Mandel, I. D., Marcus, L. S. and Waldo, A. L.: The effect of surgical procedure on salivary electrolytes, J. Oral Med., 29, 41, 1974.

Benedek-Spöt, E.: The composition of unstimulated human parotid saliva, Arch. Oral Biol., 18, 39, 1973.

Chauncey, H. H.: Salivary enzymes, J. Amer. Dent. Ass., 63, 360, 1961.

Chernick, W. S., Eichel, H. J. and Barbero, G. J.: Submaxillary salivary enzymes as a measure of glandular activity in cystic fibrosis, J. Pediat., 65, 694, 1964.

Connor, S., Iranpour, B. and Mills, J.: Alteration in parotid salivary flow in diabetes mellitus, Oral Surg., 30, 55, 1970.

Ferguson, D. B. and Fort, A.: Circadian variations in calcium and phosphate secretion from human parotid and submandibular salivary glands, Caries Res., 7, 19, 1973.

Frankel, S.: Calcium binding in saliva, J. Dent. Med., 28, 55, 1973.

Fritz, M. E., Caplan, D. B., Leever, D. and Levitt, J.: Composition of parotid saliva on different days in patients with cystic fibrosis, Amer. J. Dis. Child., 123, 116, 1972.

Gugler, E., Pallavicini, J. C., Swerdlow, H., Lipkin, I. and di Sant' Agnese, P. A.: Immunological studies of submaxillary saliva from patients with cystic fibrosis and from normal children, J. Pediat., 73, 548, 1968.

Hoerman, K. C., Chauncey, H. H., Herrold, R. D., with Veach, W. L. and Shklair, I. L.: Parotid saliva acid phosphatase in prostatic cancer, Cancer, 12, 359, 1959.

Katz, F. H. and Shannon, I. L.: Adrenal corticosteroids in submaxillary fluid, J. Dent. Res., 48, 448, 1969.

Kutscher, A. H., Mandel, I. D., Thompson, R. H. Jr., Wotman, S., Zegarelli, E. V., Fahn, B. S., Denning, C. R., Goldstein, J. A., Taubman, M. and Khotim, S.: Parotid saliva. I. Flow rate, Amer. J. Dis. Child., 110, 643, 1965.

Mandel, I., Thompson, R. H., Wotman, S., Taubman,, M., Kutscher, A. H., Zegarelli, E. V., Denning, C. R., Botwich, J. T. and Fahn, B. S.: Parotid saliva in cystic fibrosis, II Electrolytes and protein-bound carbohydrates, Amer. J. Dis. Child., 110, 646, 1965.

Mandel, I. D. and Baurmash, H.: Sialochemistry in Sjögren's syndrome, Oral Surg., 41, 182, 1976.

Puskulian, L.: Salivary electrolyte changes during the normal menstrual cycle, J. Dent. Res., 51 (Suppl.), 1212, 1972.

Schneyer, L. H., Young, J. A. and Schneyer, C. A.: Salivary secretion of electrolytes, Physiol. Rev., 52, 720, 1972.

Shannon, I. L.: Reference table for human parotid saliva collected at varying levels of exogenous stimulation, J. Dent. Res., 52, 1157, 1973.

Sproles, A. C.: Cyclic A,P concentration in saliva of normal children and children with Down's syndrome, J. Dent. Res., *52* (Suppl.), 915, 1973.

Truelove, E. L., Bixler, D. and Merritt, A. D.: Simplified method for collection of pure submandibular saliva in large volumes, J. Dent. Res., *46*, 1400, 1967.

Winer, R. A. and Chauncey, H. H.: Parotid saliva enzymes in Down's syndrome, J. Dent. Res., *54*, 62, 1975.

Wotman, S. and Mandel, I. D.: Salivary indicators of systemic disease, Postgrad. Med., *53*, 3, 1973.

Caries Activity Tests

Alban, A.: An improved Snyder test, J. Dent. Res., *49*, 641, 1970.

Bernier, J. L. and Muhler, J. C. (Eds.): *Improving Dental Practice Through Preventive Measures*, St. Louis, C. V. Mosby Co., 1966.

Sims, W.: The interpretation and use of Snyder tests and lactobacillus counts, J. Amer. Dent. Ass., *80*, 1315, 1970.

Hematology

Abbott Laboratories (North Chicago, Illinois): The use of blood, Feb., 1954.

Bowie, E. J. W., Fass, D. N., Olson, J. D. and Owen, C. A. Jr.: The spectrum of von Willebrand's disease revisited, Mayo Clin. Proc., *51*, 35, 1976.

Blecker, S. M. and Williams, A. C.: Postextraction bleeding in a patient with an acquired circulating anticoagulant against factor V, Oral Surg., *32*, 538, 1971.

Christie, R. W.: Routine admission laboratory tests in small hospitals, J. Indiana State Med. Ass., *60*, 1173, 1967.

Cohen, M. P.: Oral surgical complications with von Willebrand's disease, a case report, J. Oral Med., *30*, 115, 1975.

George, J. N. and Breckenridge, R. T.: The use of factor VIII and factor IX concentrates during surgery, J.A.M.A., *214*, 1673, 1970.

Greenberg, M. S., Miller, M. F. and Lynch, M. A.: Partial thromboplastin time as a predictor of blood loss in oral surgery patients receiving coumarin anticoagulants, J. Amer. Dent. Ass., *84*, 583, 1972.

Juniper, R. P.: The place of the erythrocyte sedimentation rate (ESR) in oral surgery, Brit. J. Oral Surg., *8*, 183, 1971.

Ray, G. C.: The ontogeny of interferon production by human leukocytes, J. Pediat., *76*, 94, 1970.

Rydell, R. O.: Blood factor XIII deficiency: review of literature and report of case, J. Oral Surg., *29*, 628, 1971.

Snyder, D. S.: Von Willebrand's disease, hemophilia A, and factor VIII, Human Path., *5*, 277, 1974.

Syracuse, E. P.: Purpura—A review, J. Oral Med., *30*, 21, 1975.

Weiss, J. I.: Thrombocytopenic purpura: the dentist's responsibility, J. Amer. Dent. Ass., *87*, 165, 1973.

White, G. E.: Oral manifestations of leukemia in children, Oral Surg., *29*, 420, 1970.

Wintrobe, M. M.: *Clinical Hematology*, 7th Ed., Philadelphia, Lea & Febiger, 1974.

Clinical Chemistry

Abildgaard, C. F., Simone, J. V., Honig, G. R., Forman, E. N., Johnson, C. A. and Seeler R. A.: Von Willebrand's disease: A comparative study of diagnostic tests, J. Pediat., *73*, 355, 1968.

Alper, C. A.: Plasma protein measurements as a diagnostic aid, New Eng. J. Med., *291*, 287, 1974.

Alsever, R. N.: Clinical problems in carbohydrate testing, Lab. Med., *6*, 31, 1975.

D'Eramo, E. M.: The significance of serum studies (SMA-12), J. Oral Surg., *31*, 795, 1973.

Didisheim, P.: Tests of blood coagulation hemostasis. II. The coagulation (clotting) time, J.A.M.A., *198*, 1299, 1966.

Elveback, L. R.: How high is high? A proposed alternative to the normal ranges, Mayo Clin. Proc., *47*, 93, 1972.

Frankel, S., Reitman, S. and Sonnenwirth, A. C. (Eds.): *Gradwohl's Clinical Laboratory Methods and Diagnosis*, 7th Ed., St. Louis, C. V. Mosby, Co., 1970.

Ghadimi, H.: Diagnosis of inborn errors of amino acid metabolism, Amer. J. Dis. Child., *114*, 433, 1967.

Guggenheimer, J. and Stiff, R. H.: Functional and teaching roles of a clinical diagnostic laboratory, J. Dent. Educ., March, 1970.

Harper, H. A.: *Review of Physiological Chemistry*, 15th Ed., Los Altos, Lange Medical Publications, 1975.

Hyman, L. R., Boner, G., Thomas, J. C. and Segar, W. E.: Immobilization hypercalcemia, Amer. J. Dis. Child., *124*, 723, 1972.

Johnson, R. H.: Clinical laboratory tests of interest to the dentist, Dent. Clin. North America, March, 1968.

Larson, P. H.: Serum proteins: Diagnostic significance of electrophoretic patterns, Human Path., *5*, 629, 1974.

Leake, D. and Deykin, D.: The diagnosis and treatment of bleeding tendencies, Oral Surg., *32*, 852, 1971.

Levinson, S. A. and MacFate, R. P.: *Clinical Laboratory Diagnosis*, 7th Ed., Philadelphia, Lea & Febiger, 1969.

McCormick, J. and Ripa, L. W.: Hypophosphatasia: review and report of case, J. Amer. Dent. Ass., *77*, 618, 1968.

Preston, J. A. and Troxel, D. B.: *Biochemical Profiling in Diagnostic Medicine*, Technicon Instruments Corporation, Tarrytown, N. Y., 1971.

Quick, A. J.: Hemostasis: theoretic and clinical aspects, Plast. Reconstruct. Surg., *26*, 321, 1960.

Rardin, T. E.: Laboratory profile screening in the family physician's office, J.A.M.A., *198*, 1253, 1966.

Reece, R. L. and Hobbie, R. K.: Computer evaluation of chemistry values. A reporting and diagnostic aid, Amer. J. Clin. Path., *57*, 664, 1972.

Shklair, I. L., Loving, R. H., Leberman, O. F. and Rau, C. F.: C-reactive protein and periodontal disease, J. Periodont., *39*, 93, 1968.

Snively, W. D. Jr.: Body fluid disturbances in dental medicine, J. Oral Med., *21*, 4, 1966.

Stimson, P. G.: Calcium metabolism in neoplastic disease, Oral Surg., *24*, 740, 1967.

Truelove, E. L., Burden, R. A. and Goebel, W. M.: Evaluation of a new chairside test for diabetes, Abstract No. 4, Program and Abstracts of Papers, 48th General Meeting, Int. Ass. for Dent. Res., New York, March 16–19, 1970.

Verne, D.: Water and electrolyte balance: a review, J. Oral Surg., *23*, 609, 1965.

Wiggins, H. E. Jr., Karian, B. K. and Smith, B. M.: A sublingual-submandibular calcific mass associated with tumoral calcinosis in a patient with suspected milk-alkali syndrome, Oral Surg., *40*, 8, 1975.

Wolf, P. L. and Williams, R.: *Practical Clinical Enzymology: Techniques and Interpretations* and Von der Muehll, E. and Wolf, P. L.: *Biochemical Profiling,* John Wiley & Sons, New York, 1973.

Zacharski, L. R., Bowie, E. J. W., Titus, J. L. and Owen, C. A. Jr.: Synthesis of antihemophiliac factor (factor VII) by leukocytes: preliminary report, Proc. Staff Meet. Mayo Clinic, *43*, 617, 1968.

Tests of Liver Function

Dacie, J. V. and Lewis, S. M.: *Practical Haematology,* London, J. and A. Churchill, 1970.

Frantzis, T. G., Sheridan, P. J., Reeve, C. M. and Young, L. L.: Oral manifestations of hemochromatosis, Oral Surg., *33*, 186, 1972.

Tietz, N. W. (Ed.): *Fundamentals of Clinical Chemistry,* Philadelphia, W. B. Saunders Co., 1970.

Examination of the Urine

D'Eramo, E. M. and McAnear, J. T.: The significance of urinalysis in treatment of hospitalized dental patients, Oral Surg., *38*, 36, 1974.

Free, A. H. and Free, H. M.: Urine sugar testing—state of the art, Lab. Med., *6*, 23, 1975.

Kory, M. and Waife, S. O. (Eds.): *Kidney and Urinary Tract Infections,* Indianapolis, Lilly Research Laboratories, 1971.

Lainson, P. A., Bjorge, T. L. and Fraleigh, C. M.: Use of the microhematocrit and urinalysis as screening tests in dental practice, J. Amer. Dent. Ass., *77*, 589, 1968.

Immunology and Serology

Beutner, E. H., *et al.*: Uses for immunofluorescence tests of skin and sera. Utilization of immunofluorescence in the diagnosis of bullous diseases, lupus erythematosus, and certain other diseases, Arch. Derm., *111*, 371, 1975.

Chang, L. W. and Tuffanelli, D. L.: The latest in serologic tests for syphilis and false-positive serologies, Med. Digest, March, 1968.

Elgart, M. L. and Higdon, R. S.: Allergic contact dermatitis to gold, Arch. Derm., *103*, 649, 1971.

Holt, L. E.: A nonallergist looks at allergy, New Eng. J. Med., *276*, 1449, 1967.

Israel, H. L. and Goldstein, R. A.: Relation of Kveim-antigen reaction to lymphadenopathy, New Eng. J. Med., *284*, 345, 1971.

Nisengard, R. J., Jablonska, S., Beutner, E. H., Shu, S., Chorzelski, T. P., Jarzabek, M., Blaszczyk, M. and Rzesa, G.: Diagnostic importance of immunofluorescence in oral bullous diseases and lupus erythematosus, Oral Surg., *40*, 365, 1975.

Shelley, W. B.: The patch test, J.A.M.A., *200*, 170, 1967.

Steigleder, G. K., Silva, A. Jr. and Nelson, C. T.: Histopathology of the Kveim test, Arch. Derm., *84*, 828, 1961.

Microbiological Examinations

Alexander, R. E.: Infectious and parasitic diseases, Oral Surg., *21*, 240, 1966.

Bell, W. A., Gamble, J. and Garrington, G. E.: North American blastomycosis with oral lesions, Oral Surg., *28*, 914, 1969.

Berger, C. J., Disque, F. C. and Topazian, R. G.: Rhinocerebral mucormycosis: Diagnosis and treatment, Oral Surg., *40*, 27, 1975.

Brewer, N. S. and Weed, L. A.: Diagnostic tissue microbiology methods, Human Path., *7*, 141, 1976.

Cohen, L.: Oral candidiasis—Its diagnosis and treatment, J. Oral Med., *27*, 7, 1972.

Furcolow, M. L., Balows, A., Menges, R. W., Rickar, D., McClellan, J. T. and Saliba, A.: Blastomycosis. An important medical problem in the central United States, J.A.M.A., *198*, 529, 1966.

Goebel, W. M. and Duquette, P.: Mycotic infections associated with complete dentures: report of three cases, J. Amer. Dent. Ass., *88*, 842, 1974.

Goldberg, M. H.: The changing biologic nature of acute dental infection, J. Amer. Dent. Ass., *80*, 1048, 1970.

Greenberg, M. S., Brightman, V. J. and Ship, I. I.: Clinical and laboratory differentiation of recurrent intraoral herpes simplex virus infections following fever, J. Dent. Res., *48*, 385, 1969.

Larato, D. C.: The antibiotic sensitivity test in dental practice, Oral Surg., *22*, 692, 1966.

Lehner, T.: Oral thrush, or acute pseudomembranous candidiasis. A clinicopathologic study of forty-four cases, Oral Surg., *18*, 27, 1964.

Lehner, T.: Immunofluorescent investigation of Candida albicans antibodies in human saliva, Arch. Oral Biol., *10*, 975, 1965.

Lennette, E. H.: Laboratory diagnosis of viral infections, Amer. J. Clin. Path., *57*, 737, 1972.

Martin, W. J. and Nichols, D. R.: Current practices in general medicine. 15. The mycoses, Proc. Staff Meet. Mayo Clinic, *35*, 149, 1960.

Nairn, R. I.: Nystatin and amphotericin B in the treatment of denture-related candidiasis, Oral Surg., *40*, 68, 1975.

Nally, F. F.: Idiopathic juvenile hypoparathyroidism with superficial moniliasis, Oral Surg., *30*, 356, 1970.

Roberts, G. D.: Laboratory diagnosis of fungal infections, Human Path., *7*, 161, 1976.

Sabiston, C. B., Grigsby, W R. and Segerstrom, N.: Bacterial study of pyogenic infections of dental origin, Oral Surg., *41*, 430, 1976.

Shuttleworth, C. W. and Gibbs, F. J.: The aetiological significance of Candida albicans in chronic angular cheilitis and its treatment with nystatin, Brit. Dent. J., *108*, 354, 1960.

Turner, J. E., Moore, D. W. and Shaw, B. S.: Prevalence and antibiotic susceptibility of organisms isolated from acute soft-tissue abscesses secondary to dental caries, Oral Surg., *39*, 848, 1975.

Weathers, D. R. and Griffin, J. W.: Intraoral ulcerations of recurrent herpes simplex and recurrent aphthae: two distinct clinical entities, J. Amer. Dent. Ass., *81*, 81, 1970.

Weinstein, L. and Chang, T-W.: Diagnosis of viral infections, Mod. Med., Jan., 83, 1958.

Young, L. L., Dolan, C. T., Sheridan, P. J. and Reeve, C. M.: Oral manifestations of histoplasmosis, Oral Surg., *33*, 191, 1972.

Tests of Endocrine Function

Albers, D. D.: Conservative treatment of oral bony lesions of hyperparathyroidism, Oral Surg., *38*, 209, 1974.

Alvarez, R. R., de and Smith, E. K.: Physiological basis for hormone therapy in the female, J.A.M.A., *168*, 489, 1958.

Bolande, R. P.: The neurocristopathies. A unifying concept of disease arising in neural crest maldevelopment, Human Path., *5*, 409, 1974.

Bull, T. R.: Taste and the chorda tympani, J. Laryngol Otol., *79*, 479, 1965.

Cheraskin, E.: The problem of diabetes mellitus in dental practice, J. Dent. Med., *15*, 67, 1960.

DeMajo, S. F. and Onativia, A.: Acromegaly and gigantism in a boy: comparison with 3 overgrown nonacromegalic children, J. Pediat., *57*, 382, 1960.

Egdahl, R. H.: Surgery of the parathyroid glands, Surg. Gynec. Obstet., *130*, 901, 1970.

Ganong, W. F.: *Review of Medical Physiology*, 7th Ed., Los Altos, Lange Medical Publications, 1975.

Gordon, G. S. and Roof, B. S.: Laboratory tests for hyperparathyroidism, J.A.M.A., *26*, 2729, 1968.

Kaplan, H.: The reagent-strip method for estimating blood glucose concentration, J. Amer. Dent. Ass., *74*, 1261, 1967.

Kay, S.: The abnormal parathyroid, Human Path., *7*, 127, 1976.

Keffer, J. H.: Thyroid diagnosis and the progressive thyroid profile, Lab. Med., *6*, 23, 1975.

Kennett, S. and Pollick, H.: Jaw lesions in familial hyperparathyroidism, Oral Surg., *31*, 502, 1971.

Kupfer, I. J.: Diabetes screening in an outpatient oral surgery clinic, New York Dent. J., *36*, 31, 1970.

Lang, E. K. and Bessler, W. T.: The roentgenologic features of acromegaly, Amer. J. Roentgen., *86*, 321, 1961.

Markel, S. F. and Johnson, R. M.: The clinical features and laboratory diagnosis of functional paraganglioma (pheochromocytoma), Lab. Med., *6*, 39, 1975.

Seed, R. W.: Changing trends in parathyroid surgery, Lab. Med., *7*, 14, 1976.

Selenkow, H. A. and Refetoff, S.: Common tests of thyroid function in serum, J.A.M.A., *202*, 153, 1967.

Snyder, M. B. and Cawson, R. A.: Jaw and pulpal metastasis of an adrenal neuroblastoma, Oral Surg., *40*, 775, 1975.

Spiegal, A. M., Marx, S. J., Ooppman, J. L., Beazley, R. M., Ketcham, A. S., Kasten, B. and Auerbach, G. D.: Intrathyroidal parathyroid adenoma or hyperplasia. An occasionally overlooked cause of surgical failure in primary hyperparathyroidism, J.A.M.A., *234*, 1029, 1975.

Thorn, G. W.: Clinical consideration in the use of corticosteroids, New Eng. J. Med., *274*, 775, 1966.

Truelove, E. L., Burden, R. and Goebel, W.: Evaluation of a new chairside test for diabetes mellitus, J. Oral Med., *26*, 139, 1971.

Watts, N.: Testing for Cushing's syndrome, Lab. Med., *6*, 45, 1975.

Weitzner, S.: Pathosis of the tongue in oculopharyngeal muscular dystrophy, report of two cases, Oral Surg., *28*, 613, 1969.

Nerve and Muscle Function Disorders

Akin, R. K., Keller, A. J. and Walters, P. J.: Myositis ossificans progressiva: a diagnostic problem. J. Oral Surg., *33*, 611, 1975.

Boddie, A. W. Jr., Guillamondegui, O. M. and Byers, R. M.: Gustatory rhinorrhea developing after radical parotidectomy—A new syndrome? Arch. Otolaryngol., *102*, 248, 1976.

Chusid, J. G. and McDonald, J. J.: *Correlative Neuroanatomy and Functional Neurology*, 15th Ed., Los Altos, Lange Medical Publications, 1973.

Diamart, H., Ekstrand, T. and Wiberg, A.: Prognosis of idiopathic Bell's palsy, Arch. Otolaryngol., *95*, 431, 1972.

Moskow, B. S.: Trichinosis in oral musculature: report of case, J. Amer. Dent. Ass., *86*, 663, 1973.

Standish, S. M.: Diseases of the muscles of the face and oral regions, in *Oral Pathology*, (Tiecke, R. W., Ed.), New York, McGraw-Hill, 1965.

Weintraub, M. I.: Facial diplegia, Arch. Otolaryngol., *102*, 311, 1976.

Section III

Recognition and Management of Oral Pathosis

This section is designed to:

1. provide a rational approach to the diagnosis of oral and facial pain (Chap. 10)

2. review representative developmental disorders of the facial structures and survey the common dermatoses of interest to the dentist (Chap. 11)

3. describe the chief pathologic conditions involving the major structures of the neck (Chap. 12)

4. discuss the diseases affecting the major and minor salivary glands (Chap. 13)

5. describe the oral soft tissues according to the presenting clinical lesion: white lesions; red lesions; pigmentations; vesicles, bullae and erosions; pustules; ulcers; cysts and cyst-like lesions; and focal and diffuse soft tissue enlargements (Chap. 14)

6. discuss the recognition and diagnosis of diseases of the jaw bones: developmental disorders; inflammatory and reactive disorders; odontogenic cysts and tumors; nonodontogenic and neoplastic-like lesions; and metabolic diseases (Chap. 15)

Chapter 10

Discomfort and Pain

The sensation of pain is difficult to clearly define and even more difficult to describe. As one of the special senses, pain must be considered physiologic as well as pathologic in nature. Additionally, the emotional aspects of pain often play a significant role in the patient's response. In certain cultures, for example, pain implies a form of chastisement for previous sins and it commonly is felt that one who has suffered pain becomes a better person for it.

While it was once thought that all sensory receptors (touch, temperature, etc) could transmit pain sensation given a sufficiently strong stimulus, it now is established that free nerve endings, which have no special receptors, register pain. These free nerve endings may additionally register pain to pressure or temperature stimuli of sufficient intensity to overcome their high threshold. For example, touch or temperature stimulation of the cornea, eardrum and dental pulp elicits only the sensation of pain. For this reason, painful pulpitis is often difficult to localize. With the development of vascular or inflammatory changes at the periapex, proprioception (position sense) permits the patient to point out the hurting tooth.

Renewed interest in pain control, acupuncture and the physiologic basis of referred pain have introduced new physiologic concepts of pain, including the so-called gate control theory of pain. Nevertheless, pain remains an enigma. Practical considerations for the prevention, diagnosis and management of pain remain a primary concern of the dentist.

SUBJECTIVE SENSATIONS AND COMPLAINTS

Pain may be described in various ways: mild, moderate or severe; acute or chronic; lancinating, pricking, sharp, burning, and aching. Colloquial or regional expressions such as the "miseries," "smarts," "quickies," and other equally vivid terms are often used by patients to describe their pain. Clearly, the severity of the pain, its frequency and distribution, and whether it is spontaneous or occurs only in response to a specific stimulus are important factors in evaluation and diagnosis (Table 10–1).

Apprehension

Fear is a universal emotion and unfortunately in the minds of many patients it is associated with thoughts of pain induced during dental care. The apprehensive patient is nervous, suspicious and distrustful. The wary eye and quiet movements of withdrawal must be recognized early so that reassurance can be given to increase the confidence of the patient.

Hysteria

This emotional upset can be extreme and the patient may be tearful, fearful and very

Table 10-1. Analysis of a Symptom.*

1. Total duration
2. Onset
   a. Date of onset
   b. Manner of onset (gradual or sudden)
   c. Precipitating and predisposing factors related to onset (emotional disturbance, physical exertion, fatigue, pregnancy, environment, injury, infection, allergy, therapeutic agents)
3. Characteristics
   a. Character (quality — burning, aching, squeezing, knife-like)
   b. Location and radiation
   c. Severity (mild, moderate, severe)
   d. Temporal character (continuous, intermittent, rhythmic, and duration of each episode)
   e. Aggravating and relieving factors
   f. Associated symptoms (e.g. chills, fever, restricted movement)
4. Course since onset
   a. Incidence
      (1) Single acute attack
      (2) Recurrent acute attacks
      (3) Periodic occurrences
      (4) Continuous chronic episode
   b. Progress (better, worse, unchanged)
   c. Effect of therapy

* Adapted from: Hochstein, E. and Rubin, A. L., *Physical Diagnosis*, New York, The Blakiston Division, McGraw-Hill Book Co., 1964.

vocal; however, this is the exception. Most patients with hysteria sublimate the outward show of their feelings and may present an apparently calm efficient appearance. Following are some of the indications of hidden hysteria. Taken alone, no single sign is indicative; however, if a few or several of these signs or symptoms are apparent, a tentative diagnosis of hysteria is justified: (1) The mouth may be scrupulously clean with the presence of cervical abrasion. (2) The patient may wear dark glasses indoors (photophobia). (3) There may be rapid fluttering of the eyelids (here it has been said that no one can blink as rapidly as an hysterical woman). (4) Often a set of what are considered by the patient to be "sinister symptoms" is presented; among these may be dizziness, palpitations, weakness and insomnia. (5) In addition there may be a history of prolonged and involved dental care, and especially recent restorative dental care which may have modified the occlusion.

Dysmorphophobia

Usually this is expressed as an abnormal fear of change in appearance, which may be presented by the patient who suffers with anesthesia, paresthesia, or the temporomandibular joint pain dysfunction syndrome.

Congenital Indifference to Pain

Bona fide examples of this are seen in cases of *familial dysautonomia* (p. 362). Carnival performers who are indifferent to the insertion of needles into their skin, or who literally may be able to walk on hot coals, may practice self-hypnotism.

Syncope (Fainting)

Fainting is not uncommonly encountered in the dental patient. While severe pain may induce syncope, most cases are associated more with apprehension than with any other truly physical reaction.

Fever

The febrile patient exhibits an intraoral temperature in excess of 98.6°F. In extreme cases, variations in body temperature can be detected by placing the palm of the hand on the patient's forehead.

Dysphagia

This is abnormal and uncomfortable swallowing or difficulty in eating.

Dyspnea

This is abnormal or difficult breathing. Apnea implies absence of breathing.

Angina

This is a painful limitation of breathing. This might result from chest pain (angina pectoris) or upper respiratory infections.

DIAGNOSIS OF ODONTALGIA

Since the complaint of toothache is the basis for the existence of the dental profession, it is surprising that our knowledge of the problems of pain has advanced so slowly. During much of the history of dentistry the treatment of toothache consisted of removing the (probable) offending tooth or teeth, often without knowing why the pain was present, and too often without knowing which tooth was involved. More recently, the establishment of the specialties of periodontics and endodontics, and the tooth-conserving efforts of such specialists, have led the dentist to a more precise definition of the need for tooth removal.

Pain as an indicator of disease is notoriously unreliable. Diagnosis would be simple if pain always indicated the inception or progress of disease, and the absence of pain indicated the absence of disease. Obviously this is not the situation, so we are forced to diagnose and treat painless and painful forms of pulpitis, periapicitis, periodontitis, and other afflictions, and differentiate them from other diseases.

Only in recent years have extensive analyses of patients with toothache been reported. Based on nearly 2,000 cases in two studies it was shown that more than half of the patients suffered pain derived from the exposed, vital dental pulp. More than one-fourth of the patients had pain arising from apical periodontitis of teeth with necrotic pulps. In about 10 percent of the cases the pain arose from the gingivae, or from the periodontium excluding the periapical region. Only a small percentage of patients complaining of toothache had pain arising from other regions (Table 10–2).

It is important not only to identify the source of pain but also to determine its severity. In these series more than 10 percent

Table 10-2. Sources of Pain.*

	No.	%
Vital pulp origin	937	57
Newly fractured tooth	10	
Pulpitis	927	
Necrotic pulp (pain of peri-apical origin; acute abscess)	502	30
	502	
Periodontal origin	177	10
Lateral abscess	131	
Acute gingivitis	16	
Pericoronitis	30	
Other	12	1
Postextraction pain	4	
Dental trauma to soft tissue	1	
Maxillary sinusitis	2	
Gingival ulcer	1	
Retained root	3	
Shedding loose tooth	1	
	Total 1628	

* From Hasler, J. F. and Mitchell, D. F.: Analysis of 1628 cases of odontalgia, J. Indianapolis Dist. Dent. Soc., January, 1963.

of the patients suffered only minor episodes of discomfort, such as is due to the stimulation of dentin uncovered by decay. Such patients certainly presented no immediate need for care, yet they were present because of "toothache."

The diagnostician now can more effectively "play the odds" in relation to the known incidences recorded above. The odds are about 3:1 that his next patient with odontalgia will have either painful pulpitis or painful periapicitis. It should be noted that many of the patients studied had suffered only slight or intermittent pain for periods ranging from a few days to several months before they sought dental care, and many patients with necrotic pulps had suffered no pain until very recently. This shows that the history of pain is unreliable as a diagnostic aid in such cases, and also indicates that painless pulpitis and painless periapicitis must occur quite frequently. Lastly, it illustrates our lack of knowledge concerning the chronology of the development of these conditions.

An *accurate diagnosis* should be made in every case of toothache, if at all possible. It is no longer feasible to extract the tooth only because it is blamed by the patient, or to guess that a given tooth is the problem and to order its removal. The adult may have 32 potential offenders, and if one or more teeth are removed wrongly injustice results. Advances in endodontics and periodontics now make it possible to save teeth formerly destined for removal.

Seldom will the practitioner be justified in waiting for difficult diagnostic cases to simplify, as was common practice in the past. It is no longer feasible for him merely to prescribe analgesics and antibiotics and hope that the diagnostic problem will resolve itself through localization to a single offending tooth. Neither is it feasible to refer all toothache patients elsewhere. It is the dentist's moral obligation to recognize this basis for the existence of his profession and to cope adequately with each case.

Pain Response of the Normal Pulp

Dentin is a unique tissue. It is vital, but it has no blood vascular system, nor is it innervated in the usual sense of the word. However, exposed dentinal tubules can carry sensory stimuli to the pulp. Occasionally a patient will complain of toothache because he has found that when he touches the neck of a tooth with his fingernail pain occurs in the pulp of that tooth. Since the sensation is new to him, he becomes apprehensive and needs to have the physiologic nature of the pain explained. If the practitioner will induce the pain with the point of a dental explorer applied to the same region, he can effectively diagnose the problem and explain it. In the same way, application of the dental bur or scaler, or even the toothbrush, may cause discomfort. Exposed dental tubules may be subject to pain from pressure during mastication. Thus a patient biting on salted celery or sugar-coated chewing gum suffers pain probably because the small crystals contact exposed dentinal tubuli. One must recognize this minor physiologic cause of "toothache" and explain it to the patient without resorting to unnecessary therapy. Special desensitizing toothpastes and agents which coagulate the exposed odontoblastic processes or sclerose these tissues often help.

Galvanic Shock

This is another relatively unimportant cause of toothache, except that it is common and must be recognized, explained, and avoided. Nearly 50 percent of a class of informed dental students who understood the nature of galvanic shock recently declared that they had experienced it.

When two dissimilar metallic restorations come into contact during mastication, a galvanic shock may result, causing pulpal pain. Thus the patient with a gold inlay in a lower tooth and a newly placed silver amalgam in an opposing upper tooth may complain of pain at the instant of closure. Once in contact, the current usually is quickly dissipated and discomfort is no longer felt. But the sharp shock may make the unknowing patient quite apprehensive unless the matter is corrected or explained.

Galvanic shock can be induced in teeth with old metallic restorations if they are suddenly touched with a "new" foreign source of metal such as a dental instrument, saliva ejector, or even a dinner fork.

Diagnosis depends upon the presence of dissimilar metals, at least one of which is a recent restoration, or upon the induction of the pain by touching one restoration with one of the prongs of cotton pliers and placing the other prong in contact with the other metallic restoration. If the pain occurs when two teeth are brought in contact during biting, it is of little use to coat one or the other

with varnish. This may give temporary relief but the varnish will soon be worn away and the problem may recur. It would be wiser to relieve one of the restorations by grinding so that contact is not established during occlusion. Educating the patient as to the cause of the pain will help him to avoid any situation which may induce it. The pain diminishes in time, with or without treatment. This presumably is due to diminishing electrical potential and increasing protection by the development of reparative or tertiary dentin. Recent evidence suggests that dissimilar metals may also contribute to the corroding of restorations and thus to their failure.

Galvanism to date has no proved relationship to diseases of the oral mucosa, despite the many references to the contrary.

Static electricity between the dentist and a patient's tooth can cause an instantaneous shock of a similar nature.

Postrestorative Discomfort Caused by Thermal Stimuli

This arises from the increased thermal conductivity of a metallic restoration. When the patient ingests something cold or hot, pain may be elicited on a physiologic basis. Since the pain is not spontaneous, it ceases immediately when the stimulus is removed. This condition has been mistermed "active hyperemia" of the pulp. The term implies that the arterial or arteriolar side of the vascular tree of the pulp is dilated and hyperemic because of the recent trauma to the dentin. There is little scientific evidence of this; it is another example of the misconception that if pain is present there must be inflammation. Even with a shallow restoration, a tooth may be hypersensitive to heat and cold for a time; yet the pulp of such a tooth would show no vasodilatation or other signs of inflammation. Moderately deep restorations may be associated with some localized inflammation and vasodilatation immediately beneath the cut dentinal tubules for a few weeks after restoration; however, postrestorative discomfort may or may not be present.

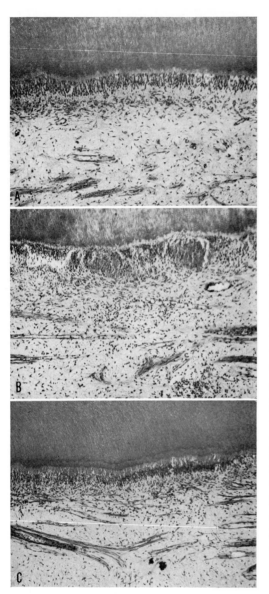

Fig. 10-1. Photomicrographs illustrating the reaction of the pulp to cavity preparation. *A*, Portion of coronal pulp of untreated tooth of young person. *B*, Disruption of odontoblasts, hemorrhage and leukocytic infiltrate beneath cut tubules 6 days after cavity preparation and temporary filling. *C*, Nine weeks. Note calciotraumatic line, reparative dentin and lack of inflammation. (Mitchell and Jensen, J. Amer. Dent. Ass., *55, 57,* 1957.)

Inflammation of this degree usually is reversible; if that were not so, many more restored teeth would be lost to pulp necrosis.

Thus it is imperative again to anticipate and explain such an occurrence. Among informed dental students more than 50 percent were found to have experienced this sensation. Most of them recalled that it had troubled them for 1 or 2 weeks after a recent restoration. On the other hand, several were sure that the problem had lasted for 6 months; and a few "knew" that it had persisted for periods of 3 to 10 years. It is not conceivable, in the light of present knowledge, that pulpal inflammation or hyperemia could persist for these prolonged periods as the result of one operative insult. Apparently the discomfort decreases as reparative dentin is deposited (Fig. 10–1*A, B, C*).

The diagnosis of pain of this variety consists essentially of recognizing that thermal shock follows the placement of metallic restorations and can frequently be avoided by the use of medicaments, varnishes, and bases under restorations when deemed necessary, especially for any patient who has complained of this phenomenon in the past. Since the recurrence of pain tends to diminish with time, a simple explanation to the patient is usually sufficient treatment. Once in a great while, if the tooth is extremely sensitive, it may be necessary to remove the metallic restoration, place an insulating base, and replace it; however, one should first look for a more serious cause for the discomfort —especially pulp exposure and pulpitis.

The "High" Restoration and Periodontal Pain

Another form of postrestorative discomfort occurs when the tooth becomes tender to occlusal pressure and percussion due to overstimulation of nerve endings in the periodontal membrane. Usually, but not necessarily, it is a vital tooth, with a recent restoration (usually cast gold) showing shiny facets of wear on its surface. Articulating paper may be used to indicate where adjustment is necessary to relieve the excessive contact.

Painful Pulpitis

Painful pulpitis is usually due to carious, traumatic, or surgical pulp exposure or to exposure caused by erosion, abrasion, or gingival recession which is so marked that auxiliary canals in the root are exposed to the gingival crevice (Figs. 10–2, 3, 4, 5). Nature's mistake of *dens in dente* frequently results in a pulp exposure (see Fig. 7–57). In such a case, infection invariably occurs and inflammation and necrosis of the pulp follow.

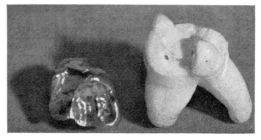

Fig. 10-4. Molar tooth removed because of symptoms of pulpitis. The restoration had been placed several weeks before under supervision in the dental school. The exposure (enlarged for the photograph) was unapparent to the student or supervisor at the time. (Mitchell, in *Endodontics* edited by Healey, courtesy of the C. V. Mosby Co., 1960.)

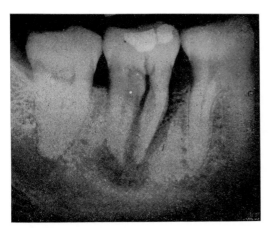

Fig. 10-2. Buccolingual fracture through the crown of a lower molar. (Mitchell, Dent. Clin. North America, November, 1957.)

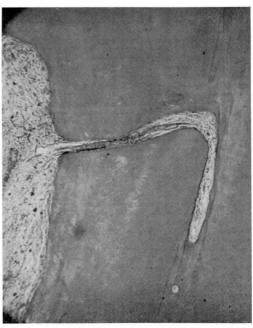

Fig. 10-5. Photomicrograph illustrating a lateral auxiliary canal connecting the interradicular periodontal tissue of a molar with the pulp. Periodontal inflammation is progressing through this canal into the pulp. (Rubach and Mitchell, J. Periodont., *36*, 34, 1965.)

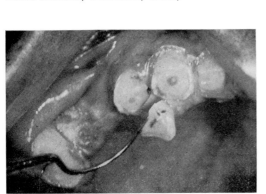

Fig. 10-3. Gross fracture of an upper bicuspid. Note the marked attrition and the undoubted associated heavy masticatory forces.

For many years investigators have attempted to correlate symptoms of painful pulpitis with microscopic findings in studies of extracted teeth. It is an unfortunate fact that several early investigators were hampered by inadequate technologic knowledge of methods to fix the pulp adequately for microscopic study. Thus much of the earlier misinformation based on artifacts of laboratory origin sometimes has been repeated and compounded by later investigators and authors.

People are reluctant to serve as experimental subjects, so that it has been difficult to obtain an adequate series of cases wherein clinical data could be compared with good histopathologic specimens obtained at the proper intervals of time. A series of such cases serves as a basis for the following conclusions and diagnostic approaches to this difficult problem (Mitchell and Tarplee) (Fig. 10–6).

Inflammation of the pulp results from exposure and concomitant infection by oral microbes. It follows that the first important step is identification of the tooth most likely to have a pulp exposure due to any of the reasons listed above. Sensitivity to percussion is an important sign since approximately 80 percent of the cases of painful pulpitis exhibit this feature to some degree. On the other hand, when the tooth is not tender, the practitioner must resort to other clinical and radiographic means to deter-

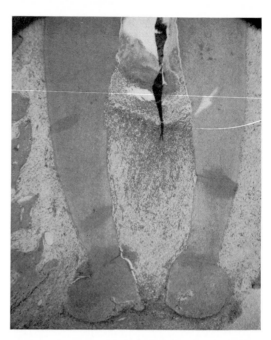

Fig. 10-7. Experimental pulpitis of the apical third of a root. The rest of the pulp is necrotic. Would such a tooth respond to electrical or thermal pulp tests? How much pulp must remain in order to respond to such tests? Would a conventional periapical radiograph be likely to show a "dentinoid" closure of the apex if the rays were directed from left to right? These questions cannot be answered at present (Camp, Thesis, Indiana University School of Dentistry, 1968.)

mine those teeth which give a vital response to the electrical test (Fig. 10–7). Electric vitality tests will reveal that the pulp is vital in such cases even though they will not indicate the degree of inflammation present. Then it is necessary to use thermal tests. Carefully performed, thermal tests, as outlined in Chapter 6, will be found to be most helpful in locating the offending tooth.

The Cracked Tooth

The "cracked tooth," or incomplete tooth fracture, may involve the pulp and result in painful or painless pulpitis. It is often difficult to demonstrate the fracture unless dyes are applied to stain the fracture line or pressure is applied to an individual cusp to test discomfort.

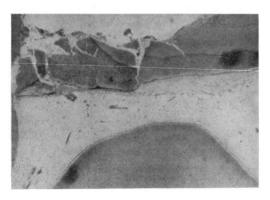

Fig. 10-6. Photomicrograph of a tooth which was presumed to have a carious exposure, pulp infection and inflammation. Diligent probing revealed hemorrhage, and yet serial sections through this tooth showed no inflammation. This illustrates the difficulty in making an accurate diagnosis of pulpitis when dealing with microns of protective dentinal floor.

Referred Systemic Pain

Pain from coronary artery insufficiency (anginal pain) may be referred to the jaws with or without associated chest or arm pain. This should be considered as a possible cause in cardiac patients or when the etiology is not obvious (see p. 295).

Non-Localized Pain

It is important to emphasize the 20 percent of the teeth with painful pulpitis in which the pain is *not* localized. Sicher has said in effect that the neurologist has less of a problem with the entire human body than does the dentist in accurately identifying the source of pain in some cases. The dentist may be dealing with 32 teeth at one time which may show no apparent cause for pain.

The phrase "atypical facial pain" is seen frequently in the dental and medical literature. It is undoubtedly true that if the dentist could discover the source of pulp pain and eradicate it, many cases of "atypical facial pain" would be cured. Such a case was reported by Rubach. Vague hemifacial pain had recurred for 18 months in this patient. Two dentists and four physicians had been consulted. Finally the hidden pulp exposure was revealed and the pulpitis was easily relieved.

If the offending tooth or teeth are not located by percussion or the thermal tests or radiographs, it may be necessary to use *selective anesthesia*. Some patients with painful pulpitis will say that the pain is distributed over half of the face and they will be unable to indicate even the jaw involved, let alone the tooth. The dentist confronted with this problem, and noting that any one of possibly 16 teeth could be involved, may elect to use a mandibular block on the affected side. If the pain is relieved, then the origin is relegated to the mandible, and further testing must await the resolution of the anesthesia. On the other hand, if the pain persists, selective periapical local infiltration anesthesia may be employed in the maxilla.

It is seldom necessary to resort to this method of diagnosis.

In extreme cases it may be necessary to wait for a day or two until symptoms are more localized. This procedure should be resorted to only in the exceptionally difficult case. In such an instance, the use of analgesics is justified.

Painless Pulpitis

There is considerable evidence that painless pulpitis is very common. Simply stated, it is an exposed, infected, and inflamed pulp without symptoms sufficient to bring it to the attention of the patient.

Several facts point up the validity of these statements. (1) Asymptomatic teeth removed in the course of other studies and subsequently sectioned have confirmed the existence of inflamed pulps with microscopic exposures. (2) Sperber's survey showed that among servicemen more than 50 percent of those requiring dental treatment denied ever having experienced dental pain. This indicated that these men had received no warning, through pain, of the presence of dental disease, even though many of them undoubtedly had exposed, inflamed dental pulps. (3) Among aviation cadets during World War II it was found that from 2 to 4 percent suffered aerodontalgia, or toothache at altitude, when subjected to decompression tests. Subsequently it was shown that most cases of aerodontalgia were due to pulpitis, painless at normal barometric pressures, but aggravated to become painful during decompression. (4) The microscopic pulp exposure is more common than is generally believed. For example, Kafrawy and Mitchell studied teeth of monkeys in which very deep Class V cavities had been prepared intentionally for the study of pulp reactions to a filling material. No clinically detected pulp exposures were noted, but serial microscopic sections showed tiny exposures in 23 of the 84 teeth. Pulpitis or pulp necrosis resulted. (5) The exposed hyperplastic pulp or pulp polyp is another form of painless pulpitis.

Seen most often in children, it occurs in teeth with crowns destroyed by caries. The pulp of the young tooth survives, inflamed but asymptomatic. (6) Internal resorption as in the "pink tooth of Mummery" is the result of proliferation of vascular, inflamed pulp tissue injured by some means. This usually is painless.

The dentist must recognize the possibility of painless pulpitis and search for possible pulp exposure. If found, the pulp must be treated in some manner or removed, or the tooth should be extracted. Whenever a tooth of strategic importance is to receive a large restoration, or is to serve as an important abutment, or is to be moved orthodontically, painless pulpitis should be ruled out before major steps are taken. Otherwise the pulpitis later may become painful, or progress to necrosis with periapicitis. A diligent search for a pulp exposure should be made. Thermal pulp tests should be used on such teeth and if the reaction is abnormal, in comparison with control teeth, the prognosis should be guarded. Hypersensitivity to cold stimuli in the absence of other symptoms is suggestive of painless pulpitis.

Hasler and Mitchell reported a study of the clinical diagnostic features of many cases of painless pulpitis. The teeth were studied microscopically and the findings confirmed those mentioned in the foregoing discussion.

Painful Periapical Disease

With one exception (see Anachoretic Periapicitis), painful periapical disease has the same etiology as pulpitis. Usually a clinical pulp exposure can be detected and the response of the pulp to an electrical test is negative because the pulp is necrotic. Once this is determined, there is no need to employ thermal tests. The bacteria or their by-products which have destroyed the pulp have caused inflammation of the apical periodontium. Such a tooth usually is tender to biting pressure or percussion, because the periodontal membrane is innervated with pain fibers.

Other diagnostic features of painful periapical disease may include visible or palpable periapical swelling and the existence of regional cellulitis or a fistula. Periapical radiolucency usually is present.

Anachoretic Periapicitis

The exception mentioned above in relation to the etiology of periapical disease is the occasion when a tooth has been traumatized by a severe blow. Anachoresis, or the anachoretic effect, occurs most commonly in youngsters, although it can occur at any age. Usually an anterior tooth is involved because these teeth are the most vulnerable to traumatic blows or falls. At the time of injury, the entering apical vessels and nerves are torn and the pulp, with little or no collateral circulation, dies. When the acute symptoms subside, the periodontal tissues may recover, and the tooth may become firm again without symptoms. This leaves the root canal filled with necrotic tissue in a warm, moist, and dark environment. This slender string of tissue may undergo a dry gangrenous change, or autolysis and liquefaction. In either event it may serve as a good bacterial culture.

There is good evidence that everyone undergoes a transient bacteremia from time to time. If bacteria in the bloodstream reach the "medium" in the non-vital pulp canal, they may grow there without effective bodily resistance because of the lack of collateral circulation of the pulp. As the bacteria proliferate, they or their by-products serve as irritants to the living apical periodontal tissues. Depending upon the virulence of the organism and the resistance of the host, periapical pathosis may develop with or without symptoms (Figs. 10–8, 9). Such an asymptomatic lesion may exist for long periods (months or even years) and suddenly become painful. Clinically the crown usually darkens with time.

Figure 10–8 illustrates the unusual occurrence of anachoretic periapicitis in a lower molar tooth. This asymptomatic non-vital

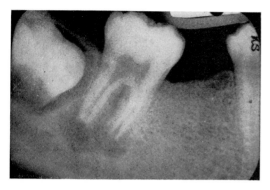

Fig. 10-8. Anachoretic periapicitis. Non-vital second molar in young patient with periapical radiolucency. Months before, the adjacent first molar had been extracted, and it can only be assumed that the second molar was elevated to such an extent that the entering apical vessels were severed and the pulp died. Subsequently during a bacteremia, the bacteria found the warm, dark, moist media within the root canal and proceeded to multiply there. The periapical radiolucency is a chronic inflammatory reaction to the bacteria and their toxins within the canal. Anachoretic periapicitis seldom is seen in a posterior tooth, but is quite common in anterior teeth subject to traumatic blows.

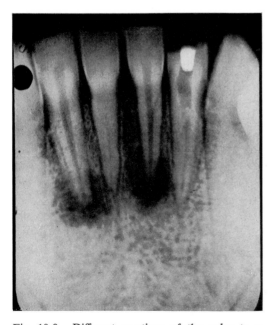

Fig. 10-9. Different reactions of the pulps to a single severe blow. The teeth were asymptomatic for a year. One lateral and one central are vital; the other lateral and central are non-vital. Which are which?

tooth was discovered with routine radiographs. Some months previously the first molar had been extracted and trauma to the second molar, by surgical elevator pressure during the operation, resulted in necrosis.

Anachoretic Pulpitis

There has been much speculation about the occurrence of "anachoretic pulpitis." Recently, additional experimental evidence that this condition occurs has become available. However, the resulting pulp infection often is overcome by the host. Whenever a moderately deep cavity is prepared, a small zone of inflammation results in the pulp immediately beneath the cut dentinal tubules. This zone is considered to be a *"locus minoris resistentiae"* or zone of lowered resistance. When bacteria of hematogenous origin reach it, an *infected* pulpitis occurs but, in light of all the successful dental restorations placed, this seems unlikely as an important cause of irreversible pulp damage (Gier and Mitchell).

Chronic Periapicitis

The histopathology of periapical lesions has not been correlated with the symptomatology. Future studies should provide information concerning the chronology of events leading to the three common forms of pathosis: the granuloma, cyst, and abscess. Only in the human being can these studies be made.

From a clinical standpoint the *granuloma* is the most common periapical lesion. Usually it is painless. Histopathologically this is a proliferating mass of granulation tissue consisting of fibroblasts, endothelial cells and new capillaries, and the cells of chronic inflammation such as lymphocytes, plasma cells, and macrophages. In addition, epithelial rests of Malassez usually are present and proliferating. This chronic inflammatory hyperplastic reaction to the irritants within the root canal requires room to grow, and osteoclastic resorption of the neighboring bone must occur. The main clinical features of the periapical granuloma then are the non-vital pulp, usually darkened or destroyed crown, and a periapical radiolucency without symptoms.

The granuloma may precede or follow *periapical abscess* formation. From a clinical standpoint the periapical abscess usually is blamed as the cause of painful periapicitis, yet it too can exist without symptoms.

The clinical diagnosis of abscess depends upon the finding of an accumulation of visible pus (suppuration). Pus may be demonstrated by opening into the pulp canal with a bur, aspiration of the radiolucent area, or incision and drainage of a palpable, periapical, or overlying soft tissue swelling, if present. While these procedures will confirm the diagnosis of periapical abscess and relieve the major symptoms temporarily, definitive treatment can only be endodontic therapy or extraction. In the event that the periapical abscess has progressed to the point of fistula formation and drainage, the lesion often becomes painless. Supportive antibiotic or other antibacterial measures (such as antiseptic irrigation) may occasionally be required to control the infection within the periapical bone and overlying mucosa or skin.

Most facial fistulas occur in connection with mandibular teeth. Young persons tend to be more prone to extraoral fistulas than are older patients. One reason for this is that the buccinator muscle attachment to the mandible often is superior to the apexes of the lower molars of young people, so that pus is diverted below the buccal sulcus, through the mandibular periosteum and onto the face. In adulthood, with normal growth and development, the attachment becomes inferior to the apical region, so that intraoral fistulas open into the buccal sulcus (see Surgical Space Infections, pp. 432–434).

Most intraoral fistulas occur on labial or buccal surfaces simply because the apices of most of the roots of most of the teeth are closer to these surfaces. Nevertheless, fistulas do sometimes occur on the lingual and palatal surfaces.

The third common periapical lesion is the apical periodontal cyst or *periapical cyst*. The epithelial rests of Malassez from odontogenic epithelium may be stimulated to proliferate and a true cyst may develop in a preexisting zone of periapicitis. The cyst is simply an epithelial-lined cavity surrounded by inflamed and proliferating fibrous tissue and multiplying capillaries which make up the "capsule." The basic irritants that caused rearrangement of preexisting tissues are still the bacteria or their by-products within the pulp canal.

It is generally conceded that the apical periodontal cyst takes considerable time to develop and most often occurs as a painless lesion. Its diagnosis depends on detection of periapical radiolucency, an associated non-vital pulp, drainage of cyst fluid from the root canal, or aspiration.

Through a radiographic study of human cadavers it was shown that, when a periapical radiolucent lesion with a diameter of more than a few millimeters was present, the odds are great that the buccal or labial cortical plate over the lesion will be resorbed or very thin (Regan and Mitchell). Thus it is usually possible to employ aspiration. If pus is obtained, the diagnosis of abscess can be made. If a clear or straw-colored fluid is obtained, then the diagnosis of cyst follows. If no fluid is obtained, either the central cavity of the lesion has been missed or the lesion is a granuloma or something else (*e.g.* periapical cemental dysplasia).

The technique of aspiration is quite simple but for some reason it is not popular among practitioners. It is simple to insert a medium-gauge needle through the overlying mucosa into such a periapical lesion, often without any need for anesthesia.

The periapical granuloma, cyst, and abscess cannot be differentiated using the radiograph alone. It follows that if more aspiration were used routinely (Fig. 6–2) to differentiate these lesions more accurately, it soon would be apparent whether each of these three conditions would respond successfully to conservative endodontic therapy. Beside the diagnostic implications of aspiration, the mere removal of the suppurative or cystic fluid might enhance the effectiveness of the therapy.

Gingival and Periodontal Pain

From 10 to 15 percent of the patients at a university dental clinic complaining of toothache were found to be suffering from gingivitis or periodontitis. Severe generalized necrotizing ulcerative gingivitis, or a localized gingivitis due to food impaction, may cause odontalgia. The ubiquitous popcorn hull is a common offender in the latter instance.

Another localized form of gingivitis is the very common *pericoronitis,* also called operculitis, because it develops under the operculum or tissue flap overlying the incompletely erupted lower third molar, most often in the 17 to 25 age group (Fig. 10–10). In such instances the tooth has "erupted," at least in part, and presents a communication from the oral cavity to the pericoronal crevice. As the inflammation progresses, a small pocket is formed between the operculum and the crown of the unerupted tooth, causing a mild local irritation or a severe pericoronal abscess. The symptoms of pericoronitis often include trismus and swelling. The pain is localized and the patient can point to the region involved. Redness and swelling of the tissues overlying the hidden tooth may be apparent. On palpation swelling may be felt, or drainage sometimes may be observed from the hidden pocket.

Emergency treatment consists of gentle exploration with a periodontal pocket probe or a more flexible gutta percha point. If suppuration is drained, relief may be almost immediate. If no suppuration is found and no foreign body is detected, then thorough irrigation with a saline solution or a dilute hydrogen peroxide solution may flush out bacteria or any hidden foreign body so that relief will occur shortly thereafter. Place-

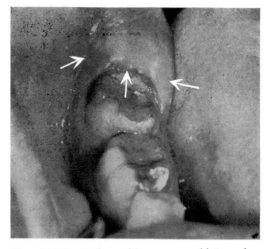

Fig. 10-10. Pericoronitis over a third molar. There is a connection between the gingival sulcus on the distal of the second molar and the pericoronal tissue over the third molar. Infection has occurred with inflammation, swelling and associated trismus.

ment of an iodoform gauze drain moistened with eugenol also is effective. If the emergency warrants, it is possible to extract an upper third molar which may be in poor position and occluding on the offending soft tissues.

Pericoronitis of comparable etiology may occur around the crown of any partially erupted tooth. This may happen during the age of the eruption of the primary dentition, or during the mixed dentition, or much later in life. For example, the unerupted or impacted maxillary canine which is either undetected or simply unremoved may be found in the maxilla of the denture-wearing patient. Resorption of overlying bone may have occurred and a small portion of the crown of the embedded tooth may be exposed to the oral cavity. It is then a likely possibility for the development of pericoronitis.

The *painful periodontal pocket* may cause vague recurring discomfort and sometimes is difficult to detect. Periodontal involvement of the palatal roots of upper molars is particularly difficult to detect radiographically or clinically unless a very flexible probe is used. Once found, irrigation with eugenol or the placement of an iodoform gauze-eugenol dressing will usually bring relief. Further periodontal care is necessary.

A deep periodontal pocket, painful or not, may form a *lateral periodontal abscess*. Because of associated gingivitis and swelling, the gingival cuff may approximate the cervix of the tooth tightly. Yet the bacterial or other irritant more apical in the pocket may cause abscess formation, swelling, pain, and even fistula formation. Diagnostic signs would include demonstrable pulp vitality, tenderness to percussion, periodontal bone loss, and detection of and release of pus by insertion of the periodontal probe through the gingival crevice to the base of the pocket (Fig. 2–15).

Sometimes periodontal discomfort may be associated with the localized development of a pyogenic granuloma (localized chronic inflammatory fibrous hyperplasia) associated with an impacted foreign body such as a popcorn hull, toothbrush bristle, or calculus. On occasion, no grossly apparent foreign body may be detectable.

Pulpal pain may result from periodontal detachment from the root of the tooth, which makes the exposed root surface sensitive to temperature change and pressure or touch through the vital dentin. One should not confuse sensitive dentin with so-called sensitive cementum. Since cementum has no innervation or vascular capacity, the pain in such a situation must arise from the stimulation of the underlying dentin through the very thin or possibly destroyed cementum.

Maxillary Sinusitis

Infection and inflammation may occur in any or all of the paranasal sinuses. Patients with sinusitis are likely to seek the help of a dentist if one of the maxillary sinuses is involved. If bilateral involvement is present, the patient is more likely to seek the help of an otorhinolaryngologist.

Maxillary sinusitis of one side may cause pain in the maxilla which the patient con-

siders to be "toothache." If the patient is asked to touch the painful region, he frequently will point to the cheek overlying the involved sinus. Palpation of this region may invoke signs of tenderness. Seldom is the sinusitis sufficient to cause erythema or cellulitis of the soft tissues overlying it. Tenderness to percussion may result from tapping any of the maxillary teeth in the entire quadrant involved (*i.e.* second premolar, first and second molars). The finding of pulp vitality in all of these teeth will give an additional clue. There may be a recent history of a common cold, and additional symptoms such as nasal phonation and a postnasal drip recognized as mucoid suppuration on the posterior wall of the nasopharynx. A Waters sinus radiograph (Fig. 10–11) and transillumination (Fig. 6–4) may help in diagnosis. The main problem for the dentist is to rule out the possibility that the patient has a true toothache, in which case the patient usually should be referred to his physician or otorhinolaryngologist.

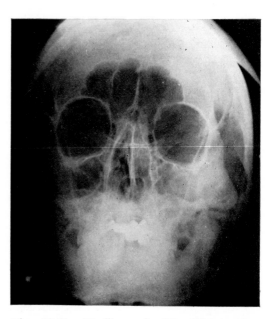

Fig. 10-11. Maxillary sinusitis (Waters sinus view). The afflicted sinus is simply more radiopaque than the opposite one. (Mitchell, in *Endodontics* edited by Healey, courtesy of the C. V. Mosby Co., 1960).

Maxillary sinusitis occasionally may result from periapical infection of maxillary posterior teeth. Sicher pointed out that the superior alveolar nerve which innervates these teeth often lies on the antral surface of bone, and stimulation of the sinus lining results in simulated pulp pain. He also stated that pulp pain may be induced by thermal shock in some cases of sinusitis.

Aerosinusitis or barotrauma afflicting a maxillary sinus may simulate odontalgia. This occurs most often during descent in aircraft (recompression) or descent in submarines (compression). For example, a pilot may have a chronic sinusitis with antral polyp formation. During descent from the rarefied atmosphere a polyp may impact in the antral opening. The resulting relative vacuum increases during further descent and pain occurs. Severe cases have been recorded in which the soft tissue lining of the sinus has been virtually stripped from the bony walls. A similar and more common phenomenon is aerotitis media, but this discomfort is not likely to be confused with any form of toothache. Occasionally aerosinusitis occurs during ascent due to increased pressure of the air unnaturally confined in a sinus.

Polyps of the wall of the maxillary sinuses are rather common in cold, humid climates. After extraction of an upper posterior tooth, they have been seen to enter an accidental antral-oral opening and be apparent in the extraction socket.

Root tips occasionally are broken off and forced into the maxillary sinus. Periapical lesions in the region may expand to invade the sinus. Occasionally benign or malignant tumors of the maxillary sinus wall invade the alveolar processes and become apparent to the dentist first (Fig. 1-19). In such instances, it is his responsibility to seek consultation and work closely with an experienced oral surgeon or otorhinolaryngologist.

Problems of the maxillary sinuses as related to dentistry are not common, but when they occur the interrelationships of dentistry and medicine often come to the fore.

Dry Socket

The "dry socket" is also referred to as post-extraction infection, alveolitis, and alveolar osteitis. The extraction wound clot is lost by mechanical action or destroyed by bacterial action. Although any extraction wound may be involved, it occurs most commonly in adults and most often after removal of impacted lower third molars. Pain occurring and increasing from the fourth to the tenth postoperative day is the chief complaint of the patient. Malodor and unpleasant taste are additional complaints. After gentle insertion of cotton or gauze into the depths of the socket, withdrawal and examination will reveal an objectionable odor of necrosis. Treatment involves gentle debridement, irrigation, and placement of a sedative dressing, repeated daily until normal healing commences. Analgesics and antibiotics may be prescribed.

Conclusions

There are many other afflictions of the head and neck that are painful, but seldom are they reported as toothache by dental patients (Fig. 10-12). These will be discussed separately.

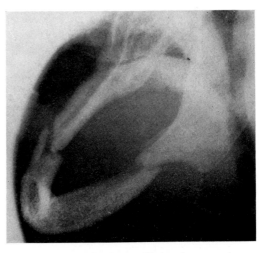

Fig. 10-12. Bilateral mandibular fractures in an edentulous male whose complaint was that his lower denture did not fit since he suffered a fall several days earlier. Pain does not always serve to warn of serious injury.

In an effort to clear up some of the confusion related to toothache diagnosis, the following points are emphasized.

1. Irreversible pulpitis (thus ultimately pulp necrosis) is usually due to pulp exposure and infection.
2. Clinically undetected (*i.e.* microscopic) pulp exposures are not uncommon in deep cavity preparations.
3. Auxiliary pulp canals opening onto lateral surfaces of roots are not uncommon. Involvement of such teeth with periodontal pockets may lead to pulpitis.
4. Painless pulpitis, which is more common than painful pulpitis, may progress to painless periapical disease, which in turn is more common than painful periapicitis. Detection of these asymptomatic forms of pulp or periapical disease presents a challenge to the practitioner.
5. The judicious use of modern instruments and techniques in cavity preparation seldom if ever causes irreversible pulp damage in the absence of pulp exposure.
6. The proper use of popular restorative materials does not cause irreversible damage to the pulp.
7. Judicious orthodontic tooth movement does not endanger the pulp.
8. Minor imbalances of occlusion, such as the presence of premature contacts during excursive movements of the mandible, do not cause pulp or periodontal tissue damage or odontalgia in the absence of other complicating conditions (*e.g.* the "high" restoration).
9. Gingival and periodontal lesions are common causes of "toothache."
10. Expansion of gases within the pulp chamber has not been shown to cause or to aggravate symptoms of odontalgia.
11. Neither vascular hypertension of the pulp nor pulp stones cause odontalgia.
12. Reliance on such terms as "causalgia," "atypical facial neuralgia" and "psychogenic pain" in the diagnosis of odontalgia should be avoided until all other possibilities have been excluded.
13. Many phrases used in the past have little diagnostic significance, for example: "cold hurts and heat relieves pulpitis"; or "heat hurts and cold relieves pulp necrosis"; or "a necrotic pulp hurts more at night"; or "a lateral abscess hurts less than a periapical abscess"; or "throbbing pain indicates a more serious infection than a dull pain."
14. The following descriptive terminology has little to support its use: "pulp atrophy," "hypersensitive cementum," "degenerating pulp," and "passive hyperemia of the pulp." Even the terms "acute," "subacute," "chronic," "serous," "purulent," "ulcerative," and "granulomatous" are of questionable value when used in association with the diagnosis of pulpitis. They have meaning only when considered as descriptive findings from a clinical endodontic standpoint, or from a microscopic standpoint, and seldom from both. When considered from the viewpoint of one seeking to induce responses to clinical objective tests, they are meaningless.

TEMPOROMANDIBULAR JOINT PAIN DYSFUNCTION SYNDROME (MYOFASCIAL PAIN-DYSFUNCTION SYNDROME)

This condition was not well defined until recent years with the advent of the textbook by Schwartz and colleagues. Many disorders of the temporomandibular joint exist but this particular syndrome is the most common problem of this region which the dentist must face. In 1934 Costen, an otolaryngologist, described patients with a set of symptoms related to this problem, and others later named it "Costen's syndrome." Costen believed that the set of symptoms which, among others, included tinnitus, hearing loss, glossodynia, vertigo, and temporomandibular joint discomfort was related to malocclusion and to mandibular overclosure in particular. With the aid of dentists, patients were treated successfully with "bite opening" devices and other appliances altering the occlusion. Through more than two decades thereafter, confusion and debate reigned and ultimately the precise set of symptoms which Costen had outlined was rejected as a true recurring syndrome, as were the earlier etiologic explanations for some of the symptoms. Nevertheless, the fact that the otolaryngologist and the dentist were mutually concerned with this general problem led to increased cooperation between the two in dealing with such cases.

Description of the Syndrome

The patient with myofascial pain dysfunction (MPD) syndrome complains of a dull, usually unilateral, pain in the region of the temporomandibular joint or preauricular area. The discomfort may radiate over the temporalis or masseter muscles or into the neck. Generally, pain cannot be elicited in the joint by palpation by way of the external auditory meatus. Rather, foci of muscle tenderness (spasm) can often be identified by palpation of one or more of the muscles of mastication, chiefly the internal pterygoid. Commonly, popping or clicking sounds may be present in the joint but these are not essential to the diagnosis since they are often found in patients without the syndrome. Limitation or deviation of jaw opening is frequently present.

Most patients are females between the ages of 30 and 50, but the condition also occurs among other age groups of both sexes. The apprehension and emotional tension which often are present in women during the fifth and later decades of life are commonly associated factors. Hysteria sometimes is present.

Thus, it appears that a person who is predisposed to suffer the pressures of day-to-day living in a stressful period of his life may become preoccupied with the occlusion of his teeth and develop the syndrome. If in addition he has noticed an annoying but usually unimportant "clicking" in the temporomandibular joint, comparable to popping knuckles, and if trismus has occurred, his fears are heightened. Often such patients have developed a sensory preoccupation with the occlusion of their teeth, especially if that occlusion has been changed recently. The oral region is exceptionally sensitive and plays a very basic role in the human being which relates to combat, the pleasures of taste, the sensual stimulation of sex, and the expressions of all emotions. If this complex neural and psychologic system is disturbed, far-reaching effects may occur. Patients with this syndrome may during careful, considerate, and time-consuming interrogation admit to cancerphobia, the use of stimulants, sedatives and tranquilizers. Serious events such as a recent death in the family and other reasons for emotional tension may be brought to light.

Excessive occlusal attrition may be observed on occasion and there may be an admission of clenching or grinding of the teeth. It is not uncommon for the spouse of the patient to be present and a history of bruxism while sleeping may be elicited.

It is important to make a thorough examination, including full-mouth radiographic surveys and radiographs of both temporomandibular joints, taken with the jaws in the open and closed positions. Very seldom are any organic changes detected which could account for the set of symptoms. Nevertheless, it is important to demonstrate this to the patient to help allay his apprehension and to gain his confidence, as well as to rule out organic abnormality (Figs. 10–13, 14).

The etiology of the discomfort thus appears to be related to prolonged involuntary overcontraction of the muscles of mastication. Since these muscles are intimate with

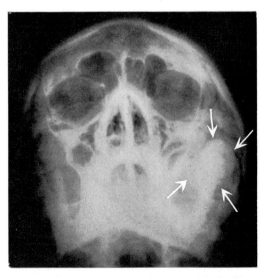

Fig. 10-13. An osteoma of the condyle is illustrated. Notice the intense radiopacity and swelling of the region. (Courtesy of Dr. Denis Forest.)

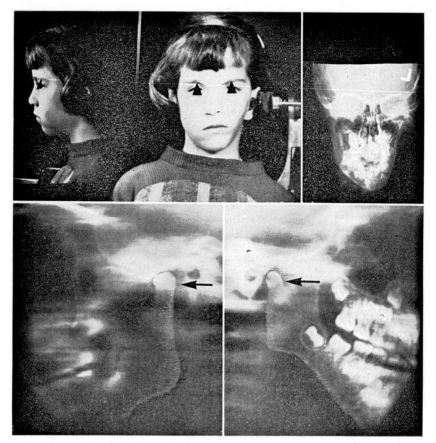

Fig. 10-14. Hypoplasia of a mandibular condyle. (Ware and Taylor, Dent. Clin. North America, March, 1968.)

the temporomandibular joint, the concentration of the pain seems to involve this structure.

Wolff has stated that sustained contraction of a muscle, such as that which occurs with emotional tension, if sufficiently prolonged will give rise to pain within that muscle. Most people recognize this truth concerned with shoulder, neck and back pains occurring in association with abnormal posture during prolonged periods of intense devotion to a task.

In most cases the minor abnormalities of the occlusion of the teeth are only contributing factors. If the extremely sensitive proprioceptive mechanism around the 32 teeth is disturbed, an unconscious and sometimes conscious preoccupation with the occlusion results. Everyone has experienced the lodgment of a small seed in an occlusal crevice which is immediately detectable by him. It is this kind of minor change superimposed on even temporary emotional instability which may result in undue clenching and grinding of the teeth and the chronic discomfort of the masticatory musculature and the syndrome. If it is not diagnosed, and if the patient is not reassured, the vicious cycle continues through apprehension to such extremes as cancerphobia and resulting insomnia and increase in the severity of symptoms.

Given any condition which is not well understood and which has a history of many different treatment methods that appear to be successful, the diagnostician should recognize that the etiology of said condition usually is unclear, and specific therapy is not known. This axiom is especially true in the temporomandibular joint pain dysfunction syndrome. Following is a list of therapeutic measures that have been tried with claimed success in previous years for this condition. Some of the more heroic methods include: condylectomy, meniscectomy, wiring of the jaws in the closed position for a long period of time, "bite raising" by removable and sometimes fixed appliances, and major orthodontic tooth movement. Other somewhat less heroic measures have included: injection of sclerosing agents within the joint capsule (though usually restricted to treating hypermobility), injections of corticoids in this region, x-ray and ultrasonic therapy, and full-mouth occlusal equilibration. More conservative measures have been reported to be successful including the topical spray of ethyl chloride on the face (to anesthetize the external masticatory muscles), heat therapy, cold therapy, massage, mouth-opening exercises (to counteract the bruxism), infrared deep heat therapy, and mock occlusal equilibration. Counseling by members of the clergy and psychiatrists and simply firm reassurance by the dentist have been shown to be valuable. Muscle relaxant drugs and tranquilizers likewise have been effective, as have sedatives.

Differential Diagnosis

It is important to rule out the following comparatively uncommon conditions which may furnish some symptoms of the syndrome: traumatic, rheumatoid, infectious, and osteoarthritis; scleroderma; condylar or fossa fracture, ankylosis; elongation or impingement of the coronoid process on adjacent soft tissues; osteoma, osteosarcoma, metastatic carcinoma, multiple myeloma, and even brain tumor. In some cases vascular neck pain (carotidynia), temporal arteritis, Eagle's syndrome, and parotitis or parotid neoplasia likewise should be considered in the differential diagnosis. Thus, it is essential to rule out organic disease, including pulpitis, before a definitive diagnosis of MPD syndrome can be established.

Treatment

Once the syndrome has been diagnosed, a conservative approach to treatment is indicated. Reassuring the patient by telling him that he has a rather common problem and not a "sinister," unknown condition sometimes is enough. Simple measures, such as opening the mouth against hand resistance, or placebo therapy, or muscle relaxants, may help. It is not certain that the muscle relaxants are pharmacologically effective in such cases, but a patient can understand the logic of such therapy and may benefit thereby.

In a severe case, consultation with the patient's physician would be wise before more potent medicaments are prescribed. It is important in early therapy *not* to alter the occlusion irreversibly. However, correction of an obvious minor discrepancy may be in order, especially if it appears to have been of recent origin, perhaps through dental treatment. Resilient "mouth guards" worn at night to discourage bruxism may prove helpful.

Extensive, time-consuming, and expensive occlusal alterations are not warranted until symptoms have subsided, and with the associated muscle hypertonicity it is difficult to assess the patient's occlusal function.

MYOSITIS

Inflammatory reactions in the oral and perioral muscles may be of infectious, functional, traumatic or metabolic origin. The affected muscle(s) is (are) tender or painful on palpation and movement and, in severe cases, muscle spasm or trismus further restricts normal function.

Suppurative Myositis

Myositis of the oral regions most commonly follows extension of pulpal or periodontal infection into the adjacent soft tissues, causing a diffuse cellulitis (p. 431).

Infiltration between muscle fibers causes considerable pain and trismus.

Trichinosis

This relatively common parasite (*Trichinella spiralis*) of striated muscle is transmitted to man by ingestion of incompletely cooked pork. In some cases, the encysted larvae may be transferred to the mouth by handling the raw meat. While sporadic outbreaks sometimes occur, public awareness of the disease, laws prohibiting the feeding of uncooked garbage to swine and deep-freezing of pork products (lethal to the organism) have reduced the incidence of this disease in recent years.

Once ingested, the larvae are freed and ultimately are carried by the bloodstream or lymphatics to the striated muscles. The patient experiences fever, nausea and diarrhea for 24 to 48 hours. Muscle pain and tenderness, sometimes accompanied by a maculopapular rash, may persist for 2 to 3 weeks. An associated eosinophilia of up to 20 percent may be present. Virtually any of the skeletal muscles may be affected: calf, diaphragm, extraocular, intercostal, cervical, masseter and tongue.

Functional Myositis

Vigorous, prolonged muscle activity may lead to muscle swelling and pain with disruption of fibers (*rhabdomyolysis*) and, in severe cases, myoglobinuria. "Shin splints" and "march myoglobinuria" are examples.

Temporal Myositis

A mild but often alarming form of functional myositis is seen in children who have chewed a large mass of bubble gum for several hours. Marked bilateral swelling and tenderness over the temporalis muscles are characteristic. With rest, the swelling subsides in 24 hours.

Traumatic Myositis

Physical injury to muscle, such as a blow or a crushing or stretch injury, induces an inflammatory response with associated tenderness. This may be followed by muscle spasm and continued pain, comparable to that seen with spasm of the internal pterygoid muscles in the myofascial pain syndrome (pp. 288–291).

Myositis Ossificans

Two forms of this disorder are recognized: traumatic myositis ossificans and generalized (progressive) myositis ossificans.

Traumatic myositis ossificans presumably follows repeated trauma or even single trauma to muscle, causing a localized and painful swelling with redness of the overlying skin and finally the development of a nodular mass. Feathery calcifications, usually with an outer radiopaque shell, appear in about two weeks. The condition is seen most frequently in the thigh muscles of football players and jockeys ("rider's bone"); in the oral regions, the masseter is commonly involved. The radiographic appearance of myositis ossificans may simulate a calcified lymph node, phlebolith or even osteosarcoma with its sunray pattern. The latter, however, is in continuity with the cortex of the underlying bone and has the least mature ossification on the periphery rather than a mature outer shell, as does myositis ossificans.

Generalized (progressive) myositis ossificans involves skeletal muscles, tendons, fascia, ligaments and aponeuroses and is unrelated to prior trauma. It is seen in children less than 10 years of age and often in the first year of life. The ossifications are first recognized in the tongue, facial and shoulder muscles as scattered nodular swellings; associated fever and joint pain may suggest rheumatic fever. In time, other muscles and connective tissues are affected with ankylosis of joints, including the TMJ, and the patient literally becomes a "petrified man."

Dermatomyositis (Polymyositis)

This form of myositis is discussed on pages 330–331.

THE NEURALGIAS

Neuritis and Neuralgia

Neuritis refers to inflammation of nerves and is characterized by pain or hypersensitivity which may progress to paresthesia or paralysis. If motor nerves are involved, loss of reflexes and muscular atrophy eventually can develop if the condition is not corrected.

Neuralgia is characterized by pain, usually of a paroxysmal character, but without a demonstrable organic lesion. Since the neuralgias involve the sensory components of the respective cranial nerves, the diagnosis is established on the basis of the nature, character and distribution of the pain. Charting of the area affected, determination of "trigger zones" if present, evaluation of psychic factors and the use of selective local anesthesia are necessary for proper evaluation.

Local factors (especially toothache) which conceivably could account for the pain directly or as a referred pain must be eliminated before a definitive diagnosis of neuralgia can be made. Obviously, a clear understanding of the anatomy and physiology of the regions involved is essential.

Typical neuralgias usually occur in older patients and are characterized by the presence of a "trigger zone" and sharp, paroxysmal pains of short duration (seconds to minutes) which are localized to the precise anatomic distribution of the involved cranial nerves. Associated signs of autonomic nervous system involvement (*e.g.* lacrimation, flushing, sweating) are not ordinarily present.

Atypical neuralgias are distinguished clinically from the typical neuralgias by pain which is poorly localized and diffuse. No trigger zone is present and the pain does not follow the anatomic distribution of a single nerve but may overlap several, even crossing the midline. Quite often there are associated autonomic nervous system signs (*e.g.* nasal congestion, lacrimation) and the patient has other neurotic traits.

The neuralgias of chief concern to the dentist involve the trigeminal (V) and glossopharyngeal (IX) nerves. Functional (sensory, autonomic, motor) disturbances are discussed on pages 261–265.

Trigeminal Neuralgia (Tic Douloureux)

Characterized by paroxysmal pain over one or more divisions of the fifth cranial nerve, trigeminal neuralgia occurs mainly in adults over 40 years of age. Stimuli (pressure, cold, movement) to a "trigger zone" on the face, lip, tongue, or gingiva activate an excruciating pain with a lightning-like or electric-shock quality which is of only a few seconds duration. Although the patient is quite comfortable between paroxysms, he may go to great extremes to protect the "trigger zone" from the wind, and men will often refuse to shave the area.

The pain on occasion may resemble a toothache, and often the patient needlessly has teeth extracted without gaining relief. Cases of pain arising from pulp, periodontal or other origins have erroneously been diagnosed as tic douloureux.

Trotter's Syndrome

A nasopharyngeal carcinoma affecting the fifth nerve in the vicinity of the foramen ovale may induce a neuralgic-like pain in the mandible, tongue and ear together with loss of soft palate function. Pain of this nature and metastasis to cervical lymph nodes will often be the first manifestations of a surprisingly small carcinoma arising high in the nasopharynx.

Paratrigeminal Syndrome (Raeder's Syndrome)

This atypical neuralgia, seen most commonly in middle-aged males, exhibits pain or headache of abrupt onset involving the fifth nerve plus ocular sympathetic paralysis.

Sphenopalatine Neuralgia (Sluder's Headache, Lower-Half Headache, Periodic Migrainous Neuralgia, "Alarm-Clock Headache")

Paroxysms of pain of several minutes' duration distributed unilaterally around the eye, maxilla and mastoid region are usual features. A trigger zone is not present although the onset of pain is frequently at the same time each day. Nasal congestion, sneezing and lacrimation accompany the attacks.

Glossodynia (Orolingual Paresthesia, "Burning Tongue," Glossopyrosis)

Painful tongue or the more extensive "burning mouth" is usually a complaint of adults in the upper age groups. In some cases, a relative xerostomia (p. 360) associated with age changes in the salivary glands may be present. Pernicious anemia, diabetes mellitus, deficiency of the vitamins B, and achlorhydria reportedly have been associated with this symptom. If this were the case, detection and treatment of the underlying ailment by the physician should lead to correction of the glossodynia. On the other hand, in many such patients, no systemic ailment or deficiency has been brought to light and some degree of emotional instability has been detected. The condition has been called a conversion reaction. In any case, many such patients become apprehensive and may develop cancerphobia if the condition is not explained to them. Thus, reassurance usually is the treatment of choice once other contributing factors have been ruled out.

Glossopharyngeal Neuralgia

In this condition, pain arises from the lateral pharyngeal wall and radiates to the side of the neck and ear. Although a precise trigger zone is not present, swallowing or coughing can stimulate an attack.

Causalgia

This term is used to describe pain in a region of prior surgery or trauma and for which there is now no apparent cause. It appears to be analogous to the "phantom pain" seen following amputation of a limb.

Usually seen in the oral regions at presumably well-healed extraction sites, burning pain may be elicited by touch or temperature stimuli. In some instances, even emotional upsets may induce the pain. The chief differential diagnosis is *traumatic neuroma* (p. 421). In any event, the diagnosis of causalgia is not justified until every effort has been made to rule out local pathosis.

Atypical Facial Neuralgia (Atypical Facial Pain)

Those conditions with signs and symptoms of the atypical neuralgias and which cannot be further categorized are lumped together under the inclusive term *atypical facial neuralgia*. The absence of a trigger zone, the non-anatomic pain distribution, associated autonomic signs and an apparent psychogenic component are usual features. The pain is diffuse, poorly localized and may persist for hours or days. While no organic basis can be established, the patient may respond temporarily to symptomatic treatment or even to a placebo. Often depressed and self-critical, these patients may actively seek surgical therapy against the advice of the dentist. Analgesics, vasoconstrictors and/or antidepressants may be effective in some cases.

Post-Herpetic Neuralgia

Herpes zoster (p. 326), seen along the distribution of sensory nerves, produces a painful vesicular eruption which may be followed by post-herpetic neuralgia. The latter is most often seen in the aged and may persist for several weeks or months. The ophthalmic division of V is commonly involved. Treatment is largely empirical.

Migraine

Severe, periodic headache accompanied by nausea is seen in migraine. This disorder often begins during the teens or early adulthood. Prodromal visual disturbances and vertigo precede the onset of headache which is often unilateral over the frontal, temporal and occipital areas.

OTHER PAINFUL CONDITIONS

A number of other situations may involve significant pain in the oral regions. In many of these, an obvious lesion of the soft tissues or bone such as an ulcer, red lesion, swelling or radiolucency is present which accounts for the pain. In this regard, certain disease entities (in addition to pulpal and periodontal disease) characteristically produce substantial pain symptoms. For example, acute infections (p. 431), traumatic neuroma (p. 421) and relatively advanced carcinoma of the tongue are typically painful lesions. Burning pain of the mucous membranes usually accompanies the erosive lesions such as chronic desquamative gingivitis, erosive lichen planus and, occasionally, geographic tongue (p. 391). Bone pain is common in acute osteomyelitis (p. 460), Paget's disease of bone (p. 489), Ewing's sarcoma (p. 485), multiple myeloma, sarcomas of bone and certain metastatic tumors. While rare in the jaws, osteoid osteoma classically produces exquisite pain. These conditions are discussed in further detail in Chapters 14 and 15.

In the following sections, several additional conditions which produce pain in the oral regions are described. For the most part, these represent situations which may be overlooked in the evaluation of the patient with a somewhat obscure source of pain. All too often, pain in the oral regions is erroneously attributed to an "atypical neuralgia" (q.v.) or to a neurosis when in fact a demonstrable causative factor exists.

Sialadenitis

The most common example of inflamed salivary glands is epidemic parotitis or mumps of childhood. Sialolithiasis, salivary gland or ductal stone formation, may be associated with adenitis and pain. Sialoliths involve Wharton's duct and/or a submaxillary salivary gland more commonly than other major glands. Occasionally an acute suppurative adenitis of bacterial origin may occur. Drainage of pus may be established by massaging the swollen gland or by probing the appropriate duct. Postsurgical parotitis has been described. Chronic, intermittent and recurrent parotitis has occurred in some adults afflicted with alcoholism, and in others with diabetes (Chap. 13). Chronic bacterial infections, though seldom painful, may lead to swelling and even induration of a major salivary gland. Sialography, in addition to ductal probing, may aid in the diagnosis of such conditions (Chap. 8).

Enlarged Bony Processes

In the older patient, elongation and enlargement of otherwise normal bony processes at sites of attachment of tendons and ligaments may bring about discomfort. The painful *styloid process (Eagle's syndrome)* may cause dysphagia or sore throat, and palpation of the tonsillar fossa and floor of the mouth in this region will induce discomfort. Lateral oblique jaw films may confirm such a diagnosis (Fig. 2–27A). Likewise, the elongated *hamular process* posterior to the tuberosity may occasionally give rise to discomfort especially in the edentulous during overclosure. Ulceration of the mucosa overlying the pterygoid hamulus is seen in Bednar's aphthae (p. 399). *Coronoid processes* of the mandible, especially in older males with heavy bites, may ultimately encroach on the internal pterygoid muscle due to a posture assumed during sleep, and thus may lead to discomfort. *Osteophytes of the cervical spine* may lead to dysphagia. Induction of the thyroid crackle may point up this uncommon condition. Though seldom uncomfortable, *elongated genial tubercles* may be detected occasionally (see Fig. 2–30).

Coronary Occlusion

Myocardial infarction may give rise to sudden chest pain which extends to the left arm and even to the left mandible on occasion.

Carotidynia

The painful carotid artery most often occurs in the adult female. The patient may complain of dysphagia or sore throat and tenderness on one side of the neck in the region of the pulsating carotid bulb. The pain may radiate upward. This is seldom severe, and subsides in a few days without treatment. It has been reported to occur following herpetic infections and aphthous ulcers. Carotid aneurysm also should be ruled out. Vascular neck pain has responded to brief courses of corticosteroids (*e.g.* prednisone, 5 mg. t.i.d. for 5 days).

Subacute Thyroiditis

Pain in the neck and jaw has been ascribed to this condition, the etiology of which is not clear (p. 342).

Temporal (Giant Cell) Arteritis

Unilateral headache and tenderness over the temple in the aged may arise secondarily to a granulomatous inflammation of the temporal artery comparable to periarteritis nodosa (p. 327). Other arteries, especially the occipital, may also be involved. Visual disturbances, sometimes leading to blindness and pain over the scalp, face, eyes and temporomandibular joint, are commonly present. Glossitis and intermittent claudication of the tongue have also been described. Other systemic signs are fever, malaise and anorexia, occasionally with generalized muscular wasting (polymyalgia rheumatica). Resection of the involved segment of the temporal artery generally eliminates the temporal pain. The steroids have been used quite effectively for both diagnosis and treatment of this condition. The disease may run a variable course from a few months to several years.

BIBLIOGRAPHY

Odontalgia

Bales, D. J.: Pain and the cracked tooth, J. Indiana Dent. Ass., *15*, 1975.
Dachi, S. F.: Rapid evaluation of the patient in pain, Dent. Clin. North America, March, 1968.
Gier, R. E. and Mitchell, D. F.: Microbiological and histopathological studies of anachoretic pulpitis, J. Dent. Res., *47*, 564, 1968.
Hasler, J. F. and Mitchell, D. F.: Painless pulpitis, J. Amer. Dent. Ass., *81*, 671, 1970.
Johnson, R. H., Dachi, S. F. and Haley, J. V.: Pulpal hyperemia—a correlation of clinical and histologic data from 706 teeth, J. Amer. Dent. Ass., *81*, 108, 1970.
Kakehashi, S., Stanley, H. R. and Fitzgerald, R. J.: The effects of surgical exposures of dental pulps in germ-free and conventional laboratory rats, Oral Surg., *20*, 340, 1965.
Kirkman, D. B.: The location and incidence of accessory pulpal canals in periodontal pockets, J. Amer. Dent. Ass., *91*, 353, 1975.
Lawson, B. F.: Odontalgia: Diagnosis and emergency treatment, Dent. Clin. North America, March, 1968.
Mitchell, D. F.: Aerodontalgia, Bulletin, U.S. Army Med. Dept., *73*, 62, 1944.
Mitchell, D. F. and Tarplee, R. E.: Painful pulpitis, a clinical and microscopic study, Oral Surg., *13*, 1360, 1960.
Natkin, E., Harrington, G. W. and Mandel, M. A.: Anginal pain referred to the teeth, Oral Surg., *40*, 678, 1975.
Reeves, R. and Stanley, H. R.: The relationship of bacterial penetration and pulpal pathosis in carious teeth, Oral Surg., *22*, 59, 1966.
Rubach, W. C.: "Atypical facial neuralgia" due to pulpitis, Oral Surg., *16*, 1039, 1963.
Rubach, W. C. and Mitchell, D. F.: Periodontal disease, accessory canals and pulp pathosis, J. Periodont., *36*, 34, 1965.
Sperber, N. D.: The unreliability of pain as a symptom of dental pathology, J. Amer. Dent. Ass., *59*, 447, 1959.
Thoma, K. H.: A comparison of clinical, roentgen, and microscopical findings in fifteen cases of infected vital pulps, J. Dent. Res., *9*, 447, 1929.
Wallace, J. R.: Pericoronitis and military dentistry, Oral Surg., *22*, 545, 1966.

Dentin and Pulp Reactions

Anderson, D. J. and Ronning, G. A.: Osmotic excitants of pain in human dentine, Arch. Oral Biol., *7*, 513, 1962.
Avery, J. K. and Rapp, R.: An investigation of the mechanism of neural impulse transmission in human teeth, Oral Surg., *12*, 190, 1959.
Baker, G. R. and Mitchell, D. F.: Topical antibiotic treatment of infected dental pulps of monkeys, J. Dent. Res., *48*, 351, 1969.

Boyd, J. B. Jr. and Mitchell, D. F.: Reaction of subcutaneous connective tissue of rats to implanted dental cements, J. Prosth. Dent., *11*, 174, 1961.

Brännström, M.: The surface of sensitive dentine, Odont. Revy, *16*, 293, 1965.

Fischer, R. M., El Kafrawy, A. H. and Mitchell, D. F.: Studies of tertiary dentin in monkey teeth using vital dyes, J. Dent. Res., *49*, 1537, 1970.

Healey, H. J., Patterson, S. S. and Van Huysen, G.: Pulp reaction to ultrasonic cavity preparation, U.S. Armed Forces Med. J., *7*, 685, 1956.

James, V. E. and Spence, J. M.: Response of human pulp to gutta percha and cavity preparation, J. Amer. Dent. Ass., *49*, 639, 1954.

Johnson, N. W., Taylor, B. R. and Bergman, D. S.: The response of deciduous dentin to caries studied by correlated light and electron microscopy, Caries Res., *3*, 348, 1969.

Johnson, R. H., Christensen, G. J., Stigers, R. W. and Laswell, H. R.: Pulpal irritation due to the phosphoric acid component of silicate cement, Oral Surg., *29*, 447, 1970.

Kafrawy, A. H. and Mitchell, D. F.: Pulp reactions to open cavities later restored with silicate cement, J. Dent. Res., *42*, 874, 1963.

Kakehashi, S., Stanley, H. R. and Fitzgerald, R.: The exposed germ-free pulp: Effects of topical corticosteroid medication and restoration, Oral Surg., *27*, 60, 1969.

Mitchell, D. F.: The irritational qualities of dental materials, J. Amer. Dent. Ass., *59*, 955, 1959.

Mitchell, D. F., Buonocore, M. G. and Shazer, S.: Pulp reaction to silicate cement and other materials: relation to cavity depth, J. Dent. Res., *41*, 591, 1962.

Patterson, S. S. and Mitchell, D. F.: Calcific metamorphosis of the dental pulp, Oral Surg., *20*, 94, 1965.

Seltzer, S.: Hypothetic mechanisms for dentine sensitivity, Oral Surg., *31*, 388, 1971.

Seltzer, S., Bender, I. B. and Kaufman, I. J.: Histologic changes in dental pulps of dogs and monkeys following application of pressure, drugs, and microorganisms on prepared cavities, Part II., Oral Surg., *14*, 856, 1961.

Shovelton, D. F. and Marsland, E. A.: A further investigation of the effect of cavity preparation on the human dental pulp, Brit. Dent. J., *105*, 16, 1958.

Shroff, F. R.: Effects of filling materials on the dental pulp, New Zeal. Dent. J., *42*, 99, 1946.

Spedding, R. H., Mitchell, D. F. and McDonald, R. E.: Formocresol and calcium hydroxide therapy, J. Dent. Res., *44*, 1023, 1965.

Truelove, E. L., Mitchell, D. F. and Phillips, R. W.: Biologic evaluation of a carboxylate cement, J. Dent. Res., *50*, 166, 1971.

Van Hassel, H. J. and Harrington, G. W.: Localization of pulpal sensation, Oral Surg., *28*, 753, 1969.

Weiss, M. B., Massler, M. and Spence, J. M.: Operative effects on adult dental pulp, Dent. Prog., *4*, 6, 1963.

Periapical Pathosis

Brynolf, I.: A histological and roentgenological study of the periapical region of human upper incisors, Odont. Revy, *18*, 176, 1967.

Genvert, H., Miller, H. and Burn, C. G.: Experimental production of apical lesions of teeth in monkeys, and their relation to systemic disease, Yale J. Biol. Med., *13*, 649, 1940–41.

Grossman, L. I.: Bacteriologic status of periapical tissue in 150 cases of infected pulpless teeth, J. Dent. Res., *38*, 101, 1959.

Kafrawy, A. H. and Mitchell, D. F.: Sequence of events following pulp exposure in monkeys, J. Dent. Res., *49*, 1181, 1970.

Melville, T. H. and Birch, R. H.: Root canal and periapical floras of infected teeth, Oral Surg., *23*, 93, 1967.

Patterson, S. S., Shafer, W. G. and Healey, H. J.: Periapical lesions associated with endodontically treated teeth, J. Amer. Dent. Ass., *68*, 191, 1964.

Regan, J. E. and Mitchell, D. F.: An evaluation of periapical radiolucencies found in cadavers, J. Amer. Dent. Ass., *66*, 529, 1963.

Seltzer, S., Turkenkopf, S., Vito, A., Green, D. and Bender, I. B.: A histologic evaluation of periapical repair following positive and negative root canal cultures, Oral Surg., *17*, 507, 1964.

Temporomandibular Joint

Blackwood, H. J. J.: Metastatic carcinoma of the mandibular condyle, Oral Surg., *9*, 1318, 1956.

Cacioppi, J. T., Morrissey, J. B. and Bacon, A. S.: Condyle destruction concomitant with advanced gout and rheumatoid arthritis, Oral Surg., *25*, 919, 1968.

Christensen, G.: The modern concept of disturbances of the temporomandibular joint, Aust. Dent. J., *1*, 249, 1956.

Cohen, B. M. and Meyers, H. A.: Multiple myeloma involving the temporomandibular joint, Oral Surg., *9*, 1274, 1956.

Costen, J. B.: Neuralgias and ear symptoms associated with disturbed function of the temporomandibular joint, J.A.M.A., *107*, 252, 1936.

Costen, J. B.: Diagnosis of mandibular joint neuralgia and its place in general head pain, Ann. Otol., *53*, 655, 1944.

Crum, R. J. and Loiselle, R. J.: Incidence of temporomandibular joint symptoms in male patients with rheumatoid arthritis, J. Amer. Dent. Ass., *81*, 129, 1970.

Goodman, P., Greene, C. S. and Laskin, D. M.: Response of patients with myofascial pain-dysfunction syndrome to mock equilibration, J. Amer. Dent. Ass., *92*:755, 1976.

Henny, F. A.: Treatment of the painful temporo-mandibular joint, J. Oral Surg., *15*, 214, 1957.

Jendresen, M. D. and Shannon, I. L.: Effect of induced occlusal disharmony on stress, USAF School of Aerospace Medicine, Aerospace Medicine Division (AFSC), Brooks Air Force Base, Texas, 1968.

Kunin, I. J.: Methocarbamol in the treatment of temporomandibular joint syndrome, Oral Surg., *14*, 296, 1961.

Kydd, W. L.: Psychosomatic aspects of temporomandibular joint dysfunction, J. Amer. Dent. Ass., *59*, 31, 1959.

Lupton, D. E.: A preliminary investigation of the personality of female temporomandibular joint dysfunction patients, Psychother. Psychosom., *14*, 199, 1966.

Lynch, B. Jr. and Hoover, D. E.: Extrapyramidal syndrome due to compazine therapy, Oral Surg., *14*, 1142, 1961.

Maddox, W. D., Gibilisco, J. A. and Steinhilber, R. M.: Movement disorders of the jaw and tongue following prochlorperazine therapy, J. Dent. Med., *17*, 10, 1962.

Marlette, R. H.: Adjunct treatment of TMJ pain with Equagesic, Military Med., *129*, 69, 1964.

Mohnac, A. M.: Bilateral coronoid osteochondromas, J. Oral Surg., *20*, 500, 1962.

Perry, H. T.: Muscular changes associated with temporomandibular joint dysfunction, J. Amer. Dent. Ass., *54*, 644, 1957.

Ramfjord, S. P.: Bruxism, a clinical and electromyographic study, J. Amer. Dent. Ass., *62*, 21, 1961.

Ricketts, R. M.: Laminagraphy in the diagnosis of temporomandibular joint disorders, J. Amer. Dent. Ass., *46*, 620, 1953.

Russell, L. A. and Bayles, T. B.: The temporomandibular joint in rheumatoid arthritis, J. Amer. Dent. Ass., *28*, 533, 1941.

Sarnat, B. G.: *The Temporomandibular Joint,* 2nd Ed., Springfield, Charles C Thomas, 1964.

Schulte, W. C.: Ankylosis of the temporomandibular joint, Oral Surg., *24*, 270, 1967.

Schwartz, L. L.: *Disorders of the Temporomandibular Joint,* Philadelphia, W. B. Saunders Co., 1959.

Sicher, H.: Anatomy and oral pathology, Oral Surg., *15*, 1264, 1962.

Ware, W. H. and Taylor, R. C.: Management of temporomandibular joint disorders, Dent. Clin. North America, March, 1968.

Williams, A. C. *et al.*: Ankylosis of the coronoid process to the zygomatic arch and maxilla, J. Oral Surg., *26*, 804, 1968.

Winter, A. A. and Yavelow, I.: Oral considerations of the myofascial pain dysfunction syndrome, Oral Surg., *40*, 720, 1975.

Wolff, H. G.: The nature and causation of headache, J. Dent. Med., *14*, 3, 1959.

Myositis, Neuralgia and Other Painful Conditions

Alling, C. C. and Burton, H. N.: Differential diagnosis of chronic orofacial pain, J. Prosthet. Dent., *31*, 66, 1974.

Balasubramanian, S.: The ossification of the stylo-hyoid ligament and its relation to facial pain, Brit. Dent. J., Feb., 1964.

Brody, H. A. and Nesbitt, W. R.: Psychosomatic oral problems, J. Oral Med., *22*, 43, 1967.

Brown, R. L.: Carotid arteritis from aphthous ulcers, Angiology, *14*, 522, 1963.

Chasens, A. I.: Facial pain—Part I, J. Oral Med., *27*, 43, 1972.

Cherrick, H. M.: Trigeminal neuralgia, Oral Surg., *34*, 714, 1972.

Chusid, J. G.: *Correlative Neuroanatomy and Functional Neurology,* 15th Ed., Los Altos, Lange Medical Publ., 1973.

Dachi, S. F. and Stein, L. I.: Diagnosis and management of orofacial pain of emotional origin, J. Oral Surg., *26*, 345, 1968.

Das, A. K. and Laskin, D. M.: Temporal arteritis of the facial artery, J. Oral Surg., *24*, 226, 1966.

Eggleston, D. J.: Periodic migrainous neuralgia, Oral Surg., *29*, 524, 1970.

Ettinger, R. L. and Hanson, J. G.: The styloid or "Eagle" syndrome: an unexpected consequence, Oral Surg., *40*, 336, 1975.

Every, R. G.: The significance of extreme mandibular movements, Lancet, July, 1960.

Facer, J. C.: Osteophytes of the cervical spine causing dysphagia, Arch. Otolaryng., *86*, 117, 1967.

Garretson, H. D. and Elvidge, A. R.: Glossopharyngeal neuralgia with asystole and seizures, Arch. Neurol., *8*, 26, 1963.

Gayford, J. J.: The aetiology of atypical facial pain and its relation to prognosis and treatment, Brit. Dent. J., *7*, 202, 1970.

Gier, R. E.: Management of neurogenic and psychogenic problems, Dent. Clin. North America, March, 1968.

Goldstein, N. P., Gibilisco, J. A. and Rushton, J. G.: Trigeminal neuropathy and neuritis, J.A.M.A., *184*, 458, 1963.

Gores, R. J.: Pain due to long hamular process in the edentulous patient, Appl. Ther., *7*, 1128, 1965.

Hilger, J.: Carotid pain, Laryngoscope, *59*, 829, 1949.

Hitch, J. M.: Dermatological manifestations of giant cell (temporal, cranial) arteritis, Arch. Derm., *101*, 409, 1970.

Kelly, R. J., Jackson, F. E., DeLove, D. P. and Dunn, J.: The Eagle syndrome. Hemocrania secondary to elongated styloid process, U.S. Navy Med., *65*, 11, 1975.

Kydd, W. L.: Cranial arteritis simulating temporo-mandibular joint arthrosis, Oral Surg., *15*, 677, 1962.

Lovshin, L. L.: Vascular neck pain—A common syndrome seldom recognized, Cleveland Clin. Quart, *27*, 5, 1960.

Norman, J. E. de B.: Facial pain and vascular disease—Some clinical observations, Brit. J. Oral Surg., *8*, 138, 1970.

Olivier, R. M.: Trotter's syndrome, Oral Surg., *15*, 527, 1962.

Robinson, M. and Slavkin, H. C.: Dental amputation neuromas, J. Amer. Dent. Ass., *70*, 662, 1965.

Rushton, J. G., Gibilisco, J. A. and Goldstein, N. P.: Atypical face pain, J.A.M.A., *171*, 545, 1959.

Sakurai, E. H. and Richardson, J. H.: Vascular neck pain. A source of odontalgia, Oral Surg., *25*, 553, 1968.

Standish, S. M.: Diseases of the muscles of the face and oral regions. In: *Oral Pathology* (R. W. Tiecke, ed.), New York, McGraw-Hill, 1965.

Stevens, H.: Conversion hysteria: A neurologic emergency, Mayo Clin. Proc., *43*, 54, 1968.

Tolman, D. E., Gibilisco, J. A. and McConahey, W. M.: Subacute thyroiditis: A diagnostic possibility for the dentist, Oral Surg., *15*, 293, 1962.

Turner, J. C. Jr., Devine, K. D. and Judd, E. S.: Auriculotemporal (Frey) syndrome after parotid surgery, Surg. Gynec. Obstet., *111*, 564, 1960 and J.A.M.A., *219*, 175, 1961.

Uppgaard, R. O.: Trigeminal neuralgia—of dental origin, Northwest Dent., *46*, 267, 1967.

Wooten, J. W., Tarsitano, J. J. and Reaves, D. K.: The pterygoid hamulus: a possible source for swelling, erythema, and pain: report of three cases, J. Amer. Dent. Ass., *81*, 688, 1970.

Chapter 11

Diseases of the Face and Skin

The thorough physical examination should include methodical evaluation of extraoral structures of the head and neck since this may reveal changes of significance to the patient's general health or aid in the diagnosis and treatment of oral diseases. Such an examination, which is not time consuming, should include the face and neck, ears, nose, eyes, hair and scalp, skin appendages and the hands and nails.

DEVELOPMENTAL ABNORMALITIES OF THE HEAD AND FACE

The routine examination should begin with a general observation of the size, contour and symmetry of the face. Although minor asymmetry of the facial structures is seen in virtually every individual, gross deviations from normal may indicate underlying soft tissue or bony change. Disturbances of growth and development of these tissues include a spectrum of defects, ranging from minor variations and anomalies to the more severe monstrosities.

Discrepancies in Dental Arch Relationships

Jaw relationships and malocclusions are commonly described according to Angle's classification:

Class I—Normal mesiodistal relation of arches
Class II—Mandible distal to normal relationship to maxillary arch
   Division 1—Protruding maxillary incisors, with mandible bilaterally distal
      Subdivision—Protruding maxillary incisors, with mandible unilaterally distal
   Division 2—Retruding maxillary incisors, with mandible bilaterally distal
      Subdivision—Retruding maxillary incisors, with mandible unilaterally distal
Class III—Mandible mesial to normal relationship with maxillary arch
   Division—Mandible bilaterally mesial to maxilla.
      Subdivision—Mandible unilaterally mesial to maxilla

While a comprehensive discussion of the several predisposing and proximate causes of malocclusion is not within the scope of this text, it may be noted these are several and varied. An accurate appraisal of discrepancies in dental arch relationships will necessarily consider such factors as eruption and exfoliation patterns of the teeth; chronologic, bone and tooth age; skeletal, cranial and facial growth patterns; possible genetic or familial traits; relationship of the jaws to the cranial base; habits or disease; variations in jaw size and dental arch relationships; or various combinations of these factors.

Agnathia

Agenesis or aplasia of the jaw, usually the mandible, is extremely rare. Congenital defects of this magnitude are usually accompanied by numerous other severe anomalies and are not compatible with life.

Micrognathia

Hypoplasia may be real or represent an apparent jaw size discrepancy because of a posterior position of the jaw in relation to the cranial base (retrognathia) or when compared to an enlarged opposing jaw. Micrognathia of the maxilla is generally characterized by a high, arched palate with reduced arch width. Cleft palate, with collapse of the lateral halves of the palate, or cleft lip extending into the premaxilla, is a common cause of micrognathia of the maxilla. Intrauterine or birth trauma may damage the condylar region and thereby hamper the growth of the mandible, with resultant hypoplasia or even ankylosis of the temporomandibular joint.

Macrognathia

Hyperplasia of the jaws is commonly seen as mandibular prognathism and a Class III malocclusion. Such conditions may result from excessive growth and development, particularly in the ramus and condylar regions, as in bilateral condylar hyperplasia. Pituitary hyperfunction (p. 253) arising prior to closure of the epiphyseal and other growth centers in the bones results in pituitary giantism with general overgrowth of all bones. Hyperfunction of the pituitary in the adult also causes increased size of several facial bones and the hands and feet even though growth centers have calcified. Enlargement of facial bones secondary to specific disease processes is discussed in Chapter 15.

Facial Hemihypertrophy, Hemiatrophy

Hemihypertrophy and hemiatrophy of the facial structures are generally of congenital origin and involve not only the superficial soft tissues of the face but underlying muscle and bone as well (Fig. 11-1*A, B*). On occasion such changes may involve the entire half of the body. Hyperplasia of the ramus or body of the mandible or condyle may result in overgrowth of the one side, producing deviation toward the non-affected side.

A number of other conditions may superficially simulate facial hemihypertrophy, and must be differentiated clinically. Atrophy of the facial musculature follows prolonged

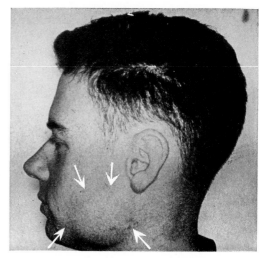

Fig. 11-2. Masseter hypertrophy. (Courtesy of N. H. Rowe.)

facial nerve paralysis (Bell's palsy, pp. 262, 358 and Fig. 7–2). A clenching habit or some other unusual functional activity has been associated with some cases of *masseter hypertrophy* (Fig. 11–2). Neoplasms, inflammation and reactive processes involving the connective tissues and/or musculature of the cheek may also resemble hemihypertrophy. Examples of such conditions would include neurofibromatosis (Fig. 14–60), lymphangioma and cystic hygroma (Fig. 14–56), erectile hemangioma in the cheek muscles (Fig. 14–54), myositis ossificans of the masseter muscle, angioneurotic edema, cellulitis of the buccal space, etc.

Facial Clefts

Other obvious gross defects of the face include a variety of *facial clefts* usually involving the oral aperture (Fig. 11–3). The most common of these is the cleft lip (hare lip) which may also extend into the alveolar ridge and palate (Fig. 4–15). Such clefts may be unilateral, bilateral or, on rare occasions, midline. Since cleft lip and palate usually are repaired within the first few weeks after birth, a scar is usually visible representing the line of closure. Because of scar

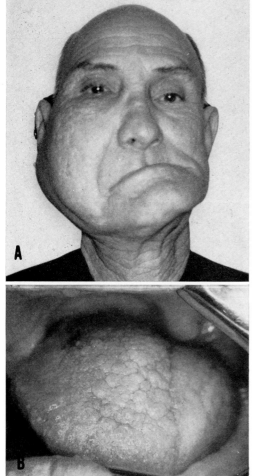

Fig. 11-1. Hemihypertrophy. The enlargement of the (*A*) face, and (*B*) tongue had been present since birth. (Rowe, Oral Surg., *15,* 572, 1962).

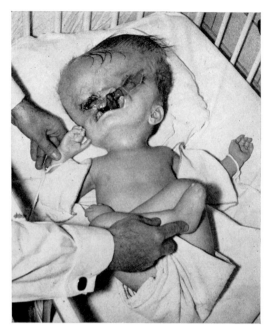

Fig. 11-3. An infant with hydrocephaly, bilateral oblique facial clefts, with clefts of alveolar process and palate, syndactyly and adactyly. (Sakurai, Mitchell and Holmes, Cleft Palate J., 3, 181, 1966.)

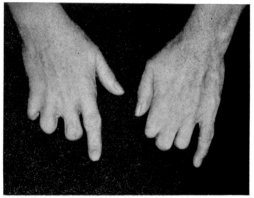

Fig. 11-4. Congenital amputations of digits. (Sakurai, Mitchell and Holmes, Cleft Palate J., 3, 181, 1966.)

contraction and subsequent growth of the jaws, there is almost always some shortening of the lip postoperatively. Defects involving the alveolar ridge and/or palate usually show concomitant disturbances in tooth development or arch form.

Some facial clefts involve the commissures of the mouth, extending along the embryonic lines of closure toward the ear (Fig. 11-3). Gross defects of this type often are repaired shortly after birth. Less severe variations in the size of the oral aperture (macrostomia, microstomia) may not require treatment. Congenital clefts frequently are associated with malformations of portions of the external ear and other structures that were developing embryologically at the time of the causative injury.

A number of syndromes have been described which exhibit multiple congenital and often hereditary defects of the jaws and facial structures. Examples of some of these are described in the following sections.

Treacher-Collins Syndrome (Mandibulofacial Dysostosis)

Treacher-Collins syndrome typically shows multiple defects, including hypoplasia of the mandible and malar bones, antimongoloid palpebral fissures, coloboma and absence of eyelashes, macrostomia, high or cleft palate, and deformities of the ears with deafness (Fig. 11–5A and B).

Crouzon's Disease (Craniofacial Dysostosis)

In craniofacial dysostosis (e.g. Crouzon's disease) there is premature synostosis of cranial sutures with resultant maxillary hypoplasia. Mandibular prognathism with protuberant frontal ridges and bosses, arched or cleft palate, parrot's beak nose, hypertelorism, and exophthalmos are typical features.

Pierre Robin Syndrome

This condition is a somewhat milder form of craniofacial dysostosis characterized by micrognathia, glossoptosis and cleft palate. The bird-face features of these patients are quite striking. In the newborn with this condition, emergency measures to avoid asphyxiation from the severe glossoptosis are sometimes required.

Orodigitofacial Dysostosis (OFD Syndrome)

This unusual syndrome appears to occur exclusively in females. Facial defects include

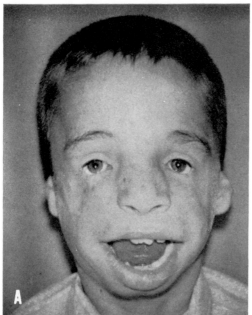

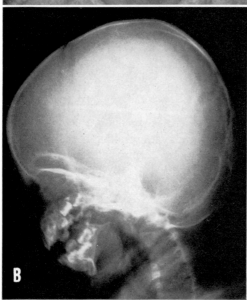

hypertelorism, median clefts of the upper lip, and short alar cartilages and columella. There are characteristic submucous clefts of the palate as well as alveolar ridge clefts involving both jaws. These latter are seen as prominent fibrous bands or freni which extend from the buccal mucosa through the cleft of the ridge.

Banti's Syndrome (Chronic Congestive Splenomegaly, Splenic Anemia)

In this condition, striking physical changes secondary to the splenic anemia, leukopenia, thrombocytopenia and liver cirrhosis are seen. Brownish discoloration of the skin, cyanosis of the nails and lips, gingival and gastrointestinal hemorrhage and clubbing of the fingers are generally seen (Fig. 11-6).

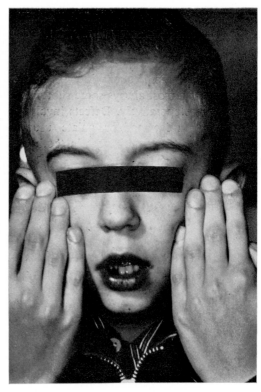

Fig. 11-5. Treacher-Collins syndrome (mandibulofacial dysostosis). *A,* Note the sunken cheek bones, macrostomia, malformed ears, broad nose and wide-set eyes characteristic of this syndrome. (Garner, Oral Surg., *23,* 320, 1967.) *B,* Radiograph of the head of a 5-year-old girl with Treacher-Collins syndrome. Note especially the underdeveloped mandible.

Fig. 11-6. Banti's syndrome. Cyanosis of the face, lips and nails was marked, and clubbing of the fingernails is apparent, due to developmental vascular defects.

Encephalotrigeminal Angiomatosis (Sturge-Weber Syndrome)

This is another striking syndrome showing hemangiomas of the soft facial and oral tissues which tend to follow the distribution of one or more divisions of the trigeminal nerve (Fig. 11–7). The angioma also involves the cortical leptomeninges on the ipsilateral side with intracranial "tram-line" calcifications seen on radiographs. Some pa-

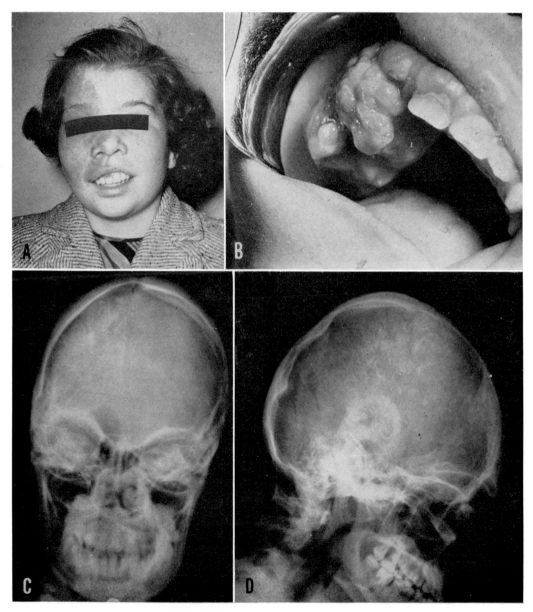

Fig. 11-7. Sturge-Weber syndrome (encephalotrigeminal angiomatosis). *A*, Red-purple facial hemangioma which extends intraorally. The gingiva on the affected side is hyperplastic. *B*, Another case with massive recurring gingival hyperplasia on the side involved with hemangioma. *C*, Another case showing meningeal calcifications in the cranial projection of one side and *D*, lateral view showing the characteristic meningeal "tram-line" calcifications of the intracranial hemangioma. (*C* and *D*, courtesy of Louis Holmes.)

tients may have epileptic seizures, mental retardation or, rarely, hemiplegia. The oral angioma is in continuity with the facial lesion and often causes marked gingival enlargement.

Angioosteohypertrophy Syndrome (Klippel-Trenaunay-Weber Syndrome, Hemangiectatic Hypertrophy)

This condition should be considered in the differential diagnosis of unilateral nevus flammeus of the face and oral cavity. It also follows the course of the trigeminal nerve but does not exhibit intracranial calcifications or neural disturbances. Typically there is bone enlargement, most commonly of the long bones but also of the jaws.

Cleidocranial Dysostosis

Cleidocranial dysostosis is an unusual syndrome which exhibits the following pathognomonic features (Fig. 11–8): retained pri-

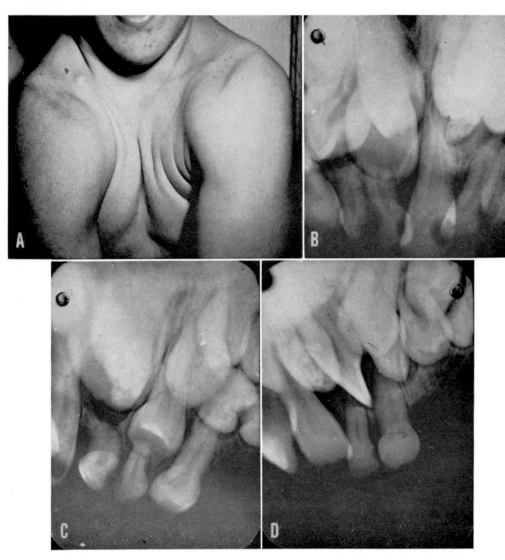

Fig. 11-8. Cleidocranial dysostosis in a young adult. *A*, Near approximation of shoulders due to clavicle deficiency. *B*, *C*, and *D*, Retained deciduous and unerupted permanent teeth and supernumerary teeth. (Courtesy of David Bixler and Arden Christen.)

mary and delayed eruption of permanent teeth, numerous supernumerary teeth; open fontanelles and sutures, and wormian bones of the skull; stunting of growth; high prominent forehead and prominent chin, small maxilla, high arched palate and retrusion of middle third of face; and partial or complete absence of clavicles. Laboratory findings are normal. Because of the absence of normal clavicles, patients have the rather dramatic ability to bring their shoulders together. No specific treatment is required other than management of the complex dental problem.

Carpenter's Syndrome

Described in 1966, this syndrome is characterized by multiple defects of the skull, face, hands and feet (Fig. 11–9).

Reference should be made to Chapter 4 for further information on genetic disorders and syndromes of the oral regions. A more exhaustive review of syndromes is found in the text by Gorlin and Pindborg.

THE SKIN

The character and consistency of the skin are usually determined by simple observation and palpation during the routine dental examination. The dentist must be familiar with the more common dermatoses, particularly those that may be infectious or a threat to the patient's health, as well as those having oral manifestations. While the dentist should not attempt to diagnose or treat dermatologic disease, he is expected to recognize abnormal changes and seek consultation when indicated.

The conditions described on the following pages represent those dermatologic lesions which may be encountered by the dentist in his practice. Considerable emphasis is placed on the precancerous dermatoses, the keratotic lesions, and the pigmentations of the skin. Some effort has been made to group the various dermatoses according to the type of presenting clinical lesion, while others are discussed according to etiology when appro-

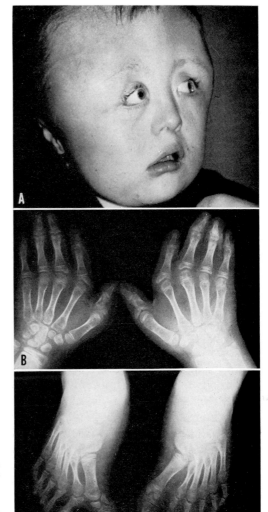

Fig. 11-9. Carpenter's syndrome (acrocephalo-polysyndactyly) is characterized by *A*, a tower skull, peculiar face, *B*, brachysyndactyly of hands, and *C*, poly- and syndactyly of feet and mental retardation (8-year-old male).

priate. A number of diseases of infrequent occurrence or of incidental interest to the dentist are listed without discussion (see Table 11–1).

Precancerous Dermatoses

Since the skin of the face and hands is rather constantly exposed to a number of

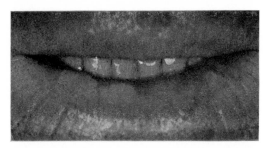

Fig. 11-10. Sailor's lip. Note the hyperkeratosis and indistinct mucocutaneous border in this aging male who has spent much of his life in the sun.

environmental factors, especially sunlight, it will reflect changes of diagnostic significance, especially in aging individuals. The so-called sailor's or farmer's skin shows a series of changes analogous to aging which consists of wrinkling, alterations in pigmentation, and hyperkeratosis. In addition, focal areas of telangiectasia or so-called crepe-paper skin may be seen. These skin changes occur more commonly in light-complexioned individuals (who have less protective melanin coloration), and are seen particularly over bony prominences of the face and the lower lip (Figs. 11–10 and 7–9). Since basal cell or squamous cell carcinoma may arise from such precancerous dermatoses, even minor changes in skin texture deserve careful examination.

Actinic Keratosis
(Solar Keratosis, Senile Keratosis)

This common precursor of skin malignancy is seen clinically as a scaly, rough and slightly erythematous lesion which may be slightly elevated above the adjacent normal skin surface. Periodic desquamation of the keratotic portion of the epithelium occurs with reformation of the scaly surface within a few days. Frequently, the patient is unaware of the lesion or does not consider it to be of serious consequence. The patient should be referred to a dermatologist for further evaluation. Senile keratosis or senile elastosis is a frequent finding on the lower

lip and may predate epidermoid carcinoma in this location.

Cutaneous Horn

This uncommon condition represents a focal piling up of keratin similar to an animal horn (Fig. 11–11). The forehead or the lower lip are typical sites on the face. Such lesions should be removed not only for cosmetic reasons but because the base of the lesion is usually identical to senile keratosis and, on occasion, undergoes malignant transformation into squamous cell carcinoma.

Radiodermatitis

Improper use of superficial radiation for such conditions as acne, hirsutism, or other minor dermatologic conditions may result in irreversible changes in the skin which become clinically significant many years following the initial therapy. The involved skin is thin and shiny with mottled areas of hypo- and hyperpigmentation. Numerous telangiectasias and scaly papules appear. Subsequent ulceration or fissuring suggests the develop-

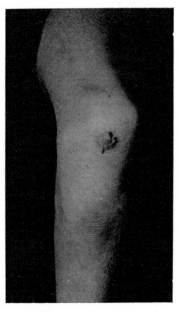

Fig. 11-11. Cutaneous horn on the knee. (Courtesy of Anand P. Chaudhry.)

ment of basal cell or squamous cell carcinoma in these areas.

Spindle cell carcinoma of the lower lip has been associated with prior radiation or trauma. This histologic variant of epidermoid carcinoma consists of pleomorphic spindle cells which are often histologically indistinguishable from malignant fibroblasts or other mesenchymal cells.

Thermal and Chemical Burns

Old thermal and chemical injuries of the skin in which there are extensive scars may undergo malignant transformation (Marjolin's ulcer), usually into squamous cell carcinoma.

Chronic Osteomyelitis

Persistent sinus tracts associated with chronic osteomyelitis, usually of the long bones, commonly become partially epithelized. In some instances, squamous cell carcinoma arises in the tract epithelium after many years of chronic drainage and periodic acute exacerbations of the infection.

Arsenical Dermatitis

Exposure to significant amounts of arsenic usually precedes the development of malignancy by many years. Although exposure to occupational arsenic may be of importance in certain industries, the majority of cases arise secondarily to the use of arsenical compounds in a variety of medications such as Fowler's solution (potassium arsenite), an agent used several years ago for the treatment of skin diseases. In recent years, an arsenic-containing preparation for the treatment of asthma has been popular. The resulting arsenical keratosis commonly manifests as multiple punctate, horny lesions of the palms of the hands and soles of the feet. Another response is characterized by mottled pigmentation with generalized dryness and scaling of the palms and soles, a form less likely to undergo malignant changes than the horny variety. Arsenical dermatosis may also involve other locations on the skin, such as the trunk, and appear as brown, scaly lesions or arise primarily as multicentric basal cell carcinomas.

Lentigo Maligna (Melanotic Freckle of Hutchinson, Circumscribed Precancerous Melanosis of Dubreuilh)

This distinctive clinical and histologic entity appears as a tan to brown to black macule, most often seen on exposed areas of the head and neck in the middle-aged to elderly. The lesions show a variegated color pattern and irregular peripheral extension and regression of the margins. This radial growth pattern may persist for as long as 40 years. The lesions range in size from less than a centimeter to several centimeters in diameter. Rapid growth, a marked increase in pigmentation and/or the appearance of a nodular growth within the macule indicate possible evolution into lentigo maligna melanoma (malignant melanoma), a form of the disease with a distinctly better prognosis than the superficial spreading melanoma arising from the junctional nevus (Fig. 14–15*B*).

Malignant Epithelial Tumors of the Skin

Malignant epithelial tumors of the skin are the basal cell carcinoma, squamous cell carcinoma, and malignant melanoma. Carcinoma should be suspected in any lesion of the skin exhibiting continued growth regardless of its clinical features. These may appear clinically as keratotic, ulcerated, or exophytic nodules. Carcinoma of the skin may occur at any age and at any site although middle-aged or older individuals, usually those with skin poorly protected by melanin pigment, are most commonly affected. Patients with a history of excessive or prolonged exposure to such carcinogenic factors as ultraviolet light, arsenic, tar, oil, and x-ray radiation are likely candidates.

Basal Cell Carcinoma (Rodent Ulcer)

The most common variety of malignant skin tumor, the basal cell carcinoma (Fig. 7–5), generally presents characteristic features which permit a reasonably accurate clinical diagnosis. Nevertheless, the diagnosis should be confirmed by histologic examination. In its early stages, the basal cell carcinoma appears as a slightly elevated, waxy nodule with a shiny or crusting surface. With further growth, it develops a central depression which subsequently ulcerates. Periods of attempted healing and desquamation characterize its progress. The borders tend to become elevated and indurated with a telangiectatic surface as growth progresses.

The vast majority of basal cell carcinomas occur in the head and neck regions, usually on bony prominences over the upper portion of the face. Most are seen in individuals of blond or light complexion and nearly all have a history of long exposure to sunlight or other carcinogenic agents. Negroes are rarely affected. Most cases occur in patients in the fifth or later decades, although the lesion is sometimes seen even in children and young adults. The age range for basal cell carcinoma is markedly greater than for squamous cell carcinoma. Further, it is not uncommon for an elderly adult to develop numerous basal cell carcinomas over a period of many years.

Considerable variation in the natural behavior of the basal cell carcinoma may be seen. Most exhibit slow or indolent growth, particularly in the early stages. In other instances, the lesion may grow rather rapidly, with marked invasion of any underlying structures, including bone and cartilage. These features are related in part to the degree of differentiation of the tumor. It is believed that basal cell carcinomas arise from skin appendages and for this reason they almost never occur on oral mucous membrane.

Basal cell carcinoma does not metastasize except on extremely rare occasions and is quite amenable to treatment by surgical excision, electrocoagulation, curettage or x-ray therapy.

Nevoid Basal Cell Carcinoma Syndrome (Jaw Cyst-Basal Cell Nevus-Bifid Rib Syndrome, Gorlin and Goltz Syndrome)

The association of nevoid basal cell carcinomas of the skin and odontogenic keratocysts of the jaws (Fig. 4–4) comprises a well-defined clinical entity. Basal cell carcinomas have their onset in childhood and are largely clustered in the facial areas about the eyes, mouth, nose and ears and on the skin of the back. "Nevoid" in the sense that they arise early in life, they remain relatively quiescent until after 10 to 12 years of age, when they show the destructive characteristics and high recurrence rate of the common "rodent ulcer." An autosomal dominant trait, the syndrome may exhibit a variety of clinical abnormalities:

Cutaneous lesions
　Nevoid basal cell carcinomas
　Dyskeratotic pitting of the palms, soles
　Ectopic soft tissue calcifications
Skeletal lesions
　Odontogenic keratocysts (p. 469)
　Rib anomalies (bifid ribs)
　Shortened metacarpals
　Vertebral anomalies
　Hypertelorism
　Prognathism
Central nervous system defects
　Medulloblastoma
　Calcification of falx cerebri
Other defects
　Ovarian fibromas
　Lymphatic mesenteric cysts

Squamous Cell Carcinoma

Squamous cell carcinoma of the skin shows a distinct predilection for older age groups with about three-fourths of the cases arising on the skin of the face and neck. Nearly one-third of these occur on the lower lip (Fig. 1–17). The remaining cases may be found on the dorsum of the hand, ears and other miscellaneous sites.

A number of squamous cell carcinomas of the skin arise in areas of senile keratosis or other precancerous dermatoses, while some appear to arise in previously normal skin. The clinical appearance may vary considerably in the early stages and appear as a verrucous lesion or as a small, flat, indurated area which subsequently develops a shallow ulcer surrounded by an elevated border. Induration of the surrounding skin reflects the invasive growth of the tumor laterally under the adjacent normal epithelium.

Treatment of epidermoid carcinoma is by wide surgical excision or radiation therapy. The cure rate can be correlated in part with the size of lesion at the time of diagnosis, the degree of differentiation, the presence or absence of metastasis, and previous treatment if any. For example, epidermoid carcinoma of the lower lip is generally an extremely well-differentiated tumor which is usually recognized early and which metastasizes late in its course and then only to regional nodes, seldom below the clavicle. Thus the cure rate of lower lip carcinoma is high.

Intraepithelial Carcinoma

Carcinoma-in-situ may occur on skin surfaces and precede the invasive tumor by varying periods of time (Fig. 11–12). The so-called *Bowen's disease* appears clinically

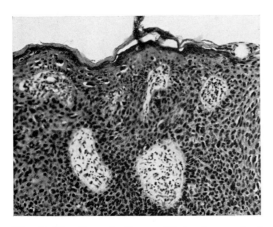

Fig. 11-12. Bowen's disease. Photomicrograph of skin showing intraepithelial carcinoma. Present are basilar hyperplasia, hyperchromatism, increased nuclear/cytoplasmic ratio and other disturbances in cellular maturation.

as a somewhat irregular but sharply outlined reddish patch which may scale. A crust may develop over the surface of the lesion which tends to spread slowly in a lateral direction. Invasive carcinoma, usually of a moderately to poorly differentiated variety, later develops.

Malignant Melanoma

In the skin, malignant melanoma may arise from malignant transformation of a junctional nevus or the melanotic freckle of Hutchinson (lentigo maligna). The melanomas exhibit a biphasic growth pattern with an often prolonged period of radial growth in which no metastasis occurs, followed by a vertical growth pattern with invasion and metastasis. Although not all junctional nevi are necessarily premalignant, it is generally believed that the malignant melanoma arises from the junctional nevus. Signs of malignant transformation may be ulceration, bleeding, an increase in pigmentation, lateral growth and/or the appearance of small satellite nodules. In some instances, the malignant melanoma may not form visible melanin (amelanotic melanoma) and thus appears clinically as a flesh-colored or red lesion. Malignant melanoma of the skin has a somewhat better prognosis than that on the oral mucous membranes (p. 383, Figs. 14–15B, 14–16).

Other Keratotic Lesions of the Skin

A number of other dermatologic lesions may appear as keratinizing defects with fairly typical clinical manifestations. Such conditions may appear either as solitary or multiple defects involving other portions of the body in addition to the face or hands. The diagnosis often may be established by correlating the clinical appearance with the frequently typical distribution of the lesions over the body surface.

Psoriasis

This rather common disease exhibits broad irregular papules or plaques which are

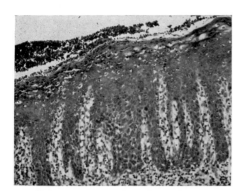

Fig. 11-13. Psoriasis. The histologic changes in psoriasis include parakeratosis, elongation and clubbing of the rete pegs, and intraepithelial micro-abscesses (Monro's abscesses). The tips of the connective tissue papillae are covered by thinned epithelium, thereby accounting for the bleeding points seen when the scales exfoliate.

dull red to brownish color and are usually covered with layers of fine silvery scales. These keratin flakes exfoliate, exposing the underlying skin surface which may show fine bleeding points (Auspitz's sign). The skin of the face and scalp is frequently involved, usually at the hairline. In some instances, psoriasis may involve much of the body surface. The disease runs a chronic course with improvement usually noted in the summer months with increased exposure to ultraviolet light. It worsens in winter with low humidity and flare-ups are sometimes seen at sites of skin injury (*Koebner phenomenon*). Patients with the skin lesions of psoriasis may, on extremely rare occasions, also exhibit oral lesions (p. 374). A few cases of oral psoriasis in the absence of coexisting skin lesions have been reported as well (Fig. 11–13).

Pachyonychia Congenita

This disease follows a hereditary pattern and exhibits hyperkeratosis chiefly on the palmar and plantar surfaces, changes in the fingernails and toenails, and hyperkeratosis of the oral mucosa (p. 378). The most prominent clinical signs are the defects of the fingernails which show marked thickening into claw-like appendages.

Keratoacanthoma

Sometimes referred to as self-healing squamous cell carcinoma, the keratoacanthoma shows rapid development within a few weeks into a conical elevation of the

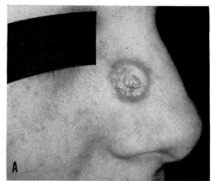

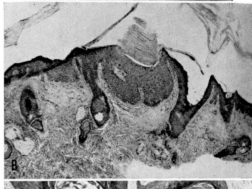

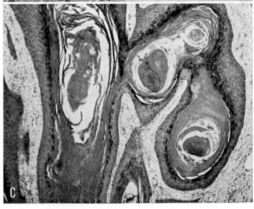

Fig. 11-14. Keratoacanthoma. *A*, Large keratoacanthoma on the nose of a young woman. (Courtesy of Abel Cardoso.) *B*, Photomicrograph of a much smaller lesion from the forehead of an adult male. Hyperkeratosis and acanthosis of the surface epithelium with an inverted growth pattern is shown. *C*, Photomicrograph showing a deeper portion of a keratoacanthoma with keratin plugs.

skin with a central keratin plug (Fig. 11–14). It has a definite predilection for the nose, lips, and cheeks as well as the hands and lower arms of middle-aged or older males. Fully developed, the lesions range from 0.5 to 2 or more centimeters in diameter. Even without treatment, the keratin plug is exfoliated and the lesion disappears except for a pale scar. Despite the characteristic history and appearance, its resemblance to carcinoma makes surgical removal preferable. The possibility exists that many so-called low-grade, well-differentiated epidermoid carcinomas of the lower lip are in fact keratoacanthomas. Some cases have been reported on the oral mucous membrane surfaces (p. 379).

Verruca Vulgaris (Wart)

The common wart of the skin is analogous to the papilloma of the oral mucosa (p. 419) and appears clinically as a rough, exophytic growth with numerous finger-like projections over the surface. Commonly found in children, it occurs especially on the fingers, palms, and occasionally about the face and lips. Warts are believed to have a viral etiology thereby accounting for their sudden appearance in crops or clusters. Many involute spontaneously, although these may be followed by an additional crop in the child. Solitary verrucae may be seen in adults also. Other varieties include plantar warts and condyloma acuminatum.

Seborrheic Keratosis

Sometimes referred to as basal cell papilloma or verruca senilis, this lesion usually occurs in patients of middle age or older and appears clinically as a raised, sharply circumscribed mass with a dark, verrucous appearance and a somewhat greasy consistency. Sometimes described as a "piece of wax," it occurs chiefly on the forehead and trunk. The mass is made up principally of basal cells which are usually pigmented (Fig. 11–15).

Molluscum Contagiosum

This mildly contagious lesion of the skin appears clinically as a firm, greyish-white elevation, often on the face and particularly the eyelids, arms, genital regions and occasionally the trunk. Of viral origin, these lesions usually occur in groups or in a linear

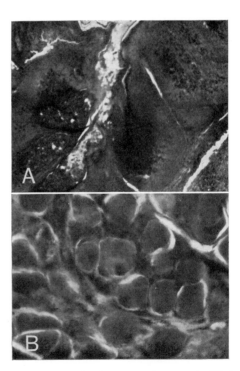

Fig. 11-16. Molluscum contagiosum. *A,* Photomicrograph showing the umbilicated pattern characteristic of this viral lesion. Molluscum bodies are seen in the acanthotic epithelium on either side of the crater. *B,* High magnification of the "brick-red" molluscum bodies.

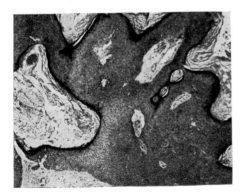

Fig. 11-15. Seborrheic keratosis.

Table 11-1. Miscellaneous Skin Diseases.

	Primary and Secondary Lesions	Distribution	Course	Etiology
Acanthosis nigricans (adult malignant type)	clinically similar to juvenile type	similar to juvenile type	associated with internal malignancy, usually adenocarcinoma	unknown
Acanthosis nigricans (benign juvenile type)	verrucoid lesions, hyperpigmentation	axilla, neck, skin folds; rarely, oral lesions of lips, tongue	arises before puberty; chronic	unknown
Acne vulgaris (pimples)	comedones, pustules, cysts, pits, scars	face, neck, back	chronic during adolescence and teenage—less severe in summer	hyperactivity of pilosebaceous units
Acrodermatitis enteropathia	eruptions, vesicles, bullae; loss of hair, diarrhea	skin, especially near body orifices; oral erosions reported	long term survival with quinoline therapy	genodermatosis (autosomal recessive)
Adenoma sebaceum (Pringle's disease)	yellowish to red papules, mental deficiency and epileptic seizures	nose, cheeks, nasolabial folds	chronic	inherited; may be associated with tuberous sclerosis of brain
Calcifying epithelioma of Malherbe	solitary; hard nodule	face, upper limbs	chronic; does not undergo malignant transformation	cf. calcifying epithelial odontogenic cyst (p. 470)
Chloasma	irregular hyper-pigmentation	sides of face, forehead, neck	slowly progressive, more apparent in summer	mark of pregnancy, or chronic illness
Chondroectodermal dysplasia (Ellis-van Creveld syndrome)	dwarfism; hidrotic ectodermal dysplasia of nails, hair, teeth; polydactyly; congenital heart defects	skin, hair, nails, teeth, long bones, heart	chronic; survival related chiefly to severity of heart defects	inherited chondrodysplasia of long bones

Condyloma acuminata ("venereal warts")	pink, raised, cauliflower-like clusters	anogenital areas; oral lesions reported	persistent; treatment with podophyllin or surgery	viral transmission, usually by sexual contact
Contact dermatitis	erythema, edema, vesicles or bullae, crusts, excoriations, secondary infection	any area of skin	short to chronic	allergens: cosmetics, poison ivy, deodorants, soaps, detergents, chemicals, etc.
Dermatitis herpetiformis (Duhring-Broeg disease)	papules, vesicles, bullae, pustules; severe pruritus; pigmentation	extremities, trunk, face, scalp; oral vesicles and erosions reported	prolonged (years), with remissions	unknown
Dermatofibroma (histiocytoma, sclerosing hemangioma)	tan to reddish brown, flat nodules, "button-like"	anterior tibial area; 1 to 2 mm; usually solitary	adults; slow growth	unknown
Dermographism	urticaria or wheals appear in areas of pressure	generalized	wheals arise immediately or up to 1 to 2 hours later	penicillin reaction, other allergies
Ehlers-Danlos syndrome (cutis hyperelastica)	fragility of skin and cutaneous blood vessels; hyperelasticity of skin; hyperextensibility of joints; nodular tumors	generalized; "fragile" oral mucosa; TMJ subject to dislocation	poor healing of wounds	hereditary (autosomal dominant)
Erysipelas	red, brawny, sharp-bordered plaque; vesicles, bullae form on plaque surface	face	fever, malaise; plaques enlarge peripherally, rapid response to antibiotics	hemolytic streptococci
Erythema infectiosum (fifth disease)	red macular rash	measles-like rash on body; flushed (slapped-face) appearance on cheeks	arises on body, spreads	probable virus

Table 11-1. Miscellaneous Skin Diseases (Continued).

	Primary and Secondary Lesions	Distribution	Course	Etiology
Folliculitis	red papules or pustules around hair follicles; crusting	scalp, beard area of face	variable	staphylococci, "Barber's itch"
Furuncle (boil)	abscess around hair follicle; carbuncles	posterior neck, buttocks, face	may be recurrent	staphylococci
Glomus tumor	solitary reddish-purple nodule; tender; paroxysmal pains	under fingernails, tips of fingers, other solitary sites	benign	arises from glomi of skin
Granuloma annulare	pale to reddish-purple with papule; peripheral enlargement, depressed center develops	dorsum of hands, fingers, ankles, neck	chronic, heals without scar in few weeks up to 2 years	unknown etiology, common in children
Hereditary ectodermal dysplasia	scanty hair; complete or partial anodontia, complete or partial absence of sweat glands, sebaceous glands; dry skin	teeth, hair, skin and skin appendages, sweat and sebaceous glands	complications from hyperthermia and absence of teeth are major problems	hereditary
Ichthyosis	dry scales ("fish-scales"); exfoliation	most of body surface	constant	hereditary
Impetigo	eroded vesicles, honey-colored serous fluid, crusts of ruptured vesicles, satellite lesions	face around nose, mouth	new lesions develop rapidly	staphylococci

Incontinentia pigmenti (Bloch-Sulzberger, Bloch-Seimens disease)	vesicular, bullous, verrucous and pigmented lesions, eosinophilia, oligodentia	extremities, ocular, CNS, teeth; arises at birth–2 years, "Zebra" or "bathing suit" pattern	chronic; pigmentation fades during 2nd, 3rd decades	congenital, probably autosomal dominant disorder, sex-limited
Keloid (hypertrophic scar) (Fig. 7-18)	overgrowth of fibrous tissue in linear or other configuration	face, neck, upper chest; common in Negroids	constant	cosmetic surgery often heals with new keloid formation
Keratosis follicularis (Darier's disease)	red papules around hair follicles; multiple, confluent crusted and ulcerated warty mass; rancid odor	seborrheic areas, face, neck, chest; genital lesions	begins in childhood; progressive; worse in summer	hereditary
Lichen planus (Figs. 7-47, 11-28, 14-4)	pruritic, shiny, violaceous papules; gray Wickham's striae on surface. Annular linear, hypertrophic, atrophic and bullous forms	symmetrical; flexor surfaces of forearms, anterior tibial areas; oral lesions (see p. 372); seen chiefly in adults	chronic, several months to years	unknown
Necrobiosis lipoidica diabeticorum	dark red plaques; flat or elevated border scaling; atrophic, yellow, depressed center as lesion enlarges	lower limbs; multiple asymmetrical	chronic	sometimes associated with diabetes mellitus
Neurodermatitis	dry scales, tiny papules, excoriation, scars	back of neck, hands, ears	severe pruritus	emotional outlet, nervous habit
Pityriasis rosea (Fig. 11-27)	"herald spot" 3 to 4 cm erythema, multiple red macules, papules	trunk mainly, facial lesions rare except in children; buccal mucosa, tongue	4 to 8 weeks; spring and fall epidemics; mildly contagious	unknown

Table 11-1. Miscellaneous Skin Diseases (Continued).

	Primary and Secondary Lesions	Distribution	Course	Etiology
Porphyria, congenital erythropoietic	photosensitivity, bullae, positive Nikolsky's sign, red staining of bones, teeth; red, fluorescent urine	generalized; skin, bones, teeth	survival unlikely past early to middle adulthood	congenital defect in porphyrin metabolism
Porphyria cutanea tarda	photosensitivity; redness, vesiculation on exposure to sun; vesicles, bullae; hyperpigmentation; atrophy, scarring of skin	exposed skin; middle-aged males	chronic	hereditary; aggravated by alcohol, barbiturates
Pseudoxanthoma elasticum	small, yellow papules in darker surrounding skin ("weathered" skin) retinal angioid streaks; GI tract bleeding	lateral neck, axilla, flexural areas	associated vascular hereditary disease; angina; intermittent claudication; aortic aneurysms	congenital defect of elastic tissue
Rheumatic nodule	fixed, firm nodules 2 to 25 mm	extensor-aspect joints, especially fingers, elbows, knees—over bony surfaces (forehead)	transient in rheumatic fever; chronic in rheumatoid arthritis	associated rheumatoid arthritis, rheumatic fever
Rosacea	erythema—papules, pustules, dilated veins, hypertrophic nose (rhinophyma)	"butterfly" area, nose	chronic	oily skin, "excess alcoholic beverages"

Disease	Appearance	Location	Course	Cause
Seborrheic dermatitis (dandruff)	scales, excoriations	scalp	chronic	
Tinea capitus (ringworm of scalp)	patchy loss of hair; crusts	scalp, chiefly in children	chronic	*Microsporum canis* and others
Tinea pedis (athlete's foot)	blisters, scabs, maceration, fissures	feet	chronic	*Trichophyton rubrum* and others
Trichoepithelioma (epithelioma adenoides cysticum)	multiple (often hundreds), small yellowish to pink nodules	face, forehead, sometimes on upper trunk	arises at puberty; may ulcerate with transition to active basal cell carcinoma	simulates hair structures, basal cell carcinoma
Urticaria (hives)	red papules	trunk	transitory in acute cases; chronic forms	drugs, heat, cold, insect bites, "nerves"
Vitiligo (Fig. 7-4)	irregular areas of depigmentation	face, dorsum of hands, body surfaces	slowly progressive, remissions frequent	unknown
Xanthelasma	multiple yellow plaques	eyelids	constant	associated with atherosclerosis or hypercholesterolemia in some cases
Xeroderma pigmentosum	photosensitivity; erythema; mottled pigmentation similar to freckles; telangiectasis; atrophy	exposed areas of skin	arises in childhood; skin carcinomas may arise from growths	hereditary

pattern and exhibit a central dark brown depression. Growth is relatively slow and the umbilicated center develops as keratinous material within the center of the lesion (Fig. 11–16). This curd-like material, composed of keratin and "molluscum bodies," may be expressed from the lesion by squeezing. It is found chiefly in children and young adults and may occur in epidemic form in institutionalized children. Rare cases of oral lesions of molluscum contagiosum have been reported.

Darier's Disease (Keratosis Follicularis, Darier-White's Disease, Benign Dyskeratosis)

This autosomal dominant dermatosis arises in childhood or adolescence with keratotic and crusty papules distributed over the face, trunk and extremities. The papules are a yellowish-brown color and are often foul smelling. Characteristic changes in the fingernails are longitudinal red and white streaks with fissuring and splintering and subungal hyperkeratosis. The oral lesions of Darier's disease appear as rough, white, keratotic papules and plaques described as having a "cobblestone" appearance (p. 379).

Other Keratoses

A number of other rare conditions of the skin which exhibit varying degrees of keratosis include *ichthyosis* and *keratosis palmaris et plantaris* (Table 11–1).

Pigmentations

A number of metabolic or foreign products may give rise to pigmented areas of the skin, especially of the face and hands. Recognition of these may have a direct bearing on the diagnosis of oral disease or, in the case of malignant melanoma, may be life-saving. Pigmentations of the skin or mucous membranes may be physiologic or pathologic and of intrinsic or extrinsic origin. Clinically, they may appear as solitary, multiple, or diffuse lesions.

Physiologic Pigmentation

Normally occurring pigments in the human are melanin, hemoglobin and hemoglobin derivatives, and the lipochromes. Of these, only melanin shows a significant variation in degree of pigmentation which is of physiologic rather than pathologic origin.

Melanin is found normally in the skin of all individuals (except albinos) but varies considerably depending upon racial extraction. The amount of the pigment will further vary within the same individual in relation to the amount of exposure to the actinic rays of the sun. Thus, racial and physiologic pigmentation is diffusely distributed in the skin with the more dense pigmentation seen in exposed areas. Racial pigmentation occurs to varying degrees on oral mucous membrane surfaces, chiefly the gingiva.

Focal areas of physiologic pigmentation are represented by the common freckle (ephelis). These small pigmented spots tend to be especially numerous in red-haired individuals and increase in number upon exposure to sunlight. The ephelis may be found on rare occasions on the vermilion border of the lips or, more rarely, on oral mucous membranes.

Pathologic Pigmentation

The abnormal pigmentations of the skin of the face and hands may be extrinsic or intrinsic in origin and be seen as focal or diffuse discolorations. Among the chief types of *extrinsic pigmentations* are those due to dyes, foreign bodies, and certain heavy metals and drugs. Deliberate implantation of various dyes into the skin in the common tattoo is seen most frequently. The decorative tattoo is of no clinical significance except in those individuals who subsequently develop a hypersensitivity to one or more of the dyes in the tattoo. Some prosthodontists have recommended tattooing as a method of permanently identifying the hinge axis of the temporomandibular joint. Foreign bodies such as cinders or graphite from a pencil lead may become implanted into the skin following traumatic injury and produce a tattoo similar to the common amalgam tattoo of the oral mucous membrane (Fig. 14–15*A*).

Extrinsic pigmentation of a diffuse distribution in the skin and mucous membrane may follow the ingestion of certain medications used in the treatment of a specific disease. Less common portals of entry may be inhalation or absorption through the skin. In either event, the pigment is eventually carried by the circulation throughout the body and becomes clinically manifest as a diffuse discoloration of the skin and mucous membranes. Some pigments of this type, particularly certain of the heavy metals such as bismuth, tend to concentrate in areas of increased vascularity. For this reason a distinct "bismuth line" appears on the gingiva, a common site of low-grade, chronic inflammation (Fig. 14–17).

Other extrinsic pigmentations of the skin include the heavy metals silver, gold, lead, arsenic, and mercury and other agents such as atabrine (an antimalarial agent) and carotene. The latter pigment is found in carrots, which when consumed in large quantities may cause a diffuse yellow coloration of the skin (carotenemia).

Intrinsic pigmentations arise from abnormal collections of pigments occurring naturally in the body, chiefly melanin, hemoglobin and hemoglobin derivatives, especially hemosiderin and bile pigments. The differential diagnosis of the pathologic pigmentations will be more accurate if the nature of the pigment can be established. Certain focal and diffuse pigmentations of a pathologic nature may simulate physiologic pigmentations. For example, the pathognomonic freckles of the *Peutz-Jegher's syndrome* (Fig. 11–17*A* and *B*) and *Addison's disease* (Fig. 11–18) clinically resemble the common ephelis except for their distribution. Although of no clinical significance, the blotchy lentigo (liver spot) seen chiefly on the hands and face of the older patient should also be differentiated from the common ephelis. The patchy areas of melanin pigmentation referred to as *café au lait* spots, while of no serious significance themselves, offer important clues in the diagnosis of such conditions as *von Recklinghausen's disease of skin (neurofibromatosis)*, or *Albright's syndrome (polyostotic fibrous dysplasia)*. Since tyrosine metabolism is under endocrine control, a pathologic increase in melanin pigmentation may occur diffusely over much of the body in Addison's disease ("bronzed disease," p. 255) and to some degree in pregnancy ("mask of pregnancy") and with the use of oral contraceptives.

Diffuse pigmentations of the skin are strongly suggestive of systemic disturbances of more serious consequence than the skin

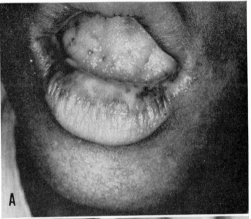

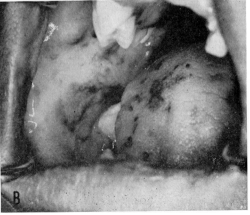

Fig. 11-17. Peutz-Jegher's syndrome. *A*, Pigmentation of lower lip. *B*, Pigmentation of tongue and cheek mucosa. (Simpson, Oral Surg., *17*, 331, 1964.)

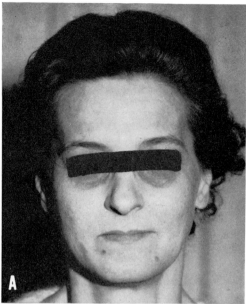

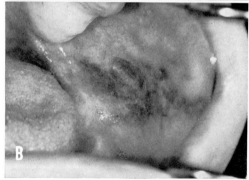

Fig. 11-18. Addison's disease. *A,* Abnormal skin pigment beneath eyes and, *B,* on inner cheek. (See also Figs. 9-22, 14-13.)

Intrinsic Pigmentations, Focal

Melanin Pigments
1. Intradermal nevus
2. Compound nevus
3. Junctional nevus
4. Blue nevus
5. Juvenile melanoma
6. Freckle of Hutchinson
7. Malignant melanoma
8. Perioral freckles of Peutz-Jegher's syndrome
9. Melanotic spots of Addison's disease
10. *Café au lait* spots of von Recklinghausen's disease of skin, and polyostotic fibrous dysplasia (Albright's syndrome)
11. Incontinentia pigmenti

Blood Pigments
1. Hemosiderin pigmentation secondary to trauma
2. Petechiae

Vascular Nevi
1. Hemangioma and hemangioendothelioma
2. Hemangioma associated with Sturge-Weber syndrome (encephalotrigeminal angiomatosis)

Intrinsic Pigmentations, Diffuse

Melanin Pigments
1. Melanosis

Blood and Bile Pigments
1. Hemosiderosis
2. Hemochromatosis
3. Jaundice
   a. Obstructive
   b. Hemolytic
   c. Erythroblastosis fetalis
4. Porphyria

pigmentation itself. On the other hand, the solitary pigmented lesion such as the nevus may represent a local neoplastic process which may undergo malignant transformation on rare occasions.

Patchy areas of *depigmentation* of the skin are seen in vitiligo (Fig. 7–4). Probably an autoimmune disorder, vitiligo is found ten times more frequently in patients with pernicious anemia than among the normal population (Grunnet *et al.*).

The more common pathologic pigmentations of intrinsic origin are listed below:

A number of other specific dermatoses may give rise to skin pigmentation of some clinical and diagnostic significance. These include Darier's disease, dyskeratosis congenita, ochronosis, xeroderma pigmentosa, incontinentia pigmenti, acanthosis nigricans and lentigo melanosis.

Cysts of the Skin

In addition to the cysts described below, which arise primarily from the skin and skin appendages, other cystic lesions may involve the skin coincidentally. For example, the branchial cleft cyst, thyroglossal tract cyst and other developmental cysts found in the neck (pp. 344–345) must be considered in the differential diagnosis of cysts in this location. Additionally, cysts of the parotid gland (papillary cystadenoma, p. 353) may produce a bulge in the overlying skin and thus be mistaken for cysts arising in the skin.

Cysts of the skin and its appendages may arise from traumatic implantation of surface epithelium (implantation, epidermal inclusion cyst), occlusion of gland ducts (sebaceous cyst), ectodermal remnants (dermoid cyst) or proliferation of epithelial buds following injury (milium).

Epidermal and Sebaceous Cysts

Proliferation of epithelial elements from skin appendages, surface epithelium, or embryonal cell remnants, blockage of a seba-

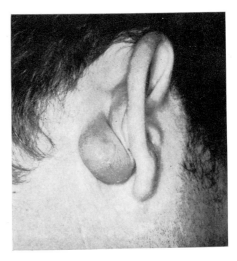

Fig. 11-20. Sebaceous cyst. (Courtesy of Frederick M. Stiren.)

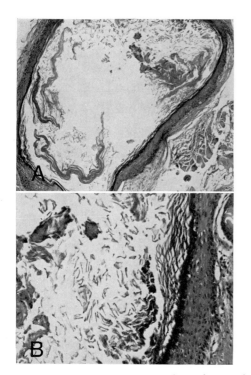

Fig. 11-19. Epidermoid cyst. *A,* Photomicrograph of a sebaceous cyst of the face in a young adult male showing a keratin-filled lumen and a portion of the epithelial lining. *B,* Higher magnification of the cyst wall and keratin-filled lumen shown in *A.*

ceous gland duct, or traumatic implantation of surface epithelium may give rise to cysts of the skin. By common usage, the terms sebaceous cyst and epidermal cyst are synonymous; however, the lesions can be differentiated on an etiologic and histologic basis. These may be filled with desquamated epithelial cells, keratin or sebum (Fig. 11–19). They are doughy or fluctuant depending upon the consistency of the contents (Fig. 11–20).

Dermoid Cysts

Embryologic enclavement of epithelial elements in the midline of the floor of the mouth and submandibular area may give rise to the dermoid cyst (Fig. 11–21). Composed of lining epithelium with varying amounts of skin appendages such as hair, sebaceous glands and sweat glands, the dermoid cyst may be located above, below or between the genioglossus, geniohyoid and mylohyoid muscles. Usually quite large, the bulging mass may protrude into the floor of the mouth and/or appear as a swelling in the submental region (Fig. 11–21). The chief differential diagnoses are ranula (Fig. 7–26), thyroglossal tract cyst, cellulitis or cystic hygroma.

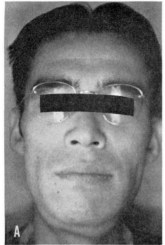

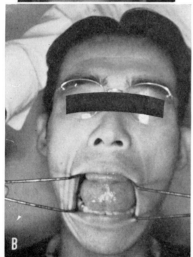

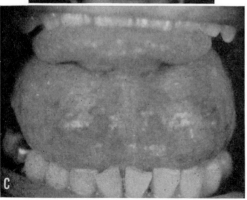

Milia

These common skin lesions appear as multiple, firm lesions of pinhead size, usually on the face. They represent foci of epithelial buds or keratin pearls found secondarily to trauma, acne or other dermatoses.

Calcifying Epithelioma of Malherbe (Pilomatrixoma)

This unusual lesion of skin is of special interest because of its histologic resemblance to the keratinizing and calcifying odontogenic cyst (Gorlin cyst, p. 470). The Malherbe appears as a hard nodule in the skin, ranging from a few millimeters to several centimeters in diameter. It is found chiefly on the skin of the face and forehead, but has appeared on other portions of the body. Most patients are less than 20 years of age, often with a history of slow growth over several years.

The mass is composed of collections of squamous cells with faint outlines (so-called shadow or ghost cells), eosinophilic material representing keratin and foci of calcification or even ossification. The lesion is treated by simple surgical excision.

Viral Dermatoses

The common viral dermatoses generally present typical primary lesions with a characteristic distribution over the skin surface. Most run a comparatively acute course with an uneventful recovery although serious complications develop on occasion. A characteristic macular rash is seen in the exanthematous diseases (measles, rubella) whereas a vesicular or macular rash followed by vesicles and finally pustules is seen in chickenpox and smallpox. Certain of the viral dermatoses such as herpes simplex; hand, foot and mouth disease; and hoof-and-mouth disease are discussed more fully

Fig. 11-21. Dermoid cyst. *A,* An enlargement is seen in the submental and submaxillary areas when the mouth is closed. *B,* The tongue is displaced palatally by the huge swelling in the floor of the mouth. Note that the swelling is no longer seen beneath the chin. *C,* Close-up view of the mass shows a relatively normal color in contrast to the usual bluish, translucent appearance of a ranula. (Courtesy of Charles Slavin.)

in Chapter 14 because of their striking oral manifestations. While verruca vulgaris and molluscum contagiosum are of viral origin they appear clinically as keratotic lesions and are discussed in that section of this chapter.

Measles (Rubeola)

This highly contagious disease is seen most frequently in school children during the early spring months. Prodromal symptoms of fever, rhinitis, conjunctivitis and a hacking cough precede the appearance of the characteristic rash by 4 or 5 days. Pathognomonic bluish white *Koplik spots* appear on the buccal mucosa (see Fig. 1–14). They persist for 1 or 2 days after the skin rash

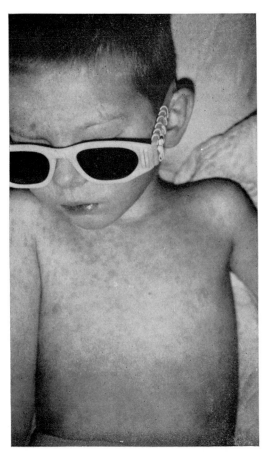

Fig. 11-22. Measles. A disseminated, macular red rash and photophobia are evident (see also Fig. 1-14). (Courtesy of John McLaughlin.)

appears. The morbilliform rash arises first over the forehead and behind the ears and then spreads over the face and neck (Fig. 11–22). Within the next 1 to 2 days it spreads over the trunk, back, and limbs. With the appearance of the rash, the patient's symptoms worsen. The early lesions are pink macules with irregular borders which blanch somewhat on pressure. The macules later become confluent and appear a deeper red or violaceous hue. In 3 to 5 days, the rash fades rapidly leaving blotchy areas which sometimes appear scaly. Complications such as myocarditis, bronchopneumonia, otitis media and measles encephalitis sometimes occur.

German Measles (Rubella)

Of interest chiefly because of the high incidence of congenital defects seen in maternal infections, rubella is a relatively mild disease. While minor epidemics do occur, it appears to be less contagious than rubeola, thereby accounting for the not infrequent occurrence in adults. Most cases appear in the early spring. The prodromal symptoms are generally mild. *Forchheimer spots,* deep red macules similar to petechiae, are seen at the junction of the hard and soft palates in some cases. The skin rash appears first on the neck and face, spreading over the chest, abdomen, back and limbs within the first 24 hours. The pink macules generally darken somewhat but, in contrast to rubeola, remain discrete and do not involve the palms of the hands and soles of the feet. The rash usually disappears in 2 to 3 days.

Pregnancies complicated by rubella during the first trimester sometimes terminate in miscarriage. Mild to severe congenital anomalies are found in approximately 10 to 15 percent of the offspring. Interventricular defects of the heart, mental retardation, deafness and cataracts are the usual findings.

Chickenpox (Varicella)

In common with the exanthematous diseases, chickenpox is a highly contagious viral infection seen commonly during the late winter or early spring in children (Fig. 1–13). The appearance of the skin lesions usually is the first sign. Occasionally, prodromal symptoms may be mild headache, fever, myalgia, malaise, and abdominal pain for 2 to 3 days prior to the outbreak of a vesicular rash on the upper trunk and spreading in lesser numbers to the face and limbs. The vesicles are thin with a clear fluid and surrounded by a broad erythematous zone. Pustules and crusts develop within 2 days. Successive crops of new lesions develop during the first several days. The lesions heal without scarring. Oral vesicles sometimes appear but promptly rupture leaving small ulcers similar to aphthous ulcers (p. 401).

Smallpox (Variola)

Because of intensive vaccination programs, smallpox has been virtually eradicated, even in undeveloped areas of the world. The prodromal symptoms are severe with headache, chills, fever, high temperature, vomiting and prostration. The early symptoms subside somewhat (2 to 4 days) and a macular rash appears, which is most prominent over the face, limbs, and palms and soles. The macules enlarge into papules; vesicle formation occurs and finally pustules develop. Severe complications, chiefly superimposed bacterial infections with septicemia, account for many of the deaths from smallpox. While severe cases of chickenpox may be confused with smallpox, the lesions of the latter tend to be deeper, symmetrically distributed and uniformly developed.

Herpes Zoster (Shingles)

The same virus is believed to cause both chickenpox and shingles. Children exposed to shingles during the first 2 or 3 days may develop chickenpox or, more rarely, adults exposed to children with chickenpox may develop shingles. The lesions are generally

unilateral and are distributed over the course of a sensory nerve. The thorax, head and neck are commonly affected. The vesicles are initially clear but soon become cloudy, and crust over after a few days. Intense pain may precede the eruption by a few days and, in aged individuals, persist for several weeks or months after the primary lesions have disappeared (post-herpetic neuralgia). Oral involvement is also seen (p. 386).

Vesicular and Bullous Dermatoses

Many of the primarily vesicular lesions of the skin are of viral origin and are discussed

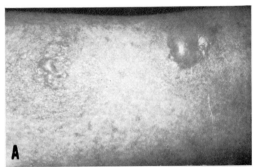

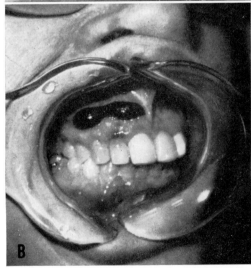

Fig. 11-23. Bullae. Transient and recurrent bullae of (A) skin and (B) oral mucosa developed suddenly in this lady. Pemphigus and other bullous diseases were ruled out. A specific antigenic agent could not be identified. (Courtesy of Dale Baker.)

in the preceding section on Viral Dermatoses.

Local bullous lesions of the skin, which are essentially large vesicles, follow local reactions to contact allergens, chemical agents or physical injuries such as burns. More extensive bullous lesions of the skin with oral lesions (Fig. 11–23A and B) include pemphigus, epidermolysis bullosa and forms of erythema multiforme. These and other vesicular, bullous and erosive lesions which frequently involve the oral mucous membranes are discussed on pages 385 to 394.

Primarily Vesicular Diseases

Herpes simplex
Herpes zoster
Herpangina
Kaposi's varicelliform eruption
Varicella
Variola
Vaccinia
Contact dermatitis
Drug eruptions
Neurodermatitis

Primarily Bullous Diseases

Pemphigus
Erythema multiforme
Epidermolysis bullosa
Familial benign chronic pemphigus
  (Hailey-Hailey)
Bullous impetigo
Dermatitis herpetiformis
Acrodermatitis enteropathica
Contact dermatitis
Bullous impetigo
Drug eruption
Acute epidermal necrolysis

The Connective Tissue (Collagen) Diseases

The so-called collagen diseases represent a loosely related group of diseases of unknown etiology which have in common a disturbance in collagen or ground substance (Table 1–1). As a group, they generally exhibit "fibrinoid" degeneration, mononuclear cell infiltration and, occasionally, a granulomatous reaction. Accumulating clinical and experimental evidence suggests that several of the so-called collagen diseases represent hypersensitivity states. The following conditions are discussed in this section: periarteritis nodosa (polyarteritis), Wegener's granulomatosis, scleroderma, lupus erythematosus, and dermatomyositis (polymyositis).

Periarteritis Nodosa (Polyarteritis)

This condition may occur at any age and in either sex although most patients are adult males. Generalized symptoms of chills, fever, headache and myalgia are common. The skin lesions of polyarteritis are commonly erythema multiforme-like lesions or other nonspecific eruptions as petechiae, purpura, bullae, urticaria or erythematous rashes. Small transitory crops of nodules of diagnostic importance are occasionally present. These represent tiny aneurysms and may pulsate. Skin and muscle biopsies of nodular lesions offer the best opportunity for diagnosis. The only available therapeutic agents are the steroids.

Wegener's Granulomatosis

This perplexing disease has many features in common with periarteritis nodosa and may represent a more disseminated manifestation of midline lethal granuloma (Fig. 14–41). The classical triad of Wegener's granulomatosis includes (1) necrotizing granulomas of upper and lower respiratory tract, (2) focal inflammatory lesions of arteries and veins, and (3) focal glomerulitis. Destructive lesions of the palatal, pharyngeal or nasal mucosa (midline lethal granuloma) are common (Fig. 11–24A). Sinusitis, nasal obstruction, ulceration and necrosis of the palate or gingiva, cough, hemoptysis or pneumonitis are early findings. Skin rash, excoriation, or other skin changes also seen in periarteritis nodosa are seen (Fig. 11–24B). Death is usually due to renal failure.

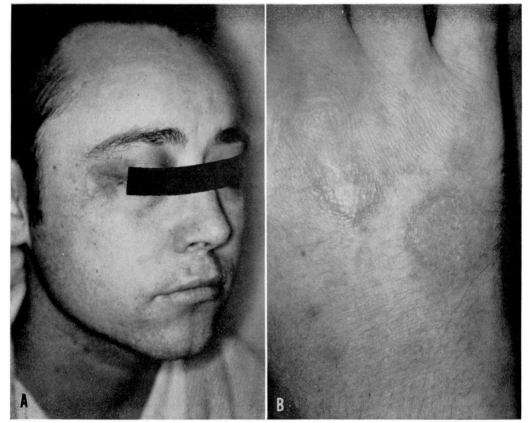

Fig. 11-24. Wegener's granulomatosis. *A,* A macular lesion is seen near the outer canthus of the eye. In addition, this patient had destruction of the nasal septum. *B,* Annular lesions are shown on the hand. Some tendency for scarring is seen.

Scleroderma

Characterized by diffuse sclerosis of the skin, scleroderma occurs in three forms: (1) circumscribed scleroderma (morphia), (2) acrosclerosis, and (3) diffuse scleroderma. Females 20 to 50 years of age are most commonly affected (Figs. 11–25*A,* 1–22).

Circumscribed scleroderma exhibits irregular, firm, inelastic, pale-yellow macules or patches with a violaceous halo on the skin. Linear bands or furrows are found on the limbs, face or scalp (*coup de sabre*). Symptoms are not marked and many lesions tend to involute after a long period of time.

Acrosclerosis represents a form of circumscribed scleroderma localized to the hands and feet with associated Raynaud's phenom-enon. The latter condition refers to a vascular disorder of the digits in which there is intermittent vasospasm with pallor and cyanosis.

Diffuse scleroderma is the most serious form of scleroderma and has a poor prognosis. The skin of the hands, feet, and face is involved early in the disease with progressive involvement of the entire skin surface. Limitation of movement occurs and the increased collagenization leads to atrophy of hair follicles and other skin appendages (Fig. 11–26). The skin is rigid and bound down with areas of calcinosis. Major organ involvement also accompanies the disease. Involvement of the tongue, soft palate, lips and pharynx accounts for dysphagia and

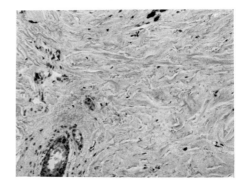

Fig. 11-26. Scleroderma. The connective tissue of the dermis is densely hyalinized with loss of skin appendages. The remnants of a hair are seen at the lower left.

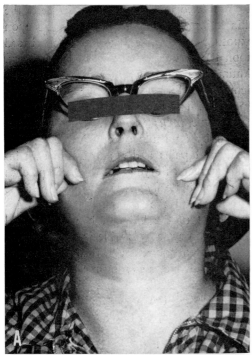

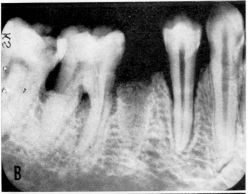

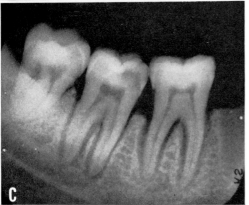

dysphonia. Thickening of the periodontal membrane space is a classic diagnostic feature (Fig. 11–25B and C).

Lupus Erythematosus

The chief forms of this disease are chronic discoid lupus erythematosus and acute disseminated (systemic) lupus erythematosus. Subacute and chronic disseminated lupus erythematosus are also recognized (Fig. 14–11). The chronic discoid form, while clinically quite different from the disseminated type, may terminate in acute disseminated lupus erythematosus on rare occasions. Both forms occur chiefly in women in the third and fourth decades.

In *chronic discoid lupus erythematosus,* the classic lesions are red, scaly patches with a pink or red elevated border over the "butterfly" area of the face and the scalp, arms and chest. The centers of the lesions are pale, atrophic and scarred. The lesions are nonsymmetrical, spread peripherally and tend to heal in the central areas. Oral lesions, usually of the buccal mucosa and lips, consist of red, atrophic areas with white

Fig. 11-25. Scleroderma. *A,* The soft tissues of the face and neck are very firm. The fingers are bent with arthritis. *B* and *C,* Radiographs of mandible reveal widened periodontal membrane spaces.

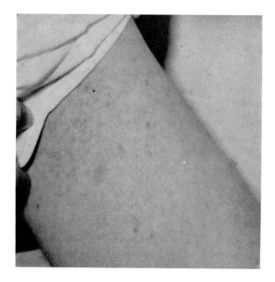

Fig. 11-27. Pityriasis rosea. The red rash shown on the leg was preceded by a "herald spot" or "target lesion" on the upper arm.

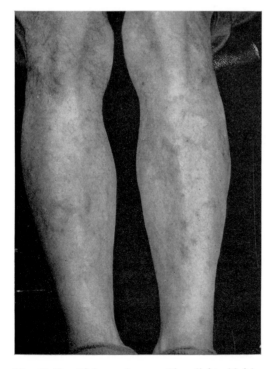

Fig. 11-28. Lichen planus. The light bluish-purple lesions on the legs were accompanied by typical striae of Wickham on the oral mucosa (see also Figs. 1-24B, 7-47, 14-4, 14-5).

keratotic borders (p. 379). When present, the oral lesions follow the appearance of the skin lesions. The skin lesions worsen upon exposure to the sun. The diagnosis is based upon the clinical features and skin biopsy. Antinuclear antibodies can occasionally be demonstrated by immunofluorescence tests (p. 234). The L.E. test is negative.

Systemic lupus erythematosus is characterized by an acute onset with fever, skin rash, joint pains and malaise. The skin lesions appear as erythematous, scaly patches over the "butterfly" area of the face, arms and legs and the fingers. Generalized involvement of the kidneys, heart, liver and other organ systems is widespread. The skin lesions are aggravated upon exposure to the sun. The diagnosis of systemic lupus erythematosus is difficult because of episodic involvement of the various organ systems. Skin biopsy is often non-specific. However, immunofluorescence tests (p. 234) show antinuclear antibodies in virtually all cases. Associated laboratory findings are leukopenia, anemia, increased sedimentation rate, and a positive L.E. test.

Dermatomyositis

This serious and often fatal disease may occur at any age but is seen chiefly in females in the 20 to 50 year age group. It involves skeletal muscles primarily (polymyositis) but commonly exhibits skin lesions as well (dermatomyositis). Facial and periorbital edema may be prominent with a lilac-colored (heliotrope) discoloration over the bridge of the nose, cheeks and forehead. An early sign may be Raynaud's phenomenon (p. 261). Muscle weakness and pain followed by atrophy is prominent in the facial, neck and other proximal muscles. Bulbar muscle involvement with dysphagia and dysphonia is present. Dermatomyositis in the elderly patient is sometimes associated with malignancy elsewhere in the body. Muscle biopsy, electromyography, and other muscle function tests are used to establish the diagnosis.

Other Skin Disorders

Included in Table 11–1 are several skin disorders that may be observed by the dentist. Even though most will not directly be related to the patient's oral problems, the dentist should have some knowledge of these for effective management. The brief listings give the essential features of the disease for general information purposes. References to dermatology texts should be made for more detailed information in suspected cases.

BIBLIOGRAPHY

Albers, G. D.: Brachial anomalies, J.A.M.A., *183*, 399, 1963.

Allen, A. C.: *The Skin. A Clinicopathologic Treatise,* 2nd Ed., New York, Grune & Stratton, 1967.

Andreasen, J. O. and Poulsen, H. E.: Oral manifestations in discoid and systemic lupus erythematosus, Acta Odont. Scand., *22*, 295, 1964 and *22*, 389, 1964.

Baer, R. L. and Harris, H.: Types of cutaneous reactions to drugs, J.A.M.A., *202*, 710, 1967.

Bergman, G., Lundström, R. and Lysell, L.: Rubella in pregnancy. Studies of the dental development of the foetus, Acta Path. Microbiol. Scand., *43*, 41, 1958.

Blank, H., Burgoon, C. F., Baldridge, C. F., McCarthy, P. L. and Urbach, F.: Cytologic smears in diagnosis of herpes simplex, herpes zoster and varicella, J.A.M.A., *146*, 1410, 1951.

Burckhardt, W. and Epstein, S.: *Atlas and Manual of Dermatology and Venereology.* 2nd Ed., Baltimore, The Williams & Wilkins Co., 1966.

Burstchi, T. A.: Herpes zoster involving the fifth and tenth cranial nerves, Oral Surg., *15*, 1434, 1962.

Dodge, P. R., and Poskanzer, D. C.: Varicella-zoster and herpes simplex antibody responses in patients with Bell's palsy, Neurology, *12*, 34, 1962.

Dummett, C. O.: The oral tissues in vitiligo, Oral Surg., *12*, 1073, 1959.

Fellner, M. J.: An immunological study of selected penicillin reactions involving the skin, Arch. Derm., *97*, 503, 1968.

Foster, S. C. and Album, M. M.: Incontinentia pigmenti: Block-Sultzburger, Block-Seimens disease, Oral Surg., *29*, 837, 1970.

Freeman, M. J. and Standish, S. M.: Facial and oral manifestations of familial disseminated neurofibromatosis, Oral Surg., *19*, 52, 1965.

Garell, D. C. and Silver, H. K.: Resistance to viral infections, Amer. J. Dis. Child., *105*, 106, 1963.

Garner, L. D.: Cephalometric analysis of Berry-Treacher-Collins syndrome, Oral Surg., *23*, 320, 1967.

Gorlin, R. J. and Pindborg, J. J.: *Syndromes of the Head and Neck,* New York, McGraw-Hill Book Co., 1964.

Grunnet, I., Howitz, J., Reymann, F. and Schwartz, M.: Vitiligo and pernicious anemia, Arch. Derm., *101*, 82, 1970.

Hall-Smith, S. P., Corrigan, M. J. and Gilkes, M. J.: Treatment of herpes simplex with 5-iodo-2-deoxyuridine (I.D.U.), Brit. Med. J. (Dec. 9) p. 1515, 1962.

Hambrick. G. W. Jr., Cox, R. P. and Senior, J. R.: Primary herpes simplex infection of fingers of medical personnel, Arch. Derm., *85*, 583, 1962.

Haring, O. M. and Lewis, F. J.: Collective review. The etiology of congenital development anomalies, Surg. Gynec. Obstet., Int. Abst. Surg., *113*, 1, 1961.

Jawetz, E.: Virus infection of interest to the dentist, Oral Surg., *8*, 1069, 1955.

Kaseff, L. G.: Investigation of congenital malformations of the ears with tomography, Plast. Reconstr. Surg., *39*, 282, 1967.

Kierland, R. R.: Cutaneous manifestations of systemic disease, Proc. Staff Meet., Mayo Clinic, *35*, 451, 1960.

Klauder, J. V.: The interrelation of some cutaneous and ocular diseases, Arch. Derm., *80*, 515, 1959.

Lever, W. F.: *Histopathology of the Skin,* 4th Ed., Philadelphia, J. B. Lippincott Co., 1967.

Lile, H. A., Rogers, J. F. and Gerald, B.: The basal cell nevus syndrome, Amer. J. Roentgen., *103*, 214, 1968.

Lundström, R., Lysell, L. and Berghagen, N.: Dental development in children following maternal rubella, Acta Pediatrica, *51*, 151, 1962.

McDonald, J. B. and Edwards, R. W.: "Wegener's granulomatosis"—a triad, J.A.M.A., *173*, 1205, 1960.

Mitchell, D. F. and Chaudhry, A. P.: Roentgenographic manifestations of scleroderma, Oral Surg., *10*, 307, 1957.

Mottlet, N. K. and Szanton, V.: Exfoliated measles giant cells in nasal secretions, Arch. Path., *72*, 439, 1961.

Oikarinen, V. J.: Neurofibromatosis (von Recklinghausen's disease) with oral involvement, Suom, hammaslaak. toim., *63*, 156, 1967.

Perry, H. O.: Skin diseases with mucocutaneous involvement, Oral Surg., *24*, 800, 1967.

Randall, P. and Royster, H. P.: First branchial cleft anomalies, Plast. Reconstr. Surg., *31*, 497, 1963.

Reisner, R. M., Cyrus, G. and Gurevitch, A. N.: Oral changes in incontinentia pigmenti, J. Amer. Dent. Ass., *76, 795,* 1968.

Rushmer, R. F., Buettner, K. J. K., Short, J. M. and Odland, G. F.: The skin, Science, *154,* 353, 1966.

Sauer, G. C.: *Manual of Skin Diseases,* Philadelphia, J. B. Lippincott Co., 1959.

Scott, A. and Rees, E. G.: The relationship of systemic lupus erythematosus and discoid lupus erythematosus, Arch. Derm., *79,* 422, 1959.

Shklar, G., Meyer, I. and Zacarian, S. A.: Oral lesions in bullous pemphigoid, Arch. Derm., *99,* 663, 1969.

Stewart, W. D., Danto, J. L. and Maddin, S.: *Synopsis of Dermatology,* St. Louis, The C. V. Mosby Co., 1966.

Wayte, D. M. and Helwig, E. G.: Melanotic freckle of Hutchinson, Cancer, *21,* 893, 1968.

Yeh, S., How, S. W. and Lin, C. S.: Arsenical cancer of skin—histologic study with special reference to Bowen's disease, Cancer, *21,* 312, 1968.

Chapter 12
Diseases of the Neck

The clinical diagnosis of swellings and other disease processes in the neck is facilitated if the primary tissue of origin can be determined. It is essential to have a working knowledge of the topographical anatomy of this region, as well as of the normal structures that can be identified by deep palpation and radiographic survey (Fig. 12–1). In particular, familiarity with the location and consistency of the cervical lymph nodes, carotid body, hyoid bone, tracheal cartilages and thyroid gland is important since these structures may be mistaken for abnormal growths, especially in the thin individual.

LYMPH NODES

The physical examination includes careful and methodical palpation of the major lymph drainage pathways of the neck (Fig. 12–2A, B and C). Techniques for examining the nodes in the anatomic subdivisions of the neck are described in Chapter 6. Since 40 to 100 lymph nodes may be identified in tissue from a normal complete neck dissection, and some are almost always palpable in healthy adults, considerable clinical judgment must be exercised in evaluating their significance. Knowledge of the anatomic region and drainage pathways is essential (Fig. 12–3).

Except for the malignant lymphomas, enlarged and/or painful lymph nodes almost always reflect a primary disease at some other site. For this reason, palpable lymph nodes should always be investigated since they may provide important clues to the diagnosis of oral and perioral disease. There should be no hesitation to refer the patient for medical consultation and node biopsy when indicated.

LYMPH NODE ENLARGEMENTS

Lymph node enlargement is the most common swelling encountered in the neck. Prominent lymph nodes are common in chil-

333

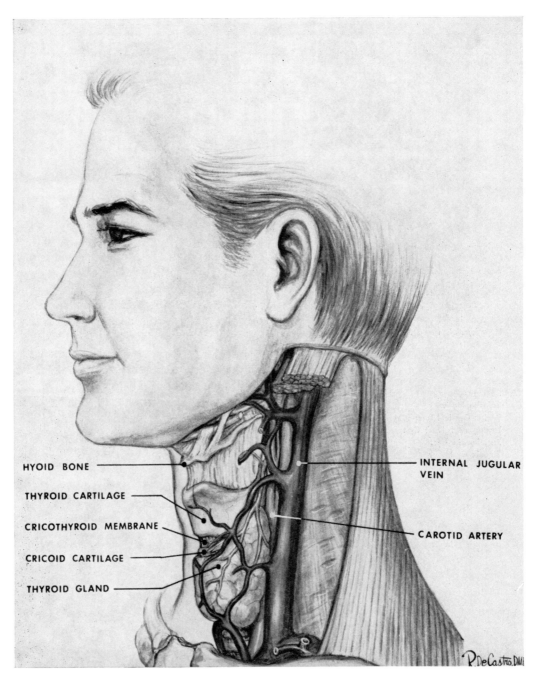

Fig. 12-1. Topographic anatomy of the neck.

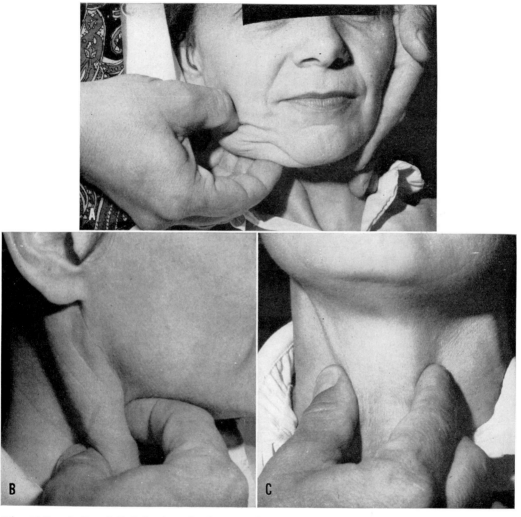

Fig. 12-2. *A*, *B* and *C*, Palpation of submandibular and neck tissues. (Fast and Forest, Dent. Clin. North America.) The technique of palpation is described in Chapter 6.

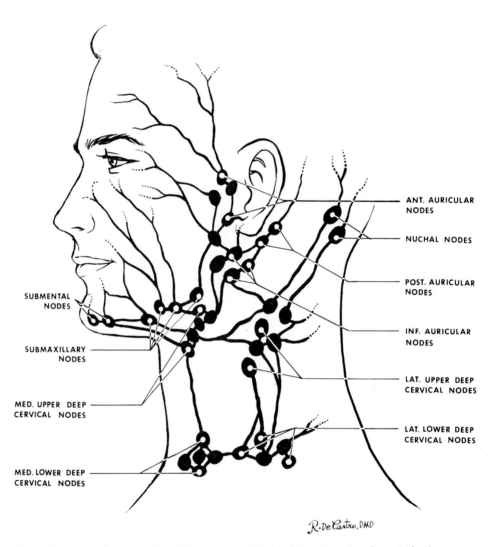

ANT. AURICULAR
NODES

NUCHAL NODES

POST. AURICULAR
NODES

INF. AURICULAR
NODES

LAT. UPPER DEEP
CERVICAL NODES

LAT. LOWER DEEP
CERVICAL NODES

SUBMENTAL
NODES

SUBMAXILLARY
NODES

MED. UPPER DEEP
CERVICAL NODES

MED. LOWER DEEP
CERVICAL NODES

R. De Castro, DMD

Fig. 12-3. The major lymph nodes of the neck and the facial and oral regions drained.

dren as are other lymphoid enlargements such as the tonsils and adenoids, since they represent a major defensive barrier against the spread of infection. The character of the nodes, *i.e.* their size, consistency, duration of the enlargement, mobility, and presence or absence of tenderness, generally permits a tentative identification of the basic pathologic process involved. Inflammatory enlargements of the cervical lymph nodes are commonly encountered in the routine examination and may vary from the small, "shotty," and only slightly tender nodes in the patient with a recent history of a cold, chronic sinusitis or similar low-grade infection, to the solitary, moderately enlarged, exquisitely tender, and occasionally suppurative node of tuberculosis (scrofula) or other specific infection.

Almost invariably, inflammatory lymph nodes are discrete, firm, tender and freely movable. Except in infectious mononucleosis and the exanthems when there is generalized lymphadenopathy, inflammatory nodes occur either singly or within a chain of enlarged nodes which drain the area of primary infection (Fig. 12–3). Low-grade infections commonly involve only the regional nodes whereas more severe infections will extend to the secondary chains as well. Generalized lymphadenitis occurs in bacteremias, viremias and infections producing potent exotoxins.

On occasion, an inflammatory (hyperplastic) node may fail to regress in size when the primary infection clears. Such "burned-out" nodes are quite firm and may even be fixed to adjacent structures by scar tissue if the original lesion was suppurative.

Neoplastic enlargement of the nodes of the neck must be considered when they are markedly enlarged, matted or fixed, indurated and occasionally painful. *Metastatic carcinoma* must be the primary consideration in such cases and a thorough search must be made for an occult tumor in the oral cavity, nasopharynx, and other areas drained by the involved nodes. Unilateral neck metas-

tasis is seen most frequently although bilateral involvement commonly occurs when the primary lesion is near the midline or in the tongue. Occasionally, a transitional cell carcinoma may be present as a small, asymptomatic lesion in the nasopharynx, undiscovered until neck metastasis has occurred.

Massive, bilateral node enlargement is characteristic of *Hodgkin's disease,* one of the malignant lymphomas. In common with the other lymphomas (*lymphosarcoma, reticulum cell sarcoma*), generalized lymph node involvement is seen chiefly in the cervical, axillary, inguinal and mediastinal nodes.

It should be recalled also that the lymph nodes not only serve as local and regional "filters" of infectious agents and malignant tumor cells but may reflect immune responses to a number of antigenic stimuli. Aberrant immunoblastic reactions frequently cause regional or generalized lymphadenopathy which may simulate malignant disease clinically and/or microscopically. Examples of such benign lymphoid hyperplasias are vaccinial lymphadenopathy, sinus histiocytosis with massive lymphadenopathy, rheumatoid arthritis and Felty's syndrome, secondary syphilis, sarcoidosis, histiocytosis X, lymphadenopathies associated with the dysproteinemias (macroglobulinemia, polyclonal gammopathies), Mikulicz's disease and Sjögren's syndrome as well as other autoimmune disorders.

Chronic Non-Specific Lymphadenitis

Regional lymphadenopathy secondary to upper respiratory infections, dental infections, or diseased tonsils is commonly encountered in the physical examination. These nodes are freely movable, firm, and painless. (Lymph nodes of this character are readily palpated in sites draining large areas of the body, such as the axilla and inguinal regions.) Usually the patient will give a history of a recent cold or other infection during which these "shotty" nodes were tender. In some instances, the nodes of the submaxillary triangle or the upper jugular chain may reach an alarming 2 cm in diameter.

The majority of enlarged nodes of chronic infectious origin regress in a few weeks or months, although occasionally they remain as "burned-out" nodes in which the lymphoid elements have been largely replaced by scar tissue. Persistent, benign, hyperplastic lymph nodes or lymphoid aggregates are occasionally encountered in the cheek mucosa or other intraoral sites.

Acute Non-Specific Lymphadenitis

Acutely inflamed lymph nodes are swollen (edematous) and tender or painful to palpation. In severe pyogenic infections the nodes may be fluctuant. Extension of the infection beyond the confines of the capsule results in redness of the overlying skin and subsequent sinus formation. After the infection is resolved, the lymph nodes regress in size and appear normal both grossly and microscopically. Those nodes with extensive architectural damage may heal by scarring.

Specific Lymphadenitis

Nearly all of the specific infectious lymphadenopathies that the dentist may encounter present primary lesions of diagnostic importance, in addition to node involvement. While the definitive diagnosis of these conditions requires identification of the causative organism, their clinical manifestations often are suggestive of the diagnosis.

Acute suppurative lymphadenitis is seen in cases of cat-scratch disease, tuberculosis, brucellosis, lymphogranuloma venereum and psittacosis. Non-pyogenic infections due to certain viruses, spirochetes or rickettsia cause marked edema but without abscess formation.

Tuberculous Lymphadenitis (Scrofula)

Regional lymph nodes are characteristically involved in nearly all of the many manifestations of tuberculosis. Tuberculosis of the tonsillar areas frequently leads to cervical lymphadenitis, often with multiple drain-

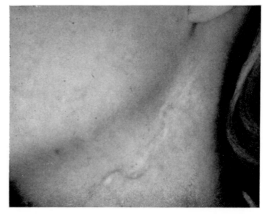

Fig. 12-4. Scrofula scar on the neck of young woman.

ing sinuses to the overlying skin (Fig. 12–4). In this form, the swollen, tender lymph nodes must be differentiated from actinomycosis, deep cervical abscesses secondary to dental infection or other specific infectious agents. Involvement of the cervical lymph nodes by the tuberculosis organism (*Mycobacterium tuberculosis*), especially as a primary infection, often results in marked scarring and calcification.

Sarcoidosis (Boeck's Sarcoid, Besnier-Beck-Schaumann Disease)

Sarcoidosis is a non-caseating granulomatous disease of unknown etiology which may involve virtually any organ or tissue of the body. It affects adults, principally in the second and third decades, and has a predilection for Negroes. Although a specific etiologic agent has not been identified in sarcoidosis, its protean manifestations suggest that it represents an anergic or hypoergic form of tuberculosis, or an atypical response to a variety of antigenic agents such as pine pollen.

The onset of the disease is often gradual with few symptoms. More often, there is cough and malaise together with other signs depending upon the particular organ systems affected. The disease most commonly affects the lymph nodes (lymphadenopathy), spleen (splenomegaly), liver (hepatomegaly), skin (multiple raised red patches), bone (radiolucent or reticulated lesions, especially of the small bones of the hands and feet), salivary glands (uveoparotitis, p. 358) and the oral mucous membranes (papules, nodules or blebs).

Lymph node involvement is characteristically seen in the hilar nodes but the cervical, submaxillary, submental, epitrochlear, preauricular and postauricular nodes (Fig. 12–3) are commonly affected. These are enlarged, firm and rubbery, but not tender or painful.

Diagnosis is based on the histologic findings (p. 358) and the Kveim test (p. 235). Additional findings of splenomegaly, uveitis or iridocyclitis, hyperglobulinemia (p. 225) and hypercalcemia (p. 226), and radiographic changes in the short bones of the hands and feet, while not diagnostic, support the diagnosis.

Infectious Mononucleosis (Glandular Fever, Kissing Disease)

Seen most commonly in young adults, infectious mononucleosis is characterized by painful enlargement of the cervical lymph nodes along with generalized symptoms of fever and chills, malaise, pharyngitis, and tonsillitis—symptoms suggesting a generalized infectious process in the early phases. Oral manifestations of stomatitis and, classically, palatal petechiae follow the general symptoms. With progression of the lymph node enlargement, frequent hepatosplenomegaly, and appearance of cutaneous petechiae or purpuric spots, leukemia may be suspected. A moderate leukocytosis (approximately 15,000 cells per mm^3 with 70 to 90 percent lymphocytes) is characteristic. The diagnosis can be established by finding the pathognomonic "atypical" lymphocytes, which are large with nuclear aberrations and a foamy cytoplasm. The Paul-Bunnell test will show a marked rise in heterophil titer (sheep red cell agglutination) even in the early stages of the disease, reaching a peak by the second or third week.

The disease runs a course of 2 to 4 weeks. Treatment is symptomatic.

Cat-Scratch Disease (Cat-Scratch Fever)

A progressive, painful enlargement of regional lymph nodes, associated fever and malaise are the chief presenting features of cat-scratch disease. A nearly healed scratch or bite may be seen on the skin of the face. Since periods of up to 3 weeks may elapse before swelling of the lymph nodes draining the injury site occurs, the association of a comparatively trivial injury from an outwardly healthy cat and the lymphadenopathy is not immediately apparent. In practically all cases, the scratch or bite shows a normal inflammatory response and heals without complications. The regional lymph nodes, however, enlarge to several centimeters in diameter and are almost invariably painful, soft and semifluctuant. The overlying skin is often red and may develop a draining sinus leading from the underlying node.

The lymphadenopathy of cat-scratch disease has many clinical features in common with other types of acute specific and nonspecific lymphadenitis, including tuberculosis, lymphogranuloma venereum, tularemia and histoplasmosis. The diagnosis can be established on the basis of the clinical history and a positive reaction to cat-scratch antigen. Biopsy of the involved lymph node shows reticuloendothelial hyperplasia and microabscesses, features suggestive of the diagnosis.

Although a viral etiology seems most likely, a causative organism has not been isolated. For this reason, no definitive treatment is available. The disease is self-limiting and runs a course of 3 weeks to 2 months.

Tumors Metastatic to Lymph Nodes

Metastatic tumor must be considered in every unexplained cervical lymph node enlargement. In most instances, the primary cancer is clinically obvious. However, failure to find the primary lesion by careful examination of the oral cavity, face and scalp does

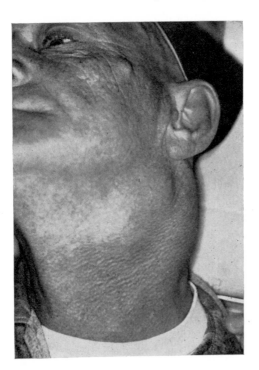

Fig. 12-5. Epidermoid carcinoma, metastatic to a neck node. The primary lesion involved the posterior mandibular gingiva and fauces.

not eliminate this possibility since carcinomas (lymphoepithelioma, transitional cell carcinoma) of the nasopharynx are typically small, difficult to find and metastasize to the regional nodes comparatively early.

Lymph nodes bearing a metastatic tumor growth are enlarged, hard, show rapid enlargement, and are frequently bound down to adjacent structures (Fig. 12–5). Some specific and non-specific infections may produce marked node enlargement that is difficult or impossible to differentiate clinically from a metastatic process. The benign, hyperplastic lymph node (q.v.) may present similar problems in diagnosis. Ordinarily, tumor-bearing lymph nodes will be localized to one side of the neck and appear as solitary enlargements, or successive nodes of one chain will be enlarged to varying degrees. Carcinomas of the tongue and nasopharynx, on the other hand, may show bilateral metastasis. Atypical metastases may

occur if there is blockage of lymphatic drainage by tumor cells. On occasion, ulceration and secondary infection of the primary lesion produce regional lymphadenitis which may mimic metastasis.

Primary Neoplasms of Lymph Nodes (Malignant Lymphoma)

Primary neoplastic diseases of the lymphoid system are referred to collectively as malignant lymphomas. Several types are recognized on the basis of the specific cell involved, i.e. the lymphocyte and histiocyte (reticulum) cell. One commonly used classification of malignant lymphoma is that given below. It should be noted, however, that other histologic classifications have been devised by Lukes, Gall and Rappaport, and others.

Leukemia is also considered to be a form of malignant lymphoma, differing from the above in the fact that the malignant cells are found in the circulating blood (p. 411). Palpable cervical nodes are present in about two-thirds of the cases of acute leukemia in children.

Giant Follicle Lymphoma

This form of malignant lymphoma occurs ordinarily in adults 40 years of age or older. The least malignant form of the lymphomas, it exhibits massive solitary or multiple lymph node enlargement. The disease runs a chronic course and many patients survive for long periods. Unfortunately, it may undergo transition to reticulum cell sarcoma or lymphosarcoma. Histologically, the disease must be differentiated from Hodgkin's disease and from a number of inflammatory hyperplasias of lymph nodes.

Reticulum Cell Sarcoma

Reticulum cells or their derivatives, the histiocytes, are ubiquitous in connective tissues throughout the body. For this reason reticulum cell sarcoma may be found not only in lymph nodes but in other connective tissues such as the pharynx, gingiva, and oral mucosa, as well as in bone.

Since reticulum cell sarcoma of bone has an entirely different prognosis, a distinction should be made. The soft tissue reticulum cell sarcoma involves chiefly men in older age groups and shows marked enlargement of multiple lymph nodes or soft tissues. Symptoms exhibited by the patient generally depend upon the primary site of the disease. In contrast, *reticulum cell sarcoma of bone* occurs in a considerably younger group, involves chiefly males, and appears as a poorly defined osteolytic defect (p. 485). The majority of the patients are under 40 years of age and up to a third are under 20 years of age. The prognosis of reticulum cell sarcoma of bone is considerably better than that of the soft tissue, with half of the patients surviving 10 years or longer.

Lymphosarcoma

This form of malignant lymphoma arises mainly in lymph nodes or lymphoid aggregates. In common with other forms of malignant lymphoma, the disease is characterized by marked enlargement of multiple nodes in the neck and other groups. The disease is seen chiefly in older men and in children. Lymphosarcoma in children has a poor prognosis, whereas the same disease process occurring in the aged patient will follow a markedly prolonged course.

Burkitt's (African) lymphoma is a form of lymphosarcoma seen chiefly in African (Kenya, Uganda) children although additional cases have been reported in other parts of the world (see p. 66). The disease is of special interest because of the frequency of jaw involvement and the association of a virus (EBV) with a malignant neoplasm in man.

Hodgkin's Disease

Hodgkin's disease is seen predominantly in males in the 20 to 40 age group. Clinical signs which would be apparent to the dentist include painless, enlarged cervical lymph nodes initially. Those of the axilla, groin, spleen, bone marrow and gastrointestinal tract become involved subsequently. The disease is extremely rare in the oral tissues proper, although involvement of the tonsillar areas has been reported. Patients frequently exhibit fever, leukocytosis (eosinophilia), anemia and other features suggestive of a viral disease.

In most instances the lymph node enlargement becomes massive with extreme enlargement of the neck and other areas in the late stages. The diagnosis is based on histologic examination of affected nodes, which show a mixture of lymphocytes, reticulum cells and the pathognomonic Dorothy Reed cells. Several histologic types have been described, depending upon certain of the microscopic features found. The prognosis of Hodgkin's disease depends upon the extent of regional node involvement.

Mycosis fungoides represents a special manifestation of malignant lymphoma which involves the skin and arises initially in multiple erythematous areas which rapidly coalesce to form plaques and finally numerous tumors scattered over much of the body surface. Histologically, mycosis fungoides shows features consistent with reticulum cell sarcoma or Hodgkin's disease. Surprisingly, patients with mycosis fungoides may survive for periods of 10 years or longer.

THYROID GLAND

Examination of the region of the thyroid gland is routinely included in the physical examination of the dental patient. The normal gland is rarely distinctly palpable. Recognition of thyroid gland enlargement may be of considerable clinical significance to the dentist, particularly if the patient is already receiving specific therapy (*e.g.* thyroxin, propylthiouracil) for the condition.

In addition to the clinical findings and medical history, a number of laboratory tests may be used in establishing the diagnosis (p. 243). In some cases microscopic examination is required, particularly when malig-

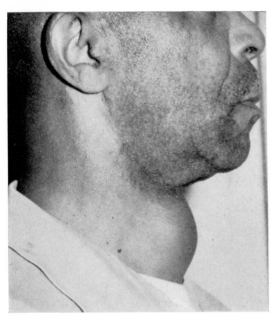

Fig. 12-6. Goiter present for many years. The patient is euthyroid.

nancy is suspected. Nevertheless, the character of the enlargement together with the clinical signs and symptoms often will provide sufficient evidence for patient counseling and medical referral.

Swellings of the thyroid gland may be diffuse or nodular, and may involve one or both lobes or the isthmus of the gland. Dependent upon the functional status of the gland, these enlargements (goiter) may be manifest clinically as hyperthyroidism, hypothyroidism or euthyroidism (Fig. 12–6). Basically, goiters are functional or nonfunctional, and of inflammatory or neoplastic origin.

Hypothyroidism (Cretinism, Myxedema)

Hypofunction of the thyroid during childhood and adulthood is termed, respectively, cretinism and myxedema. Both conditions may, under certain conditions, show thyroid enlargement. *Cretinism* ordinarily results from aplasia or hypoplasia of the thyroid gland. The cretin exhibits lack of skeletal growth, delayed eruption of teeth, low met-

abolic rate, coarse and edematous skin, and failure of sexual and mental development.

Myxedema develops most commonly without known cause. Other cases occur secondarily to exhaustion of the gland in hyperthyroidism, total or subtotal thyroidectomy, or deficiency of thyrotropic hormone. Thus, thyroid enlargement is seen in myxedema only in those cases of exhaustion of the diffuse goiter with hyperthyroidism. Clinically, the patient with myxedema is lethargic (low metabolic rate) and mentally dull, and has a dry, coarse skin. The subcutaneous tissues are thickened by a mucoid material resulting in the so-called non-pitting edema.

Thyroiditis (Inflammatory Goiter)

Inflammatory enlargements of the thyroid are rare and may follow direct trauma, radiation or extension of infection from neighboring structures. On the other hand, they may represent unique types of thyroiditis which are of unknown etiology but may represent autoimmune disorders (Table 1–1). Differentiation of these forms of thyroiditis is difficult and depends upon a variety of laboratory tests as well as microscopic examinations. Specific types of thyroiditis are subacute (granulomatous) thyroiditis (Fig. 12–7), lymphadenoid goiter (Hashimoto's struma lymphomatosa), Reidel's struma (struma fibrosa) and lymphocytic (lymphoid) thyroiditis.

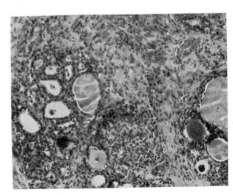

Fig. 12-7. Granulomatous thyroiditis. Thyroid follicles have been largely replaced by scar and inflammation.

Thyroid Adenomas

While the adenomas represent distinct histologic entities (follicular, embryonal Hürthle cell adenomas), they are not readily differentiated clinically from each other. Inasmuch as the adenomas are encapsulated, show an expansile growth pattern, often at the expense of the adjacent normal gland tissue, and are usually solitary nodules, these features constitute the chief criteria for clinical evaluation. Discovery of a thyroid adenoma may be of vital importance to the patient since approximately 10 percent of the adenomas of the thyroid undergo malignant transformation.

Malignant Neoplasms of the Thyroid Gland

Malignant neoplasia of the thyroid gland must be considered in every case of nodular enlargement, especially in young individuals. The solitary nodule is particularly suspect, regardless of the age of the patient. The usual signs of recent rapid growth, fixation to adjacent structures, or involvement of the recurrent laryngeal nerve (with hoarseness and non-productive cough) are important indications.

Carcinomas of the thyroid gland are of the following histologic types: papillary, follicular, medullary and anaplastic. The supporting stroma of the gland may also give rise to sarcomas.

Medullary Carcinoma

This tumor of the thyroid is of significance to the dentist since it may occur in conjunction with the neuropolyendocrine syndrome (mucosal neuroma syndrome, Sipple's syndrome, pp. 257, 421). The tumor may occur at any age but is most commonly seen in the fifth and sixth decades. However, when seen in association with Sipple's syndrome, it generally arises at a much younger age. It is often multifocal in the gland and contains calcitonin-producing C-cells. For this reason, compensatory parathyroid hyperplasia or adenoma may occur in response to the serum calcium-lowering effect of calcitonin.

The tumor grows rather slowly but metastasizes to the cervical lymph nodes in about one-half of cases. Nevertheless, the prognosis is more favorable than other anaplastic carcinomas of the thyroid.

PARATHYROID GLAND

Enlargement of the parathyroid gland due to hyperplasia or adenoma is rarely clinically detected. Since a normal parathyroid weighs about 30 mg (about the size of a small pea) and most parathyroid adenomas weigh less than 250 mg, the possibility of identifying such a lesion on the initial examination is quite remote. In most instances, clinical and radiographic evidence of von Recklinghausen's disease of bone or of renal disease (de Fanconi syndrome, tubular reabsorption defects, renal rickets, secondary hyperparathyroidism) suggests a lesion of the parathyroid gland (pp. 249, 464). However, asymptomatic cases of hyperparathyroidism are being identified with greater frequency with the increased use of multichannel chemical analyzers in hospitalized patients (see the Biochemical Profile, p. 220).

Most adenomas of the parathyroid gland occur as solitary nodules, usually in one of the lower two glands, which are found in the connective tissue adjacent to the carotid sheaths (Fig. 12–8). Parathyroid hyperplasia, on the other hand, generally involves all four glands. Since they are ordinarily quite small, they are generally not detected

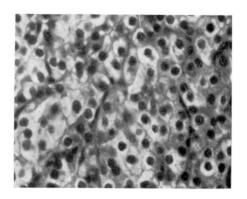

Fig. 12-8. Parathyroid adenoma.

except on surgical exploration or by angiography. The upper pair of glands is located on the superior poles of the thyroid itself. Thus, a clinically palpable nodule might easily be mistaken for a thyroid nodule. Further, ectopic parathyroid tissue may occur in the mediastinum or other aberrant location.

CAROTID SINUS

The carotid sinus is the widened portion of the internal carotid artery which is located immediately adjacent to the bifurcation of the common carotid artery. This bifurcation occurs just inferior to the angle of the mandible. Palpation of the carotid bulb elicits moderate pain. It is frequently mistaken for a swollen, inflamed lymph node, but can be differentiated from a lymph node by its distinct pulsation. In the course of examining the neck, this structure should be located and its size should be compared bilaterally. The dentist should gain experience in palpating this structure so that he has some idea of its normal size and consistency.

Bilateral pressure on the carotid bodies (the "sleeper hold" used by wrestlers) causes a drop in blood pressure and even syncope. Palpation and manipulation of the carotid sinuses are used in therapeutics to control auricular tachycardias, anginal pain and other vascular problems; however, this is not within the realm of the dentist.

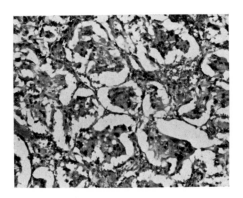

Fig. 12-9. Carotid body tumor (chemodectoma, non-chromaffin paraganglioma).

The carotid sinus may be extended or enlarged due to extreme hypertension, carotid body tumors (Fig. 12–9), aneurysms of the carotid artery and conditions such as carotidynia (p. 296).

CYSTS OF THE NECK

Cysts in the neck include those arising from the skin and its appendages (pp. 322–324), embryonic structures and remnants, and the parenchymatous organs of the neck. The parenchymal cysts are those which arise from the parenchymatous organs or their primordia (thyroglossal tract cyst, parathyroid cyst, thymic cyst and bronchogenic cyst).

Benign Cervical Lymphoepithelial Cyst (Branchial Cleft Cyst, Lateral Cervical Cyst, Benign Cystic Lymph Node)

This cyst, commonly known as the branchial cleft cyst, is usually found in the lateral aspect of the neck anterior to the sternomastoid muscle in children or young adults. Some cases are also found in the submandibular or preauricular (parotid) areas as well as the floor of the mouth (oral lymphoepithelial cyst, p. 404). It appears as an asymptomatic, soft, movable swelling which must be differentiated from sebaceous cyst, lymphadenopathy, focal parotid gland enlargement and other benign tumors.

The lymphoepithelial cysts are composed of a central lining of stratified squamous epithelium or, rarely, pseudostratified columnar epithelium and a wall of lymphoid tissue, often with germinal centers (Fig. 12–10). These features would suggest an origin from epithelium entrapped in the lymph node during embryologic development (cf. Warthin's Tumor, p. 353) versus the usual explanation of origin from remnants of the branchial arches or pharyngeal pouches. Some cases develop a fistulous tract onto the overlying surface or, rarely, the pharynx. Rare epidermoid carcinomas arising in branchial cleft cysts have been reported.

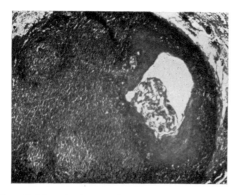

Fig. 12-10. Benign cystic lymph node. An epithelial-lined cavity is shown with reactive germinal centers in the left half of the field (cf. Lingual Tonsil, Fig. 14-67).

Presumed metastatic tumor to a cervical lymph node but without a demonstrable primary carcinoma in the oral cavity or nasopharynx may represent such instances.

Thyroglossal Tract Cyst

This uncommon cyst arises from embryologic remnants of the thyroglossal tract which runs from the region of the foramen caecum to the thyroid gland. Accordingly, the thyroglossal tract cyst is seen typically in the midline of the anterior neck as a simple swelling. Occasional cases are located higher along the original tract, sometimes near the foramen caecum where they cause intraoral swelling and dysphagia. Fistula formation on the skin or mucous membrane surface may complicate some cases. On rare occasions, carcinoma may arise from thyroglossal tract remnants or in the wall of these cysts.

Parathyroid Cyst

The parathyroid cyst is a rare anomaly which appears as a solitary swelling in the inferior lobe of the thyroid gland, generally in middle-aged adults. Most of these cysts induce deviation of the trachea and cause symptoms of respiratory distress or hoarseness with pressure on the recurrent laryngeal nerve. The cyst is lined by flattened epithelium and contains parathyroid gland tissue in its wall.

Thymic Cyst

These extremely rare cysts arise from remnants of thymic tissue left behind along the path of descent of the paired gland primordia from the third pharyngeal pouch into the superior mediastinum. Solid thymic tissue or cysts arising from these structures may thus occur anywhere along a line from the angle of the mandible to the midline of the neck at the sternal notch. Thymic cysts occur chiefly in young children through puberty (the period of greatest thymus activity) and may reach several centimeters in size. Symptoms are uncommon except in those occasional cases which are inflamed. They consist of lining epithelium, thymic tissue and, occasionally, cholesterol and a foreign body reaction.

Bronchogenic Cyst

This unusual cyst arises at birth or shortly thereafter as a slowly enlarging, fluctuant swelling or a draining sinus in the region of the suprasternal notch. It results from proliferation or budding of the respiratory tree during embryologic development and consists of respiratory epithelium with cilia and mucous cells, smooth muscle and, at times, cartilage. The chief differential diagnosis is the thyroglossal tract cyst which also occurs in the midline of the neck; however, it rarely extends as low as the suprasternal notch and is quite unlikely to be present at birth. Confirmation of the clinical diagnosis must be based on histologic examination.

MUSCULATURE OF THE NECK

The muscles of the neck are of obvious functional importance in posture, movements of the head, mastication and, to some extent, swallowing and respiration.

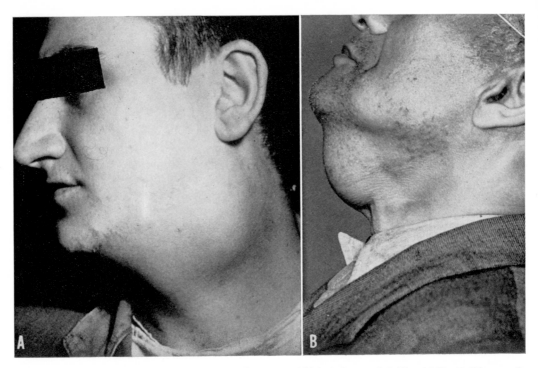

Fig. 12-11. *A* and *B*, Enlargements in the neck. *A*, Branchial cleft cyst (cf. Fig. 12-5). *B*, Lipoma. It was of soft consistency and had been present for many years (cf. Fig. 12-6).

The sternomastoid muscle is the most prominent muscle of the neck and provides a good landmark in locating lymph node chains, the carotid sinus, major vessels and other adjacent structures (Fig. 12-2*B*).

The sternocleidomastoid muscle is affected in *torticollis,* or "wry neck," with deviation of the head toward the affected side.

While few diseases affect the muscles of the neck preferentially, it is of interest that *rhabdomyosarcoma* of the head and neck regions is one of the most common malignant connective tissue neoplasms seen in children. Certain primary myopathies, notably facioscapulohumeral (mild restricted) muscular dystrophy, may involve the neck and facial muscles, causing weakness and atrophy. Weakness of the neck musculature may be marked in *myasthenia gravis,* appearing early in the disease along with ptosis of the eyelids and weakness of the muscles of mastication. (Refer to pages 257–265 and 291 *et seq.* for additional discussion of nerve and muscle function disturbances.)

BIBLIOGRAPHY

Anderson, W. A. D.: *Pathology,* 4th Ed., St. Louis, The C. V. Mosby Co., 1961.

Belfrage, S.: Infectious mononucleosis, Acta Med. Scand., *171,* 531, 1962.

Bhaskar, S. N. and Bernier, J. L.: Histogenesis of branchial cysts. A report of 468 cases, Amer. J. Path., *34,* 407, 1959.

Dodds, W. J. and Powell, M. R.: Lingual thyroid scanned with technetium 99^{m} pertechnetate, report of two cases, Amer. J. Roentgen., p. 786, 1967.

Hamner, J. E., III and Scofield, H. H.: Cervical lymphadenopathy and parotid gland swelling in sarcoidosis: a study of 31 cases, J. Amer. Dent. Ass., *74,* 1224, 1967.

Hardin, J. Jr.: Office diagnosis of cancer of the head and neck, Amer. J. Surg., *97,* 300, 1959.

Knewitz, K. W., Devine, K. D. and Waite, D. E.: Differential diagnosis of cervicofacial swellings, Oral Surg., *25,* 43, 1968.

Kramer, W. M.: Association of parathyroid hyperplasia with neoplasia, Amer. J. Clin. Path., *53,* 275, 1970.

Larson, D. L., Lewis, S. R. and Rappaport, A. S.: Lymphatics of the mouth and neck, Amer. J. Surg., *110,* 525, 1965.

Lederer, F. L. and Soboroff, B. J.: Significance and management of orbital, facial and neck swellings, Ann. Otol., *70,* 651, 1961.

Little, J. W. and Rickles, N. H.: The histogenesis of the branchial cyst, Amer. J. Path., *50,* 533, 1967.

Reich, N. E.: Carotid sinus in diagnosis and therapy, Mod. Med., *67,* 1958.

Rickles, N. H. and Bernier, J.: Cat-scratch disease, Oral. Surg., *13,* 282, 1960.

Rickles, N. H. and Little, J. W.: The histogenesis of the branchial cyst, Amer. J. Path., *50,* 765, 1967.

Robbins, S. L.: *Textbook of Pathology with Clinical Application,* Philadelphia, W. B. Saunders Co., 1962, pp. 509–526.

Sage, H. H.: Palpable cervical lymph nodes, J.A.M.A., *168,* 496, 1958.

Steg, R. F., Dahlin, D. C. and Gores, R. J.: Malignant lymphoma of the mandible and maxillary region, Oral Surg., *12,* 128, 1959.

Chapter 13

Diseases of the Major and Minor Salivary Glands

The major and minor (accessory) salivary glands are subject to a variety of developmental, inflammatory, infectious, metabolic and neoplastic diseases. In the major glands particularly, these disease states commonly manifest themselves as focal or diffuse gland enlargements which may or may not be accompanied by disturbances in function (xerostomia, sialorrhea). The accessory salivary glands are, with few exceptions, subject to the same pathologic processes as the major glands. However, because the accessory glands are distributed throughout the oral mucosa (excepting the gingiva) as simple glands, non-neoplastic enlargements (sialadenoses) are not ordinarily clinically obvious. Nevertheless, the accessory glands as well as the major glands exhibit characteristic histologic changes of certain metabolic, inflammatory and infectious disease processes such as cystic fibrosis (p. 359), benign lymphoepithelial lesion (p. 358), sarcoidosis (p. 358) and sialadenitis (pp. 355, 361). A clinical and histologic variation of the latter condition, necrotizing sialometaplasia, seems to be unique to the accessory glands, where it appears as an ulceration, usually on the palate (p. 399).

Except perhaps for the deep lobe of the parotid, the major salivary glands are rapidly examined by palpation. Bimanual palpation is essential for adequate examination of the submaxillary and sublingual glands (Fig. 2-9). Inasmuch as some asymptomatic parenchymatous enlargements may have the consistency of the normal gland, asymmetry may be the only gross evidence of disease. Normal flow of saliva from Stensen's and Wharton's ducts should be confirmed visually (pp. 28, 113).

Examination of the accessory glands is accomplished simply by drying the mucosa of the palate and inner surfaces of the lips and observing the duct orifices for secretion. It should be recalled, however, that except for the gingiva these glands are distributed throughout the oral mucosa, on the antero-ventral surface of the tongue (glands of Blandin-Nuhn) and in association with the circumvallate papillae (glands of Ebner). Uncommonly, ectopic salivary glands may be incorporated within the mandible during development or, more frequently, occur as lobules of the submaxillary gland in a bony depression on the lingual aspect of the mandible (latent bone cyst, developmental lingual salivary gland depression, Fig. 15-15).

SALIVARY GLAND ENLARGEMENTS

A great many conditions have been reported to manifest human salivary gland enlargement: neoplastic disease and benign lymphoepithelial lesions; duct blockage; specific and non-specific infections such as epidemic parotitis, ancylostomiasis, uveoparotid fever (Heerfordt's syndrome), "surgical mumps," and other primary and retrograde infections; drug-induced enlargements such as "iodide mumps," and following triiodothyronine therapy; such hereditary, systemic, or metabolic diseases as mucoviscidosis, hepatic cirrhosis, hyperlipoproteinemia, and diabetes; premenstruation, pregnancy and lactation; obesity and fat infiltration; alcoholism and malnutrition.

These conditions present a varied pathogenesis and histologic appearance and most represent either neoplastic or inflammatory responses; however, those enlargements of endocrine or neurogenic origin may on occasion appear as parenchymatous hyperplasias or hypertrophies (sialadenoses). Despite the complexity of salivary gland patho-

physiology, the clinical manifestations of most are sufficiently characteristic to establish a working diagnosis with reasonable accuracy. In some instances (chiefly the generalized enlargements) a definitive diagnosis can be made almost entirely on the basis of the medical history and/or examination.

The differential diagnosis of major salivary gland enlargement must be based on the clinical history, gross appearance and consistency, extent of the enlargement, signs and symptoms, and past medical history. The list of possible diagnoses can be considerably reduced by determining whether the enlargement involves all the major glands simultaneously or is confined to a single gland, or to a nodule in an otherwise normal gland.

It may be generally assumed that diffuse swellings which involve all major glands to some degree are most likely to be of general or systemic origin. On the other hand, a solitary mass in a gland is apt to be a developmental, focal inflammatory, or neoplastic process. Lesions of the submaxillary and sublingual gland are relatively uncommon, except for submaxillary duct blockage (sialolithiasis), ranula and secondary involvement in submaxillary space infections. The parotid gland, however, is subject to several specific disease states, some of which appear to be unique in that gland.

SOLITARY NODULES IN THE SALIVARY GLANDS

A solitary, discrete nodule or mass in the substance of a salivary gland, even in the absence of any presenting symptoms, must be investigated thoroughly. Difficulty may sometimes be encountered in differentiating clinically between a hyperplastic or neoplastic lymph node within the substance of the gland and lesions arising from the gland proper. Interestingly, the benign lymphoepithelial lesion and Warthin's tumor, traditionally classified with the salivary gland neoplasms, might be regarded as develop-

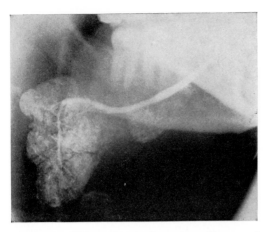

Fig. 13-1. Sialograph of the submaxillary and sublingual salivary glands. A uniform filling pattern is seen. (Fast and Forest, Dent. Clin. North America.)

mental inclusions of salivary gland tissue in lymph nodes.

Clinical evaluation of the solitary salivary gland nodule should establish as clearly as possible: (1) duration; (2) pertinent historic information including previous infections, trauma, or drug therapy; (3) related symptoms such as pain or tenderness; (4) growth rate or change in size; (5) functional disturbances involving salivary flow and consistency or facial muscle paralysis or paresthesia; and (6) the gross characteristics of the nodule. Palpation of the mass will reveal its shape, size, consistency, fixation to the skin or adjacent structures, and pain or tenderness. Sialography (p. 190) is a particularly valuable diagnostic tool (Fig. 13–1). In most instances, the information obtained will suggest the underlying pathologic process (developmental, inflammatory, metabolic, neoplastic) and often provide significant clues for a working diagnosis.

NEOPLASMS OF SALIVARY GLAND ORIGIN

With certain exceptions, tumors of the major salivary glands are similar in type and behavior to their intraoral counterparts. Differences noted appear to be related mostly to anatomic site and duration prior to removal. For obvious reasons, patients with intraoral tumors generally seek treatment earlier than those with extraoral tumors. The distinguishing clinical features of the intraoral salivary gland tumors are described on pages 424–425.

The clinical manifestations and natural behavior of the major salivary neoplasms are fairly predictable and are therefore of diagnostic importance. The parotid gland represents the chief site of occurrence of these tumors (approximately 87 percent of the cases). The submaxillary gland is involved infrequently (12 percent), whereas the sublingual is only rarely affected (1 percent). Further, approximately two-thirds of the major gland tumors will be benign, chiefly the benign mixed tumor (pleomorphic adenoma). In Foote and Frazell's series of 836 cases, however, over one-half of the submaxillary tumors (101 cases) and all (6 cases) of the sublingual gland tumors were malignant.

Clinical features useful in distinguishing benign and malignant salivary gland tumors must be applied to each individual case. The benign tumors will usually have a history of indolent or slow growth of several months' or even years' duration. For the most part, the benign salivary gland tumor will be firm or rubbery (rather than hard), freely movable, and asymptomatic. On the other hand, the malignant tumor will have exhibited recent rapid growth, be stony hard, be fixed to underlying or adjacent structures, and often have associated symptoms of pain, paresthesia, or facial nerve paralysis. Salivary gland tumors as a group may occur at any age and in either sex. Most, however, occur in the middle decades with the malignant varieties seen in the slightly older groups. The definitive diagnosis of salivary gland neoplasms can be established only upon microscopic examination.

The following classification of salivary gland tumors includes the chief histologic types.

Benign Salivary Gland Neoplasms
1. Pleomorphic adenoma
   (benign mixed tumor)
2. Oncocytoma (oxyphilic adenoma)
3. Sebaceous adenoma
4. Papillary cystadenoma lymphomatosum
   (Warthin's tumor)
5. Benign stromal tumors

Malignant Salivary Gland Neoplasms
1. Malignant pleomorphic adenoma
   (malignant mixed tumor)
2. Adenoid cystic carcinoma
   (cylindroma, basaloid mixed tumor)
3. Mucoepidermoid carcinoma
4. Adenosquamous carcinoma
5. Acinic cell adenocarcinoma
6. Adenocarcinoma, miscellaneous forms
7. Epidermoid carcinoma
8. Malignant stromal tumors

It should be noted that numerous histologic variants of these tumors are being reported with increasing frequency. For example, variants of the so-called *monomorphic adenoma* include the tubular or canalicular adenoma, basal cell adenoma, clear cell adenoma, glycogen-rich clear cell adenoma, ductal papilloma, sialadenoma papilliferum, etc. While these lesions appear to be distinct histologic entities, there is little evidence at present to indicate that their clinical behavior is significantly different from other benign salivary gland neoplasms.

Since the oncocytoma, Warthin's tumor and hemangioma of the parotid occur bilaterally with some frequency, they can be considered as developmental or hamartomatous growths rather than autonomous neoplasms. In this regard, Warthin's tumor and sebaceous lymphadenoma are "non-neoplastic tumors" arising as adnexal structures in lymph nodes. Likewise, the benign lymphoepithelial lesions (Mikulicz's disease, Sjögren's syndrome) are benign "non-neoplastic enlargements" which simulate neoplasia.

Benign Salivary Gland Neoplasms

Pleomorphic Adenoma (Benign Mixed Tumor)

The pleomorphic adenoma is seen clinically in the parotid gland as a rounded, firm mass which is freely movable and painless. Occasionally, vague symptoms of discomfort may direct attention to deep-seated tumors in the parotid which are less discrete to palpation in their early stages. The growth pattern is slow with periods of apparent inactivity. Spurts of growth, development of facial nerve paralysis, or breakdown of the overlying skin are ominous signs since they may indicate malignant transformation in a previously benign tumor. Untreated, this tumor may grow to a huge size, sometimes to 20 pounds or more. The clinical diagnosis must be confirmed by histologic examination of all portions of the mass (Fig. 13–2).

Pleomorphic adenomas of the submaxillary gland present essentially the same gross characteristics as those of the parotid. Since virtually the entire submaxillary gland can be examined by bimanual palpation, masses in this site can easily be discovered. If the physical examination, including sialography, indicates that the mass is indeed in the submaxillary gland proper rather than in a submaxillary lymph node, a tentative diagnosis of pleomorphic adenoma can be made only if all other features of this tumor are present. In the absence of any knowledge of its duration, the possibility of a malignant neoplasm must be kept in mind.

Sialography is a useful diagnostic aid since it will often distinguish between the expansile growth of the benign lesion and the infiltrative growth pattern of the malignant tumor of the salivary gland. Aspiration biopsy may demonstrate tumor cells, although this method rarely provides enough representative tissue for a definitive microscopic diagnosis. Frozen sections should be prepared at the time of excision of major gland lesions, particularly if there is any possibility of malignancy.

Surgical excision, including a wide margin of adjacent normal gland (or the entire involved lobe or gland) is indicated for the treatment of pleomorphic adenoma. Recurrence rates for pleomorphic adenomas of the parotid gland have been quite high, but im-

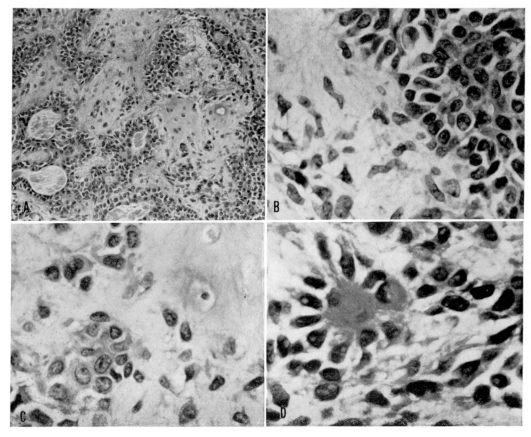

Fig. 13-2. Pleomorphic adenoma (mixed tumor). *A,* Low-power photomicrograph showing proliferating ductal epithelium intermixed with areas of chondroid stroma. *B,* Higher magnification showing sheet of epithelial cells adjacent to myxomatous supporting tissue. *C,* An area of chondroid stroma and collections of epithelial cells. *D,* Epithelial cells in collections and loose strands. (See also Fig. 1-18.)

proved surgical techniques and knowledge of the growth characteristics of this tumor are improving the cure rates and reducing the number of cases of postoperative facial nerve paralysis.

Oncocytoma (Oxyphilic Adenoma)

The oncocytoma is a rare tumor which occurs almost exclusively in the parotid gland. Generally seen in elderly patients, these tumors seldom exceed 3 to 5 cm in diameter and cannot be distinguished clinically from the pleomorphic adenoma (Fig. 13–3). They do not tend to recur following surgical removal.

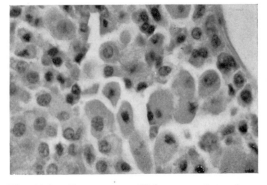

Fig. 13-3. Oncocytoma. High-power photomicrograph showing closely packed cells with an abundant eosinophilic cytoplasm. Oncocytes are commonly found lining parotid salivary ducts of elderly persons.

Sebaceous Adenoma

This extremely rare tumor, exclusive to the parotid gland, undoubtedly represents a choristoma rather than a true neoplasm since it is composed of heterotopic sebaceous glands within the salivary gland parenchyma. Surgical excision results in cure.

Papillary Cystadenoma Lymphomatosum (Warthin's Tumor)

This lesion is seen clinically as a firm to soft (or occasionally fluctuant) swelling of the parotid gland. Located in the peripheral portion of the gland just beneath the capsule, the tumor produces a distinct bulge in the overlying skin and rarely is larger than 3 cm in diameter. It exhibits a distinct predilection for men and occasionally occurs bilaterally. Its limited growth potential, occasional bilateral occurrence and distinctive histologic appearance are not typical of a true neoplasm (Fig. 13-4). It has been proposed that these tumors arise from salivary gland inclusions in cervical or parotid lymph nodes.

Benign Stromal Tumors

The supporting connective tissues of the salivary glands may give rise to benign tumors which may be mistaken clinically for parenchymal tumors because of their location. Examples of this variety include neurofibroma, neurilemmoma, lipoma and hemangioma.

Malignant Salivary Gland Neoplasms

Except for differences in incidence, the malignant tumors of the major salivary glands are identical to those of the accessory salivary glands.

Malignant Mixed Tumor (Malignant Pleomorphic Adenoma)

The term "malignant mixed tumor" implies malignant transformation in a previously benign pleomorphic adenoma. These lesions will be clinically similar to the benign variety except for additional features such as recent rapid enlargement, pain, facial nerve paralysis, fixation to underlying structures and/or poorly defined margins. Multiple sections throughout the specimen will show one or more foci of adenocarcinoma or squamous cell carcinoma. Surgical removal of the entire gland bearing the tumor, as well as associated palpable lymph nodes, is the treatment of choice.

Adenoid Cystic Carcinoma (Cylindroma, Basaloid Mixed Tumor)

The so-called cylindroma is a relatively slow-growing tumor which has a remarkable ability to infiltrate adjacent tissues by way of the perineural lymphatic vessels (Fig. 13–5). It involves the parotid and submaxillary glands with nearly equal frequency. Some studies indicate that the accessory glands, especially those on the palate, are more commonly involved than the major glands (Fig. 7–32). The tumor occurs most commonly in the fifth or sixth decades and is characterized by a mass which is usually painful and fixed. Wide surgical excision is mandatory. Even so, these tumors typically exhibit multiple recurrences and eventual widespread metastases.

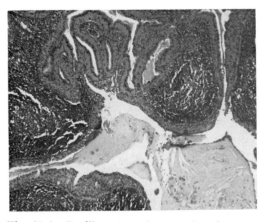

Fig. 13-4. Papillary cystadenoma lymphomatosum (Warthin's tumor). Photomicrograph showing multiple papillary projections with a double row of columnar cells lining a lumen. The lymphoid tissue contains germinal centers.

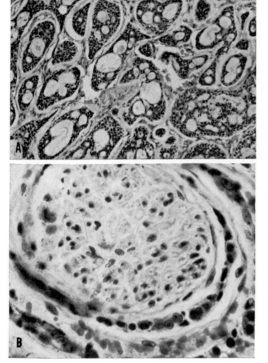

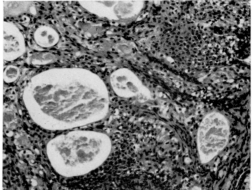

Fig. 13-6. Mucoepidermoid carcinoma. Low-power photomicrograph showing squamous epithelium, pale-staining mucus-producing cells and smaller intermediate cells. Large duct-like structures distended with mucus are present.

Fig. 13-5. Adenoid cystic carcinoma (cylindroma). *A*, Low-power photomicrograph showing the "Swiss-cheese" pattern and duct-like structures of this neoplasm. These epithelial cells resemble basal cells in their morphology and staining properties. *B*, High-power photomicrograph showing the perineural invasion characteristic of the tumor.

Mucoepidermoid Carcinoma

In 1945, Stewart, Foote and Becker described an entity composed of varying proportions of squamous, mucus-producing, and intermediate cell types (Fig. 13–6). On the basis of the clinical and histologic features, these tumors were divided into benign (mucoepidermoid tumor) and malignant (mucoepidermoid carcinoma) types. While these lesions vary considerably in their aggressiveness and tendency to metastasize, many pathologists feel that they should all be considered malignant and subclassified into low-grade, intermediate or high-grade types.

In direct contrast to the low-grade type, the high-grade type may exhibit early pain or paralysis; it grows rapidly, becomes fixed to adjacent structures, and metastasizes to regional lymph nodes or distant sites. Treatment is by surgical excision.

Adenosquamous Carcinoma

This aggressive and highly malignant tumor appears clinically as a small nodule or ulcer, generally less than 1 cm in diameter. Cases have been reported in the floor of the mouth, tongue, palate and lip, and in the nasal cavity and larynx. Histologically, the growth shows squamous carcinoma of the surface epithelium plus carcinoma in situ of underlying duct epithelium with transition into adenocarcinoma. Thus, the tumor appears to be a composite of squamous carcinoma and adenocarcinoma. Metastasis occurs early and the cure rate is extremely poor. Treatment is by radical surgical excision.

Acinic Cell Adenocarcinoma

Generally of low-grade malignancy, the acinic cell adenocarcinoma may simulate the pleomorphic adenoma clinically (Fig. 13–7). Most arise in the parotid gland although a few cases have been reported in other sites. Wide surgical excision is indicated.

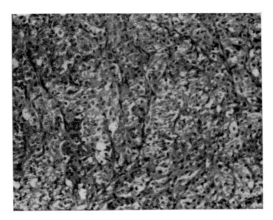

Fig. 13-7. Acinic cell adenocarcinoma. Neoplastic proliferation of the acinar elements of the gland is shown.

Adenocarcinoma, Miscellaneous

These salivary gland tumors, represented by several ill-defined histologic patterns (adamantine, canalicular, etc.), are usually of high-grade malignancy and metastasize widely.

Epidermoid Carcinoma

This highly aggressive, malignant tumor of the salivary gland is presumed to be of ductal origin. It appears to represent a separate entity and should be differentiated from the malignant pleomorphic adenoma and high-grade mucoepidermoid carcinomas, both of which may contain large areas of squamous cells. Combined radical surgery and irradiation is the treatment of choice.

Malignant Stromal Tumors

The malignant stromal tumors arising in salivary glands usually cannot be differentiated clinically from tumors arising from the gland parenchyma. Examples of malignant stromal salivary gland tumors include malignant melanoma, rhabdomyosarcoma, malignant lymphoma and hemangiosarcoma. Invasion of the gland by direct extension of malignant tumors arising in adjacent structures may occur, and a few cases of tumors metastatic to the salivary glands have been described.

DIFFUSE ENLARGEMENTS (SINGLE GLANDS)

In contrast to the circumscribed masses which characterize salivary gland neoplasms, a number of conditions may exhibit diffuse enlargement, involving one or more lobules of a gland or the entire gland. Among the diffuse enlargements of this nature are sialadenitis, sialolithiasis, ranula and retrograde infections.

Sialadenitis

In general, partial blockage of the excretory duct to a major or minor salivary gland results in loss of acini, ductal ectasia and a moderate to severe lymphocytic infiltration (Fig. 13–12). Such changes are characteristically seen in chronic *sclerosing sialadenitis,* mucocele (p. 404), and sialolithiasis.

When the blood supply to the gland is compromised, the resulting ulceration, necrosis (infarction) and squamous metaplasia of residual ducts (termed *necrotizing sialometaplasia,* p. 399) may be mistaken both clinically and microscopically for epidermoid carcinoma or mucoepidermoid carcinoma.

Complete or total blockage of the excretory duct to a gland results in eventual atrophy of the gland.

Both specific and non-specific infectious processes may result in sialadenitis. Inflammation and transient swelling of the salivary glands may also occur secondarily to therapeutic radiation of the gland.

Sialolithiasis

Salivary duct stones, or sialoliths, occur most commonly in the major gland ducts but they are occasionally recognized by histologic examination in the accessory gland ducts as well. The submaxillary gland is involved about twice as frequently as the parotid. The stone, which forms about a nidus of bacterial or desquamated epithelial cells, serves to partially block salivary flow. In the case of a sialolith in a major gland duct (Figs. 13–8 to 13–11), interference with the flow of saliva causes periodic swelling

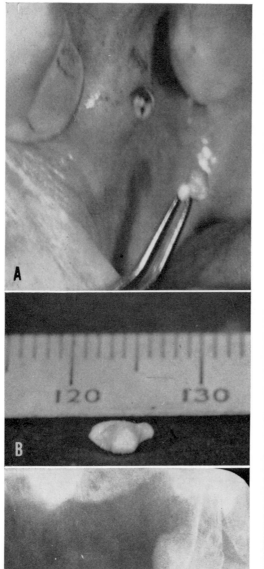

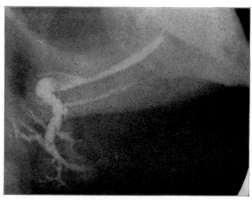

Fig. 13-9. Sialolith. Sialogram of the submaxillary gland showing ductal dilatation proximal to a faintly opaque sialolith in Wharton's duct. The acinar filling is suggestive of sialodochitis.

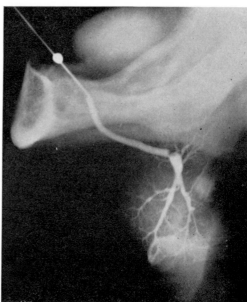

Fig. 13-10. Sialolith. Sialogram showing ductal dilatation proximal to a radiolucent stone in Wharton's duct. (Courtesy of George Blozis.) (See also Figs. 2-27, 6-3A, 8-29.)

Fig. 13-8. Sialoliths of Stensen's duct. *A,* A sialolith has been removed and another protrudes from the orifice. *B,* The sialolith shown in (*A*) above. *C,* Periapical radiograph showing 2 small sialoliths near the lower edge of the radiograph and other semi-opaque stones superimposed over the maxillary sinus and coronoid process.

of the proximal portion of the duct and gland, usually most severe at mealtimes. On occasion, stones near the terminal portion of the duct may be palpated manually or probed by inserting a lacrimal probe through the duct orifice (Fig. 6–3). In some cases, they may be "milked" out of the duct (Fig. 13–8*A*). Sialoliths may also be demonstrated on routine radiographs (Figs. 2–27*A*, 13–8*B*) or by sialography (Figs. 13–9 to 13–11). In some cases, however, sialoliths will be radiolucent and thus not visualized on the radiograph. Sialography will frequently confirm the presence of the stone.

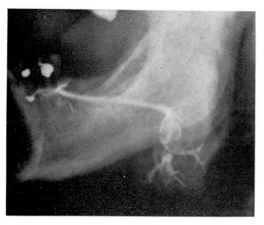

Fig. 13-11. Sialolith. Sialogram of sialolith in Wharton's duct. (Courtesy of George Blozis.)

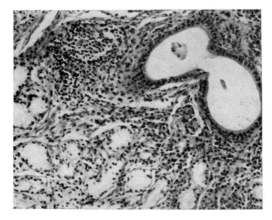

Fig. 13-12. Sialadenitis. Photomicrograph showing a chronic inflammatory cell infiltrate with ductal dilatation and breakdown of acini.

Ranula

The ranula or mucous retention cyst typically occurs in the floor of the mouth because of blockage of the submaxillary gland duct (Fig. 7–26). There is marked dilatation of the duct which is seen clinically as a rounded swelling on either side of the midline in the anterior portion of the floor of the mouth. Because of the marked distention of the overlying mucosa, the mucous membrane looks pale to bluish. In some instances mucus may have escaped from the injured duct into the surrounding connective tissue in the same manner as is seen in the ordinary mucocele of accessory glands (p. 404). Treatment of the ranula may be either marsupialization or excision of the entire fluid-filled mass. To avoid collapse of the mass upon incision, some dentists inject the ranula with alginate impression material prior to operation.

Retrograde Infection

Secondary or retrograde infections of the salivary glands result from extension of microorganisms up the major excretory duct. Since this condition usually follows reduced salivary gland function, most cases are bilateral. Extension of infection into the substance of the salivary gland from contiguous structures may occur in various forms of cellulitis. This condition occurs most frequently in the submaxillary gland space and in the space of the parotid gland.

DIFFUSE ENLARGEMENTS (MULTIPLE GLANDS)

Diffuse enlargements involving the salivary glands represent both local and systemic disease processes. Diffuse enlargements of multiple salivary glands of chief concern to the dentist include epidemic parotitis, enlargement secondary to drug therapy and metabolic disease processes, and the so-called benign lymphoepithelial lesions.

Epidemic Parotitis (Mumps)

This common childhood disease is seen clinically as a diffuse, tender swelling of the salivary glands, chiefly the parotid and submaxillary glands. The patient exhibits pain on salivation and will generally give a history of previous exposure to a person with the disease. In some instances, unilateral involvement may suggest a simple sialadenitis or ranula secondary to a salivary stone. However, the history of the 2- or 3-week incubation period and sudden onset with symptoms of fever and malaise is usually sufficient to make the diagnosis.

The diagnosis of mumps may be difficult when only the submaxillary or sublingual glands are affected. In such cases, complement-fixation tests which have been devised will usually show an elevation in antibody titer and the serum amylase will be elevated. For the complement-fixation test, two samples of blood should be obtained, one at the beginning when the disease is first suspected and another after 10 or more days.

"Chemical Mumps"

Diffuse salivary gland enlargement may occasionally follow the administration of therapeutic iodine and is referred to as "iodine mumps."

Surgical Mumps

This unusual enlargement of the salivary glands usually involves the parotid gland and may be unilateral or bilateral. In general, the condition occurs subsequent to surgery requiring a general anesthetic. Thus, it may be associated with a period of xerostomia, dehydration, and/or local trauma to the major glands. These combined factors may permit retrograde invasion of the salivary gland by bacteria from the mouth. There is acute swelling and tenderness of the gland, often with erythema and edema of the overlying skin, and purulent material can be expressed from Stensen's duct.

Uveoparotid Fever (Uveoparotitis, Heerfordt's Syndrome)

Uveoparotitis is characterized by painless, bilateral parotid enlargement, inflammation of the uveal tract of the eyes, low-grade fever and, often, cranial nerve involvement. On occasion, the submaxillary, sublingual and lacrimal glands are also enlarged; this, together with the associated xerostomia, may simulate Mikulicz's disease or Sjögren's syndrome. The cranial nerve involvement is most commonly a seventh nerve paralysis (Bell's palsy, p. 262), although other neuropathies such as trigeminal paresthesia, soft palate paralysis or ptosis may be present.

Salivary gland biopsy reveals non-caseating granulomas (tubercles) with epithelioid cells and multinucleated giant cells replacing much of the gland parenchyma. Since acid-fast microorganisms are not present, the histologic features resemble those seen in sarcoidosis (p. 338).

There is no definitive treatment for uveoparotitis although the steroids are often helpful in the early acute stages. Because of the visual impairment which follows the uveitis, management of the eye lesions should be undertaken by an ophthalmologist. The disease runs a protracted course over several months or even years, and subsides often with some residual gland enlargement and vision defects.

Benign Lymphoepithelial Lesions

This disease is characterized by multiple diffuse enlargements of the salivary glands as well as other associated glands such as the lacrimal gland and pharyngeal mucous glands (Fig. 13–13). For the most part the disease occurs in middle-aged or older adults, usually females, and is characterized by a diffuse enlargement of these glands, along with marked xerostomia. Although they very probably may represent the same basic pathologic process, *Mikulicz's disease* and *Sjögren's syndrome* are commonly used to designate two different forms of benign lympho-

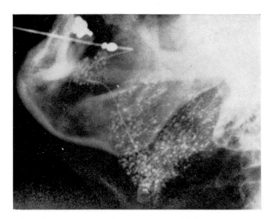

Fig. 13-13. Sjögren's syndrome. Sialogram showing abnormal filling defects diffusely distributed throughout both the submaxillary and sublingual glands. (Courtesy of George Blozis.)

epithelial lesions. In Mikulicz's disease bilateral enlargement of salivary glands and marked xerostomia occur. In Sjögren's syndrome, involvement of the salivary, lacrimal and pharyngeal glands and associated rheumatoid arthritis are seen. Both conditions are characterized by marked xerostomia (sicca syndrome) and, if other glands are involved, dryness of the eyes and throat as well. In some instances, the major glands may exhibit eventual scarring and atrophy. Both surgery and radiation treatment have been used. Recent evidence indicates that Sjögren's syndrome represents an autoimmune disease such as Hashimoto's thyroiditis and disseminated lupus erythematosus (p. 330).

Mucoviscidosis (Cystic Fibrosis of the Pancreas)

Diffuse salivary gland enlargement may be seen in cystic fibrosis of the pancreas, a hereditary disease which involves duct structures of the pancreas primarily as well as other glands in the body. In recent years, clinical studies have established that the diagnosis of cystic fibrosis may be confirmed by salivary analyses (p. 208) and by biopsy of the salivary glands, particularly the accessory glands of the lip. This disease is char-

acterized by the formation of mucinous plugs within the duct of the salivary glands as well as those of the pancreas.

DISTURBANCES IN SALIVARY GLAND FUNCTION

Functional disturbances involving the major and minor salivary glands are reflected by changes in the physical properties (volume, viscosity, pH) and/or composition (proteins, enzymes, electrolytes, water) of the saliva (pp. 208–209). Since the control of salivary secretion is through the autonomic nervous system, transient alterations in flow and composition commonly occur reflexly under conditions of stress (fear), oral stimulation (*e.g.* manipulation of oral tissues, new prosthetic appliances), or dehydration associated with fever, pain stimuli, etc. However, functional disturbances of prolonged duration, particularly reduced salivary volume, often have profound effects on the health of the mucous membranes and teeth and may cause aberrations in taste, deglutition and phonation. Since such signs and symptoms may reflect some other basic underlying disease process, complaints of altered salivary function should be investigated thoroughly (p. 208). The changes in physical properties and composition of saliva which have been associated with a variety of systemic and metabolic conditions are discussed in the section Examination of the Saliva (pp. 208–209). Xerostomia and sialorrhea are discussed in the following sections.

Xerostomia

Dry mouth, or xerostomia, represents a symptom complex of salivary gland dysfunction which may be of developmental, degenerative, inflammatory, metabolic, neurologic, iatrogenic or idiopathic origin. In transient xerostomia, the patient complains of "dry mouth" but there are few overt clinical signs since some salivary function is generally present. However, prolonged xerostomia typically results in a dry, red and shiny mucosal surface, loss of papillae on the tongue and fissuring and cracking of the lips. The patient may complain of painful or burning mucous membrane, especially of the tongue. Denture wearers may have difficulties with retention of their appliances. Since taste sensation requires solvent action of saliva on the food, decreased taste acuity (hypogeusia) or perverted taste (hyposmia) may be the patient's primary concern, along with speech and swallowing difficulties. Increased caries activity, especially root caries, is a common sequela of xerostomia (Figs. 1–4, 2–2 and 2–3).

In evaluating a patient's complaint of dry mouth, the examiner should attempt to establish the time of onset, duration and severity of the xerostomia as well as current and past medications, associated major salivary gland enlargement (or atrophy), co-existing systemic diseases or conditions and the patient's emotional status. The amount of salivary flow should be evaluated by observation of the major salivary gland duct openings. Their patency can be established by the use of a lacrimal probe (p. 115). Accessory salivary gland function can be easily assessed by drying the palate and observing salivary flow from the duct orifices for a few moments. Specific sialogogues (nicotinic acid, pilocarpine) can be administered as a diagnostic measure.

Conditions Sometimes Associated with Transient or Prolonged Xerostomia

Psychogenic factors
  Fear
  Stress
Age changes, senility
Fever, dehydration
Neurologic disturbances
  Psychoses
  Anxiety states
  Manic depressive states
Developmental disturbances
  Salivary gland aplasia
  Salivary gland duct atresia
  Sialolithiasis
Sialadenitis (p. 355)
  Mumps (epidemic parotitis) (p. 358)

Sarcoidosis (uveoparotid fever, Heerfordt's syndrome) (p. 358)
  Non-specific sialadenitis
Metabolic conditions
  Megaloblastic anemia (p. 408)
  Iron deficiency anemia (p. 408)
  Diabetes mellitus (p. 247)
  Diabetes insipidus (p. 253)
  Pregnancy
  Vitamin A deficiency
Autoimmune diseases
  Sicca syndrome (Sjögren's syndrome, Mikulicz's disease, p. 358)
  Felty's syndrome (rheumatoid arthritis, splenic neutropenia, anemia and keratoconjunctivitis sicca)
  Waldenstrom's macroglobulinemia (p. 225)
  Lupus erythematosus (p. 329)
Drug-induced xerostomia (pp. 14, 361)
  Atropine
  Antihistamines
  Tranquilizers
  Amphetamines
Radiation-induced xerostomia

Age Change and Senility

Some reduction of salivary secretion occurs as a natural sequence with age change in most patients. Because of the importance of saliva in the retention of dentures, even a moderate reduction in salivary flow is apt to be noted by the full denture wearer. In these cases, careful examination will generally demonstrate some degree of salivary gland function, although it may be less than optimum. Lozenges or other agents may be recommended to increase physiologic stimulation of the glands or, in severe cases, sialogogues (*e.g.* pilocarpine) may be prescribed with caution.

Salivary Gland Aplasia, Ductal Atresia

Agenesis or aplasia of the salivary glands is a rare condition in which the major and minor salivary glands fail to develop (Fig. 1–4). In most instances, other ectodermal structures such as teeth and hair may be defective or missing. The lack of saliva with its detergent and antibacterial action results in the rampant caries characteristic of this condition.

Radiation-Induced Xerostomia

Therapeutic doses of x-ray irradiation to the major salivary glands result in virtual elimination of the salivary gland function. In general, patients receiving sufficient doses of x ray to the parotid gland and the side of the face will subsequently develop "radiation caries" on the side of the mouth receiving the treatment. While other factors may be partly responsible for this effect, it is generally believed that salivary dysfunction is the main factor in the development of carious lesions in these individuals. For the most part, the lesions occur along the cervical areas of the teeth. Because of the possible complications (osteoradionecrosis, Fig. 15–23) following tooth extraction in individuals who have had heavy x-ray irradiation, it is essential that teeth be kept in repair.

Sialadenitis

Inflammation of the interstitial tissues of salivary glands (sialadenitis) generally results in reduced secretion and discomfort (p. 355, Fig. 13–12). Unless there is diffuse involvement of all of the salivary glands with severe inflammation, this is generally not of sufficient magnitude to be a problem.

Drug-Induced Xerostomia

Commonly used drugs such as the tranquilizers and antihistamines may cause xerostomia according to dosage and individual drug response (Fig. 2–3). Since the patient may not consider such routine use of drugs significant, this information may not be reported except under direct questioning (p. 90).

Fever and Dehydration

Loss of body fluids secondary to fever, vomiting, hemorrhage, diarrhea or other causes results in an attempted compensatory reduction of salivary flow. Thirst increases because of the altered water balance and the desire to relieve the dry mouth.

Autoimmune Diseases

The xerostomias (sicca syndrome) of Mikulicz's disease and Sjögren's syndrome (benign lymphoepithelial lesion) are described on page 358. Replacement of gland parenchyma with lymphocytes accounts for the reduced flow. The mechanism of reduced flow in the other autoimmune diseases is less obvious.

Metabolic Conditions

Both diabetes mellitus and diabetes insipidus are characterized by polyuria and polydipsia (increased thirst). The associated xerostomia probably represents a compensatory mechanism comparable to that seen in dehydration.

Vitamin A Deficiency

Severe deficiency of vitamin A in experimental animals is known to induce squamous metaplasia in salivary gland duct epithelium and other specialized epithelium. While these changes have not been clearly established in man, it is presumed that comparable functional changes occur.

Sialorrhea

Increased salivary volume, or sialorrhea, is seen most commonly in dental practice as a result of simple manipulation of the oral tissues or during the course of minor operative procedures. For example, marked sialorrhea in infants and young children is almost invariably encountered during oral examination. Reflex stimulation of salivary flow may be quite marked but transitory in the patient wearing dentures for the first time.

Sialorrhea of a prolonged nature may arise from a variety of causes, both local and systemic. The patient usually complains of the need to swallow the excess saliva at frequent intervals and there may be constant drooling of saliva from the mouth, with resultant maceration at the commissures (angular cheilitis).

Conditions Sometimes Associated with Transient or Prolonged Sialorrhea

Psychogenic factors
  Sight of food
  Nasal stimuli
  Nausea
  Sexual stimuli, etc.
Oral stimulation
  Manipulation of oral tissues
  Taste stimuli
  Pain, etc.
Oral inflammation
  Aphthous stomatitis (p. 401)
  "Teething"
  Erythema multiforme (p. 387)
  Foot-and-mouth disease (p. 387)
Neurologic disturbances
  Epilepsy
  Cerebral palsy
  Parkinson's disease
  Mental retardation
  Rabies
Psychiatric disturbances
  Schizophrenia
Mercury exposure
  Hg toxicity
  Hg sensitivity
  Acrodynia
Familial dysautonomia (Riley-Day syndrome)
Periodic sialorrhea
Esophageal and gastric disturbances
  Salivary reflex, water brash
  Esophageal spasm, ulcer, carcinoma
  Gastric ulcer, gastritis
  Pancreatitis
Pregnancy (variable)
Certain atypical neuralgias
  Sphenopalatine neuralgia (p. 293)
Drug therapy
  Sympathomimetic drugs (p. 208)
    Epinephrine
    Norepinephrine
  Parasympathomimetic drugs (p. 208)
    Acetylcholine
    Methacholine
    Pilocarpine

As noted in the previous section, the control of salivary secretion is under autonomic nervous system control and thus is responsive to various neurologic, psychogenic and metabolic stimuli as well as vegetative needs. With stimulation of the parasympathetic system, there is an increased volume of rather watery saliva, whereas sympathetic stimulation causes increased organic content but less volume increase. Reflex stimulation of salivary flow through psychogenic, touch, taste, hunger or pain stimuli is a normal physiologic response; however, abnormal reflex stimulation of salivary flow is seen in a number of conditions involving the gastrointestinal tract, *e.g.*, esophageal spasm, ulcer or carcinoma as well as gastric ulcer and pancreatitis, and may induce sialorrhea via the esophageal-salivary reflex.

Water brash, the reflex gushing of saliva which has accumulated above the cardiac sphincter in cardiospasm, may be associated with such cases.

Acrodynia (Pink Disease, Swift's Disease)

This condition is of special interest to the dentist because of the associated premature exfoliation of the deciduous teeth. Seen chiefly in the young infant as a result of mercury toxicity or idiosyncrasy to mercury preparations such as teething lotions, mercury ointment or bichloride of mercury disinfectant, the disease is characterized by pruritic erythema of the skin, stomatitis, increased sweating, sialorrhea, tachycardia, hypertension, exfoliation of the teeth and hair and other signs of generalized systemic involvement.

Familial Dysautonomia (Riley-Day Syndrome, Familial Autonomic Dysfunction)

This congenital disorder of the autonomic nervous system is characterized by postural hypotension, stress hypertension, indifference to pain, defective speech, emotional problems, hyperhidrosis, lack of tears and sialorrhea. The condition occurs chiefly in Jewish children as an autosomal recessive trait. Most affected individuals do not survive to adulthood.

Periodic Sialorrhea

This rare autosomal dominant trait is characterized by salivary gland enlargement and associated sialorrhea which recurs at regular intervals, usually weekly or monthly. Seen chiefly in women, the condition represents one of the "periodic diseases" and frequently occurs in conjunction with periodic abdominalgia or cyclic neutropenia.

BIBLIOGRAPHY

General

Beahrs, O. H. and Woolner, L. B.: Surgical treatment of diseases of salivary gland, J. Oral Surg., 27, 119, 1969.

Dhawan, I. K., Bhargava, S., Nayak, N. C. and Gupta, R. K.: Central salivary gland tumors of jaws, Cancer, 26, 211, 1970.

Evans, R. W. and Cruickshank, A. H.: Epithelial Tumors of the Salivary Glands (Vol. 1 in Major Problems in Pathology, Bennington, J. L., Consulting Ed.), Philadelphia, W. B. Saunders Co., 1970.

Eversole, L. R.: Histogenic classification of salivary tumors, Arch. Path., 92, 433, 1971.

Foote, F. W. Jr. and Frazell, E. L.: Tumors of the major salivary glands, Cancer, 6, 1065, 1953.

Hall, H. D.: Diagnosis of diseases of the salivary glands, J. Oral Surg., 27, 15, 1969.

Hamperl, H.: Benign and malignant oncocytoma, Cancer, 15, 1019, 1962.

Krolls, S. O., Trodahl, J. N. and Boyers, R. C.: Salivary gland lesions in children. A survey of 340 cases, Cancer, 30, 459, 1972.

Krugman, S. and Ward, R.: Infectious Diseases of Children, St. Louis, The C. V. Mosby Co., 1960, p. 194.

Ollerenshaw, R. and Rose, S.: Siaolgraphy, a valuable diagnostic method, Dent. Radiogr. Photogr., 29, 37, 1956.

Shafer, W. G., Hine, M. K. and Levy, B. M.: A Textbook of Oral Pathology, 2nd Ed., Philadelphia, W. B. Saunders Co., 1963.

Spiro, R. H., Koss, L. G., Hajdu, S. I. and Strong, E. W.: Tumors of minor salivary gland origin, A clinicopathologic study of 492 cases, Cancer, 31, 117, 1973.

Vellios, F. and Davidson, D.: The natural history of tumors peculiar to the salivary glands, Amer. J. Clin. Path., 25, 147, 1955.

Whinery, J. G.: Inflammatory salivary gland disease, J. Oral Surg., 22, 488, 1964.

Salivary Gland Enlargements

Albright, E. C., Larson, F. C. and Deiss, W. P.: Hypertrophy of salivary glands during treatment of myxedema with triiodothyronine, J. Lab. Clin. Med., 44, 762, 1954.

Barbero, G. J. and Sibinga, M. S.: Enlargement of the submaxillary salivary glands in cystic fibrosis, Pediatrics, 29, 788, 1962.

Bernier, J. L. and Bhaskar, S. N.: Lymphoepithelial lesions of salivary glands, histogenesis and classification based on 186 cases, Cancer, 11, 1156, 1958.

Biggam, A. G. and Ghalioungui, P.: Ancylostoma anemia and its treatment by iron, Lancet, 2, 299, 1934.

Bonnin, H., Moretti, G. and Geyer, A.: Le grosses parotides des cirrhoses alcooliques, Presse Med., 62, 1419, 1954.

Borsanyi, S. and Blanchard, C. L.: Asymptomatic enlargement of the parotid glands, J.A.M.A., 174, 20, 1960.

Brodkin, R. H. et al.: Generalized cytomegalic inclusion disease, Arch. Derm., 84, 650, 1961.

Carter, J. E.: Iodide "mumps," New Eng. J. Med., 274, 987, 1961.

Daniels, T. E., Silverman, S. Jr., Michalski, J. P., Greenspan, J. S., Sylvester, R. A. and Talel, N.: The oral component of Sjögren's syndrome, Oral Surg., 39, 875, 1975.

Davies, J. N. P.: Essential pathology of kwashiorkor, Lancet, 1, 317, 1948.

Dobreff, M.: Compensatory hypertrophy of the parotid gland in presence of hypofunction of pancreatic islands, Deutsch. Med. Wschr., 62, 67, 1936.

Dunlap, C. L. and Barker, B. F.: Necrotizing sialometaplasia. Report of five additional cases, Oral Surg., 37, 722, 1974.

Epker, B. N.: Obstructive and inflammatory diseases of the major salivary glands, Oral Surg., 33, 2, 1972.

Font, R. L., Yanoff, M. and Zimmerman, L. E.: Benign lymphoepithelial lesion of the lacrimal gland and its relationship to Sjögren's syndrome, Amer. J. Clin. Path., 48, 365, 1967.

Gillman, J., Gilbert, C. and Gillman, T.: The Bantu salivary gland in chronic malnutrition, with a brief consideration of the parenchyma-interstitial tissue relationship, S. Afr. J. Med. Sci., 12, 99, 1947.

Gilman, R. A., Schwartz, M. and Gilman, J. S.: Fatty infiltration of the parotid gland, J.A.M.A., 160, 48, 1956.

Goldberg, M. H. and Harrigan, W. F.: Acute suppurative parotitis, Oral Surg., 20, 281, 1965.

Jansen, H. H.: Parotisverunderungen bei Labercirrhose, Verh. Deutsch. Ges. Path., 42, 252, 1959.

Kaltreider, H. B.: Bilateral parotid gland enlargement and hyperlipoproteinemia, J.A.M.A., 210, 2067, 1969.

Langlais, R. P. and Kasle, M. J.: Sialolithiasis: the radiolucent ones, Oral Surg., 40, 686, 1975.

Leban, S. G. and Stratigos, G. T.: Benign lymphoepithelial sialadenopathies. The Mikulicz/Sjögren controversy, Oral Surg., 38, 735, 1974.

Mandel, L. and Baurmash, H.: Parotid enlargement due to alcoholism, J. Amer. Dent. Ass., 82, 369, 1971.

Phillips, L. G.: Parotid swelling associated with lactation: with report of a case, Amer. J. Obstet. Gynec., *22,* 434, 1935.

Racine, W.: Le syndrome salivaire pre-menstrual, Schweiz. Med. Wschr., *69,* 1204, 1939.

Sandstead, H. R., Koehn, C. J. and Session, S. M.: Enlargement of the parotid gland in malnutrition, Amer. J. Clin. Nutr., *3,* 198, 1955.

Schwartz, A. W., Devine, K. D. and Beahrs, O. H.: Acute postoperative mumps ("surgical mumps"), Plast. Reconstr. Surg., *35,* 51, 1960.

Sprinzels, H.: Parotisvergrosserung bei Fettleibigen, Wein Klin. Wschr., *25,* 1901, 1912.

Standish, S. M. and Shafer, W. G.: The mucous retention phenomenon, J. Oral Surg., *16,* 15, 1959.

Thompson, W. C.: Uveoparotitis, Arch. Intern. Med., *59,* 646, 1937.

Tarpley, T. M. Jr., Anderson, L. G. and White, C. L.: Minor salivary gland involvement in Sjögren's syndrome, Oral Surg., *37,* 64, 1974.

Wolfe, S. J., Summerskill, W. H. and Davidson, C. S.: Parotid swelling, alcoholism and cirrhosis, New Eng. J. Med., *256,* 491, 1957.

Wong, T. and Warner, N. E.: Cytomegalic inclusion disease in adults, Arch. Path., *74,* 403, 1962.

Benign Salivary Gland Neoplasms

Christ, T. F. and Crocker, D.: Basal cell adenoma of minor salivary gland origin, Cancer, *30,* 214, 1972.

Eneroth, C.-M. and Zajicek, J.: Aspiration biopsy of salivary gland tumors. III. Morphologic studies on smears and histologic sections from 368 mixed tumors, Acta Cytol., *10,* 440, 1966.

Goldman, R. L. and Klein, H. L.: Glycogen-rich adenoma of the parotid gland. An uncommon benign clear-cell tumor resembling certain clear-cell carcinomas of salivary origin, Cancer, *30,* 749, 1972.

Krolls, S. O. and Boyers, R. C.: Mixed tumors of salivary glands. Long-term follow-up, Cancer, *30,* 276, 1972.

Lathrop, F. D.: Benign tumors of the parotid gland: A twenty-five year review, Laryngoscope, *72,* 992, 1962.

Matteson, S. R., Cutler, L. S. and Herman, P. A.: Warthin's tumor. Report of a case and survey of 205 salivary gland neoplasms, Oral Surg., *41,* 129, 1976.

Miller, A. S. and McCrea, M. W.: Sebaceous gland adenoma of the buccal mucosa: report of a case, J. Oral Surg., *26,* 593, 1968.

Min, B. H., Miller, A. S., Leifer, C. and Putong, P. B.: Basal cell adenoma of the parotid gland, Arch. Otolaryngol., *99,* 38, 1974.

Saksela, E., Tarkkanen, J. and Wartiovaara, J.: Parotid clear cell adenoma of possible myoepithelial origin, Cancer, *30,* 742, 1972.

Malignant Salivary Gland Neoplasms

Abrams, A. M., Cornyn, J., Scofield, H. H. and Hansen, L. S.: Acinic cell adenocarcinoma of the major salivary glands, a clinicopathologic study of 77 cases, Cancer, *18,* 1145, 1965.

Bhaskar, S. N. and Bernier, J. L.: Mucoepidermoid tumors of major and minor salivary glands, clinical features, histology, variations, natural history and results of treatment for 144 cases, Cancer, *15,* 801, 1962.

Eby, L. S., Johnson, D. S. and Baker, H. W.: Adenoid cystic carcinoma of the head and neck, Cancer, *29,* 1160, 1972.

Gadient, S. E. and Kalfayan, B.: Mucoepidermoid carcinoma arising within a Warthin's tumor, Oral Surg., *40,* 391, 1975.

Gerughty, R. M., Hennigar, G. R. and Brown, F. M.: Adenosquamous carcinoma of the nasal, oral and laryngeal cavities. A clinicopathologic survey of ten cases, Cancer, *22,* 1140, 1968.

Gerughty, R. M., Scofield, H. H., Brown, F. M. and Hennigar, G. R.: Malignant mixed tumors of salivary gland origin, Cancer, *24,* 471, 1969.

Gravanis, M. B. and Giansanti, J. S.: Malignant histopathologic counterpart of the benign lymphoepithelial lesion, Cancer, *26,* 1332, 1970.

Greene, G. W. Jr. and Bernier, J. L.: Primary malignant melanomas of the parotid gland, Oral Surg., *14,* 108, 1961.

Hyman, G. A. and Wolff, M.: Malignant lymphomas of the salivary glands. Review of the literature and report of 33 new cases, including four cases associated with the lymphoepithelial lesion, Amer. J. Clin. Path., *65,* 421, 1976.

Melrose, R. J., Abrams, A. M. and Howell, F. V.: Mucoepidermoid tumors of the intraoral minor salivary glands: A clinicopathologic study of 54 cases, J. Oral Path., *2,* 314, 1973.

Moran, J. J., Becker, S. M., Brady, L. W. and Rambo, B. V.: Adenoid cystic carcinoma, Cancer, *14,* 1235, 1961.

Smith, L. C., Lane, N. and Rankow, R. M.: Cylindroma (adenoid cystic carcinoma). A report of fifty-eight cases, Amer. J. Surg., *110,* 519, 1965.

Stewart, F. S., Foote, F. W. Jr. and Becker, W. F.: Muco-epidermoid tumors of salivary glands, Ann. Surg., *122,* 820, 1945.

Tarpley, T. M. Jr. and Giansanti, J. S.: Adenoid cystic carcinoma. Analysis of fifty oral cases, Oral Surg., *41,* 484, 1976.

Disturbances in Salivary Gland Function

Afonsky, D.: *Saliva and its Relation to Oral Health: A Survey of the Literature,* Birmingham, University of Alabama Press, 1961, pp. 296–297.

Bahn, S. L.: Drug-related dental destruction, Oral Surg., *33*, 49, 1972.

Bertram, U.: Xerostomia—clinical aspects, pathology and pathogenesis, Acta Odont. Scand., *25*, 126, 1967.

Brown, L. R., Dreizen, S., Rider, L. J. and Johnston, D. A.: The effect of radiation-induced xerostomia on saliva and serum lysozyme and immunoglobin levels, Oral Surg., *41*, 83, 1976.

Conner, S., Iranpour, B. and Mills, J.: Alteration in parotid salivary flow in diabetes mellitus, Oral Surg., *30*, 55, 1970.

Greenspan, J. S., Daniels, T. E., Talal, N. and Sylvester, R. A.: The histopathology of Sjögren's syndrome in labial salivary gland biopsies, Oral Surg., *37*, 217, 1974.

Kashima, H., Kirkham, W. R. and Andrews, R. J.: Postirradiation sialadenitis: A study of the clinical features, histopathologic changes and serum enzyme variations following irradiation of human salivary glands, Amer. J. Roentgen., *94*, 271, 1965.

Kley, W.: Munch. Med. Wschr., *101*, 997, 1959 (or Seifert, G.: Pathologie und atiologie der speicheldrusenschwellunger, Deutsch. Zahnarztebl., *14*, 784, 1960).

Schall, G. L., Anderson, L. G., Wolf, R. O., Herdt, J. R., Tarpley, T. M. Jr., Cummings, N. A., Zeiger, L. S. and Talal, N.: Xerostomia in Sjögren's syndrome. Evaluation by sequential salivary scintography, J.A.M.A., *216*, 2109, 1971.

Standish, S. M. and Shafer, W. G.: Serial histologic effects of rat submaxillary and sublingual gland duct and blood vessel ligation, J. Dent. Res., *36*, 866, 1957.

Westcott, W. B., Starcke, E. N. and Shannon, I. L.: Chemical protection against postirradiation dental caries, Oral Surg., *40*, 709, 1975.

Chapter 14

Diseases of the Intraoral Soft Tissues

Syphilitic Ulcer
Vincent's Ulcer
Aphthous Ulcer
Periadenitis Mucosa Necrotica Recurrens
Other Infectious Ulcers
Midline Lethal Granuloma
Noma
Cysts and Cyst-like Lesions
Palatal Cyst of the Newborn
Dental Lamina Cyst of the Newborn
Gingival Cyst of the Adult
Cyst of the Incisive Papilla
Nasolabial Cyst
Dermoid Cyst
Oral Lymphoepithelial Cyst
Heterotopic Oral Gastrointestinal Cyst
Extraosseous Calcifying Epithelial Odontogenic Cyst
Mucocele
Ranula
Antral Mucocele
Epithelial Inclusion Cyst
Hemorrhagic and Vascular Lesions
General Features
Oral Manifestations
Red Blood Cell Disorders
Polycythemia
Anemia
White Blood Cell Disorders
Agranulocytosis
Cyclic Neutropenia
Leukemia
Infectious Mononucleosis
Differentiation of Platelet, Coagulation and Vascular
Integrity Disorders
Platelet Disorders
Thrombocytopenia
Thrombocythemia
Thrombocytopathia
Thrombocytasthenia
Disorders of Vascular Integrity
Hereditary Hemorrhagic Telangiectasia
Vitamin C Deficiency
Other Vascular Integrity Disorders
Hereditary Coagulation Disorders
Hemophilia A
von Willebrand's Disease
Hemophilia B
Hemophilia C
Other Hereditary Coagulation Disorders
Acquired Coagulation Disorders
Vitamin K Deficiency
Liver Disease
Anticoagulant Therapy
Circulating Anticoagulants
Disseminated Intravascular Coagulation
Fibrinolysis
Lesions of Blood and Lymph Vessels
Hemangioma
Nevus Flammeus
Hemangioendothelioma
Kaposi's Sarcoma
Sturge-Weber Syndrome
Juvenile Nasopharyngeal Angiofibroma

Vascular Anomalies
Lymphangioma
Soft Tissue Enlargements
Focal Soft Tissue Enlargements
Papilloma
Fibroma
Scar
Focal Epithelial Hyperplasia
Lipoma
Verruciform Xanthoma
Traumatic Neuroma
Multiple Mucosal Neuroma
Neurofibroma
Neurolemmoma
Congenital Epulis of the Newborn
Granular Cell Myoblastoma
Osteoma Mucosae
Accessory Salivary Gland Tumors
Pyogenic Granuloma
Peripheral Giant Cell Granuloma
Peripheral Odontogenic Fibroma
Lingual Tonsil
Lingual Thyroid
Diffuse Soft Tissue Enlargements
Inflammatory Fibrous Hyperplasia
Inflammatory Papillary Hyperplasia
Crohn's Disease
Condyloma Acuminata
Neurofibromatosis
Locally Aggressive Fibrous Lesions
Lymphoproliferative Disease of the Hard Palate
Diffuse Gingival Enlargements
Macrocheilia
Cheilitis Glandularis Apostematosa
Cheilitis Granulomatosa
Macroglossia
Diffuse Cellulitis
Surgical Space Infection
Buccal Space Infection
Infraorbital Space Infection
Submandibular Space Infection
Ludwig's Angina
Pterygomandibular Space Infection
Cavernous Sinus Thrombosis

THE APPROACH TO CLINICAL DIAGNOSIS

The clinical diagnosis of oral soft tissue lesions is predicated upon a carefully executed examination. The lesion must be found and recognized as abnormal, and all pertinent information must be collected and evaluated. It should be recognized that the diagnostic significance of isolated observations made in the preliminary stages of the examination may not be readily apparent. For this reason, an orderly and systematic approach to the clinical examination has been stressed to assure that no important findings are inadvertently missed.

Establishment of a definitive, provisional or differential diagnosis presupposes a working knowledge of the etiology, clinical features and pathologic basis of oral disease. It follows that the correlation of basic concepts of disease with the results of the physical examination, together with the utilization of indicated laboratory procedures, should provide a reasonable basis for diagnosis of even uncommon lesions. Although many oral lesions are sufficiently characteristic to permit a *definitive diagnosis* based solely on their clinical features, others require the use of special diagnostic methods. In such cases it is convenient to establish a *differential diagnosis* and proceed to deal with the various possibilities with additional tests. If the clinical evidence strongly suggests a given entity, the tentative working or *provisional diagnosis* then provides a sound basis for further investigation or even a clinical trial of some definitive treament.

CLINICAL MANIFESTATIONS OF DISEASE OF THE ORAL SOFT TISSUES

Knowledge of the natural behavior of disease entities that involve the oral tissues, together with an understanding of basic tissue responses in diseased states, will give a sound basis for clinical diagnosis.

Living tissues react to injury or disease in only a limited number of ways. These pathologic responses are *aplasia, hypoplasia, degeneration, atrophy, inflammation, hyperplasia, neoplasia* or combinations of these. The clinical manifestations of these responses may occur singly or in combination. For example, a clinical lesion characterized by necrosis, desquamation, ulceration, redness, change in consistency, swelling, or proliferation of tissue can be a manifestation of inflammation. Since the gross clinical lesion is a reflection of the basic pathologic process, it frequently is responsible for many of the patient's subjective symptoms and almost invariably represents the major ob-

jective sign upon which the differential diagnosis is predicated.

The Clinical Lesion

The clinical lesion may appear as an enlargement, ulcer, erosion, macule, papule, pustule, white, red or pigmented area, vesicle, bulla, or as various combinations of these reactions. The reactions may be focal or diffuse, solitary or multiple, painful or nonpainful, and primary or recurrent. For example, the pyogenic granuloma is a focal soft tissue enlargement and occasionally may be ulcerated. On the other hand, epidermoid carcinoma may occur as an indurated ulcer, a focal swelling with or without ulceration, a white (keratotic) patch, or an exophytic growth. In an early stage (carcinoma in situ), an innocuous-appearing, red, velvety lesion (erythroplakia, p. 380) is seen. Because of this overlap of basic pathologic responses (*e.g.* neoplasm with secondary infection), some knowledge of the variants that may be encountered clinically is necessary.

Correlation of Clinical Findings

In dealing with a lesion of obscure origin an effort should be made to categorize the reaction as a probable developmental, degenerative, inflammatory, infectious, metabolic, neoplastic or other basic disease process if possible. Thus, if a given lesion appears to be infectious in nature, a reasonably direct approach to establishment of a definitive diagnosis can be taken by the use of microbiologic tests or antibacterial therapy.

In more difficult cases the lesion must be evaluated in reference to the several known diseases or conditions which characteristically demonstrate similar features. For example, a chronic crateriform ulcer of the lateral border of the tongue in an adult commonly will resist accurate classification according to basic pathologic process, since such a lesion will present features suggestive of inflammatory and infectious as well as neoplastic disease. Since the primary lesion is an ulcer, first consideration in the differential diagnosis must be given to those conditions characterized by ulcers and specifically to those which tend to involve the lateral border of the tongue. This mental list of "ulcers" may be further shortened on the basis of the information obtained up to this point in the examination. The remaining possibilities may then be systematically investigated, beginning with the common, and therefore more likely, conditions first.

In the example given, such conditions as aphthous ulcer, periadenitis mucosa necrotica recurrens or chancre might reasonably be discarded as likely possibilities simply on the basis of the findings mentioned. On the other hand, traumatic (decubitus) ulcer, epidermoid carcinoma or a specific granulomatous infection such as tuberculosis would be more likely possibilities (differential diagnosis). Since these lesions cannot be further differentiated on a clinical basis alone, biopsy would then be mandatory in order to establish a definitive diagnosis.

WHITE LESIONS

The white lesions of the oral mucosa comprise a rather large group of conditions which can appear in a variety of clinical forms. These may be smooth, folded, shaggy, elevated, lacy or annular. Each of these may be, in turn, fissured, ulcerated, eroded or inflamed and occur as solitary, multiple, focal or diffuse lesions. The majority represent a disturbance of the covering epithelium, usually with an increased thickness of one or more layers. In other instances coagulation necrosis of the epithelium resulting from the escharotic effect of chemical agents, or associated with superimposed colonies of *Candida* organisms, may cause the mucosa to appear white. On rare occasions, increased collagenization of the subepithelial connective tissue with reduction in blood supply as in scleroderma and submucous fibrosis will result in a white appearance. Although a fibrinous exudate can often resemble a white

patch, careful probing will reveal an underlying ulcer or erosion.

Leukoplakia (White Plaque)

This term designates a white, tough, adherent patch on the mucosa which cannot be rubbed off and which is not diagnosable as any other disease entity. Histologic examination of such areas may show changes ranging from hyperkeratosis through malignant transformation. Inasmuch as the term leukoplakia has been used both in the clinical sense and as a microscopic term, the precise meaning in communications should be clearly understood. Since a number of specific entities such as lichen planus, white sponge nevus and candidosis also appear as white patches, the term leukoplakia should be restricted to mean a white keratotic patch other than such specific disease entities on the mucous membrane.

Disturbances in epithelial maturation occasionally seen in biopsies of leukoplakic areas imply that some cases conceivably might undergo malignant transformation after some undetermined period of time. For example, a white patch due entirely to thick-

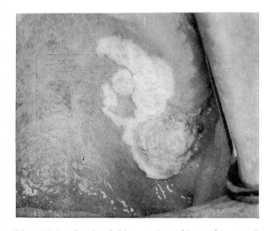

Fig. 14-1. Leukoplakia and epidermoid carcinoma. This elderly male developed epidermoid carcinoma in the maxillary tuberosity area. The area of leukoplakia seen clinically on the palate showed hyperkeratosis and acanthosis with foci of epithelial dysplasia microscopically. Another area of leukoplakia is seen on the soft palate posterior to the post-dam area of the patient's denture.

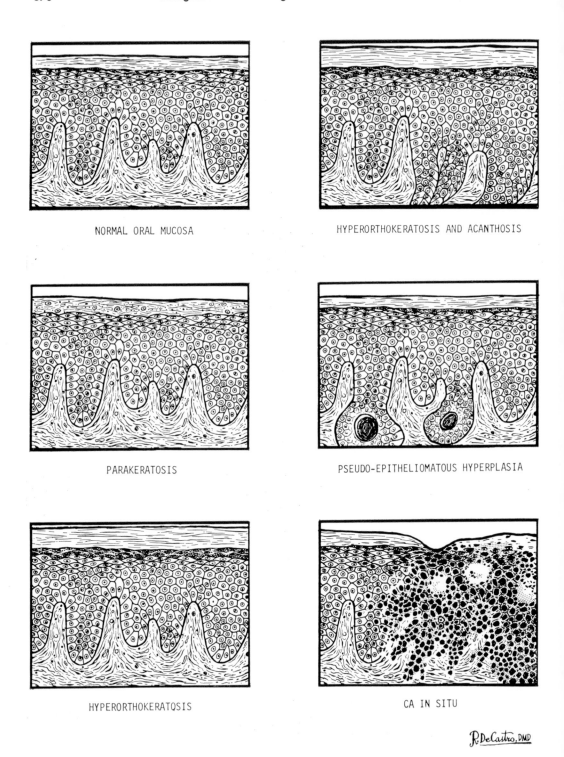

NORMAL ORAL MUCOSA

HYPERORTHOKERATOSIS AND ACANTHOSIS

PARAKERATOSIS

PSEUDO-EPITHELIOMATOUS HYPERPLASIA

HYPERORTHOKERATOSIS

CA IN SITU

R. DeCastro, DMD

Fig. 14-2.   Diagrammatic representation of histologic changes in oral epithelium.

ening of the keratin layer will be of less serious concern than a case showing maturation disturbances in the deeper layers of the epithelial cells. Once a microscopic diagnosis of some epithelial dysplasia has been obtained, the dentist must then exercise considerable clinical judgment in evaluating any remaining lesions and the need for proper follow-up.

Simple hyperorthokeratosis of the mucous membrane will appear pearly-white and will feel relatively smooth and flexible. Areas of cracking, bleeding or piling up of keratin into horny masses are somewhat more serious clinical signs (Figs. 14–1, 14–2). Areas of induration, ulceration or red-velvety erythematous areas (speckled leukoplakia, erythroplakia) scattered throughout the white portions are ominous features requiring biopsy. The initial biopsy should be chosen so that representative specimens are obtained from the involved areas. Multiple specimens are generally of greater value than one large sample. Each specimen should be identified according to site and placed in a separate bottle of fixative (see pp. 199–204).

A number of microscopic terms are used to designate the several epithelial changes which may be seen in the white lesions of the oral mucosa (Fig. 14–2).

Parakeratosis

The term parakeratin refers to the presence of viable nuclei at the epithelial surface without actual keratin formation. If the parakeratin layer is thickened (hyperparakeratosis) to any degree, the epithelium becomes more opaque, giving a white appearance.

Hyperorthokeratosis

Keratinization reflects an effort of the epithelium to build up a protective layer on the surface similar to that seen in a skin callus. Some keratinization of the gingiva and palatal mucosa is considered normal. Hyperorthokeratosis of the oral mucosa indicates a thickening beyond the normal.

Acanthosis

The spinous layer of the epithelium is composed of pavement-like cells which become progressively flatter toward the surface. Acanthosis is an increased thickness of the spinous layer and implies considerably greater epithelial activity prior to final maturation of the cells and formation of keratin.

Basilar Hyperplasia

This change implies unusual proliferative activity of the basal layer extending throughout much of the thickness of the covering epithelium. Thus, cells in the spinous layer will resemble basal or parabasilar cells.

Dyskeratosis

This term implies literally abnormal keratinization, often of individual epithelial cells in the deeper layers of the epithelium. Ordinarily, the term is used to indicate a number of individual cytologic alterations essentially identical to those seen in epithelial dysplasias.

Epithelial Dysplasia (Atypia)

Disturbances in maturation of epithelial cells somewhat less severe than carcinoma in situ are referred to as epithelial dysplasias or atypias. For example, hyperchromatism, increased mitotic activity or increased nuclear/cytoplasmic ratio may be seen in scattered cells in the deeper cells of the epithelium. This diagnosis requires careful examination of other areas of the epithelium as well as frequent postoperative checkups. Rebiopsy of adjacent areas may be necessary and in many instances surgical stripping (e.g. "lip shave") will be indicated.

Carcinoma in Situ

This histologic diagnosis indicates that malignant epithelial cells are present (usually at all levels in the epithelium) but do not exhibit actual invasion of the underlying connective tissue. The cells individually show pleomorphism, hyperchromatism, clumping of chromatin, increased nuclear cytoplasmic ratio, abnormal mitoses, or other changes characteristic of malignant cells. The diagnosis of preinvasive carcinoma does not rule out the possibility of invasive carcinoma in other areas of the lesion not examined microscopically.

Epidermoid Carcinoma

This term indicates invasion of subjacent connective tissues by malignant epithelial cells. Usually the pathology report will give the degree of differentiation and indicate whether or not the margins of the specimen are free of tumor (see pp. 65–67, 310, 395–397 for additional discussion of epidermoid carcinoma).

Leukoedema

Clinically, this is a diffuse, translucent, bluish-white area on the buccal mucosa opposite the molar teeth (Fig. 14–3). Recognized most readily in Negroid patients, the condition is bilateral and asymptomatic. The white appearance of the mucosa is caused by parakeratosis, acanthosis and intraepithelial edema of the upper layers of the epithelium. The condition requires no treatment and is of no clinical significance.

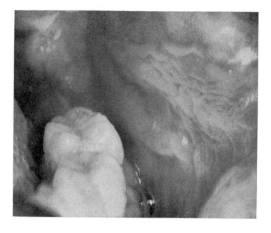

Fig. 14-3. Leukoedema. The buccal mucosa appears wrinkled and white to bluish-grey in the relaxed state. When the tissue is drawn taut, the whitish appearance disappears.

Lichen Planus

Lichen planus is a relatively common disease of unknown etiology which affects the mucous membrane of the mouth but may occur either independently or concomitantly with skin lesions. The oral lesions of the most common form of lichen planus appear as bluish-white lines (striae of Wickham) arranged in a net-like (reticular), or lacy pattern on the buccal mucosa (Fig. 1–24). Cases with this clinical appearance can be diagnosed with considerable confidence on clinical grounds alone. Similar lesions occur less commonly on the ventral surface of the tongue, floor of the mouth and lips (Fig. 14–4A, E).

At other sites, oral lichen planus may appear as thick, elevated white plaques. These occur on the dorsum of the tongue, the hard palate and gingivae (Fig. 14–4B, C). If these are unaccompanied by reticular lesions elsewhere, clinical diagnosis is difficult since they resemble hyperkeratosis or other epithelial dysplasias.

An erosive form of lichen planus is much less common. This appears as a raw or eroded area usually on the buccal mucosa and may not be readily recognized clinically. Careful examination of the surrounding intact mucosa may reveal peripheral striae of Wickham. In some cases, vesicles or bullae occur (bullous lichen planus) (Fig. 14–22). As with most vesicles or bullae of the oral mucous membranes, these promptly rupture, leaving a patch of desquamation and erosion. Histologic examination is often necessary to rule out other erosive and vesiculobullous diseases if no reticular pattern of white lines is present (see pp. 385–394).

The skin lesions of lichen planus appear as discrete macules or papules with a scaly, keratinized surface (Fig. 11–28). Near the periphery, the lesions present a violaceous or reddish to dark brown hue. Striae of Wickham, while not especially prominent in the skin lesions, may be observed upon careful examination (Fig. 14–4F). Often, there is marked pruritus or itching.

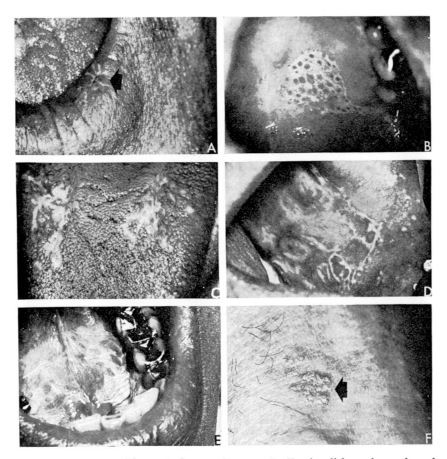

Fig. 14-4.   Lichen planus. *A,* Lip. *B,* Palate. *C,* Tongue. *D,* Erosive lichen planus, buccal mucosa. *E,* Plaque-type lichen planus, floor of mouth. *F,* Lichen planus, skin. (Silverman, Dent. Clin. North America, March, 1968). (See also Figs. 1-24*A,B,* 7-47, 11-28, 14-5*A,B,C,* 14-22.)

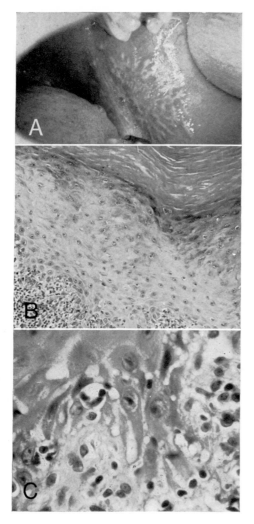

Fig. 14-5. Lichen planus. *A,* Typical striae of Wickham present on the buccal mucosa. *B.* Photomicrograph showing hyperkeratosis, acanthosis, spiking of rete pegs and a subepithelial lymphocytic infiltrate. *C,* Dissolution of the basal layer shown in this higher magnification of *B.*

Although the etiology of lichen planus is unknown, the most common associated factor involved is nervous tension or stress. In many instances, however, the patient appears to be a stable individual who will deny any particular emotional problem. Nevertheless, it can be assumed at least that lichen planus may represent a particular manifestation of tension which in other individuals could manifest clinically as neurodermatitis or some other psychosomatic condition.

Lichen planus has been observed to occur with some frequency in association with diabetes mellitus and vascular hypertension, a triad of features referred to as *Grinspan's syndrome.*

No definitive treament for lichen planus is known. The duration is quite variable, from a few months to several years. Except for the erosive and bullous forms, no particular symptoms are associated with the oral lesions. Often, the most effective treatment is reassurance that the disease is of no serious consequence. Since the erosive lesions may cause discomfort, bland mouthwashes and topical applications of protective ointments may offer some relief. The skin lesions of lichen planus likewise require no particular therapy, although a dermatologist should be consulted to confirm the diagnosis.

Psoriasis

This common skin disorder (p. 311, Fig. 11–13) involves the oral mucosa only on extremely rare occasions. While its existence on mucosal surfaces has been questioned, several reports have demonstrated lesions histologically identical to skin psoriasis. In some cases, the patient also had typical skin lesions. The clinical lesion of oral psoriasis ranges from a silvery white, somewhat scaly lesion to irregular, erythematous lesions with a whitish border. The reported cases have involved the lips, gingiva, buccal mucosa and floor of the mouth.

Fordyce's Granules (Ectopic Sebaceous Glands)

Ectopic sebaceous glands are commonly found on the buccal and labial mucosa (Figs. 7–13, 14–6). Uncommon in young children, they increase in number at about the time of puberty and after. They are seen clinically as white or yellowish granules which are sometimes slightly elevated above the surface of the adjacent mucosa. They consist of sebaceous glands, identical to the sebaceous glands in the skin, except that the excretory ducts of the latter open around a hair shaft.

Although the diagnosis of this common condition is made readily by clinical examination, the patient who discovers it in his own mouth may fear that he has cancer. Because of the uncommon occurrence in other locations of the mouth, Fordyce's granules may not be recognized immediately when they occur on the tongue or palate. No symptoms are associated with them and no treatment is indicated.

Chemical and Thermal Burns

A number of chemical agents deliberately or inadvertently placed on the oral mucosa coagulate the covering epithelium, creating a necrotic slough with a white appearance (Figs. 14–27 and 28). The white area may be mistaken for leukoplakia or, if the area of necrosis is deep enough, for carcinoma. The most common chemical agents responsible for chemical burns in the oral cavity are aspirin (acetylsalicylic acid), phenol, trichloroacetic acid, silver nitrate, sodium perborate, and other similar agents.

Aspirin burns are induced most commonly by topical application of the drug as a home remedy for toothache (Fig. 14–7). The onset is sudden, and healing generally occurs within a week to 10 days without unusual complications. A palliative antibacterial ointment may be useful. If aspirin is prescribed,

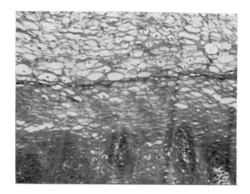

Fig. 14-7. Aspirin burn. The upper pale cells of the epithelium show coagulation necrosis which is sharply demarcated from the viable spinous cells at deeper levels of the mucosa.

it should be made clear to the patient that it should be swallowed.

Other burns occur due to the ingestion of hot liquids and foods such as pizza. Iatrogenic burns have occurred following contact of the anesthetized mucosa with an overheated contra-angle, wax, gutta percha or other materials (Fig. 14–35).

The so-called cotton roll burn, which is not actually a thermal or chemical burn, may cause rather extensive necrosis in some patients (Fig. 14–36). The mucosa, which sometimes sticks to a dry cotton roll, may be stripped off when the cotton roll is removed from the mouth. Coating the mucosa with petroleum jelly before inserting the cotton roll is said to prevent this type of injury.

Stomatitis Nicotina

This condition is seen clinically as multiple white and slightly elevated nodules with red umbilicated centers on the posterior hard palate and soft palate. Seen almost exclusively in pipe smokers, this condition reflects hyperkeratosis around and inflammation of the palatal salivary duct orifices (Fig. 7–28). The red center represents the orifice of an accessory salivary gland duct which is irritated by the pipe smoking and yet protected by the mucous flow. If the patient wears a full upper denture, the lesions will be re-

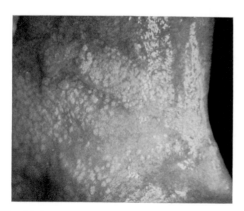

Fig. 14-6. Fordyce's granules of the buccal mucosa.

stricted to palatal tissue posterior to the prosthesis. While the condition is of no serious consequence, the patient should be informed of the condition and its relationship to smoking.

Many users of snuff, a form of tobacco, habitually place the material in the lower labial sulcus (Fig. 7–10). A typical wrinkled hyperkeratosis results in time and may eventually undergo malignant transformation. This undesirable condition should be pointed out to the patient.

Pathomimia

The *linea alba* appears as a white somewhat elevated and occasionally scalloped line corresponding to line of occlusion. More severe factitial injuries from biting habits (*pathomimia mucosae oris*) may appear as whitish lesions with increased keratinization and other epithelial changes or, occasionally, ulceration (Fig. 14–8). These habits have also been referred to as *morsicatio labiorum* (lip biting) and *morsicatio buccarum* (cheek biting).

Candidosis (Candidiasis, Moniliasis, Thrush)

A superficial infection of the oral mucous membranes due to *Candida albicans,* candidosis occurs as a profuse white plaque (often

described as "milk-curds") on the mucous membrane surface which ordinarily can be peeled off without difficulty (Fig. 14–9*A* to *D*). The underlying mucosa presents a raw bleeding surface since the active organisms infiltrate the covering epithelium. In other cases, the involved mucosa is predominately raw and erythematous-appearing, with only scattered white areas. Less commonly, advanced cases may exhibit a tough and adherent white membrane with indurated margins. Biopsy may reveal only chronic inflammation unless candidosis is suspected and a concerted effort made to demonstrate the microorganisms (Fig. 14–9*B*). Therapeutic trial of topical fungicides may control the condition, aiding the diagnosis.

It should be noted that although *Candida albicans* is a common organism of the oral flora, it seldom causes candidosis except in the very young (thrush), the aged or those debilitated by chronic diseases. Cases which fail to respond to treatment should be evaluated for diabetes or other endocrine disease (p. 248).

Microscopic smears or cultures grown on special media are useful in confirming the diagnosis (p. 240, Fig. 9–12). Rarely, candidosis may involve other epithelial tissues of the body, including the skin, nails, geni-

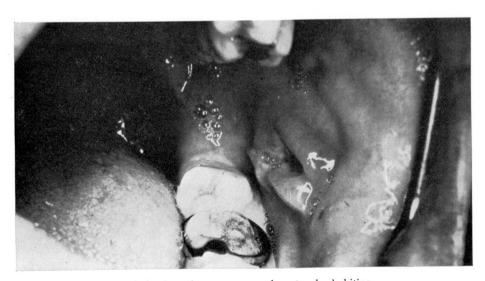

Fig. 14-8. Factitial injury of the buccal mucosa secondary to cheek biting.

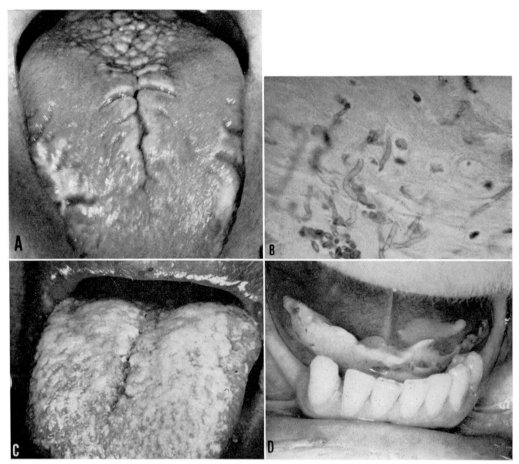

Fig. 14-9. Candidosis. *A*, The white material in this case is very tough and adherent. *B*, Photomicrograph of biopsy specimen from tongue showing *Candida* within the epithelium. *C*, Candidosis of the tongue of a middle-aged male with leukemia. The white material is softer and more readily removed than in the previous case. Patients with refractory moniliasis should be investigated for diabetes mellitus or other systemic disease. (Courtesy of Charles Waldron.) *D*, Candidosis in the floor of the mouth. (Courtesy of Francis Howell.)

talia, lungs, and intestinal tract, occasionally resulting in death.

Mucous Patch

The secondary stage of syphilis follows the appearance of the primary lesion or chancre (p. 400) by 6 to 8 weeks. Generalized eruptions of the skin, lymphadenopathy and oral mucous membrane lesions are found. Diffuse inflammation of the mouth and pharynx, often with areas of pseudomembrane formation, may be present with the classical mucous patch. The mucous patch is essentially an erosion which is covered with a greyish-white membrane. Stripping off the membrane shows an underlying erythematous base. Less distinctive erythematous macules are also seen in the mouth, chiefly on the palate. "Split papules" may also be present at the commissures of the mouth. The oral lesions of secondary syphilis contain large numbers of spirochetes and must be considered contagious. A healed tertiary lesion (gumma) of the palate is shown in Figure 2–4.

White Sponge Nevus (White Folded Gingivostomatitis, Cannon's Disease)

This hereditary condition appears clinically as a diffuse, white thickening of the oral mucosa, but may also affect other mucosal surfaces including the vagina and rectum (Fig. 14–10). Commonly described as having a "parboiled" appearance, the mucosa is thickened and presents a folded or corrugated surface extending over the buccal mucosa, floor of the mouth and sometimes the palate. Several members of the same family are usually affected, often from birth.

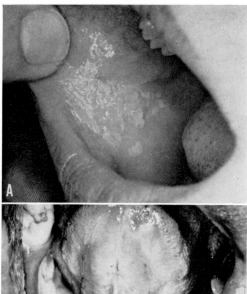

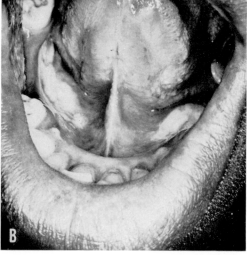

Fig. 14-10. *A,* White sponge nevus. Diffuse white lesions are shown on the buccal mucosa of a 40-year-old woman. *B,* Symmetrical lesions are seen in the floor of the mouth in a 23-year-old woman. (See also Fig. 4-19.)

While the diagnosis can be made with considerable assurance on a clinical basis (especially in the young), biopsy is diagnostic. The lesions are asymptomatic and no treatment is indicated.

Hereditary Benign Intraepithelial Dyskeratosis (Witkop's Disease, The Red Eye)

An hereditary syndrome affecting the oral mucosa and conjunctiva, hereditary benign intraepithelial dyskeratosis occurs only in a racial isolate found in North Carolina. The oral lesions are clinically and microscopically similar to white sponge nevus. The eye lesion occurs as a gelatinous plaque on the bulbar conjunctiva and may involve the cornea. These plaques are generally shed in the late summer or fall. Blindness often occurs in older patients due to corneal involvement.

Dyskeratosis Congenita (Linsser-Engman-Cole Syndrome)

A rare inherited disorder, dyskeratosis congenita is characterized by oral leukoplakia, dystrophy of the fingernails and toenails and skin pigmentation. The disease appears to be a recessive and possibly sex-linked trait, inasmuch as all reported cases have been in males. The oral lesions arise in childhood or adolescence and precede the onset of the other features of the syndrome. Interestingly, oral vesicles and bullae appear on the mucosa during the early stages of the disease. Later, these areas become atrophic and finally thickened and white. The skin shows marked epithelial atrophy with melanin deposition in a reticulated pattern. Thymic dysplasia and aplastic anemia are also part of the syndrome.

Pachyonychia Congenita

Diffuse congenital hyperkeratosis of the oral mucosa, chiefly the tongue and buccal mucosa, together with palmar and plantar hyperkeratosis and dystrophic changes in the nails are diagnostic of pachyonychia congenita.

Darier's Disease
(Keratosis Follicularis)

The characteristic oral lesions of Darier's disease (p. 320) appear to correspond to the severity of the skin disease and range from a few scattered keratotic papules seen chiefly on the palate to numerous "cobblestone" lesions over much of the oral cavity. The diagnosis of Darier's disease is made on the basis of the clinical findings of widespread skin lesions and biopsy. As noted, the histology is identical to the solitary lesion of warty dyskeratoma.

Warty Dyskeratoma
(Isolated Keratosis Follicularis)

This lesion, seen with greater frequency on the skin of the head or neck, is a small whitish cratiform lesion, most commonly on the attached mucosa. The oral lesions are histologically identical to the skin lesions of both warty dyskeratoma and the generalized Darier's disease (keratosis follicularis). The term oral focal acantholytic dyskeratosis has also been suggested for this entity.

Squamous Acanthoma

This recently described histologic entity appears clinically as a well-circumscribed, white, flat to elevated lesion on the oral mucosa. It appears to represent the terminal stage of a spectrum of changes in the epithelium, ranging from pseudoepitheliomatous hyperplasia to the mature form, squamous acanthoma. The cases reported to date have occurred chiefly in older males. They are presumed to be of traumatic origin.

Keratoacanthoma

Most cases of keratoacanthoma occur on the hair-bearing areas of the skin, although rare cases have been reported on mucous membrane surfaces such as the lip, palate and conjunctiva. Clinically they are raised, usually white, and umbilicated lesions. Patients with xeroderma pigmentosa,

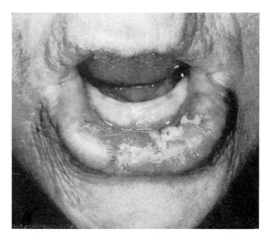

Fig. 14-11. Chronic disseminated lupus erythematosus in a middle-aged woman. Note the scarring about the lips and the chronic cheilitis. (Courtesy of Ralph Beatty.)

an inherited skin disease, appear to have a higher frequency of keratoacanthomas as well as a predisposition to basal cell and squamous cell carcinoma.

Chronic Discoid Lupus Erythematosus

The most characteristic features of chronic discoid lupus erythematosus are seen on the skin of the face (p. 329). Oral mucous membrane involvement also occurs in some of these patients as a patchy keratosis (Fig. 14–11).

Oral Submucous Fibrosis

Seen chiefly in India, oral submucous fibrosis exhibits a blanched, opaque-white appearance of the mucous membrane, chiefly of the palate, uvula, tonsillar pillars, buccal mucosa and tongue. Dense fibrous bands often form causing trismus. Frequently, inflammation with vesicle formation precedes the later changes of "stiffening" of the tissues. There is atrophy of papillae and inability to protrude the tongue. The patients will often show an elevated erythrocyte sedimentation rate and anemia. Of unknown etiology, oral submucous fibrosis is currently thought to be associated with prolonged exposure to irritating food (chili) or possibly to betel nuts.

RED LESIONS

A number of disease entities may manifest themselves by either primary or secondary red lesions of the oral mucosa. In this section, only those conditions appearing primarily as focal or diffuse red macules with intact surface epithelium are discussed. The secondary red lesions, seen frequently with rupture of vesicles and bullae, in erosive disorders, in vascular and hematologic disorders and in certain infections such as candidosis, are covered in following sections.

Erythroplakia

This term is used to denote a red macule or plaque on the mucosa which does not represent any other specific clinical entity. In this sense, erythroplakia is analogous to leukoplakia and thus may demonstrate upon microscopic examination a rather broad spectrum of histologic changes in the covering epithelium, ranging from epithelial dysplasia to carcinoma in situ or invasive epidermoid carcinoma. It is particularly significant that, while erythroplakia may appear clinically innocuous, a substantial number of cases are serious or potentially serious. Shafer and Waldron have reported that 91 percent of 65 biopsies described clinically as erythroplakia showed either epithelial dysplasia, carcinoma in situ or invasive carcinoma.

The clinical lesion of erythroplakia may appear homogeneously red and velvety, as a red lesion with multiple patches of leukoplakia, or as an area of erythroplakia speckled with white ("speckled erythroplakia"). Erythroplakia may occur on any area of the mucosa and range in size from a few millimeters to several centimeters in diameter. Since the character of the epithelial changes in erythroplakia cannot be judged clinically, and in view of the surprisingly high incidence of dysplastic and neoplastic changes, such lesions should be subjected to biopsy.

Plasma Cell Gingivitis
(Allergic Gingivostomatitis)

This unusual disorder of the free and attached gingiva was observed with considerable frequency during a 3- or 4-year period beginning about 1968. At that time, numerous cases were observed with boggy, erythematous and edematous gingiva, angular cheilitis and a bald and fissured tongue (Fig. 14–12). There was a rather sudden onset and gingival biopsy showed a diffuse plasma cell infiltration of the connective tissue with intact overlying stratified squamous epithelium. As suggested by Kerr *et al.*, the condition represented an allergic response to some component of chewing gum which was used by affected patients. This condition seems to have disappeared altogether, apparently after chewing gum manufacturers altered

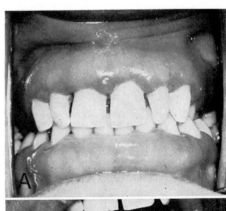

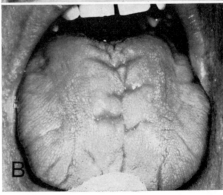

Fig. 14-12. Plasma cell gingivitis. *A,* Diffuse erythematous involvement of both the free and attached gingiva in a young male. *B,* Bald fissured tongue in the patient shown in *A.* (Courtesy of Dr. Charles E. Tomich.)

some component of the product. Although plasma cell gingivitis is hopefully now only of historical interest, it does illustrate a rather classic example of contact stomatitis to a commonly encountered agent and the application of historical and laboratory studies in its diagnosis.

Allergy

The clinical manifestations of allergy and hypersensitivity reactions to various allergens are referred to on pages 392–393. As noted with plasma cell gingivitis, such conditions may induce a red lesion at the interface of the allergen and the mucosa or subsequent to the systemic ingestion of the causative agent.

Specific Infectious Agents

Certain microorganisms, most notably the erythrogenic streptococci, may produce erythematous lesions of the skin and sometimes of the oral mucosa. The signs and symptoms of rash, fever and malaise generally suggest the diagnosis of an acute or subacute infectious process. Other specific infections may have associated red lesions of the oral mucosa and oropharynx, notably the exanthematous diseases of childhood. Less commonly, histoplasmosis, candidiasis and tuberculosis will show erythematous macules with intact surface mucosa.

Non-specific Inflammation

Chronic irritation from dental appliances, rough or jagged teeth, smoking and other habits may produce focal or diffuse red lesions of the mucosa. Generally, a careful oral examination and thorough health history will demonstrate the correct etiology.

Red lesions involving the gingival mucosa can usually be attributed to some form of periodontal disease, most commonly local irritation. For the most part, these will be confined largely to the free gingiva in relation to an overhanging margin, food impaction, poor oral hygiene, calculus, periodontal pocket or other irritant. More diffusely distributed primary red lesions involving both the free and attached gingiva frequently indicate a more generalized disorder, possibly of allergic, endocrine, metabolic or hematologic origin. Clearly, those cases which do not respond promptly to therapy must be reevaluated and consideration given in the differential diagnosis to stomatitis venenata, stomatitis medicamentosa (p. 392), plasma cell gingivitis (*q.v.*), puberty gingivitis, pregnancy gingivitis, diabetes mellitus (pp. 245–249), scurvy or other deficiencies and certain blood dyscrasias (p. 405). Additionally, primary herpetic gingivostomatitis must be considered in the young patient, since the onset of the more diagnostic vesicles may be preceded by a diffuse inflammation of the oral mucosa and pharynx (p. 385).

Erythema of the soft palate has been described secondary to the trauma of fellatio. Petechial hemorrhages have also been noted in some cases, presumably caused by reflex spasm of the palatal muscles and the negative pressures created during this sex act.

Erythema of the oral mucous membranes, most notably of the soft palate, is also frequently seen as a result of chronic marihuana smoking.

PIGMENTATIONS

Extrinsic and intrinsic pigmentations of the skin are discussed on page 320 *et seq.* It should be apparent that the skin pigmentary disorders described commonly have counterpart lesions of the oral cavity, usually pigmentations of the same nature. In some instances the skin pigmentations are dermatologic "markers" helpful in the diagnosis of other lesions in the mouth. For example, the skin *cafe-au-lait* spots of von Recklinghausen's disease and Albright's syndrome (seen rarely on the mucous membranes) may point to the diagnosis of oral neurofibroma and fibrous dysplasia of bone, respectively. In other cases, the oral pigmentation may be more clinically obvious than in the skin, as in Addison's disease and certain of the heavy metals such as bismuth

gingivitis. Finally, it should be noted that oral pigmentary disorders may account for intrinsic and extrinsic staining of the teeth, as described on pages 153–156.

In this section, the clinical oral manifestations of the generalized pigmentary disorders as well as those unique to the oral cavity are briefly discussed.

Intrinsic Pigmentations

Physiologic Pigmentation of the Gingiva

Negroids and many brunette Caucasoids exhibit physiologic pigmentation of the gingiva. Usually, the free and a portion of the attached gingiva will show diffuse melanin pigmentation which is of no clinical significance. Occasionally isolated macules are found on the buccal mucosa or on the inner surface of the lip as well. The histologic findings show dermal and/or epidermal melanosis.

Ephelis, Lentigo

The ephelis, or freckle, is seen occasionally on the vermilion border of the lip or on the mucosal surface of the lip. Lentigo ("liver spots"), seen commonly on the hands and face of older persons, may also occur as solitary pigmented macules on the lips.

Peutz-Jeghers Syndrome

Distinguished from the ordinary ephelides by their peculiar distribution on and around the lips and on the buccal mucosa, gingiva, and hands and feet, this finding justifies further medical workup for intestinal polyposis (p. 321).

Addison's Disease

The oral pigmentation associated with Addison's disease appears as irregular areas of yellow-brown to bluish pigment distributed on the anterior gingiva, lips, cheeks, palate and other areas of the mouth (Fig. 14–13). While the development of intraoral pigmentation of this nature may suggest the possi-

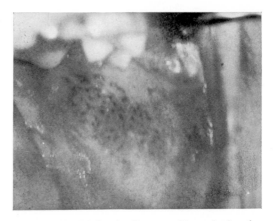

Fig. 14-13. Addison's disease with melanin pigmentation of the inner surface of the cheek. (See also Fig. 11-18A,B.)

bility of Addison's disease, the diagnosis is established by other findings (p. 255).

Pigmented Nevi

The benign neoplasms in this category are the intradermal, junctional, compound and blue (Jadassohn-Tieche) nevi, Hutchinson's freckle (p. 309), and the juvenile melanoma (spindle cell and epithelioid cell nevi). The malignant forms include the malignant melanoma, lentigo maligna melanoma (p. 311) and the malignant blue nevus.

The intradermal, junctional and compound nevi are seen rarely on the oral mucous membranes as innocuous-appearing tan to brown colored macules (Fig. 7–3). The

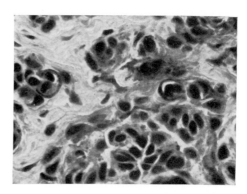

Fig. 14-14. Intradermal nevus. The theques of nevus cells are shown together with scattered granules of melanin pigment.

overlying mucosa is intact. The three types can only be distinguished histologically (Fig. 14–14). Since the junctional nevus has some potential to undergo malignant transformation, excisional biopsy is indicated.

Blue Nevi

Extremely rare in the mouth, the reported cases have occurred mainly in the palate. Clinically, these have appeared as small, smooth, slightly raised lesions with a dark blue color. The blue nevus undergoes malignant transformation only on rare occasions.

Juvenile Melanoma
(Spindle Cell Nevus, Epithelioid Cell Nevus)

Seen in the child, this lesion has several histologic criteria of malignancy, *i.e.* malignant melanoma, but a benign clinical behavior. It presents a difficult diagnostic problem, especially when it is seen in the teenager, since malignant melanoma does occur rarely in children.

Malignant Melanoma

In the oral mucosa, malignant melanoma generally appears clinically as a darkly pigmented area, usually on the alveolar ridge and palate (Fig. 14–15*B*). (Pigmentation is not seen, however, in the amelanotic melanoma.) As for pigmented lesions of the skin, recent increases in pigmentation, increases in size, appearance of satellite lesions, bleeding or ulceration are ominous signs. In contrast to melanoma of the skin, the oral melanoma tends to occur in older adults, shows a slight predilection for males and has a worse prognosis (Fig. 14–16).

Melanotic Neuroectodermal Tumor of Infancy

This unusual tumor appears as a darkly pigmented nodule, chiefly on the anterior ridge of newborn infants. Known formerly as melanotic prognoma, pigmented ameloblastoma and other terms, the tumor is perfectly benign despite its ominous clinical appearance (see p. 484).

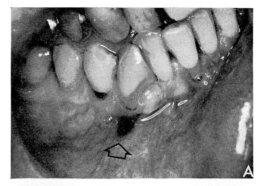
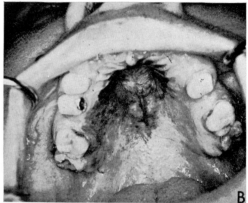

Fig. 14-15. Extrinsic and intrinsic pathologic pigmentations. *A,* Amalgam tattoo, gingiva. *B,* Malignant melanoma, palate. (Silverman, Dent. Clin. North America, March, 1968.)

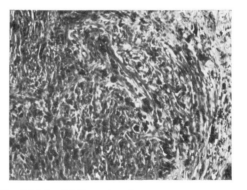

Fig. 14-16. Malignant melanoma.

Other Rare Forms of
Intrinsic Pigmentation

Oral pigmentations of intrinsic origin have been reported to occur in conjunction with a variety of other disease states. For the most part, these are rare and unusual associations observed coincidentally and not of diagnostic importance in view of the patient's other signs and symptoms. For example, intraoral melanin pigmentation is rarely seen in *von Recklinghausen's disease* and *Albright's syndrome* whereas the *cafe-au-lait* spots on the skin together with the characteristic neurofibromas and osseous lesions are typical. Likewise, jaundice is occasionally recognized as a color change on the undersurface of the tongue; however, the sclera of the eyes and the skin of the anterior chest show the most obvious changes. The conditions listed below represent unusual forms of intrinsic pigmentation which sometimes occur on the oral mucosa. Brief discussion of these conditions may be found on the pages indicated.

> von Recklinghausen's disease of skin (p. 421)
> Albright's syndrome (p. 457)
> Jaundice (p. 230)
> Submucous fibrosis (p. 379)
> Hemosiderosis (p. 231)
> Hemochromatosis (p. 231)
> Ochronosis (alkaptonuria) (p. 18t)
> Porphyria (p. 154)
> Acanthosis nigrans (p. 314)
> Xeroderma pigmentosa (p. 319)
> Incontinentia pigmenti (p. 317)
> Riehl's melanosis (p. 322t)
> Darier's disease (p. 320)

Extrinsic Pigmentations

Amalgam Tattoo

Fragments of silver amalgam filling materials are seen on frequent occasions in the oral mucous membranes or alveolar bone (Fig. 14–15*A*). Particles of filling material may fall into an extraction wound, or can be accidentally embedded in the tissues by a rotating dental instrument. Radiopaque particles without any surrounding tissue response may be detected. The amalgam tattoo may be confused clinically with a pigmented nevus or melanoma (Fig. 14–15*B*). Since amalgam in the tissues is essentially inert, no treatment is required.

Other Foreign Materials

Numerous other particles of exogenous origin may be accidentally embedded in the soft tissues and appear clinically as apparent pigmented areas of the mucosa. For example, fragments of carborundum discs and broken dental burs may be forced into the soft tissues during operative procedures and not recovered. Frequently, the mucosa heals without incident and the foreign material in the submucous membrane gives a dark or pigmented appearance. It is not unusual for children to puncture the mucosa with the point of a pencil held in the mouth. The pencil point of graphite or carbon remains embedded in the tissues as a black, pigmented area.

Heavy Metal Pigmentation

Bismuth, copper, silver, lead, gold and mercury ingested accidentally or therapeutically in sufficient quantities may induce diffuse or focal discolorations in the oral mucosa and skin (p. 320). Bismuth and lead tend to accumulate in areas of chronic inflammation (anachoresis) such as the gingiva, producing a blue-black bismuth or lead "line" (Fig. 14–17). Lead, mercury and silver (argyria) may also cause a generalized dusky-grey color of the mucous membranes and skin.

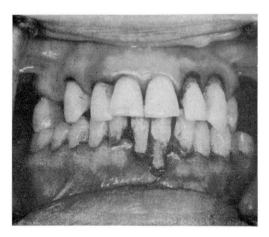

Fig. 14-17.   Bismuth line on the gingiva.

Black Hairy Tongue

In this condition, there is elongation of the filiform papillae of the tongue, presenting a "furry" appearance (Figs. 7–21 and 7–30). These commonly take on a black or greenish coloration, depending on the diet or medications (*e.g.* oral antibiotics) of the patient as well as on the specific microorganisms growing in the tangled masses of papillae.

Other Extrinsic Pigmentations

A number of other extrinsic substances have been reported to produce oral pigmentation on rare occasions: charcoal dentifrices, arsenic, phenolphthalein, antimalarial agents (quinacrine, chloroquine, amodiaquine), inorganic mercury compounds (diuretics), oral contraceptives, and progesterone-estrogen agents.

VESICLES, BULLAE AND EROSIONS

A number of specific disease entities appear as vesicles, bullae or desquamative lesions of the oral mucous membranes. Several of these pose difficult problems in diagnosis, both from the clinical and the laboratory standpoint, since they exhibit many features in common.

Vesiculobullous and erosive lesions may be produced by viruses, chemical and physical agents, hereditary factors, allergens and drug sensitivities. In addition, a substantial number of diseases having these features are of unknown etiology (Fig. 14–18*A* and *B*). Inasmuch as many vesicles and bullae, at least in the oral cavity, rupture soon after their formation, often only an eroded area is seen. An attempt can be made in suspected cases of chronic desquamative gingivitis or pemphigus to induce blister formation or desquamation by rubbing the mucosa (Nikolsky's sign).

The number, distribution and duration of the lesions as well as the age at onset are important observations. The lesions may be solitary or multiple and with or without involvement of other mucosal surfaces (con-

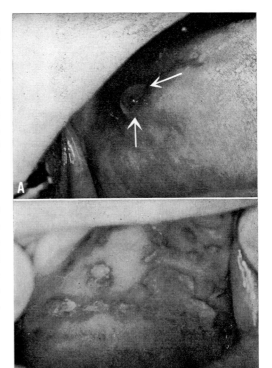

Fig. 14-18. Benign mucous membrane pemphigoid. *A,* A larger vesicle is seen on the lateral border of the tongue. *B,* Multiple ulcers on the palate of the patient shown in *A.* These were preceded by the formation of vesicles and bullae which ruptured. (Blozis, Dent. Clin. North America, March, 1968.)

junctiva, genital mucosa) and the skin. The character of the intact mucous membrane surrounding the lesion should be determined since this may suggest a specific agent such as a virus if it is erythematous, or a generalized dermatologic disease if it is of normal color.

Primary Herpes Simplex

The initial exposure to the herpes simplex virus produces a mild or subclinical infection with resultant immunity in most individuals. In some cases, however, an acute, febrile infection occurs which may involve the oral cavity (acute herpetic gingivostomatitis), the skin (Kaposi's varicelliform eruption) or the central nervous system (herpetic meningoencephalitis). Most cases occur in small children, usually 2 to 5 years of age, although older children and occasionally adults may be affected (Fig. 7–45). On the oral mucous membranes, an acute gingivitis is seen along with numerous, scattered vesicles in various parts of the mouth and lips. These rupture quickly leaving small ulcers. The patient experiences pain, gingival bleeding, fever, malaise, foul breath and difficulty in eating because of the sore mouth. New vesicle formation usually continues over a 4- or 5-day period. The ulcerated areas heal in approximately 2 weeks without scar formation.

Generally, the diagnosis can be established entirely on the clinical findings. Cytologic smears from the base of an intact vesicle show characteristic multinucleated cells and, with biopsy, inclusion bodies (Lipshutz bodies) are found (see p. 242).

Recurrent Herpes Simplex

Secondary herpetic infections typically involve the lips (rather than the oral mucous membranes), often following illness, trauma, prolonged exposure to the sun or emotional disturbances. Frequently, the mild trauma to the lips during prolonged dental treatment will trigger an attack of "cold sores" or "fever blisters." Many susceptible patients can predict their appearance by itching, burning or pain which is followed in a few hours by several tiny vesicles. At this stage, the vesicles may be ruptured and a heterotricyclic dye (neutral red) applied to the base and exposed to fluorescent light for 15 minutes (photodynamic inactivation technique). This treatment appears to promote healing and delay recurrences.

Recurrent intraoral herpes simplex is seen almost invariably on mucosa supported by bone, i.e., hard palate, gingiva and alveolar ridge. The lesions are found in crops of tiny vesicles, 1 mm or less in diameter, which soon rupture, leaving small punctate ulcerations with a red base and, often, a red halo.

Herpes Zoster (Shingles)

This disease most commonly involves the skin over the distribution of the intercostal sensory spinal nerves (p. 326). Other skin sites as well as oral mucous membrane involvement are seen on occasion, sometimes over the distribution of the sensory division of the trigeminal nerve. The outstanding symptom of herpes zoster is pain followed by the development of tiny vesicles over the terminal receptor of the sensory nerve in the skin or mucous membrane. In the mouth, the vesicles quickly rupture leaving ulcers. Postherpetic pain may be most uncomfortable. No specific treatment is known and the lesions heal without residual scar.

Herpangina

Caused by the Coxsackie group A virus, herpangina is a relatively common disease of young children which often occurs in mild epidemics during the late summer months (cf. Hand-foot-and-mouth Disease). The prodromal symptoms of fever, intestinal upset, headache and sore throat precede the appearance of tiny vesicles on the soft palate, pharynx and occasionally the tongue. These promptly rupture leaving miniature ulcers with erythematous borders resembling petechiae. The clinical appearance is quite similar to that of primary herpetic gingivostomatitis except for its different anatomic distribution. Several children in the same family may be affected at the same time. Although a lasting immunity to a specific strain of the Coxsackie virus results, the same individual may develop the disease several times upon exposure to other strains.

Dermatitis Herpetiformis

This dermatologic disorder (Table 11–1) may rarely occur with oral vesicular lesions up to 10 mm in diameter at various sites on the mucous membrane. Since the skin lesions are quite extensive and characterized by intense pruritus, patients ordinarily consult a dermatologist for the initial diagnosis; nevertheless, the dentist should be aware of

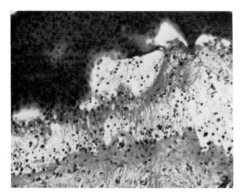

Fig. 14-19. Dermatitis herpetiformis. Epithelial separation with the formation of a fluid-filled vesicle. Neutrophils and eosinophils are prominent.

the various manifestations of the disease. The skin lesions are vesiculobullous and symmetrically distributed over the scalp, shoulders, arms, thighs and sacral areas. Because the itching is relieved by scratching and rupture of the vesicles, secondary excoriations are present, often with hyperpigmentation. The vesicles show a subepidermal split and are filled with edema fluid, eosinophils and neutrophils. The histologic findings, coupled with the clinical features, are diagnostic (Fig. 14–19). Fluorescent antibody tests (p. 234) show IgA deposits in the region of the epithelial separation. An eosinophilia of 10 percent or more is characteristic; however, despite the name, no association with a herpes virus or other etiologic agent has been established. The disease occurs 2 to 3 times more frequently in males than in females and may persist for many years with periods of remission. Unlike many other dermatoses, it does not respond to corticosteroid treatment; rather, sulfapyridine appears to be specific in controlling the disease.

Hand-foot-and-mouth Disease

A common Coxsackie virus infection, hand-foot-and-mouth disease occurs in epidemic form, chiefly in young children during the summer months. Adult members of the same family, or even the consulting physician or dentist, may contract the disease, which is spread by droplet infection or direct contact. It presents only mild prodromal symptoms of malaise, fever or sore throat. Vesicular and ulcerative lesions of the palate, buccal mucosa, floor of mouth and tongue and the tonsillar pillars and pharynx quickly develop in all cases, often preceding the appearance of the skin lesions by 1 to 3 days. Typical vesicles or red, maculopapular lesions are distributed over the palms and dorsal surfaces of the hands and the lateral and dorsal surfaces of the feet. Occasionally, additional lesions are seen on the buttocks, extremities and face. The disease regresses in 10 days to 2 weeks and ordinarily requires only symptomatic treatment.

Hoof-and-mouth Disease (Foot-and-mouth Disease, Aphthous Fever, Epizootic Fever)

A viral disease more commonly seen in cattle and other cloven-hoofed animals, foot-and-mouth disease occasionally is transmitted to humans. Stringent laws on importation of animals, however, have virtually eliminated this disease in the United States. Following an incubation period of 2 to 5 days, the patient complains of fever, headache and excessive salivation. These symptoms are followed in a few days by vesicles in various areas of the mouth, and on the palms of the hands, soles of the feet and the interdigital surfaces of the fingers and toes. Other mucosal surfaces, especially the conjunctiva and genitalia, are sometimes involved. The mucosal vesicles enlarge and rupture leaving irregular eroded areas. The diagnosis is based on the clinical findings, history of exposure, and the use of cultures, animal inoculations and serologic (complement-fixation) test. The acute phase with fever persists for a week or more, after which the lesions gradually heal during an additional 2-week period. Treatment is largely symptomatic.

Erythema Multiforme

Both skin and mucous membranes are involved in this disease (p. 327). It occurs chiefly in young adults and probably represents an allergic or hypersensitivity response, although a viral etiology cannot be ruled out. Frequently the patients will give a history of a preceding viral infection or exposure to a variety of drugs including salicylates or certain antibiotics.

Erythematous macules appear, develop into vesicles or bullae and promptly rupture leaving a raw surface. The oral lesions are usually seen after the vesicles have ruptured and show desquamation or a raw erythematous surface with an erythematous border ("target lesions," "iris lesions"). Lesions of the skin, chiefly the lips, tend to weep a clear exudate and ultimately develop crusts over the surface. Oral lesions generally follow the development of the skin lesions.

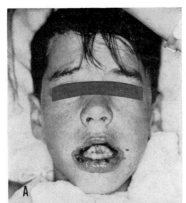

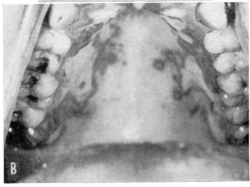

Fig. 14-20. Stevens-Johnson syndrome. *A*, Ulcerating and crusting lesions of the lips are shown. The patient has conjunctivitis and photophobia. Genital lesions were also present. *B*, The multiform red lesions on the palate surround areas of ulceration with a whitish, fibrinous exudate.

Involvement of other tissues in a symptom complex (mucocutaneous-ocular syndrome) is seen in several variations of erythema multiforme including Stevens-Johnson syndrome, Behcet's syndrome and Reiter's syndrome. These conditions all show various combinations of oral, skin, eye and genital lesions. Additionally, arthritis is seen in Behcet's and Reiter's syndromes. The most common of these, Stevens-Johnson syndrome, shows the characteristic oral lesions along with severe conjunctivitis and genital lesions (Fig. 14–20*A* and *B*).

The treatment of erythema multiforme and its variants is largely symptomatic. The use of steroids may alleviate the inflammatory phases of the reactions. Elimination of possible antigenic agents should be attempted. Healing of the skin and mucous membrane lesions occurs without scar formation although involvement of the cornea and conjunctival lesions may have serious consequences. The duration of the disease usually is a matter of weeks.

Acute Epidermal Necrolysis (Lyell's Syndrome, Ritter's Disease)

Characterized by large, transient bullae and peeling of the skin, often with mucous membrane involvement, two clinically similar forms of acute epidermal necrolysis are seen: Lyell's syndrome (toxic epidermal necrolysis) and Ritter's disease (*staphylococcal scalded-skin syndrome*). The former, seen mostly in adults, is often drug-related with several features in common with erythema multiforme. Ritter's disease, on the other hand, affects children primarily, and is associated with coagulase-positive staphylococci.

Chronic Desquamative Gingivitis (Gingivosis)

Seen in apparently healthy individuals of all ages, chronic desquamative gingivitis most commonly occurs in women about the age of menopause. This erosive disease may involve both the free and attached gingiva

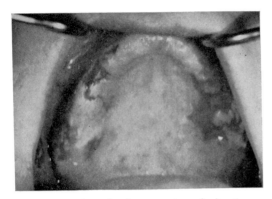

Fig. 14-21. Chronic desquamative gingivostomatitis in an edentulous middle-aged woman. Irregular areas of desquamation involved the alveolar ridge areas chiefly but extended into the mucobuccal fold and onto the buccal mucosa. Separation of the epithelium from the underlying connective tissue could be induced by heavy finger pressure. The patient did not wear artificial dentures.

or extend to other areas of the mucosa; if so, the condition might more properly be called chronic desquamative stomatitis (Fig. 14–21) and must be differentiated from erosive lichen planus and benign mucous membrane pemphigoid. In fact, several investigators believe that these conditions are all variants of the same disease process.

Chronic desquamative gingivitis appears clinically with irregular, raw red areas on both the free and attached gingiva (in contrast to marginal gingivitis). In some areas, a white surface representing remnants of desquamated epithelium can be seen. The diagnosis is based on the distribution of the lesions and the presence of a positive Nikolsky sign. Rubbing the gingiva with the finger or using a blast of compressed air from a syringe (Fig. 2–14) is usually sufficient to separate the epithelium from the underlying connective tissue.

The patient almost invariably complains of the tender areas of the mucosa and is unduly concerned that the disease could become cancer. This prospect should be firmly denied. In most instances these patients have exceptionally clean and well-cared-for mouths. The condition itself appears to have no relationship to local irritation although

the possibilities of nutritional or hormonal disturbances have been suggested.

Treatment is largely symptomatic. The use of surface protectants may provide some temporary relief. A wide variety of specific agents have been tried with varying success, including massive doses of vitamin A both systemically and topically, various steroids and other agents. The condition should be differentiated from other erosive and bullous lesions of the mucous membrane including erythema multiforme, benign mucous membrane pemphigus (pemphigoid), and pemphigus.

The prognosis of gingivosis is uncertain. Spontaneous recovery may occur, or the condition may persist for many years. The patient must be reassured that the development of other serious problems is highly unlikely.

Erosive and Bullous Lichen Planus

Erosive and bullous forms of lichen planus (Fig. 14–22) may simulate other conditions, especially chronic desquamative gingivitis (stomatitis) and benign mucous membrane

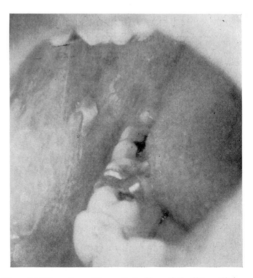

Fig. 14-22. A collapsed bulla of bullous lichen planus is shown on the buccal mucosa. There was bilateral involvement of the buccal mucosa and mucobuccal fold. Striae with annular lesions typical of lichen planus are also seen. (See also Figs. 1-24 A, B, 7-47, 11-28.)

pemphigoid. A more detailed discussion of lichen planus is given elsewhere.

Benign Mucous Membrane Pemphigoid

This rare condition is seen clinically with raw eroded surfaces which arise initially as vesicles or bullae (Fig. 14–18). Involvement is limited mainly to the mucous membranes and conjunctivae, usually in the older adult female. Histologically, the epithelial separation is subepidermal and thus is similar to the findings in chronic desquamative gingivitis, bullous pemphigoid and bullous erythema multiforme. Basement membrane antibodies may be demonstrated by immunofluorescent tests (p. 234). Although it may persist for years, this disease has a remarkably better prognosis than pemphigus and skin lesions do not develop at any stage. Intralesional injections of triamcinolone acetonide have been effective in promoting healing but do not prevent recurrences.

Bullous Pemphigoid

Seen chiefly in the elderly patient, this chronic and generally self-limiting disease exhibits large, somewhat tough and tense bullae located most often in the axilla, groin, lower abdomen and flexor surfaces of the arms. Vesicular oral lesions, which occur in approximately one-third of the cases, break down to form eroded areas similar both clinically and histologically to chronic desquamative gingivitis or benign mucous membrane pemphigoid. However, epidermal basement membrane antibodies can be demonstrated with fluorescent antibody tests (p. 234) in bullous pemphigoid.

Benign Familial Chronic Pemphigus (Hailey-Hailey Disease)

This rare, generally familial, disorder arises in adolescents or young adults as crops of vesicles chiefly on the neck and in the axilla. The vesicles rupture and secondary eroded and crusty lesions appear. Oral lesions resemble the skin lesions but are an uncommon feature of the disease.

Epidermolysis Bullosa

A rare hereditary disease, epidermolysis bullosa is characterized chiefly by the formation of bullae of the skin and mucous membranes following mild to moderate trauma. Areas subject to frequent mild trauma such as the elbows and knees develop bullae and subsequently rupture. In the milder type of the disease (epidermolysis bullosa simplex), healing takes place without scarring. In more severe types (epidermolysis bullosa dystrophica) mutilating, atrophic scars form. The former generally improves at about puberty, whereas the latter are progressive and involve the mouth and pharynx as well. Dental treatment of these patients is extremely difficult since inadvertent pressure on the lips and oral tissues causes a bullous lesion or ulcer to form. In the severest form, death occurs in the first weeks of life. No definitive treatment is known.

Pemphigus

This uncommon disease is characterized by bullae formation on any portion of the skin, mucous membrane of the oral cavity, throat or genitalia. Since the oral lesions of pemphigus may precede the appearance of the skin lesions by several weeks or months, it is particularly important, perhaps even lifesaving, that the dentist in consultation with the dermatologist establish the diagnosis and initiate treatment early.

Pemphigus is rarely encountered in patients under 30 years of age and does not exhibit any particular sex predilection. Several types of true pemphigus are recognized: pemphigus vulgaris, pemphigus vegetans, pemphigus foliaceus and pemphigus erythematosus (Senear-Usher disease).

Tense and fluid-filled, the bullae can be induced at will by heavy pressure or rubbing of the mucous membrane or skin surface (Nikolsky's sign). Lesions can also be induced as a diagnostic procedure in previously uninvolved skin within 24 hours by exposure to an erythema dose of ultraviolet

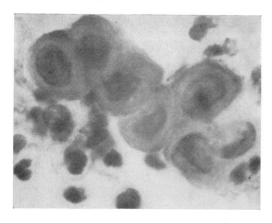

Fig. 14-23. Tzanck cells obtained from an intact bulla in a case of pemphigus. The swollen nuclei and marked hyperchromatism ("fried-egg cells") are strongly suggestive of the diagnosis which must be confirmed by other clinical and laboratory findings.

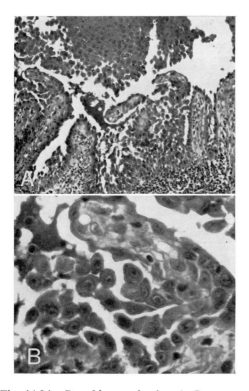

Fig. 14-24. Pemphigus vulgaris. *A*, Low-power photomicrograph showing vesicle formation and the suprabasilar split characteristic of pemphigus. Numerous acantholytic cells are present. *B*, High-power photomicrograph showing acantholytic cells at the level of the suprabasilar split.

light. Cytologic smears of material obtained from an intact vesicle exhibit Tzanck cells which are characteristic of pemphigus as well as certain other vesicular diseases (Fig. 14–23). The biopsy of an early lesion will show a suprabasilar split of the epithelium with the formation of an intraepithelial vesicle (Fig. 14–24*A, B*). Because the epithelial cells have lost cohesiveness, numerous Tzanck cells are seen within the vesicle. Intercellular antibodies may be demonstrated by immunofluorescent serology and immunohistology (p. 234).

Pemphigus generally responds to treatment with the steroids. Prior to the use of these drugs, it was almost invariably fatal.

Geographic Tongue (Benign Migratory Glossitis)

This condition is seen clinically as irregular erosive red patches on the dorsum and lateral borders of the tongue representing desquamation of the filiform papillae (Fig. 14–25). The borders of the eroded areas are slightly raised and white. The patient seldom experiences symptoms, but occasionally the reddened surfaces may be sensitive to extremes of hot and cold or to spicy food products. The irregular configuration and the tendency to heal in some areas and desquamate in others with a changing pattern over a period of days or weeks are sufficient to make the diagnosis. Some cases have been followed for many years. More commonly

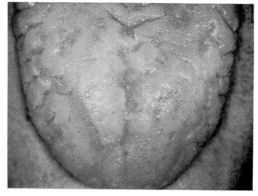

Fig. 14-25. Geographic and fissured tongue. (Courtesy of Southern P. Hooker.) (See also Figs. 7-24, 7-25.)

seen in young adults, often females, the condition is thought to be related to psychosomatic or neurogenic factors. No effective treatment is available but the nature of the condition and its possible cause should be explained to the patient. Reassurance that it is not of any serious clinical significance should be given.

Stomatitis Areata Migrans ("Ectopic Geographic Tongue," Erythema Migrans, Annulus Migrans, Migratory Stomatitis, etc.)

Lesions clinically and histologically similar to geographic tongue but occurring elsewhere on the oral mucosa are occasionally seen. They may be found in association with geographic tongue, extending onto the ventral surface of the tongue or floor of the mouth (Fig. 7–24 *C* and *D*) or separately on the buccal mucosa or lip (Fig. 7–25).

Reiter's Syndrome

This disease of young males exhibits the classic features of urethritis, arthritis, conjunctivitis and mucocutaneous lesions. The skin lesions are similar to psoriasis and the oral lesions, where present, are erythematous with a white circinate border. Because Reiter's syndrome and geographic tongue, stomatitis areata migrans and psoriasis have many clinical and histologic features in common, Weathers *et al.* have referred to them collectively as *"psoriasiform lesions."*

Stomatitis Medicamentosa

Untoward reactions of the oral mucosa to systemically administered drugs is called stomatitis medicamentosa. Drug reactions may occur because of the inherent toxicity of the drug, intolerance or idiosyncrasy to the drug or the development of an allergic response to the drug (see also p. 25).

The tissue reactions seen in stomatitis medicamentosa are quite variable and frequently non-specific. Erythematous lesions, vesicles, bullae, erosions, ulcers, secondary mycotic infections, hyperplasias or granulomatous lesions may occur depending upon the nature of the causative agent and the individual response. In addition to the oral lesions, involvement of other tissue and organ systems occurs, most notably the skin (p. 104) and the hematopoietic systems (p. 213). Because a significant number of the oral lesions are vesiculobullous or erosive, the approach to diagnosis of suspected cases of stomatitis medicamentosa is discussed here. Other types of reactions such as Dilantin hyperplasia (Fig. 7–40), bismuth gingivitis (Fig. 14–17), agranulocytosis (Fig. 14–50), angioneurotic edema (Fig. 7–14) and arsenical keratosis (p. 309) are discussed in other sections.

General features of stomatitis medicamentosa useful in establishing a diagnosis are: (1) sudden appearance of the lesions; (2) frequent involvement of other tissues and systems; (3) history of other allergies; (4) appearance of lesions subsequent to the administration of suspect drugs or medication; and (5) dissimilarity to other specific disease entities.

Considerable judgment is required in making a clinical diagnosis of stomatitis medicamentosa inasmuch as it may simulate a number of other specific disease processes. Also, withdrawal of the suspected drug for short periods does not necessarily result in the prompt improvement expected and so the tentative diagnosis is discarded. Needless to say, withdrawal of the drug should be undertaken only with the approval of the practitioner who prescribed it originally. If the primary disease being treated is of a serious nature, an effective substitute drug should be sought.

As noted, the vesiculobullous and erosive lesions of the oral cavity which follow systemic drug administration are not in themselves pathognomonic. Examples of drugs known to produce lesions of this nature in susceptible individuals are listed below.

Antibiotics, sulfa drugs
Antipyretics
Arsenic
Ataractics

Iodides, bromides
Phenolphthalein
Salicylates
Quinine, atabrine

Stomatitis Venenata

The local reaction of drugs or other substances coming in direct contact with the oral tissues is called stomatitis venenata. The

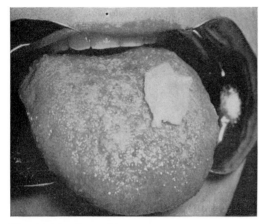

Fig. 14-26. Stomatitis venenata due to extreme overdosage of penicillin troches. When the patient appeared, the tongue was completely covered with a loose white plaque which could be peeled away readily. One piece has been placed on the tongue for illustrative purposes. Candidiasis was expected, but the material proved to be fibrin. (Mitchell and Chaudhry, J. Amer. Dent. Ass., *53,* 714, 1956.)

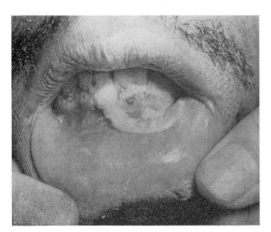

Fig. 14-27. Aspirin burn. Ulceration followed the placement of an aspirin tablet on the gingiva opposite an aching tooth. Fibrinous exudate and necrosis extended over the gingival mucosa into the mucobuccal fold of the lower lip. (See also Fig. 14-7).

agent may cause local injury directly due to its physical, chemical or toxic nature or induce an allergic response (Figs. 14–26 to 14–29). In the latter instance, the response is delayed for a time until sensitization has become established. As in stomatitis medicamentosa, the erosion induced is variable and rarely typical for a given agent.

The diagnosis is based largely on a history of exposure to a suspect agent prior to the appearance of the lesion and the ruling out of other specific disease entities. Elimination of the suspected agent should result in recovery.

A number of drugs, dental materials and cosmetic preparations used by either the dentist or the patient may occasionally give

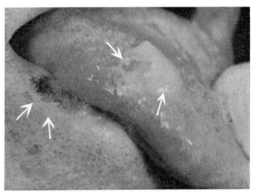

Fig. 14-28. Chemical injury (phenol burn) of tongue and lip accidentally caused by the dentist.

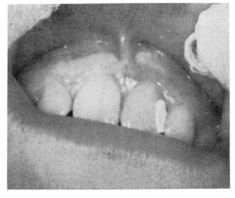

Fig. 14-29. Phenol burn. The white coagulated area on the gingival mucosa above the upper right central incisor occurred when phenol seeped under the rubber dam during root canal therapy.

rise to vesiculobullous, erosive or other oral lesions upon contact with the oral tissues. A list of some commonly used substances or drugs known to cause stomatitis venenata in susceptible individuals is given below.

> Amalgam
> Methylmethacrylate
> Anesthetic agents (injected and topical)
> Silver nitrate
> Aspirin
> Trichloroacetic acid
> Phenol
> Sodium perborate
> Lipstick
> Toothpaste, tooth powder
> Mouthwashes
> Antibiotic lozenges

PUSTULES

Pustules comparable to those seen on the skin are rarely found on the mucosa.

Parulis (Gumboil)

An abscess emerging from an underlying periapical or lateral periodontal abscess is essentially a pustule prior to opening and drainage. These appear clinically as fluctuant elevations of the soft tissue with a pe-ripheral erythematous halo. A yellow center ("point") appears just prior to spontaneous drainage (Fig. 2–15).

Chickenpox (Varicella)

Solitary pustules of chickenpox are occasionally seen on the mucous membranes along with the more characteristic skin lesions (Fig. 1–13).

Pyostomatitis Vegetans

Multiple tiny and often confluent abscesses or pustules of the oral mucous membranes and lips, followed by proliferative excrescences of the surface, characterize this unusual disease (Fig. 14–30A and B). While only a very limited number of cases have been described, nearly all such patients have had concomitant ulcerative colitis. No specific treatment of the oral lesion is known; however, treatment of the colitis is indicated.

ULCERS

For purposes of differential diagnosis, a clinical distinction should be made between ulcers and other conditions in which the cov-

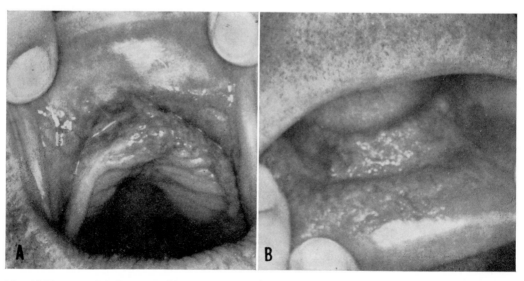

Fig. 14-30. *A* and *B*, Pyostomatitis vegetans. Roughened, erythematous areas arose under the patient's denture and spread progressively to involve the inner surfaces of the cheeks and lips. Biopsy revealed chronic inflammation and microabscesses associated with the tiny papillary projections. (Courtesy of G. Thomas Childes.)

ering epithelium may be lost, such as erosions, vesicles and bullae. Although these latter conditions may appear as ulcers at the time of examination, the clinical history and examination will generally establish their basic nature. In like manner, swellings and enlargements may ulcerate following even minor trauma, secondary infection or interference with blood supply. For example, malignant salivary gland tumors involving the hard palate typically appear as enlargements with ulceration of the surface (p. 425). Those conditions which are basically erosions, vesiculobullous diseases or enlargements, even though they exhibit ulcerated surfaces, are discussed in other sections.

Ulcers are defined as open sores. Loss of the integrity of the covering stratified squamous epithelium may follow trauma or tissue necrosis induced by infectious agents or foreign bodies.

From whatever cause, exposure of the underlying connective tissue results in inflammation with exudation of tissue fluids and accumulation of a fibrinous exudate over the surface. The exudate appears as a filmy white material which can be removed, and a bleeding surface is exposed.

Clinical evaluation of the ulcer must take into account the gross characteristics of the ulcer and surrounding mucous membranes, and the nature of the underlying tissue. The clinical history may provide important clues and should reveal duration, previous episodes of similar lesions, history of allergy or hypersensitivity reactions, concurrent diseases, previous or current drug therapy, previous radiation therapy and the patient's general systemic health.

The presenting symptoms, in particular the character of any pain, paresthesia, functional disturbance or prodromal symptom, should be recorded. These features plus the character of the ulcer itself may suggest a working diagnosis. The thickness of the fibrinous exudate and the ease with which it can be stripped from the underlying tissue should be determined. For example, the

pseudomembrane of ulceromembranous gingivitis is rather easily wiped off the surface revealing raw, dark red tissue with oozing of blood. If the exudate can be stripped cleanly from the underlying connective tissue, the character of the tissue reaction can often be estimated. Organizing granulation tissue underneath will be soft, bright red, and show a finely granular surface. On the other hand, if removal of the fibrinous exudate reveals additional tissue necrosis, foreign body or suppurative material, a specific inflammatory or infectious process is likely.

The character of the tissue surrounding the ulcer proper should be carefully examined. A number of bacterial infections will show varying degrees of erythema and edema of the surrounding mucous membrane. Viral infections in particular will show a bright red halo around a relatively small central ulceration. The margins of ulcers, especially those of long standing, are generally elevated and rolled. Such features are characteristic of epidermoid carcinoma as well as other chronic ulcers. This response represents an attempt of the epithelium to proliferate and cover the exposed connective tissue surface. If the reparative potential is reduced or the infectious agent, foreign body, neoplasm or other cause is still operative, reepithelialization will not take place.

It is imperative that all ulcers which fail to heal be investigated thoroughly and a diagnosis be established. The conditions discussed in this section are restricted to those that appear clinically as relatively uncomplicated ulcers.

Epidermoid Carcinoma

Intraoral epidermoid carcinoma is the most common malignant tumor of the oral cavity (p. 65). The dentist has a continuing responsibility to detect oral cancer at its earliest possible stage since he is trained in the examination of the oral tissues and the recognition of oral diseases. Because many patients visit the dentist on a regular basis, the dental office can be an effective detec-

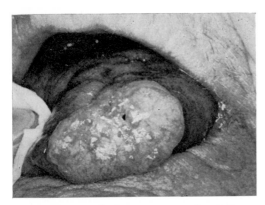

Fig. 14-31. Exophytic squamous cell carcinoma of the tip of the tongue of an 84-year-old female. The tongue is nearly hidden by the lesion.

tion center for oral cancer and skin cancer as well (p. 307).

Intraoral epidermoid carcinoma (excluding the lips) is found on the *tongue* in about one-half of the cases. In most instances, it arises on the lateral border at the posterior or the middle one-third (Fig. 7–17). It may appear as indurated ulcer, an exophytic mass, or an infiltrating mass with minimal surface changes (Fig. 14–31). Direct visual examination of the posterior lateral border of the tongue is accomplished by grasping the tongue with gauze and pulling it forward and laterally. This area of the tongue should be palpated as well.

While no single etiologic factor has been proposed for carcinoma of the tongue, poor oral hygiene, chronic trauma, alcohol and tobacco addiction, and syphilis have been associated with many cases. It is of interest that carcinoma of the dorsum of the tongue is rarely seen except when it arises in syphilitic glossitis.

Carcinoma of the floor of the mouth is the second most common site for intraoral carcinoma. Frequently, carcinoma in this location extends to involve the alveolar mucosa and the base of the tongue.

Carcinoma of the alveolar mucosa and gingiva often presents difficult diagnostic problems inasmuch as the early lesions may be mistaken for periodontal disease or other inflammatory or infectious conditions (Fig. 2–6). The gingiva may be involved primarily or by direct extension of carcinoma of the floor of the mouth or the buccal mucosa.

Carcinoma of the palate is seen most commonly on the soft palate or at the junction of the hard and soft palates. In general, ulcerated lesions that involve the hard palate represent malignant salivary gland tumors (Fig. 7–32).

Carcinoma of the buccal mucosa is found along the line of occlusion or in the mucobuccal fold. In general, the more posterior the primary site of the carcinoma in the buccal mucosa, the more highly undifferentiated the tumor. A significant number of cases of carcinoma involving the lower mucobuccal fold arise in areas of leukoplakia secondary to the use of snuff or other tobacco products (Fig. 14–32).

An interesting variety of epidermoid carcinoma which should be clinically and microscopically differentiated is the so-called *verrucous carcinoma*. These appear clinically as roughened papillary growths, often on the buccal mucosa or gingiva of middle-aged to elderly males, and are often considered to be papillomas or papillary hyper-

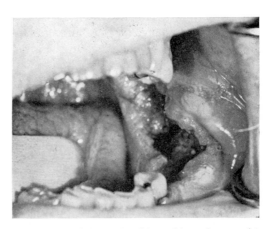

Fig. 14-32. Advanced epidermoid carcinoma with deep ulceration and indurated borders. The ulcer is full of chewing tobacco. The lesion was asymptomatic. The patient came to the dentist because of a toothache on the opposite side of the mouth. (See also Figs. 1-17, 1-19, 2-6, 7-17, 7-30, 9-3, 14-1, 14-31.)

plasias. Because they are well-differentiated lesions, the microscopic diagnosis of verrucous carcinoma is often difficult. The correlation of a diffuse, broad-based, papillary lesion with a somewhat "dirty" appearance together with comparable histologic findings would suggest the diagnosis. This variety of carcinoma shows a relatively slow growth with little tendency to invade the underlying tissues or metastasize to regional lymph nodes until late in its course. In most instances, wide surgical excision is the treatment of choice. Some reports indicate that verrucous carcinoma may undergo transition to a less well-differentiated form following radiation therapy.

Adenoid Squamous Cell Carcinoma (Adenoacanthoma, Pseudoglandular Squamous Cell Carcinoma)

This lesion occurs most commonly on the skin of the head and neck, usually in the older male patient with solar-damaged (or susceptible) skin. The tumor also may occur on the lower lip and occasionally on the upper lip. It appears typically as a hyperkeratotic or ulcerated granular lesion which may be somewhat nodular. Histologically, the lesion shows downgrowth of dysplastic epithelium with formation of tube- or duct-like structures in the deeper areas and acantholytic cells (Fig. 14–33). The tumor thus appears to be a histologic variant of the squamous cell carcinoma with a strong predilection for sun-damaged skin and lip tissue. Treatment is by surgical excision. Metastasis may occur on rare occasions.

Traumatic Ulcer

The traumatic or decubitus ulcer of the oral mucous membrane is seen most frequently in the patient with artificial dentures. Typically, these are linear ulcers with a grey, fibrinous exudate over the surface. If chronic, ulcers of this type may show a considerable amount of induration of the surrounding tissue and simulate epidermoid carcinoma. Relief of the denture or its re-

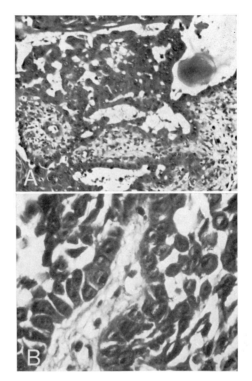

Fig. 14-33. Adenoid squamous cell carcinoma. *A,* Both squamous and duct-like epithelium are present. *B,* High-power photomicrograph of *A* showing a portion of a duct-like area with acantholytic cells.

moval entirely results in uneventful healing. It is fruitless and dangerous, however, to continue such adjustments on the ill-fitting denture indefinitely.

Traumatic ulcers seen typically along the lateral border of the tongue comprise a special group inasmuch as they frequently present difficult diagnostic problems (Fig. 7–1). Occasionally, trauma from a broken tooth or from biting the tongue will result in a large chronic ulcer which fails to heal (Fig. 14–34). The ulcer persists despite continued proliferation of the surrounding epithelium in an abortive effort to reepithelialize the surface. This results in a marked induration of the surrounding mucosal surface remarkably similar to epidermoid carcinoma. This same response may also be seen in a number of the specific granulomatous infections, particularly tuberculosis.

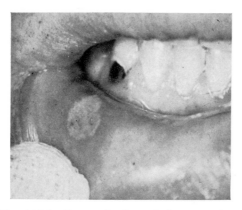

Fig. 14-34. Traumatic ulcer of the mucosal surface of the lower lip. The sharp edges of the carious lesion in lower canine oppose the ulcer.

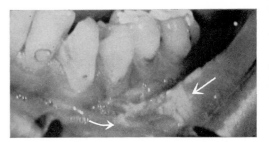

Fig. 14-36. "Cotton roll burn." The mucosa was stripped in removing a cotton roll.

patient protect it long enough for healing to take place.

Ischemic or Trophic Ulcer

Ulceration and necrosis may follow interference with blood supply to an organ or tissue. The most common ulcer of this type seen in the oral cavity occurs at the site of injection of a local anesthetic (Fig. 14–37). A large volume of the anesthetic introduced rapidly in the tissue may produce local necrosis and possibly thrombosis of local blood vessels. Because of interference of blood supply, the overlying mucosa breaks down

Quite often, the traumatic ulcer may be large and show severe induration. Although the patient may have recognized its presence for some period of time, pain or discomfort is not a significant feature. If a local irritating factor is present which can be reasonably assumed to be the cause, a short "watch and wait period" may be justified (Figs. 14–35 and 36). Even so, some traumatic ulcers will not heal even though the initial causative factor is removed. Early biopsy of the lesion is therefore justified to rule out the possibility of epidermoid carcinoma or a specific granulomatous infection. Quite often, surgical manipulation of the traumatic ulcer is sufficient to trigger the healing process even though the entire lesion was not removed. If the lesion is factitial, the operation and subsequent soreness may make the

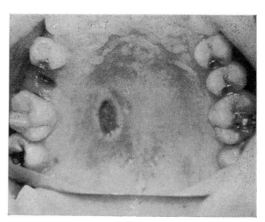

Fig. 14-37. Ischemic ulcer of the palate. This ulcer appeared following extraction of the second premolar tooth (note healing extraction site). Because of the firm, rolled border and its failure to heal, the lesion was scraped with a tongue blade and a cytologic smear prepared. The cytology report was negative for malignant cells. Healing was stimulated by the scraping procedure. The lesion was believed due to interference of blood supply by the palatal injection. (Courtesy of Walter J. Dean.)

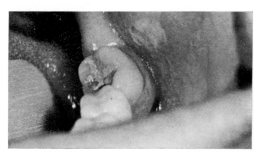

Fig. 14-35. Contact of the mucosa with an overheated contra-angle during cavity preparation resulted in a burn and subsequent ulceration.

with the formation of an ulcer. While these lesions are seen sometimes in the mucobuccal fold, a more common site is the hard palate following routine palatal injection. The volume of the anesthetic deposited in this location is frequently sufficient to lift the firm mucosa away from the bone, resulting in breakdown of the tissue. The appearance of the ulcer a few days following the operative procedure is generally sufficient evidence for the diagnosis of the ischemic ulcer. Since this lesion also may fail to heal spontaneously, a biopsy is indicated, partly to stimulate healing and partially to confirm the clinical diagnosis. In some instances, the stimulus induced by simply taking a cytologic smear is sufficient to trigger the healing process.

Necrotizing Sialometaplasia

This condition appears typically as a persistent, crateriform ulcer on the hard palate. Both the clinical features and the histologic findings may be confused with epidermoid carcinoma or mucoepidermoid carcinoma. However, the features of squamous metaplasia of the underlying salivary gland ducts (Fig. 14–38*A*) and infarction with spillage of mucus (Fig. 14–38*B*) suggest an inflammatory (traumatic) origin, probably associated with interruption of the vascular blood supply to the gland. Surgical excision, even when incomplete, results in cure.

Bednar's Aphthae (Pterygoid Aphthae)

Ulceration of the posterior palate overlying the pterygoid hamulus in infants has been referred to as Bednar's aphthae or pterygoid aphthae. Often bilateral, the lesions have been associated with thumb sucking or, at times, trauma to the region when the obstetrician clears the newborn infant's mouth and throat of mucus. Similar ulcers may occur in adults following trauma to the area, especially if the hamulus is especially prominent, or with marked alveolar ridge resorption in the edentulous patient.

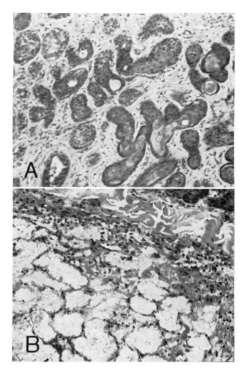

Fig. 14-38. Necrotizing sialometaplasia. *A*, An area of ductal squamous metaplasia of the palate. *B*, Necrosis and spillage of mucus are seen in this photomicrograph of another area of the lesion shown in *A*.

Riga-Fede Syndrome
(Riga's Aphthae, Cardarelli's Aphthae)

This condition refers to a form of traumatic ulcer seen on the ventral surface of the tip of the tongue, usually in infants or young children. A factitial injury, it is caused by abrasion of the tongue against the lower incisor teeth. Habit may play a role in some cases; in others, uncontrolled coughing as in whooping cough may produce the injury.

Tuberculous Ulcer

A number of specific granulomatous infections of the oral tissues may be seen clinically as non-healing ulcers. They behave as chronic disease processes characterized by the exuberant production of granulomatous tissue (pp. 53, 338, Fig. 12–4). The infectious agent induces breakdown of the overlying epithelium and the development of a chronic ulcer with a raised and rolled border. Several other specific infections such as syphilis (chancre), blastomycosis, and histoplasmosis as well as tuberculosis can exhibit these features.

Tuberculous infections occur most frequently in individuals with active pulmonary disease in which a large number of *Mycobacterium tuberculosis* organisms are present in the sputum. Thus, minor abrasions of the mucous membrane or an extraction site may serve as a point of reinfection. Hematogenous spread to the oral tissues is also possible. The typical tuberculous ulcer occurs on the lateral border of the tongue and presents a clinical appearance similar to that described for traumatic ulcer and epidermoid carcinoma. Although the history of tuberculosis may suggest the possibility of a tuberculous ulcer in the oral cavity, this cannot be established on a clinical basis. Biopsy is therefore mandatory.

As in the lungs and other sites, tuberculosis of the oral tissues may exhibit a gamut of histologic features ranging from the typical tubercle to non-specific granulomatous response, or even acute inflammation. Demonstration of acid-fast microorganisms in the histologic section is virtually diagnostic, inasmuch as other pathogenic acid-fast microorganisms are rarely found in the oral tissues. Nevertheless, chest x-ray films, sputum examination and other specific laboratory tests are indicated if the clinical diagnosis of active tuberculosis has not been made previously.

Syphilitic Ulcer (Chancre)

The primary lesion of syphilis is the chancre which occurs most commonly on the genitalia but also may occur on the lips, tongue or palate (p. 53). It is an indurated and elevated ulcer with associated unilateral lymphadenopathy. A brown crust or scab forms on the lip lesions, while in the moist environment of the mouth a whitish exudate is found over the surface. The lesions are not painful unless secondarily infected. They may last a few weeks. The rapid appearance, demonstration of *Treponema pallidum* by dark-field examination, and corroborating positive serology serve to differentiate the disease from other specific infections or carcinoma (p. 235).

Vincent's Ulcer (Vincent's Angina, Acute Necrotizing Ulceromembranous Gingivitis, ANUG)

Large, irregular, dirty-grey ulcers of the lips (Fig. 14–39), buccal mucosa or the tonsillar pillars and pharynx (Vincent's angina) may uncommonly follow the onset of acute necrotizing ulceromembranous gingivitis (p. 144). The clinical diagnosis of Vincents ulcer is supported if the characteristic pseudomembranous necrosis of the gingiva is present. Ordinarily, this is quite severe and the diagnosis is obvious. Rarely, only a single incubation zone, which will suggest the diagnosis, may be found in an interproximal space.

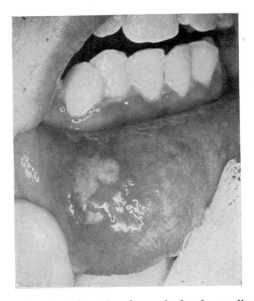

Fig. 14-39. Vincent's ulcer of the lower lip. Acute necrotizing ulceromembranous gingivitis is present along the free gingival margin. Trauma to the lip from the malposed canine resulted in an ulcer with superimposed Vincent's infection.

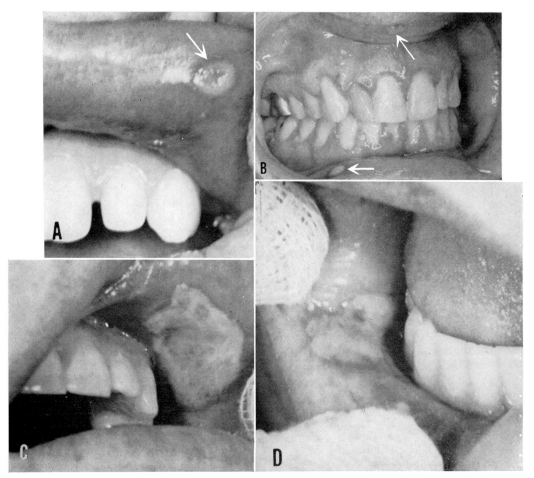

Fig. 14-40. Aphthous ulcers. *A,* Ulcer on the upper lip. *B,* Ulcers on the lips with an associated gingivitis (aphthous stomatitis). (Courtesy of H. M. Swenson and M. Gerhard.) Both cases show a typical white fibrin-coated ulcer surrounded by an erythematous halo. *C* and *D,* Large recurrent ulcers in the mouth of a young woman.

Aphthous Ulcer

The aphthous ulcer presents a typical clinical history and appearance. In most instances, patients with aphthous ulcers will report that similar ulcers have occurred with some regularity, often following minor illnesses or local trauma. These ulcers may appear as either solitary or multiple lesions, often in the floor of the mouth, the mucobuccal fold, or the ventral surface of the tongue (Fig. 14–40*A* to *D*). Less frequently, they are found on the palate or buccal mucosa (Fig. 7–33). Covered by a yellowish-white fibrinous exudate, the aphthous ulcer is generally less than 0.5 cm in diameter with a depressed center and an erythematous periphery. Many patients are able to recognize prodromal symptoms such as burning, itching or tenderness which precede the appearance of the ulcer (cf. Recurrent Herpes Simplex, p. 386).

Periadenitis Mucosa Necrotica Recurrens (Mikulicz's Aphthae, Recurrent Scarring Aphthae, Sutton's Disease, Major Aphthae)

This condition differs from the more common aphthous ulcer in that the ulcers tend to be larger and more painful, and heal by scarring. In many instances, the patient is never completely free of lesions, having at least one active ulcer at all times.

Other Infectious Ulcers

A number of other specific microorganisms may on rare occasions involve the oral tissues as ulcerations. These include diphtheria (*Corynebacterium diphtheriae*), tularemia or rabbit fever (*Pasteurella tularensis*), granuloma venereum or granuloma inguinale (*Donovania granulomatis*), histoplasmosis (*Histoplasma capsulatum*, p. 241), cryptococcosis *(Cryptococcus neoformans,* p. 240), coccidiomycosis or San Joaquin Valley fever (*Coccidioides immitis*, p. 240), and sporotrichosis (*Sporotrichium schenkii*).

In view of the increased incidence of venereal disease in recent years (see Chap. 3), *gonococcal stomatitis* must be considered in erythematous and ulcerative lesions of obscure origin. This infection, caused by the gram-negative diplococcus (*Neisseria gonorrhoeae*), may simulate major aphthae, herpetic stomatitis, Stevens-Johnson syndrome or Behcet's syndrome.

Midline Lethal Granuloma

A destructive process involving the palate, nasal cavity or face, the midline lethal granuloma has certain features in common with the collagen and autoimmune diseases. Patients may complain of stuffiness of the nose for a long time prior to actual tissue breakdown. Ulceration with deep necrosis, often arising in the posterior palate, is seen (Fig. 14–41). The differential diagnosis includes specific infections (tuberculosis, tertiary syphilis, mycotic infections), malignant lymphoma, carcinoma and noma. Histologic examination shows non-specific inflammation, vasculitis and necrosis. The disease runs a variable course with death occurring in a few weeks or months or, in some cases, after several years. The relationship to Wegener's granulomatosis (Fig. 11–24) is discussed on page 327.

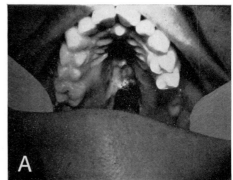
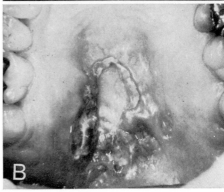

Fig. 14-41. Midline lethal granuloma. *A,* In this case, perforation of the hard palate has occurred. *B,* Another case shows ragged ulceration of the hard and soft palates. (Courtesy of William Hohlt.)

Noma (Cancrum Oris, Gangrenous Stomatitis)

Severely debilitated children, and occasionally adults, may develop a progressive necrosis of the oral soft and hard tissues which ultimately destroys large areas, perforates the cheek and often results in death from pneumonia or septicemia. Of rare occurrence, noma is readily recognized by the rapidly spreading necrosis, severe pain and odor. A mixed population of microorganisms (including oral fusospirochetes as well as others common to the oral cavity) rather than a single, specific agent is present. Broad-spectrum antibiotics, debridement, and intensive supportive care which must include correction of nutritional imbalances and systemic problems are required for effective treatment.

CYSTS AND CYST-LIKE LESIONS

Cysts are pathologic epithelial lined cavities in soft tissue or bone filled with fluid or occasionally a caseous material such as keratin or sebum.

The diagnosis of any cyst is based on the anatomic knowledge of the sites in which epithelium can be found. Most often there is no particular history involved as far as the patient is concerned. Sometimes a history of slow asymptomatic swelling is given. On occasion a cyst becomes infected and develops into an abscess which can be painful.

Diagnostic information may be obtained by aspiration, incision, exploration, excision and gross and microscopic examination of the specimen. Palpation of a cyst not covered by bone may reveal fluctuation and the rebound phenomenon. If an intrabony cyst has a thin cortical bone covering, crepitus may be felt. Syringe aspiration of the fluid content of a cyst is of considerable importance in diagnosis (Fig. 6–2). The appearance of the fluid may range from a water-clear to a straw-colored solution, or to a blood-tinged mixture. If the contents are caseous, aspiration usually is not possible. Examination of cytologic smears of the cells of the aspirate spun down in a centrifuge may be helpful.

Only the cysts and cyst-like lesions involving the oral soft tissues will be discussed in the following paragraphs. Reference should be made to appropriate sections for descriptions of other cystic lesions such as the odontogenic cysts (pp. 465–470), fissural and developmental cysts (pp. 453–455), cysts in the skin (pp. 322–324) and cystic lesions of the neck (pp. 344–345).

Palatal Cyst of the Newborn

Cystic, keratin-filled nodules are sometimes found on the alveolar ridges and hard palates of newborn infants. Those located along the midpalatine raphe and near the junction of the hard and soft palate are referred to as palatal cysts of the newborn. Presumed to be related to the development of accessory salivary gland ducts in these areas, they are distinguished from the dental lamina cysts of the newborn (p. 467).

Dental Lamina Cyst of the Newborn

These cysts occur in the alveolar ridge. The lesions have been referred to as Epstein's pearls or Bohn's nodules. No treatment is required inasmuch as they exfoliate spontaneously.

Gingival Cyst of the Adult

These cysts of the gingiva or alveolar mucosa arise from odontogenic epithelial remnants but, unlike the dental lamina cysts of the newborn, are seen in adults (see p. 467).

Cyst of the Incisive Papilla

Epithelial remnants of the nasopalatine duct most commonly give rise to cysts within the bony confines of the canal (p. 454). In some instances, however, the cyst will be located within the incisive or palatine papilla overlying the canal and may or may not be associated with cystic enlargement of the canal. In this situation, the cyst will appear as a palatal soft tissue swelling overlying the incisive foramen.

Nasolabial (Nasoalveolar, Klestadt's) Cyst

This uncommon developmental cyst is recognized by its presence in the mucobuccal fold and soft tissue of the upper lip just beneath the ala of the nose. It is treated by surgical excision.

Dermoid (Epidermoid) Cyst

The rare dermoid cyst is found in the midline of the neck or floor of the mouth as a fluid-filled swelling which may elevate the tongue much like the ranula or, if it is more deeply situated in relation to the adjacent muscle groups, appear as a rounded swelling under the chin (Fig. 11–21). Ectodermal structures found within these cysts include squamous epithelium, sebaceous glands and other skin appendages. The development of the dermoid cyst coincides with the development of the skin appendages. An analogous lesion is the so-called dermoid cyst (teratoma) of the ovary which contains structures from all embryonic layers, including teeth.

Oral Lymphoepithelial Cyst

The intraoral counterpart of the benign cervical lymphoepithelial cyst seen in the lateral neck (p. 344), this lesion is a yellowish nodule, usually in the floor of the mouth or the ventral surface of the tongue. It is composed of a cystic cavity lined by squamous epithelium contained within a lymphoid nodule. The lymphoid tissue commonly exhibits typical follicles with germinal centers. Comparable collections of lymphoid aggregates with cystic inclusions or crypts similar to the palatine tonsils are found on the lateral aspects of the tongue (Foliate Papillitis, p. 427).

Heterotopic Oral Gastrointestinal Cyst

On rare occasion misplaced (heterotopic) gastric mucosa gives rise to cystic lesions in the tongue or floor of the mouth. Such lesions represent a choriostoma (*i.e.* a developmental tumor consisting of tissues not native to the area) and are composed of gastric mucosa with parietal and chief cells much like the stomach, often with a muscularis mucosa present. Similar heterotopic cysts have been reported in the esophagus and pancreas as well.

Extraosseous Calcifying Epithelial Odontogenic Cyst (Gorlin Cyst)

Approximately one-fourth of the cases of Gorlin cyst are extraosseous lesions on the gingiva without bone involvement. In this location, they appear as firm nodules which may be secondarily inflamed or ulcerated. The histologic features and clinical behavior of the extraosseous lesions are identical to those occurring in the jaw bones.

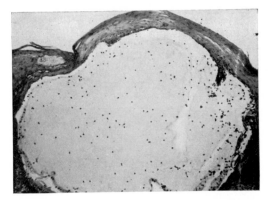

Fig. 14-42. Mucous retention phenomenon (mucocele). A mucous pool is shown distending the overlying epithelium. (Standish and Shafer, J. Oral Surg., *16,* 15, 1959.)

Mucocele (Mucous Retention Phenomenon, Mucous Retention Cyst)

Minor injury or blockage of salivary gland ducts with escape of mucus into the surrounding connective tissue gives rise to the mucocele (Fig. 1–5). The majority are not lined by epithelium but by a granulation tissue wall (Fig. 14–42). Mucocele is encountered most frequently on the inner surface of the lower lip but may occur at any site in the oral cavity where accessory salivary glands are found. If located deep in connective tissue, it may simply be represented by a swelling. When larger and nearer to the surface, the thin mucosa may be slightly bluish, translucent and obviously raised by fluid. It is usually painless.

Ranula

The ranula is a mucous retention cyst associated with Wharton's duct (Fig. 7–26). A large translucent to bluish swelling in the floor of the mouth on one side is the major diagnostic feature. The phrase "belly of a frog" is an apt clinical description. An occlusal radiograph sometimes reveals the presence of a sialolith which has blocked the duct and caused the phenomenon (Figs. 13–8 to 11). The use of the lacrimal or salivary gland duct probe (p. 115) may help locate the obstruction.

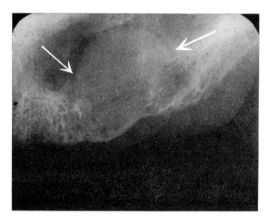

Fig. 14-43.   Retention cyst of the maxillary sinus. Most cases are discovered on routine radiographic examination. They are usually asymptomatic and require no treatment.

Antral Mucocele
(Retention Cyst of the Maxillary Sinus)

Lesions analogous to the oral mucocele may develop in the antrum. Most cases are recognized coincidentally by routine dental radiographs as dome-shaped, soft-tissue densities (Fig. 14–43). Ordinarily, the lesions are asymptomatic and frequently disappear spontaneously.

Epithelial Inclusion (Implantation) Cyst

The *inclusion* or *implantation* cyst may occur in soft or hard tissue following the surgical implantation of epithelium during an operation (Fig. 11–19). While not common, a particular type of inclusion cyst of this nature is the *surgical ciliated cyst* induced during Caldwell-Luc operations for intraoral entry to the maxillary sinus (see p. 460).

HEMORRHAGIC AND VASCULAR LESIONS

The vascular and hematologic disorders often exhibit oral lesions of diagnostic importance. Inasmuch as a number of these diseases are extremely serious, most notably the hemorrhagic diatheses and the leukemias, they must be differentiated from the several inflammatory, traumatic, infectious, and other local conditions known to exhibit similar signs and symptoms. In some cases, a limited period of local therapy may be undertaken but, if a prompt response is not obtained, appropriate laboratory tests or other diagnostic methods should be performed without further delay (pp. 216–219 and 411–412).

General Features

Considerable reliance must be placed on the history, the distribution of the lesions and the general physical condition of the patient in deciding whether the oral changes are of local or systemic origin.

A *history* of anemia or other previously diagnosed blood dyscrasia would of course strongly support but not confirm a provisional diagnosis of vascular or hematologic disease. Intensive questioning of the patient regarding previous or current drugs taken is often profitable in the clinical diagnosis of suspected blood disease, since it is not unusual for a patient to be under active treatment for a condition of which he is not aware. For example, anticoagulant therapy (coumarin derivatives, heparin, indandione derivatives) is most commonly employed in cases of thromboembolic diseases (p. 415) such as myocardial infarction, thrombophlebitis, suspected pulmonary embolism and cerebral thrombosis. Iron, vitamin B_{12} or folic acid therapy would suggest that the patient probably is being treated for iron-deficiency anemia, pernicious anemia or a malabsorption syndrome such as sprue. Antimetabolites (methotrexate, mercaptopurine, 5-flurouracil); alkylating agents (nitrogen mustard, triethylene melamine, and cytotoxin); steroid hormones (cortisone, ACTH, estrogen, androgen); certain antibiotics (actinomycin D, streptomycin) or radioisotope treatment are most commonly employed in leukemia or other malignant lymphomas, other disseminated or inoperable malignant diseases and certain thyroid diseases.

Several of the antimetabolites, especially methotrexate, cause oral ulcerations. The onset of the ulcers is used as a guide to determine the maximum tolerable dose of the agent. In addition, several drugs used in the treatment of a number of unrelated conditions cause agranulocytosis, thrombocytopenia or aplastic anemia (p. 408). Common offenders are certain antipyretic agents (aminopyrine, phenylbutazone), tranquilizers (chlorpromazine, other phenothiazine compounds), antithyroid drugs (thiourea derivatives), some antibiotics (chloramphenicol, streptomycin) and the sulfonamides.

A history of chronic blood loss (bleeding peptic ulcer, hemorrhoids, abnormal menstrual bleeding) or recent severe hemorrhage may be obtained in iron-deficiency anemia. Prolonged hemorrhage or delayed healing following simple wounds, while not pathognomonic of a particular disorder, must be investigated prior to definitive treatment. Frequently, excessive bleeding reported by a patient following previous tooth extraction is due to local causes; however, the examining dentist cannot safely make this assumption.

The *distribution of the lesions* in the mouth is often helpful in ruling out local inflammatory or vascular disease. For the most part, diffuse involvement of the gingiva or other areas of the oral cavity is suggestive of a generalized disease process, whereas the solitary lesion is most apt to be due to local disease.

The overall *physical condition of the patient* can sometimes provide a basis for judgment of the oral lesions in suspected generalized vascular or hematologic disorders. Excessive fatigue, shortness of breath, hypertension, pallor, a flushed or ruddy complexion, telangiectasia, ecchymoses or petechiae, clubbing of the fingers, or cyanosis justify referral for a physical examination.

Oral Manifestations

Pallor, redness, petechiae, purpura, hemorrhage, hyperplasia, ulceration or necrosis of the oral mucous membranes are the clinical lesions seen most commonly in the vascular and hematologic disorders. As has been noted, such lesions are not in themselves pathognomonic since other disease entities may show similar changes. Each of the above is discussed in the following paragraphs with this point in mind.

Pallor of the mucous membranes is not generally obvious on casual oral inspection. Usually, attention is directed first to paleness of the skin. Iron-deficiency anemia, aplastic anemia and the leukemias frequently cause pallor of the oral mucous membranes. Patients with congestive heart failure and congenital cardiac defects may also show oral pallor, marked cyanosis of the lips, shortness of breath and clubbing of the fingers.

Redness of the mucous membranes along with marked ruddiness of the skin is seen in polycythemia vera. The tremendous numbers of circulating red blood cells and the associated vascular congestion account for the redness (p. 408). Localized erythematous lesions such as erythroplasia, simple inflammation and the predominantly vascular lesions (*e.g.* pyogenic granuloma, peripheral giant cell reparative granuloma and hemangioma) are not likely to be confused with polycythemia since these tend to be focal. Hunter's glossitis, seen in pernicious anemia, is characterized by a red, shiny and bald tongue.

Petechial hemorrhages accompany a reduction in platelets (which plug minor breaks in the capillary walls) or disturbances in vascular integrity (Figs. 14–44, 45). Petechiae

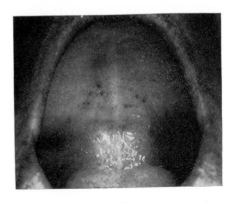

Fig. 14-44. **Palatal petechiae.**

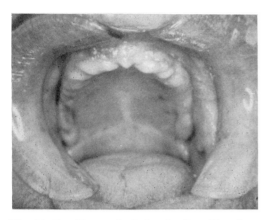

Fig. 14-45. Monocytic leukemia. Petechiae (secondary to thrombocytopenia) and ulcers (secondary to chemotherapy) developed beneath patient's denture. The patient died of the disease 1 month later. (Courtesy of Joe G. White.)

appear clinically as punctate spots representing minute extravasations of blood from capillaries (Fig. 7-31).

Petechial hemorrhages are typically seen in primary and secondary thrombocytopenia, thrombocythemia, thrombocytopathia, thrombocytasthenia, scurvy, hereditary hemorrhagic telangiectasia, certain connective disorders and infectious mononucleosis (Fig. 14-46).

Purpura or ecchymoses represent a more severe extravasation of blood into the tissue spaces and may be seen in many of the diseases exhibiting petechial hemorrhage. (Hematoma, which is usually of traumatic ori-

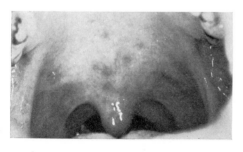

Fig. 14-46. Infectious mononucleosis ("kissing disease"). Palatal petechiae, lymphadenopathy (p. 339), gingivitis, occasional oral ulcers and systemic symptoms (fever, chills, malaise, etc.) are suggestive of the diagnosis. The Paul-Bunnell test (p. 234) was positive.

gin, represents a mass or swelling composed of extravasated blood.) It follows therefore that abnormal hemorrhage of this nature may indicate a disturbance in platelets, an abnormality of the vascular wall or a defect in the blood clotting mechanism. Spontaneous hemorrhage, hematoma or excessive postextraction hemorrhage is commonly seen in polycythemia, scurvy, thrombocytopenia, the acute leukemias, aplastic and pernicious anemia and hemophilia (Fig. 1-20). Other hemorrhagic diseases may be caused by disturbances or deficiencies of any of the recognized blood clotting factors described on pages 215–217.

Hyperplasia of the gingival tissues is seen in certain of the vascular and hematologic disorders, chiefly the leukemias, polycythemia, aplastic anemia and scurvy. In general, the enlargement is due to the increased blood cell infiltrate and/or an abnormal repair response to injury. Differentiation from simple hyperplastic gingivitis may be difficult (Fig. 7-41). Failure of the tissues to respond to adequate periodontal treatment within a reasonable period makes additional diagnostic procedures mandatory. Other forms of gingival hyperplasia, such as Dilantin gingivitis (Fig. 7-40) or hereditary gingival fibromatosis (Fig. 7-39), are more easily differentiated on the basis of the history and the absence of a significant inflammatory component.

Ulceration and *necrosis* of the oral tissues, especially the gingiva, are characteristic of agranulocytosis (Fig. 14-50), aplastic anemia and leukemic gingivitis. In each of these conditions there are inadequate numbers of mature neutrophils present to respond normally to minor injury and infection. In contrast, noma (cancrum oris) and midline lethal granuloma (Fig. 14-41) generally involve the buccal mucosa or palate as large but discrete destructive processes. Vincent's infection (ulceromembranous gingivitis) typically involves the interdental areas and free gingiva (Fig. 7-43) although other tissues, commonly the tonsillar regions, may exhibit pseudomembrane formation and necrosis (Fig. 2–11).

Red Blood Cell Disorders

Polycythemia

Persistent elevation of the circulating red blood cells occurs secondarily to reduced oxygen tension (secondary polycythemia) in individuals living at high altitudes, or primarily (polycythemia vera) as a neoplastic proliferation of red blood cells analogous to leukemia. Polycythemia vera is more commonly found in adult males. Its onset is gradual and the duration of the disease may be as long as 10 to 20 years. Myelogenous leukemia may further complicate the disease in its terminal stages. It is characterized clinically by the ruddy, congested appearance of the skin and mucous membranes and associated symptoms of dizziness and fatigue. The red blood count may show elevations as high as 10 million or more cells per cubic millimeter. In addition to the thrombocytopenia usually present, the platelets are presumably abnormal thereby accounting in part for the spontaneous gingival hemorrhage seen. Thrombosis is a common complication.

The treatment consists of phlebotomy and/or depression of bone marrow activity by radiation or antimetabolites.

Anemia

Several types of anemia may exhibit oral lesions, chiefly pallor, glossitis and atrophy of the mucosal surface (Fig. 14–47).

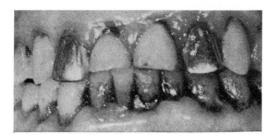

Fig. 14-47. Anemia. Spontaneous gingival hemorrhage is widespread throughout the mouth.

Iron-deficiency Anemia

The most common type of anemia, iron-deficiency anemia, occurs typically in middle-aged women. In addition to the generalized pallor of the skin and mucosa, there is patchy loss of tongue papillae. Severe cases exhibit a painful, burning tongue.

Plummer-Vinson Syndrome

Seen most frequently in women at or past menopause, Plummer-Vinson syndrome consists of a hypochromic-microcytic (iron-deficiency) anemia, achlorhydria, and atrophy of the oral and pharyngeal mucous membranes (p. 66). The patients complain of dysphagia, xerostomia, and angular cheilosis, and the tongue is smooth and red. A lemon-yellow pallor of the skin is present and there is koilonychia (spoon-shaped fingernails). A higher incidence of oral and pharyngeal epidermoid carcinoma is seen in such patients than in unaffected patients.

Pernicious Anemia

This form of anemia is a macrocytic hyperchromic anemia seen chiefly in middle-aged adults. Glossitis, weakness, pallor and neurologic disturbances are the usual presenting signs and symptoms. The tongue is fiery red and shows loss of papillae, with erosion and ulcers on occasion. Tingling or paresthesia of the limbs accompanies the other signs and is helpful in ruling out nutritional deficiencies such as pellagra or the other macrocytic anemias such as *sprue* (steatorrhea). Sprue shows oral manifestations similar to pernicious anemia; however, it may occur in children as well as adults and is improved with folic acid therapy. Pernicious anemia is treated with vitamin B_{12}.

Aplastic Anemia

Aplastic anemia follows depression of bone marrow activity and therefore shows a reduction in all the formed elements of the blood. Accordingly, anemia, leukopenia and thrombocytopenia are present and account for the features of pallor, weakness, purpura, hemorrhage and necrosis of the mucous membranes.

Sickle-cell Anemia

A hereditary (dominant, non-sex-linked) form of anemia seen chiefly in Negroes, sickle-cell anemia (and sickle-cell trait) is characterized by red blood cells which assume bizarre (sickle or moon-shaped) forms when exposed to low oxygen tension (Fig. 9–5). The red cells undergo some hemolysis since they are quite fragile. The sickle-cell trait (heterozygotes) is found in about 1 of 10 Negroes who generally show no clinical symptoms. Of those with the abnormal hemoglobin, only about 5 percent have sickle-cell anemia (homozygotes). In addition to malaise, pallor, easy fatigability and jaundice, individuals with sickle-cell anemia have an increased tendency for thrombus formation and exhibit bizarre radiographic changes, chiefly a widening of the diploe or a "hair-on-end" radiographic change of the outer table of the calvaria (Fig. 14–48). Some reduction in trabeculation in the jaw bones also occurs. Widening of the marrow cavity in the long bones occurs with thinning of the cortex, perhaps as a result of hyper-

plasia of the bone marrow. This form of anemia has a generally good prognosis although occasional transfusions may be required.

Thalassemia (Erythroblastic, Mediterranean, Cooley's Anemia)

Seen chiefly in children of Italian, Greek, or Mediterranean nationalities, erythroblastic anemia follows an autosomal recessive hereditary pattern. Depending upon the pattern of inheritance, the disease may be manifest in a severe, usually fatal form (thalassemia major) or a mild, often asymptomatic

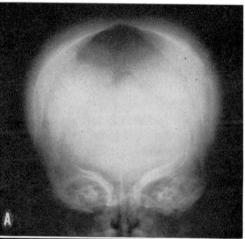

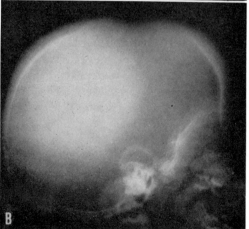

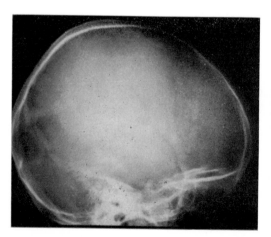

Fig. 14-48. Sickle-cell anemia. Widening of the diploe of the cranium is shown. Erythropoietic activity of the marrow may produce the changes shown or the classical "hair-on-end" effect. (Courtesy of Franklin S. Weine.)

Fig. 14-49. Thalassemia. *A,* AP radiograph showing changes in the diploe. *B,* Lateral headplate showing distortion of the cranium. Marrow activity in the maxilla and zygomatic bones causes enlargement of the middle portions of the face. (Courtesy of Franklin S. Weine.)

form (thalassemia minor). Generally, the children exhibit pallor, weakness and other signs of anemia. An associated hepatosplenomegaly may accompany the disease. Prominent malar bones, depression of the bridge of the nose and protuberance of the premaxilla give the child a mongoloid facial appearance. The long bones have a widened marrow cavity with a thin cortex due to hyperactivity of the hematopoietic marrow. The jaws also show some alterations in trabecular pattern but the most dramatic changes are those seen in the calvaria with widened diploe or "hair-on-end" effect similar to that seen in sickle-cell anemia (Fig. 14–49). The laboratory findings show a microcytic hypochromic type of anemia with "target cells," characteristic "safety-pin" cells, and an associated leukocytosis.

Erythroblastosis Fetalis

A congenital hemolytic anemia due to Rh factor sensitivity, erythroblastosis fetalis occurs in infants born of an Rh positive male parent and Rh negative female parent. The Rh positive blood factor of the child acts as an antigen to sensitize the mother through transfer through the placenta. While the first child is generally not affected, with subsequent pregnancies the anti-Rh agglutinins of the mother may hemolyze the red blood cells of the infant. The child demonstrates ascites and jaundice with blood and bile pigmentation of various tissues including the brain (kernicterus) and teeth. The teeth show a brownish-green discoloration. A newborn with this condition has large numbers of circulating immature red blood cells (in an attempt to maintain a normal RBC count) and exhibits extramedullary hematopoiesis in the liver and spleen.

White Blood Cell Disorders

Agranulocytosis

A marked reduction of circulating granulocytes characterizes agranulocytosis. The condition may arise secondarily to drug idio-

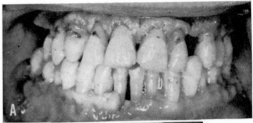
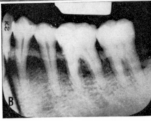

Fig. 14-50. Agranulocytosis. *A,* Severe gingivostomatitis resulted in the loss of soft gingival tissues and exposure of alveolar bone. The necrotic bone has been removed from the lower left quadrant. *B,* Radiograph from the same case showing a "splint" of sequestrating bone. (Swenson, Redish and Manne, J. Periodont., *36,* 466, 1965.)

syncrasy, or to ingestion of toxic chemical agents, or may follow overwhelming infections. Less commonly, cases arise primarily and without apparent cause. The most outstanding clinical feature of agranulocytosis is severe ulceration and necrosis of the mucous membranes (Fig. 14–50). Because of the reduced numbers of neutrophils, minor injuries fail to heal and bacterial invasion occurs. Similar infections can also develop on the skin.

Cyclic Neutropenia

This unusual condition involves a periodic and precipitous drop in the circulating neutrophils approximately every 21 days. At this time, severe inflammation of the gingiva and other oral tissues occurs and persists until the neutrophil count rises. Since the period of neutropenia is relatively short, necrosis is not ordinarily seen. The recurring nature of the disease suggests the diagnosis, which must be confirmed by white cell counts taken at intervals throughout the cycle.

Leukemia

The appearance of malignant cells of the leukocyte series in the circulating blood is called leukemia. Acute and chronic forms occur. The leukemias may be further classified as *myelogenous, lymphocytic* and *monocytic,* depending upon the primary cell type involved. Highly undifferentiated forms are called *stem cell leukemia.* The leukemias are generally classified as malignant lymphomas and differ chiefly from lymphosarcoma, reticulum cell sarcoma and Hodgkin's disease in that the malignant cells are found in the circulating blood in the former and are confined mainly to lymph nodes in the latter diseases (p. 340).

Since the massive proliferation of the malignant white blood cells in the marrow crowds out the red blood cells and platelets, patients with leukemia commonly exhibit anemia and thrombocytopenia as well. Hemorrhage, necrosis and marked gingival hyperplasia (leukemic gingivitis) are frequently seen in acute leukemia, particularly monocytic leukemia. Gingival involvement (Fig. 14–51) is usually less marked in the chronic forms of the disease.

The diagnosis is established by peripheral white blood cell count and bone marrow studies (p. 215). In *aleukemic leukemia,* the peripheral blood count may be normal or even subnormal; however, atypical precursor cells are found in the marrow.

The prognosis of the leukemias is poor, particularly for the acute forms of the disease. On the other hand, the elderly patient with chronic lymphocytic leukemia may survive for several years.

Infectious Mononucleosis ("Kissing Disease")

The oral lesions of infectious mononucleosis consist of palatal petechiae, erythematous areas of the oropharynx, and occasional generalized stomatitis with necrosis similar to that seen in agranulocytosis (Fig. 14–46). Common in teenagers and young adults, the disease exhibits features of a generalized infectious process with associated lymphadenopathy (p. 339). Atypical circulating lymphocytes and a positive heterophile agglutination (Paul Bunnell) test confirm the diagnosis (p. 234).

Differentiation of the Platelet, Coagulation and Vascular Integrity Disorders

The recognition of potential hemorrhagic problems in the dental patient must be made in advance of definitive therapy in order to avoid serious and sometimes life-threatening complications. Evaluation is based on the clinical findings, history and, where indicated, selected screening tests for the hemorrhagic diatheses (Table 9–3, p. 219). Fundamental to the diagnosis is a basic understanding of the blood coagulation mechanism (Fig. 9–7) and the recognition of pathognomonic features characteristic of disorders of this system.

Platelets of adequate number and quality physically plug breaks in the vessell wall and form the early hemostatic plug. The stability of the plug is dependent in part on the integrity of the vessel wall (endothelial cells, cement substance, perivascular connective tissue) and its ability to contract. The clotting factors are activated through a cascade reaction to produce the fibrin clot. Ultimately, the clot is lysed through action of the fibrinolytic system. If these basic points are kept in mind, it can usually be determined from a synthesis of the clinical findings and history whether the disorder is an essentially *physical* bleeding defect (involving platelets

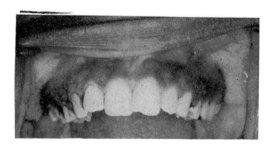

Fig. 14-51. Leukemia in a 17-year-old female with spontaneous gingival hemorrhage.

or vascular integrity) or a *biochemical* defect (involving the clotting factors). *Disorders of the platelets or vascular disturbances* characteristically show petechiae, especially on mucosal surfaces, and multiple small superficial ecchymoses. Persistent and frequently profuse bleeding may occur from simple cuts. Acquired platelet defects may have a history of drug therapy. The *coagulation disorders (coagulopathies)*, on the other hand, commonly exhibit delayed bleeding from wounds such as extraction sites, extensive hematomas, deep bleeding into joint spaces and large, superficial ecchymoses. Bleeding from small scratches or cuts is generally minimal. The hereditary coagulation defects occur in males and there is typically a family history of a bleeding tendency. Acquired coagulation defects may have a history of anticoagulant therapy or liver disease.

Platelet Disorders

Thrombocytopenia (Thrombocytopenic Purpura)

Abnormal reductions in the number of circulating platelets occur in (1) primary thrombocytopenia (Werlhof's disease, purpura hemorrhagica, idiopathic purpura), probably an autoimmune disease, and (2) secondary thrombocytopenia, a disease of multiple etiologies.

The diagnosis of idiopathic or primary thrombocytopenia is made by exclusion of a causative factor for the reduced numbers of platelets (less than 60,000/mm³). Among the more common etiologic factors in secondary thrombocytopenia are drug sensitivity or idiosyncrasy, myelophthisis, (replacement of bone marrow by leukemic cells, tumor cells metastatic to the bone marrow, osteopetrosis or myelofibrosis), certain systemic infections (*e.g.* tuberculosis, measles, infectious hepatitis, infectious mononucleosis, etc.), x-radiation or radiomimetic (chemotherapeutic) agents and hypersplenism.

Since adequate numbers of platelets are necessary to physically plug minor breaks in the capillary walls, both forms of thrombocytopenia are accompanied by petechial hemorrhages, especially of the palate and skin, and ecchymoses. Gingival bleeding, epistaxis and hematuria are common.

Thrombocythemia

Increased numbers of circulating blood platelets may occur as a transitory reactive thrombocytosis or secondary thrombocythemia in response to exercise, surgery, infections or other demands on the hematopoietic system. Primary or "essential" thrombocythemia, of unknown etiology, is characterized by platelet counts 10 to 15 times normal with epistaxis, gastrointestinal hemorrhage and thrombosis. Most patients exhibit splenomegaly. Gingival bleeding is characteristic and post-extraction hemorrhage may be severe.

The basis for the bleeding problems in thrombocythemia is not clear, although it has been proposed that the excessive numbers of platelets interfere in some way with thromboplastin release.

Thrombocytopathia (Thrombocytopathic Purpura)

One of the disorders of platelet function, thrombocytopathia, is characterized by epistaxis, ecchymoses, gastrointestinal tract bleeding and spontaneous gingival bleeding. Bruises on the skin occur readily and women with this disorder may experience severe menstrual bleeding. The platelet count is normal; however, the bleeding time is prolonged, probably because of defective platelet aggregation and release of platelet factor III (PF-3).

Thrombocytasthenia (Glanzmann's Thrombasthenia, Familial Thrombasthenia)

This qualitative defect of platelets exhibits a normal platelet count and clotting time but both bleeding time and clot retraction time are markedly prolonged. The disorder is caused by defective ADP-induced platelet aggregation. The clincial features are similar to those seen in thrombocytopathia.

Disorders of Vascular Integrity

Hereditary Hemorrhagic Telangiectasia (Rendu-Osler-Weber Disease)

This familial disorder is characterized by spider-like telangiectasias which appear over the face, neck, lips and nasal and oral mucous membranes, beginning about puberty (Figs. 7–8, 14–52). Because of the fragility of the small capillary walls and/or the perivascular connective tissue, hemorrhage from the nose (epistaxis) or the gingival tissue is common. Bleeding from the spider nevi may be surprisingly difficult to control. Bleeding and clotting times are normal (p. 217).

Vitamin C Deficiency (Scurvy)

The classical signs of scurvy have been known for several centuries: gingival bleeding with hyperplasia and ulceration, foul breath, loosening and exfoliation of the teeth, poor bone and soft tissue wound healing, and subcutaneous and subperiosteal hemorrhages.

Petechiae are seen in the skin, particularly around hair follicles and the inner surface of thighs, and on the palate. Bleeding is due to poorly formed collagen and intercellular

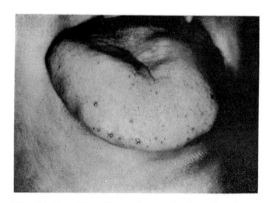

Fig. 14-52. Hereditary hemorrhagic telangiectasia. The lesions blanch under pressure but do not disappear completely. Epistaxis is the most common symptom. The vascular nevi were also present on the palate, buccal mucosa and hands (see Fig. 7-8).

cementing substance, resulting in defective perivascular supporting tissues and endothelial lining.

Other Vascular Integrity Disorders

Numerous other conditions, collectively referred to as the *non-thrombocytopenic purpuras*, may cause bleeding diatheses. Purpuras associated with vascular abnormalities (adapted from Wintrobe) are listed below, with representative examples.

> Autoimmune vascular purpuras
> Allergic purpuras (anaphylactoid purpura, Henoch-Schönlein purpura)
> Drug-induced vascular purpura
> Phenacetin, aspirin, iodides, penicillin, etc.
> Infections
> Scarlet fever, endocarditis, measles, etc.
> Structural malformations
> Hereditary hemorrhagic telangiectasia, osteogenesis imperfecta, Ehlers-Danlos syndrome, other connective tissue disorders
> Senile purpura
> Miscellaneous
> Paraproteinemias (Waldenstrom's macroglobulinemia, p. 225)
> Autoerythrocyte sensitization
> Vicarious bleeding, stigmata

Hereditary Coagulation Disorders

Recognized for centuries as "bleeder's disease," "disease of kings" or "disease of the Hapsburgs," hemophilia is the most common of the several hereditary coagulation disorders. Manifest in males and transmitted by unaffected females as a sex-linked recessive trait, it is of serious concern to the dentist and patient. Fortunately, most patients are aware of their disease and inform the dentist in advance of any anticipated operative procedures. If tooth extraction or other surgical procedure is planned, the patient should be hospitalized, the precise clotting factor deficiency determined and appropriate sera made available.

With certain exceptions, the various types of hemophilia as well as other clotting factor disorders show generally similar clinical signs and symptoms (p. 219).

Hemophilia A (AHG Deficiency, Factor VIII Deficiency)

Patients with this disease exhibit persistent bleeding which may be spontaneous or follow even minor injury. Subcutaneous hemorrhage or hematoma, ecchymosis and painful hemarthrosis, including the temporomandibular joint, are characteristic. The eruption and exfoliation of teeth may be accompanied by hemorrhage persisting for several days or even weeks. Primary hemostasis of minor surgical procedures generally is normal but delayed bleeding may occur after several hours or days. Thus, tooth extraction, tonsillectomy or other procedures are hazardous unless appropriate hematologic therapy is employed.

A tentative diagnosis of hemophilia may be established by the history, clinical features and selected screening tests (Table 9–3). In such cases of "presumptive" hemophilia, more definitive coagulation factor tests may be run to confirm the diagnosis.

von Willebrand's Disease (Vascular Hemophilia, Pseudohemophilia)

The most common of the hereditary coagulation disorders, von Willebrand's disease is frequently discovered in the male infant at the time of circumcision and in the female at puberty with the onset of unusually heavy menses. This sex-linked autosomal dominant trait differs from hemophilia in several respects. It occurs in both males and females and may be transmitted by either sex. Prolonged bleeding time, mild to moderate deficiency of factor VIII and alteration of platelet adhesiveness to glass are frequent findings. An important diagnostic feature is the unusual increase in factor VIII levels following administration of normal plasma, indicating a defect in a precursor form.

Hemophilia B (Christmas Disease)

A factor IX (PTC) deficiency, this disorder is similar to hemophilia A in both its genetic transmission (X-linked recessive) and its clinical features.

Hemophilia C

Hemophilia C is due to factor XI (PTA) deficiency and is autosomal recessive. For the most part, its clinical manifestations are less severe than other forms of hemophilia in that spontaneous hemorrhage and hemarthrosis are uncommon; however, postoperative bleeding may be quite severe.

Other Hereditary Coagulation Disorders

Other hereditary factor deficiencies are listed in Table 9–3.

Acquired Coagulation Disorders

In contrast to the hereditary disorders in which the deficiency nearly always is of a single factor, the acquired coagulation disorders may be combination defects of perhaps several clotting factors and/or platelets and vessels as well.

Biosynthesis by the liver of the vitamin K-dependent factors prothrombin, VII, IX and X may be impaired by vitamin K deficiency or functional liver disease. Related coagulopathies also occur with anticoagulant therapy, pathologic circulating anticoagulants, "consumption coagulopathy" and, additionally, exaggerated fibrinolysis.

Vitamin K Deficiency

Vitamin K is fat soluble, synthesized in part by normal intestinal flora and absorbed from the gut, along with vitamins A and D, through the action of bile salts. Thus, vitamin K deficiency of varying degrees may occur with impaired bacterial synthesis (secondary to antibiotic and sulfonamide therapy) and in the *"malabsorption syndromes,"* sprue, celiac disease, cystic fibrosis and biliary obstructions.

Liver Disease

Biosynthesis of clotting factors prothrombin, VII, IX and X, bile production for absorption of vitamin K, and clearance of intrinsic activators of fibrinolysin are normal liver functions. These mechanisms may be impaired in cirrhosis, hepatitis, obstructive liver disease or congenital malformations of the biliary tree.

Anticoagulant Therapy

Anticoagulants (chiefly coumarin), heparin, thrombolytic drugs and inhibitors of platelet function are used in the control of thromboembolic disease states. Coumarin, a competitive inhibitor of vitamin K, produces deficiencies (or abnormal forms) of prothrombin and factors VII, IX and X. Heparin, given parenterally in acute pulmonary embolism, does not affect synthesis of blood clotting factors but does interfere directly with several reactions of blood clotting in the intrinsic and common pathways (Table 9–3). The thrombolytic agents are proteolytic enzymes which activate plasminogen (p. 216). Inhibitors of platelet function, such as aspirin and dextran, modify platelet aggregation and release of platelet factors.

Bleeding due to the use of anticoagulants may complicate oral surgical procedures unless appropriate control measures are taken in cooperation with the patient's physician to monitor the anticoagulant dosage. For example, the return of clotting factor levels to normal after discontinuation of coumarin may require several days. However, if vitamin K is given, the levels may return to normal by 48 hours. The risk of thromboembolism, particularly in the patient with an artificial heart valve, must be assessed if the patient's anticoagulant therapy is to be modified.

Circulating Anticoagulants

Pathologic inhibitors of coagulation, present in several clinical conditions, may compromise the hemostasis mechanism. Antibodies to factor VIII and more rarely factors IX, V, XI and XIII are recognized as well as a factor X antibody associated with lupus erythematosus (p. 329). Patients with liver disease, multiple myeloma and other paraproteinemias may produce antithrombins as well.

Disseminated Intravascular Coagulation (DIC, Consumption Coagulopathy)

This complex and poorly understood disorder represents a disturbance in normal intravascular coagulation and fibrinolytic balance. Under normal circumstances platelets continuously plug tiny breaks in the vessel walls and fibrin strands are continuously deposited on the vessel walls. These minute "clots" are simultaneously lysed by the fibrinolytic system. DIC may occur when this balance is altered. For example, a generalized vasculitis with its widespread endothelial injury triggers extensive platelet aggregation and fibrin deposition. Thus, platelets and fibrin are used up or "consumed" at a rapid rate with resulting hemorrhagic complications. Over 50 diseases and conditions have been associated with DIC, notably obstetric complications, infections, neoplasms (prostate, lung, pancreas, etc.), transfusion of incompatible blood, anaphylaxis and vascular disorders. Nalbandian *et al.* propose that consumption coagulopathy may manifest itself clinically as one of three types: predominately with activation of coagulation, predominately with activation of fibrinolysis or with simultaneous coagulation and fibrinolysis. These types can be recognized by appropriate laboratory tests and, once the specific type of DIC is identified, lifesaving measures can be instituted.

Fibrinolysis

Factor XIII, or fibrin stabilizing factor, polymerizes the fibrin clot into a stable structure. Clot lysis is mediated by the plasminogen (fibrinolytic) system. Abnormal clot lysis, causing delayed postoperative bleeding, may be associated with endogenous activation of fibrinolysin (stress, catecholamine release, aspirin administration, etc.) or absence of anti-plasmin (liver disease). Treatment is by administration of ϵ aminocaproic acid.

Lesions of Blood and Lymph Vessels

Hemangioma

The best known of the predominately vascular lesions seen in the oral cavity is the hemangioma which may be either of a capillary or cavernous type, depending upon the size of the vascular spaces present (Figs. 1–16 and 7–27). Many cases are present at birth and behave more as hyperplastic growths or hamartomas than neoplasms. Some of these undergo involution. Others become clinically manifest at later ages. Hemangioma of bone is discussed on page 483.

The hemangiomas may be flat and diffuse or circumscribed and elevated above the adjacent mucosal surface. They have a soft consistency, are red to bluish-purple and blanch upon palpation. Thrombus formation sometimes occurs within the vascular mass (Figs. 14–54, 7–27). The lips, tongue and cheek are common intraoral sites for the hemangioma (Figs. 14–53, 14–57B). Large lesions of the lips and tongue may interfere seriously with speech or deglutition (see Macrocheilia, p. 430; Macroglossia, p. 431). The smaller hemangiomas can usually be safely removed by surgical excision, while the larger, diffuse cases are often treated with sclerosing agents, cryotherapy or irradiation.

Nevus Flammeus

The *nevus flammeus* or "port-wine stain" is a superficial hemangioma seen commonly

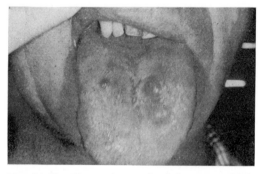

Fig. 14-53. Hemangiomatosis of the tongue. Multiple bluish-purple lesions are present over the dorsal surface of the tongue.

on the skin of newborn infants. Such birthmarks are quite disfiguring, particularly when they occur on the face. In the past, these have been treated by radiation therapy. Even though the lesion responds dramatically to this treatment, the radiation unfortunately may arrest tooth formation on the exposed side. In recent years, it has been common practice to defer treatment of any kind until the child is 5 or 6 years of age. Within that period many of the hemangiomas regress or disappear altogether.

Hemangioendothelioma

The *juvenile hemangioendothelioma* is a benign tumor mass composed chiefly of proliferating cells and some capillary spaces. For this reason, it may be of normal color or bright red, depending upon the number of patent vessels present. A similar clinical finding is seen with the adult form of the hemangioendothelioma and the hemangiopericytoma, both of which frequently behave as low-grade malignancies.

Kaposi's Sarcoma (Multiple, Idiopathic Hemorrhagic Sarcoma of Kaposi, Angioreticuloendothelioma)

This neoplasm occurs typically on the skin of older men, usually outdoor workers. The feet and legs are commonly involved with other lesions sometimes found on the face or, more rarely, in the oral cavity. The skin tumors, which are usually multiple, appear as reddish-brown nodules up to a centimeter or more in diameter. The main differential diagnosis is malignant melanoma (p. 311). Some cases arise concomitantly with malignant lymphoma. The lesions are slowly progressive and respond well to radiation therapy.

Sturge-Weber Syndrome (Encephalotrigeminal Angiomatosis)

The peculiar distribution of a diffuse hemangioma over the approximate course of the trigeminal nerve is suggestive of this syndrome (Fig. 11–7). Intracranial calcifications and mental retardation may be evident (p. 305).

Juvenile Nasopharyngeal Angiofibroma

Seen most commonly in the nasopharyngeal regions of teenaged males, this tumor is composed of a highly vascularized, fibrous connective tissue stroma with an expansile and infiltrative growth pattern. Nasal stuffiness, epistaxis, sinusitis, anterior bowing of the posterior wall of the maxillary sinus and bulging of the face or palate are common features. It often appears in the mouth as a resilient bulge of the hard palate or protrudes into the oropharynx from above. While it frequently exhibits spontaneous hemorrhage, it may not be recognized as a vascular lesion on clinical examination and thus must be included in the differential diagnosis of diffuse soft tissue enlargements (p. 428). Biopsy may be followed by profuse hemorrhage and the cut section appears as a "bloody sponge." Rarely, cases arise intraorally in the soft tissues or, even more rarely, in the jaw bones. Radiation therapy and surgical excision are usually employed in treatment.

Vascular Anomalies

Varices, dilated and tortuous veins, are commonly seen as purple, somewhat elevated blebs on the inner surfaces of the lips or as multiple areas on undersurface or lateral borders of the tongue (*lingual varicositis*) (Fig. 7–22). Considered an age change in the oral tissues, they are of no clinical significance other than their occasional tendency to develop thrombi (Fig. 14–54).

"Cherry spots," "venous lakes" or *"microcherry" venous anomalies* are somewhat comparable to varices. These appear as tiny blue or purple spots on the lips of elderly people.

Arteriovenous aneurysms (A-V anomalies, A-V fistulae) represents direct communications between an artery and vein which may be developmental in origin or represent atypical repair following injury. They clini-

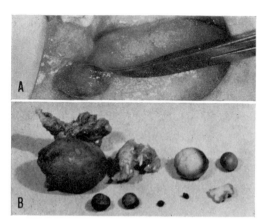

Fig. 14-54. Hyalinized thrombi of the cheeks. Several firm masses were palpated in the cheek of an elderly woman who exhibited swelling of the face. Radiographs showed multiple radiodense bodies. *A,* An incision has been made and one of the masses is being removed surgically. *B,* Multiple, hard bodies which cut with difficulty were found. Histologic examination established the diagnosis of hyalinized thrombi. (Ewbank, Standish, and Mitchell, J. Oral Surg., *22,* 456, 1964.)

cally resemble the hemangioma and may be the source of unexplained localized hemorrhage of the gingiva. Usual locations are the lips, palate and alveolar ridge or gingiva. Rarely, they are seen centrally in the jaw.

Lymphangioma

The superficial vascular lesions of the lymphatic vessels appear as tiny, soft blebs of normal or pale color on the mucosal surface. The proliferating lymphatic vessels are located mainly in the connective tissue papillae just beneath the surface epithelium, thereby accounting for its pale, soft character (Fig. 14–55). The small, superficial lymphangiomas may be removed surgically.

More deep-seated lymphangiomas cause a diffuse enlargement and are boggy on palpation (Fig. 14–56). The neck, tongue and floor of the mouth of the newborn infant are sometimes involved with massive lymphangioma (*cystic colli hygroma*) which is extremely difficult to manage because of its diffuse infiltration of major structures in the neck and floor of the mouth.

Other highly vascular lesions which must be differentiated clinically and microscopically from the angiomatous lesions are the pyogenic granuloma (p. 425), the so-called pregnancy tumor, and the peripheral giant cell granuloma (p. 427).

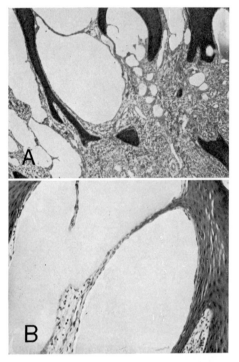

Fig. 14-55. Lymphangioma. *A,* Large lymphatic spaces are shown in the papillary layer of the connective tissue, between the epithelial rete pegs. *B,* High-power photomicrograph of *A.*

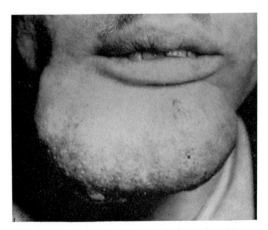

Fig. 14-56. Lymphangioma of the chin. (Courtesy of Pedro Tinoco.)

SOFT TISSUE ENLARGEMENTS

Most soft tissue swellings encountered by the dentist are of inflammatory or infectious origin. These may range from swelling secondary to the edema of inflammation to reactive, hyperplastic processes such as those seen adjacent to ill-fitting dentures. Solitary enlargements of this nature are associated in most instances with a specific etiologic factor such as dental infection, other specific infectious agents, or an obvious physical irritant such as a denture, rough edge of a clasp or fractured tooth, cheek biting or other habits producing chronic injury.

Other soft tissue enlargements may be neoplastic in origin. Seen more rarely are diffuse enlargements due to hereditary or congenital defects (*e.g.* hereditary gingival fibromatosis, Fig. 7–39) and metabolic or endocrine disturbances (*e.g.* macroglossia of cretinism and acromegaly, pp. 253, 431).

The clinical diagnosis of inflammatory soft tissue enlargements of the oral cavity can generally be made with considerable accuracy (Fig. 14–57*A*). Full use of all appropriate clinical and laboratory methods of diagnosis (usually biopsy) should be employed since swellings of this nature may be confused with other less innocuous processes. The oral physical examination obviously must include careful palpation of the lesion and a thorough search for other similar lesions in the mouth. The general consistency and color will frequently determine the primary tissue (epithelium, fibrous connective tissue, blood vessels, fat, etc.) which has increased in size. The presence of ulceration over the surface, the relative vascularity of the swelling, possible association with infected teeth or periodontal pockets, evidence of trauma or other irritating factors, time of appearance, rate of growth, symptoms or signs, and location will often provide clues for a working diagnosis.

The clinical and radiographic examination should determine whether or not the enlargement is confined to the soft tissue or also involves the underlying bone. The gen-

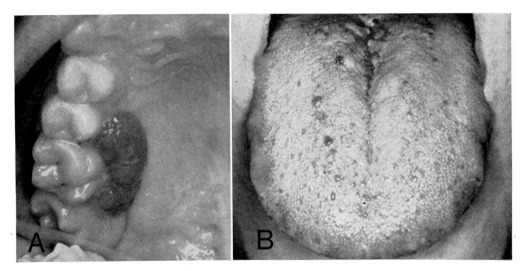

Fig. 14-57. *A,* Pyogenic granuloma. *B,* Angiomatosis of the tongue.

eral consistency of the lesion and the patient's description of its rate of growth will permit some evaluation of its tissue of origin and growth potential. In most instances, the definitive diagnosis must be based on microscopic examination of a biopsy specimen. In a few instances, other diagnostic laboratory procedures (*e.g.* microbiologic) are indicated.

Focal Soft Tissue Enlargements

Most of the focal, discrete enlargements seen on the oral mucosa are benign processes, either inflammatory/reactive or benign neoplasms.

These clinical lesions appear as well-defined, relatively homogenous, tumor-like growths. The surface may be smooth, papillary, keratotic or ulcerated with a fibrinous exudate. The consistency of these focal enlargements may be quite firm (suggesting fibroma or benign connective tissue neoplasm) or soft and granulomatous (suggesting an inflammatory or reactive process). Occasionally, extraosseous odontogenic tumors arise as lumps on the gingiva (see Chap. 15) and one, the peripheral odontogenic fibroma, occurs only on the gingiva.

In some cases, multiple focal enlargements occur as in Heck's disease, multiple

mucosal neuroma syndrome or, occasionally, granular cell myoblastoma.

Papilloma

The intraoral counterpart of the verruca vulgaris of the skin (p. 313) is the papilloma. It appears clinically as an exophytic growth attached by a narrow stalk to the mucosa (Fig. 7–46). The surface of the mass has numerous finger-like projections which may be elongated and resemble a palm frond or appear rough and cauliflower-like (Fig. 14–58). It may occur anywhere on the mucous membrane surface, especially the gingiva, tongue, lips and palate. In contrast to the common wart on the skin, which is

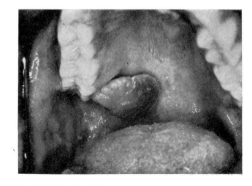

Fig. 14-58. Papilloma.

seen most commonly on the hands of children and is of viral etiology, the oral papilloma does not demonstrate viral inclusion bodies. It is of interest, however, that canine oral papillomatosis is of proven viral origin.

Fibroma (Irritation Fibroma, Focal Fibrous Hyperplasia)

The fibroma is a focal, well-circumscribed overgrowth of fibrous connective tissue which is seen clinically as a more or less firm swelling beneath the oral mucous membrane. Commonly seen on the lips, buccal mucosa and gingiva, the fibroma represents a reaction to chronic injury and therefore is more logically classified as a hyperplasia rather than as a true neoplasm (Fig. 2–5). While the etiologic agent or injury may be identified in some instances, usually the primary injury occurred at some previous date. For this reason, the terms "traumatic fibroma," "irritation fibroma" or "focal inflammatory fibrous hyperplasia" are commonly used.

The consistency of the fibroma may be either soft or hard depending upon the relative density of the collagen fibers which make up the bulk of the lesion. Because they are prominent and protuberant masses, fibromas are subject to secondary trauma and occasionally may become ulcerated. Treatment is by surgical excision.

Scar

Surgical scar tissue may appear as a pale, slightly elevated, usually linear lesion of the oral tissues or more commonly may be palpated as a firm mass below the surface of the mucosa (Fig. 7–18). Traumatic scars are most commonly encountered in the lips. Postsurgical scar tissue filling in a bony defect is common in the anterior maxilla (p. 459). A counterpart of the keloid of the skin (hyperplastic scar tissue) has not been described in the oral tissues. A history of previous traumatic injury or surgery in the area is strongly suggestive of the diagnosis. Discrete nodules of apparent scar tissue should be biopsied since the clinical diagnosis may be in error.

Focal Epithelial Hyperplasia (Heck's Disease)

Heck's disease exhibits multiple, focal nodules with a sessile base distributed on the lips, buccal mucosa, gingiva and tongue. It is seen in various Indian and Eskimo groups from several parts of the world, particularly Navajos, Eskimos of Greenland and Alaska and several Indian tribes in Central and South America. There is some evidence to suggest the condition is of viral origin although this has not been confirmed. The lesion is composed of benign, acanthomatous epithelium and supporting connective tissue. Some lesions regress without treatment.

Lipoma

This benign tumor of mature adipose tissue appears clinically as a soft nodule or tumor mass, often with a distinct yellow color (Fig. 7–35). Deeper-seated lesions and those with a prominent fibrous connective tissue component (lipofibroma) may be firmer and of normal color. Unless traumatized, the covering epithelium is intact. They are found on the lips, buccal mucosa or other sites (Figs. 7–29 and 12–11B).

Verruciform Xanthoma

This recently described entity appears on the mucosa as a solitary lesion with a sessile base and a red or keratotic cobblestone or pebbly surface. It ranges in size from a few millimeters to over a centimeter in diameter. Most cases occur in older adults, usually on the alveolar mucosa, palate, floor of mouth or lip. The covering epithelial surface shows a verrucoid pattern with parakeratin plugging of the crypts between the epithelial "fingers" (Fig. 14–59A). The underlying connective tissue papillae contain numerous lipid-filled histiocytes (xan-

The overlying mucous membrane is of a normal or sometimes pale color and a peripheral lesion grossly resembles the fibroma. A previous history of injury together with the pain symptoms are suggestive of the diagnosis. The clinical diagnosis should be confirmed by microscopic examination.

Multiple Mucosal Neuromas (Sipple's Syndrome, Neuropolyendocrine Syndrome)

Multiple mucosal neuromas are seen as elevated, sessile nodules on the tongue and lips (p. 257). The lips may also be diffusely thickened (Macrocheilia, p. 430) with numerous submucosal neuromas and small nodules may be found on the margins of the eyelids. The tumors, which represent tangled masses of nerve with thickened perineurium similar to the traumatic neuroma, may be present at birth or appear during the first year of life. Early recognition of Sipple's syndrome may be lifesaving since it permits earlier recognition of the associated adrenal pheochromocytoma and medullary carcinoma of the thyroid (p. 343).

Neurofibroma

The neurofibroma, seen most commonly on the skin surface, may also involve the oral mucous membranes (Fig. 14–60A to D). They look like soft or somewhat rubbery overgrowths of tissue which are pale to normal color. Multiple neurofibromas and *café-au-lait* spots are found in neurofibromatosis or von Recklinghausen's disease of skin (p. 321). The neurofibroma may undergo malignant transformation into *neurogenic sarcoma.*

Neurilemmoma

Neurilemmoma is a benign tumor of nerve sheath origin (Fig. 14–61). It is a somewhat firm mass which does not undergo malignant transformation. The diagnosis is established by histologic examination.

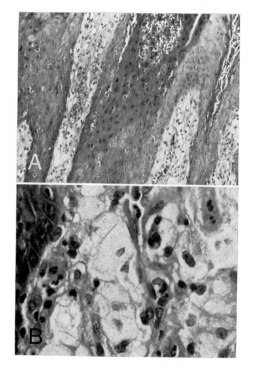

Fig. 14-59. Verruciform xanthoma. *A,* The papillary epithelial pattern seen histologically accounts for the pebbly surface seen clinically. *B,* Foam cells shown under higher magnification of *A* predominate in the connective tissue papillae.

thoma or "foam" cells) (Fig. 14–59*B*). The lesion is benign and treated by surgical excision.

Traumatic Neuroma (Amputation Neuroma)

The traumatic neuroma arises secondarily to peripheral nerve injury and appears clinically as a soft to firm and almost invariably painful enlargement. Transection of a peripheral nerve ordinarily results in regeneration of the axis cylinder down the original neurilemmal sheath. If the severed ends of the nerve trunk are displaced or if scar tissue forms between them, the regenerating fibers will sometimes continue to proliferate forming a tangled mass of nerve and dense fibrous conective tissue. Since these neurofibrils still react to stimuli, the traumatic neuroma is often extremely painful to touch.

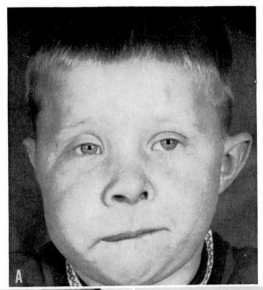

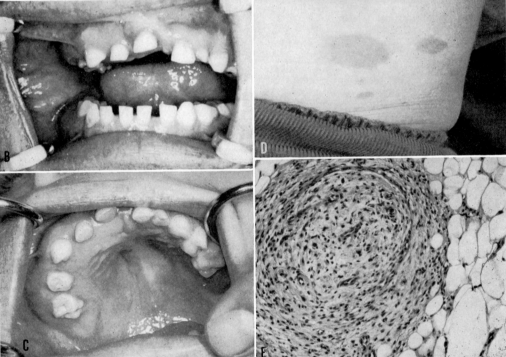

Fig. 14-60.   Multiple neurofibromatosis. *A,* Marked facial asymmetry due to plexiform neurofibroma of the cheek. *B,* Intraoral view showing enlargement of the inner aspect of the cheek. *C,* Occlusal view of the maxilla showing enlargement of the alveolar ridge and spacing of the teeth. Radiographs show widened alveolar spaces in the bone. *D, Cafe-au-lait* spots on the skin of the abdomen. (Freeman and Standish, Oral Surg., *19,* 52, 1965.) *E,* Plexiform neurofibroma. Photomicrograph showing one of the several histologic patterns of neurofibromas and adjacent normal adipose tissue.

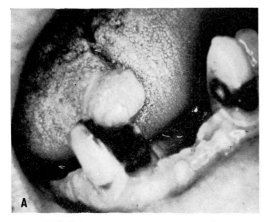

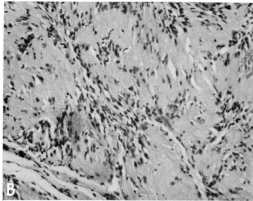

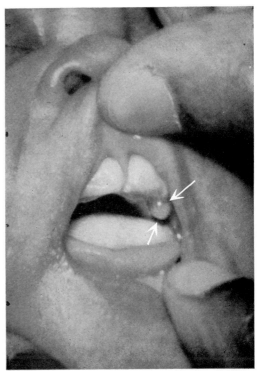

Fig. 14-62. Congenital epulis of the newborn. (Courtesy of Arthur S. Miller.)

Fig. 14-61. Neurilemmoma. *A,* **This solitary nodule** of the anterior portion of the tongue had been present for several years. *B,* Photomicrograph showing palisaded nuclei of Antoni type A tissue. (Courtesy of Robert Eubank.)

Congenital Epulis of the Newborn

Seen on the anterior alveolar ridge in newborn infants (Fig. 14–62), the congenital epulis appears as a smooth-surfaced or lobulated soft tissue mass. It is seen most commonly on the maxilla and is differentiated clinically from the neuroectodermal tumor of infancy (p. 484) by the marked melanin pigmentation of the latter. Histologically similar to the granular cell myoblastoma, the congenital epulis is also benign and treated by simple surgical excision.

Granular Cell Myoblastoma
(Myoblastic Myoma)

This enlargement appears as a well-circumscribed mass which may be elevated

or deep seated, usually within the musculature of the tongue (Fig. 14–63). Less common locations are the lip, buccal mucosa, and floor of the mouth and, rarely, near the openings of the submaxillary salivary gland ducts. Extraoral sites are chiefly the skin, breast and larynx. Most of the oral cases are discovered in early adulthood. Except for its long duration and characteristic location in the musculature of the tongue, it presents no significant clinical features suggestive of the diagnosis. Its consistency is that of scar tissue or fibroma. The surface of the lesion may be of normal color or pale and keratotic if it is subject to chronic irritation. A positive diagnosis can be made only by microscopic examination. Since nearly half of the granular cell myoblastomas of the tongue will exhibit pseudoepitheliomatous hyperplasia of the covering epithelium, an erroneous diagnosis of well-differentiated epider-

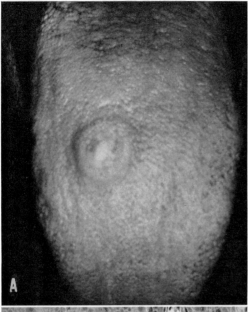

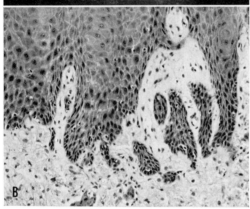

Fig. 14-63. Granular cell myoblastoma. *A*, Myoblastoma on the dorsum of the tongue. (Courtesy of Ralph E. Beatty.) *B*, Photomicrograph showing pseudoepitheliomatous hyperplasia (PEH) and subjacent granular cells.

moid carcinoma is sometimes made. Although the cell origin of myoblastoma is in dispute, its clinical behavior is benign and recurrence following removal is highly unlikely.

Osteoma Mucosae (Osseous Choristoma)

This unusual lesion appears as a hard nodule in the soft tissues, chiefly the tongue or buccal mucosa. Radiographs of the soft tissue show a discrete radiopacity with well-defined trabeculae of bone which are confirmed by histologic examination. Comparable lesions with cartilage (*cartilaginous choristoma, chondroma, osteochondroma*) have also been reported in the tongue.

Accessory Salivary Gland Tumors

With certain exceptions, the same types of benign and malignant salivary gland neoplasms involve both the major and accessory salivary glands (p. 350). The oncocytoma, Warthin's tumor and sebaceous adenoma occur almost exclusively in the parotid gland with but single cases of Warthin's tumor and sebaceous adenoma reported in the palate and buccal mucosa, respectively. On the other hand, the adenosquamous carcinoma occurs in the mucous membranes of the oral cavity, nasal cavity and larynx. A corresponding tumor has not been reported in the major salivary glands.

Neoplasms of the accessory salivary glands account for approximately one-fourth of all salivary gland tumors. It is of significance that a substantial number, perhaps as high as 50 percent, of all intraoral salivary gland tumors are malignant.

The palate is the most common location for accessory salivary gland tumors with the upper lip, buccal mucosa and retromolar area being the next most common sites. More rarely, they are found in the tongue, the lower lip and within the mandible. It is of some clinical diagnostic importance that salivary gland lesions involving the lower lip are almost always mucoceles, whereas salivary gland lesions of the upper lip are most commonly neoplasms. Inasmuch as normal glandular tissue is not found in the free or attached gingiva, salivary gland tumors arising primarily in this location are not seen.

The clinical manifestations, histologic features, and treatment of the accessory salivary gland tumors are essentially as described for those seen in the major glands. While descriptions of individual tumors will not be repeated in this section, some general considerations of the intraoral lesions will be emphasized.

Because of their relatively superficial location, accessory salivary gland neoplasms appear clinically as distinct, dome-shaped swellings which may occasionally be ulcerated. As a general rule, the benign salivary gland tumors (pleomorphic adenoma, cystadenoma and cellular adenoma) present an intact mucosal surface without radiographic evidence of bone destruction (Fig. 1–18). On the other hand, the malignant salivary gland tumors (adenocystic basal cell carcinoma, acinic cell adenocarcinoma and mucoepidermoid carcinoma) tend to be ulcerated and invasive, especially those located on the palate (Fig. 7–32).

Salivary gland tumors of the palate are generally located on the posterior hard palate, approximately halfway between the alveolar process and the midline, overlying the posterior palatine vessels and nerves. Although epidermoid carcinoma may also occur on the palate, the majority will be at the junction of the hard and soft or on the soft palate proper (Fig. 7–30).

Salivary gland neoplasms are far more common on the upper than the lower lip. Such lesions at this site tend to be well circumscribed, freely movable and benign, usually histologic variants of the pleomorphic adenoma such as the canalicular adenoma or cellular (monomorphic) adenoma. The differential diagnosis of nodules involving the upper lip would include fibroma, scar, foreign body, pleomorphic adenoma, nasoalveolar cyst and granular cell myoblastoma.

The mandibular retromolar areas are fairly common sites for salivary gland neoplasms, chiefly mucoepidermoid carcinoma (Fig. 13–6). Accordingly, a clinical swelling in these regions should be considered a malignant salivary gland tumor until proven otherwise.

Salivary gland neoplasms of the tongue are uncommon, but do occur. For the most part, these are mucoepidermoid carcinomas

and adenoid cystic basal cell carcinomas (pp. 353, 354).

Rare cases of intrabony salivary gland tumors such as pleomorphic adenoma, adenoid cystic carcinoma and, more commonly, mucoepidermoid carcinoma have been reported in the posterior mandible. It has been theorized that salivary gland tissue entrapped during development of the mandible has the same potential for neoplastic transformation as salivary gland tissues in any other location (p. 487).

Because of the physical inconvenience of an enlargement of the intraoral soft tissues, the patient is likely to seek professional attention much earlier than for corresponding lesions of the major salivary glands.

Pyogenic Granuloma

The pyogenic granuloma occurs most commonly on the gingiva and, less frequently, at other sites in the oral cavity and on the skin (Figs. 1–8 and 7–44). It presumably arises secondarily to minor injury and/or infection which stimulates the formation of an exuberant overgrowth of young, highly vascular granulation tissue. Despite its name, it is not pus-producing nor can specific microorganisms be identified in the tissue. Those lesions occurring on the gingiva are often associated with impacted food or a fragment of calculus which may be presumed to be the causative agent. The pyogenic granuloma is histologically similar to the capillary hemangioma and, on the gingiva, is clinically and microscopically identical to the so-called pregnancy tumor (Fig. 14–64B).

Because of its vascular component, the pyogenic granuloma is red with a somewhat spongy consistency and bleeds readily following minor trauma (Fig. 14–57A). The gingival lesions typically have an ulcerated surface, particularly along that portion of the surface in contact with adjacent or occluding teeth (Fig. 14–64A). As might be expected, a thick fibrinous exudate over the

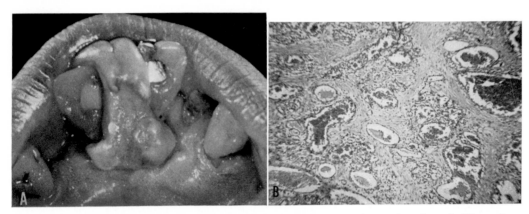

Fig. 14-64. *A*, Large pyogenic granuloma of the gingiva. Note the ulcerated surface. *B*, Photomicrograph showing numerous vascular spaces and proliferating endothelial cells characteristic of the pyogenic granuloma. (See also Figs. 1-8, 14-57.)

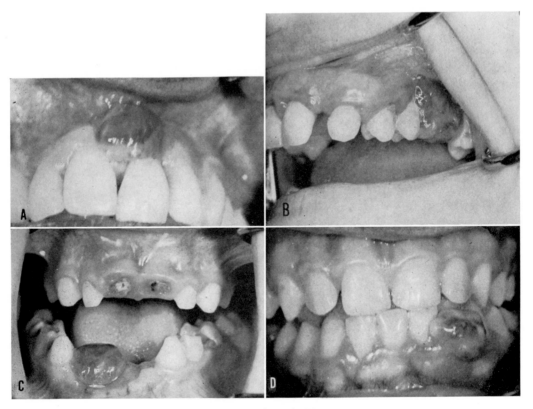

Fig. 14-65. Peripheral giant cell granulomas (*A* through *D*).

surface of the ulcer gives a whitish appearance to that area.

In most instances, the pyogenic granuloma shows initial rapid growth and then remains relatively static. It may vary considerably in size from a small hyperplastic mass on a gingival papilla to a 2- or 3-cm tumescence nearly covering adjacent teeth and extending both labially and lingually (Fig. 14–64A). At other sites on the oral mucous membrane such as the tongue or lips, it appears as a red, dome-shaped elevation with an ulcerated surface. Pain or tenderness is not significant.

Treatment of the pyogenic granuloma is by surgical excision. Recurrence is not common except in those gingival lesions in which the local irritant was not removed from the adjacent teeth at the time of surgery.

Peripheral Giant Cell Granuloma

Clinically quite similar to the pyogenic granuloma, the lesion appears as a purple to red, highly vascular soft tissue mass on the gingiva, usually anterior to the first molar teeth (Figs. 14–65, 14–66). It tends to bleed easily and often a thin fibrinous exudate overlying a superficial ulcer is present. Radiographs show some evidence of resorption of the underlying bone. When it is seen in edentulous areas, characteristic "cuffing" of the alveolar bone is seen.

Peripheral Odontogenic (Ossifying) Fibroma

This common tumor, believed to be of periodontal ligament origin, is listed here since it has several clinical features in common with the other focal gingival enlargements. Thus, pyogenic granuloma, peripheral giant cell granuloma and peripheral odontogenic fibroma must be considered in the differential diagnosis of such gingival lesions. The peripheral odontogenic fibroma is discussed on page 473.

Lingual Tonsil (Foliate Papillitis)

Lymphoid tissues, representing a portion of Waldeyer's ring, occurring as lymphocytic aggregates on the posterolateral borders of the tongue are called lingual tonsil (Fig. 14–67). They are usually bilateral and oc-

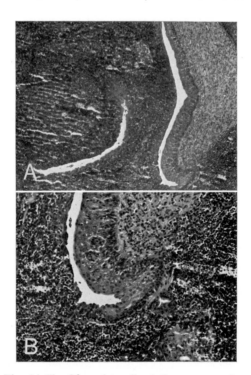

Fig. 14-67. Lingual tonsil. A, Low-power micrograph showing epithelial lined crypts and associated lymphoid tissues. B, High magnification of A showing the base of a crypt with scattered taste buds in the lining epithelium.

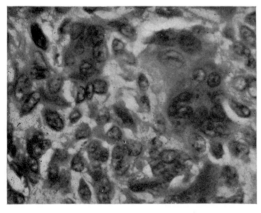

Fig. 14-66. Peripheral giant cell granuloma. Photomicrograph showing multinucleated giant cells.

casionally enlarge and ulcerate. If unrecognized they may be confused with other more serious lesions, most notably epidermoid carcinoma.

Surgical removal and histologic examination are indicated for those areas which appear atypical, unilateral, infected, or if a firm clinical diagnosis cannot be established.

Lingual Thyroid

Residual thyroid tissue on the posterior dorsum and posterolateral borders of the tongue rarely may appear as small nodules. Surgical excision is indicated only for those that are subject to trauma. Because the lingual thyroid may be the only active thyroid tissue the patient has, an ^{131}I scan should always be done prior to surgery. This will establish the diagnosis if functional thyroid tissue is present.

Diffuse Soft Tissue Enlargements

The diffuse, poorly defined enlargements of the oral soft tissues are most commonly of inflammatory origin, chiefly related to ill-fitting dentures. On occasion, diffuse enlargements induced by blood or lymph vascular lesions (Sturge-Weber syndrome, p. 305, Fig. 11–7; lymphangioma, p. 417; nasopharyngeal angiofibroma, p. 417) or developmental disorders of the facial structures (hemihypertrophy) must be considered in the differential diagnosis. Diffuse enlargements due to infection (cellulitis) and those which preferentially affect the gingiva, lips and tongue are discussed in following sections.

Inflammatory Fibrous Hyperplasia
(Denture Hyperplasia, Epulis Fissuratum)

This common response to low-grade chronic irritation over a long period of time results in diffuse enlargement of the tissue (redundant tissue, epulis fissuratum, granuloma fissuratum). This commonly occurs under or along the borders of an old, ill-fitting denture. With resorption of the alveolar ridges, an unequal distribution of forces upon the supporting tissues occurs. This injury causes inflammation often with ulceration (decubital ulcer, traumatic ulcer). In those areas where the denture is not supported by contact with the tissues, soft tissues proliferate to fill in the void. Repeated injury, inflammation, tissue breakdown, formation of granulation tissue, reepithelialization and repetition of the cycle over a long period account for the often remarkable increase in volume of soft tissue seen. In cases of long standing the denture literally "floats" in large flaps or folds of soft tissue overlapping the denture borders.

Inflammatory fibrous hyperplasia associated with denture injury varies considerably in its color and consistency, even in the same patient. Areas of recent injury or secondary infection may show a linear ulcer and chronic inflammation. Most of this redundant tissue will be soft and flabby. Portions that have been relatively free from inflammation and "healed" with the formation of dense collagen will be quite firm in consistency and of normal color.

Removal of the denture for an extended period of time will result in some clinical improvement in the color and consistency. Unfortunately, the excess tissue is reduced in size only to the degree that edema was present.

Surgical excision and recontouring of the tissues are recommended prior to the construction of new dentures.

Inflammatory Papillary Hyperplasia
(Papillomatosis)

This condition occurs on the hard palate beneath full maxillary dentures with excessive "relief chambers," excessive lateral movement, improper contact with the palatal mucosa and/or poor oral hygiene. Proliferation of new tissue to fill in the void under the denture results in a shiny, pebbly-surfaced overgrowth of soft tissue (Fig. 14–68). This tissue is generally red and inflamed and feels spongy to palpation. Ulceration is not commonly seen.

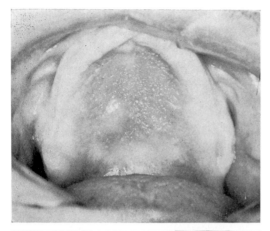

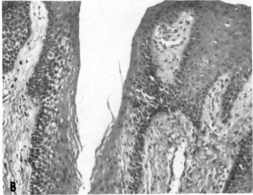

Fig. 14-68. Papillomatosis (papillary hyperplasia). *A*, Red, edematous palatal mucosa in a patient who had worn the same denture for many years. *B*, Photomicrograph showing the characteristic papillary hyperplasia of the mucosa shown in *A*. Portions of two of the papillary projections are shown.

Although in the past some investigators were of the opinion that papillomatosis is a premalignant lesion, it seems more likely that epidermoid carcinoma arising in an area of papillomatosis occurs coincidentally. The comparatively low incidence of epidermoid carcinoma of the palate seems unrelated to the large number of denture wearers with papillomatosis.

Removal of the denture results in some reduction in size corresponding to the reduced inflammation and edema. Special "tissue conditioners" placed in the palatal vault of the old denture have also been recommended in some cases. Surgical removal with microscopic examination of the resected tissue is usually indicated prior to construction of the new dentures.

Crohn's Disease

This non-specific, chronic granulomatous disease of the terminal ileum (regional ileitis) may exhibit associated lesions throughout the gastrointestinal tract, including the oral cavity. The oral lesion generally appears as a poorly circumscribed, nodular or "cobblestone" swelling, often with ulceration. The histologic features show a granulomatous reaction with epithelioid cells and multinucleated giant cells comparable to sarcoidosis. However, the Kveim test (*q.v.*) is negative and specific microorganisms cannot be identified. The diagnosis is based on the exclusion of sarcoidosis or infectious agents and the confirmation of the diagnosis of regional ileitis. It should be noted, however, that some cases have been reported in which the oral lesions preceded the gastrointestinal tract disease by several months or even years.

Condyloma Acuminata (Venereal Wart)

This viral disease occurs most commonly in the anogenital areas; however, rare cases have been recognized in the oral cavity, chiefly involving the gingival and alveolar mucosa. It appears as a diffuse overgrowth of bulbous or papillomatous tissue made up largely of parakeratotic and acanthomatous epithelium. The oral lesion is treated by excision; podophyllin is frequently used to treat the anogenital lesions.

Neurofibromatosis (Multiple Neurofibromatosis, von Recklinghausen's Disease of Skin)

Neurofibroma of the oral mucosa may appear as a focal enlargement (p. 421) or, in severe cases, as diffuse enlargements (Fig. 14–60) in the fully developed syndrome. If other stigmata of the disease are present, the diagnosis is readily made (p. 321).

Locally Aggressive Fibrous Lesions

A number of locally aggressive but benign fibrous connective tissue lesions are recognized as histologically and clinically distinct entities: *nodular fasciitis, aggressive fibromatosis* (extra-abdominal desmoid), *fibrous histiocytoma* (fibroxanthoma), *proliferative myositis* and *desmoplastic fibroma of bone* (p. 483). With the exception of the latter, they are found chiefly in the dermis with rare cases described in the oral soft tissues such as the tongue. Desmoid tumors involving the sternomastoid muscle produce *torticollis* or wry neck. Desmoid tumors of the skin are a feature of Gardner's syndrome (p. 482). In the past, these conditions were sometimes diagnosed as "low-grade fibrosarcoma" or "non-metastasizing fibrosarcoma." They appear clinically as exuberant overgrowths of tissue with poorly defined margins and a fibrous consistency. While their rapid growth and "fleshy" consistency may suggest a fibrous connective tissue neoplasm, possibly sarcoma, there are few distinguishing features upon which to base a clinical diagnosis. Their rapid infiltrative growth and tendency to recur locally make their clinical management difficult.

Lymphoproliferative Disease of the Hard Palate

This recently described entity occurs chiefly in the elderly as a diffuse, somewhat soft, swelling of the hard palate. The involved mucosa is usually of normal color although it may sometimes appear red or dusky. The swelling usually is unilateral in the region of the greater palatine foramen, with occasional extension onto the soft palate. The lesion represents a lymphocytic lymphoma which may or may not be accompanied by disseminated disease. Once the diagnosis is established by biopsy and appropriate medical workup (CBC, bone marrow biopsy, etc., Chap. 9), the patient should be treated by irradiation or chemotherapy. In 21 cases reported by Tomich and Shafer, the patients averaged 70 years

of age and 8 of 14 (for which follow-up information was available) died of disseminated disease, 3 were alive with disease and 3 were free of disease.

Diffuse Gingival Enlargements

Diffuse or generalized enlargements of the gingiva are discussed elsewhere (see pp. 141, 407). Representative forms are simply listed here for purposes of establishing a differential diagnosis for this common group of soft tissue enlargements: hyperplastic gingivitis (Fig. 7–41), pregnancy gingivitis, Dilantin hyperplasia (Fig. 7–40), leukemic gingivitis (Figs. 1–20, 14–51), and fibromatosis gingivae (Fig. 7–39).

Macrocheilia

Diffuse enlargement of one or both lips is commonly seen as a familial or racial trait, and *double-lip* is not unusual (Fig. 7–11). *Lymphangioma* and *hemangioma,* when extensive, may cause marked enlargement of the lip (Fig. 1–16). Diffuse enlargements of the lips of sudden onset are seen following severe *trauma,* in *acute cellulitis* and in *angioneurotic edema* (Figs. 1–11 and 7–14).

Cheilitis Glandularis Apostematosa

This is a rare condition in which there is diffuse, nodular enlargement of the lower lip. The lip is firm with numerous palpable masses which represent hypertrophy and inflammation of the lip mucous glands and their associated ducts. Thick mucoid or even purulent material can be expressed from the duct orifices. Electrocoagulation of the duct orifices or surgical excision has been tried with some success.

Cheilitis Granulomatosa

This condition also affects chiefly the lower lip as a chronic, diffuse and rubbery enlargement. Histologic examination suggests that the condition is basically a granulomatous reaction although a specific microorganism cannot be identified. No effective treatment is known for this rare condition.

The combined features of cheilitis granulomatosa, facial paralysis and congenital fissured tongue are called the *Melkersson-Rosenthal syndrome* (p. 262).

Macrocheilia of varying severity is occasionally seen in *myxedema, acromegaly, leprosy* and *filariasis*. Diffuse enlargement of the lips, and elevated nodules, are frequently present in Sipple's syndrome (pp. 257, 421).

Macroglossia

Diffuse enlargement of the tongue may arise primarily from structures normally present which undergo hyperplasia or neoplasia or secondarily from infiltration of the tissues by cells or fluids. Edentulous patients who do not wear dentures have a broad flat tongue which may be mistaken for macroglossia. After functional dentures are constructed, the tongue assumes its normal shape.

With the exception of *lymphangioma,* most neoplasms of the tongue present a solitary tumescence. *Hemangioma* and *neurofibroma,* however, may be multiple in some cases (Fig. 14–69).

Macroglossia is a frequent finding in *cretinism* or *infantile myxedema* (p. 245), *mongolism* (Fig. 4–13), *gargoylism, acromegaly* (Fig. 1–21, p. 253), *glycogen storage disease* and *Beckwith's hypoglycemic syndrome*. The latter condition exhibits marked macroglossia, neonatal hypoglycemia, hepatosplenomegaly, microcephaly, and somatic giantism. *Amyloid* infiltration, either primary or secondary, of the tongue may cause moderate enlargement. Diffuse unilateral enlargement of the tongue is seen in hemihypertrophy (Fig. 11–1*B*.).

Marked swelling of the tongue with elevation against the palate and interference with breathing is found in *Ludwig's angina* (p. 433).

Diffuse Cellulitis (Phlegmon)

Acute infections arising from the teeth or periodontal tissues may spread widely in the tissue spaces, causing diffuse swelling (Fig. 1–11). Generally, the patients are in some distress and complain of moderate to severe pain. In most instances, reactions of this nature arise from periapical or periodontal infections.

The spread of infection can generally be followed fairly accurately on the basis of the patient's history, beginning with pain in a tooth. As the periapical tissues become involved, sensitivity to percussion develops. If a productive apical abscess forms, the infection spreads within the marrow space producing moderately severe pain. With perforation of the bony cortex, pain becomes extremely severe due to elevation of the sensitive periosteum from the underlying bone. Once the infection perforates through the periosteum, the pain subsides remarkably. Depending upon the adjacent anatomic structures, a "gumboil" (parulis, p. 394) may appear on the alveolar mucosa or a diffuse swelling of associated anatomic or surgical spaces develops. In any event, the severe pain subsides concomitantly with extension of the infection into the less confining soft tissues.

The spread of infection in the soft tissue spaces is restricted by bone, muscle and, to some degree, fascial planes. Because of the rather loose areolar tissue around arteries, veins, nerves and salivary gland ducts, infections (and neoplasms) tend to spread along these structures into adjacent spaces. The

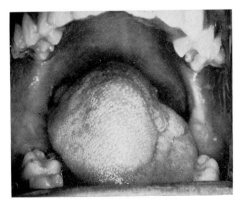

Fig. 14-69. Macroglossia secondary to neurofibroma. (Courtesy of Gerald E. Albert.)

severity of the infection and the degree of swelling are further modified by the potency of the microorganisms, the "resistance" of the host and the treatment instituted. Organisms such as the streptococci which release significant amounts of hyaluronidase (spreading factor) tend to extend widely.

Cellulitis of the face or neck may open through the skin (Fig. 1–12). Once the acute phase of the infection subsides, the patient may not seek further treatment. The opening through the skin alternately closes over and reopens as suppurative material builds up. With the proliferation of granulomatous tissue, a mass forms which may be mistaken for a superficial dermatologic infection or even neoplasm. Removal of the source of infection usually results in healing of the skin lesion. In some cases, excision of the residual lesion on the skin is necessary for cosmetic reasons.

Surgical Space Infections

As noted above, infections arising from the teeth and jaws may extend into the adjacent soft tissues where (depending upon the relative severity of the infectious process) the spread is limited chiefly by the surrounding anatomic structures. The classical "anatomic spaces," bounded by fascial planes, muscles and other structures, are only potential spaces. Since many of the fascial boundaries of these spaces are thin and ineffective barriers to infection, it is considered more appropriate to speak of the *surgical spaces* of the head and neck.

Periapical or periodontal infections which extend through the bony cortex into the nearby soft tissues cause characteristic soft tissue swellings. The diagnostic features of some of the more common surgical space infections will be described here. Reference should be made to oral surgery and anatomy texts for additional details.

Infection arising from the periapex of a tooth, if uncontrolled by body defenses, antibiotic treatment or drainage through the root canal or extraction site, usually "points"

through the nearest bony wall. It follows, therefore, that in the jaws such infection usually perforates the facial plates of bone because most tooth apices are nearest this cortical surface. Less commonly, in the case of the upper lateral incisors, the mandibular second and third molars and the palatal roots of the upper posterior teeth, lingual plate perforation occurs. On rare occasions, the maxillary sinus and nasal cavity may be involved.

Buccal Space Infection

Muscle attachments on the jaws play a major role in determining the direction in which the infection initially spreads. The buccinator muscle attachment to the maxilla and mandible is often coronal to the apices of the posterior teeth and therefore forces infection into the *buccal space*. Infections here are found laterally to the buccinator muscle and buccopharyngeal fascia, medially to the subcutaneous tissue and skin of the face, and limited superiorly by the zygomatic arch and lower border of the mandible, respectively. The posterior limit of the buccal space is the anterior border of the masseter muscle. Buccal space infections appear as rounded swellings of the cheek which do not extend below the lower border of the mandible.

The attachment of the mentalis muscle to the mandible exerts a similar effect on infections arising from the lower anterior teeth. If the infection perforates the cortical bone inferior to the mentalis attachment, the swelling appears low on the point of the chin. On the other hand, if it opens above the attachment, swelling occurs on the alveolar mucosa or in the mucobuccal fold.

Infraorbital Space Infection

These infections arise following the entrapment of infection between the caninus and infraorbital heads of the quadratus labii superioris muscles. Since each of these muscles converges to insert into the orbicularis oris muscle, the infection is forced upward toward the inner canthus of the eye. Infraorbital space infections appear as anterior facial swellings with obliteration of the nasolabial fold. The eye may be swollen shut and drainage near the inner canthus may occur.

Submandibular Space Infection

These infections are most commonly associated with partially impacted or infected mandibular third molars. The thick, external oblique ridge in this region and the nearness of the third molar apices to the lingual cortex favor extension of the infection lingually. Further, the mylohyoid ridge and muscle attachment is located coronally to the tooth apex, thereby permitting the infection to enter the submandibular space. Palpation of the posterior floor of the mouth reveals marked tenderness and swelling bounded laterally by the medial aspect of the body of the mandible, medially by the hyoglossus muscle, superiorly by the mylohyoid muscle, and inferiorly by the digastric muscle. A triangular-shaped swelling can be seen beneath the mandible on the affected side.

Since the mylohyoid ridge runs anteriorly and inferiorly along the medial surface of the mandible, the apices of the premolar and canine teeth are located superiorly to the ridge. Infection arising from a mandibular first molar tooth is said to have about equal chances of pointing either buccally or lingually. If the infection opens toward the lingual, the chances are again about equal that it will open above or below the mylohyoid muscle.

Sublingual Space Infection

These infections usually arise from infected mandibular premolar or first molar teeth. Submandibular space infections may extend along Wharton's duct around the posterior border of the mylohyoid muscle and into the sublingual space. Injuries to the anterior floor of the mouth may also give rise to sublingual space infection. This space is bounded inferiorly by the mylohyoid muscle, laterally by the mandible, medially by the hyoglossus and intrinsic muscles of the tongue, and superiorly by the mucous membrane. Thus, a sublingual space infection causes bulging of the anterior floor of the mouth on either side of the tongue.

Ludwig's Angina

As mentioned above, infection may spread from the submandibular space to the sublingual space. From here it may extend anteriorly to the hyoglossus muscle to the opposite side of the mouth. It may further dissect between the genioglossus, geniohyoid and intrinsic muscles of the tongue, elevating the tongue against the roof of the mouth and interfering with respiration. In this case, all of the spaces of the floor of the mouth (submandibular, sublingual, submental) are involved and the condition is called Ludwig's angina.

Pterygomandibular Space Infection

The pterygomandibular space is bounded laterally by the medial aspect of the mandibular ramus, medially by the internal pterygoid muscle, anteriorly by the pterygomandibular raphe, and posteriorly by the deep lobe of the parotid gland. Infection may be carried into this space during a mandibular infection. Mandibular molar infections may enter this space below the attachment of the pterygomandibular raphe to the mandible or maxillary infections may involve it from above. Pterygomandibular space infections cause swelling, marked trismus and tenderness of the oropharynx opposite the medial surface of the mandibular ramus.

Infections from the pterygomandibular space may extend posteriorly into the *parapharyngeal space, retropharyngeal space* or *parotid space*. The fascia covering the deep lobe of the parotid is particularly thin and offers little resistance to infection arising from within the gland proper or from adjacent areas. A parotid abscess thus may point through the skin or, in severe cases, involve deeper adjacent spaces.

Cavernous Sinus Thrombosis

This is an extremely serious condition which may occur following comparatively minor facial or dental infection. Communication is by way of the pterygoid plexus or through the anterior facial vein via the inferior or superior ophthalmic veins. The patient with cavernous sinus thrombosis shows a high spiking temperature, malaise, fever and other features of toxemia. Venous obstruction accounts for the marked periorbital edema, exophthalmos, lacrimation, dilated pupil and photophobia. Cranial nerves (III, IV, V_2, VI) in close proximity to the cavernous sinus are affected. Later the optic nerve is involved and, as the thrombus extends, the contralateral eye is affected. Subdural abscess and meningitis appear in the terminal stages of the infection.

BIBLIOGRAPHY

General

Bartels, H. A., Cohen, G. and Scopp, I. W.: The tongue: appearance and ecology in systemic diseases and chemotherapy, J. Periodont., *38*, 449, 1967.

Bhaskar, S. N.: Oral lesions in infants and new born, Dent. Clin. North America, July, 421, 1966.

Goldberg, L. C. and Diamond, A.: Letterer-Siwe disease, Arch. Derm., *92*, 561, 1965.

Gorlin, R. J. and Pindborg, J. J.: *Syndromes of the Head and Neck,* New York, McGraw-Hill Book Co., 1964.

Halperin, V., Kolas, S., Jefferis, K. R., Huddleston, S. O. and Robinson, H. B. G.: The occurrence of Fordyce spots, benign migratory glossitis, median rhomboid glossitis and fissured tongue, in 2,478 dental patients. The occurrence of torus palatinus and torus mandibularis in 2,478 dental patients, Oral Surg., *6*, 1072, 1134, 1953.

Harrison, T. R., Adams, R. D., Bennett, I. L. Jr., Resnik, W. H., Thorn, G. W. and Wintrobe, M. M., Eds.: *Principles of Internal Medicine,* 5th Ed., New York, McGraw-Hill Book Co., 1966.

Hayward, J. R.: Foreign body simulating a palatal lesion: report of case, J. Amer. Dent. Ass., *76*, 826, 1968.

Kutscher, A. H., Zegarelli, E. V. and Hyman, G. A., Eds.: *Pharmacotherapeutics of Oral Disease,* New York, McGraw-Hill Book Co., 1964.

Little, J. W. and Bartlett, R. C.: Differentiation of common local and systemic disease in oral soft tissues, Dent. Clin. North America, March, 141, 1968.

McCarthy, P. L. and Shklar, G.: *Diseases of the Oral Mucosa,* New York, McGraw-Hill Book Co., 1964.

McKusick, V. A.: Genetic factors in intestinal polyposis, J.A.M.A., *182*, 271, 1962.

McLean, D. M.: Virus infections of the mouth and throat, J. Canad. Dent. Ass., *26*, 650, 1960.

Meyer, I. and Shklar, G.: The oral manifestations of acquired syphilis, Oral Surg., *23*, 45, 1967.

Mitchell, D. F.: Some diagnostic problems associated with denture prostheses, J. Indiana Dent. Ass., *37*, 8, 1958.

Pindborg, J. J.: *Atlas of Diseases of the Oral Mucosa,* Philadelphia, W. B. Saunders Co., 1968.

Porterfield, H. W. and Trabue, J. C.: Submucous cleft palate, Plast. Reconstr. Surg., *35*, 45, 1965.

Shafer, W. G.: Initial mismanagement and delay in diagnosis of oral cancer, J. Amer. Dent. Ass., *90*, 1262, 1975.

Shafer, W. G., Hine, M. K. and Levy, B. M.: *A Textbook of Oral Pathology,* Philadelphia, W. B. Saunders Co., 1974.

Sharp, G. S. and Fister, H. W.: The etiology and treatment of the sore mouth, J. Prosth. Dent., *16*, 855, 1966.

Witkop, C. J., Jr. and Gorlin, R. J.: Four hereditary mucosal syndromes, Arch. Derm., *84*, 762, 1961.

White Lesions

Andreasen, J. O.: Oral lichen planus. I. A clinical evaluation of 115 cases, Oral Surg., *25*, 31, 1968.

Andreasen, J. O.: Oral lichen planus. II. A histologic evaluation of ninety-seven cases, Oral Surg., *25*, 158, 1968.

Andreasen, J. O. and Pindborg, J. J.: Cancercudvikling i oral lichen planus, Saertryk fra Nordisk Medicin, *70*, 861, 1963.

Azaz, B. and Lustmann, J.: Keratoacanthoma of the lower lip. Review of the literature and report of a case, Oral Surg., *38*, 918, 1974.

Cannell, H.: Dyskeratosis congenita, Brit. Dent. J., *9*, 8, 1971.

DeGregori, G., Pippen, R. and Davies, E.: Psoriasis of the gingiva and tongue: Report of a case, J. Periodont., *42*, 97, 1971.

El-Labban, N. G. and Kramer, I. R. H.: Civatte bodies and the actively dividing epithelial cells in oral lichen planus, Brit. J. Derm., *90*, 13, 1974.

Giunta, J. L., Gomez, L. S. A. and Greer, R. O.: Oral focal acantholytic dyskeratosis (warty dyskeratoma), Oral Surg., *39*, 474, 1975.

Hamner, III, J. E., Looney, P. D. and Chusea, T. M.: Submucous fibrosis, Oral Surg., *37*, 412, 1974.

Jasoway, J. R., Nelson, J. F. and Boyers, R. C.: Adenoid squamous cell carcinoma (adenoacanthoma) of the oral labial mucosa. A clinicopathologic study of fifteen cases, Oral Surg., *32*, 44, 1971.

Krolls, S. O. and Hoffman, S.: Squamous cell carcinoma of the oral soft tissues: a statistical analysis of 14,253 cases by age, sex, and race of patients, J. Amer. Dent. Ass., *92*, 571, 1976.

McCarthy, P. L. and Shklar, G.: The oral lesions in lichen planus: observation on 100 cases, Oral Surg., *14*, 164, 1961.

Martin, J. L. and Crump, E. P.: Leukoedema of the buccal mucosa in Negro children and youth, Oral Surg., *34*, 49, 1972.

Miles, A. E. W.: Sebaceous glands in the lip and cheek mucosa of man, Brit. Dent. J., *105*, 235, 1958.

Norins, A. and Yaffee, H.: Psoriasis of the hard palate, Arch. Derm., *76*, 357, 1957.

Ortega, J. A., Swanson, N. L., Landing, B. H. and Hammond, G. D.: Congenital dyskeratosis. Zinsser-Engman-Cole syndrome with thymic dysplasia and aplastic anemia, Amer. J. Dis. Child., *124*, 701, 1972.

Payne, T. F.: Why are white lesions white? Oral Surg., *40*, 652, 1975.

Pindborg, J. J., Chawla, T. N., Srivastava, A. N., Gupta, D. and Mohrotra, M. L.: Clinical aspects of submucous fibrosis, Acta Odont. Scand., *22*, 679, 1964.

Pindborg, J. J., Joist, O., Renstrup, G. and Roed-Petersen, B.: Studies in oral leukoplakia: a preliminary report on the period prevalence of malignant transformation in leukoplakia based on a follow-up study of 248 patients, J. Amer. Dent. Ass., *76*, 767, 1968.

Pisanty, S. and Ship, I. I.: Oral psoriasis, Oral Surg., *30*, 351, 1970.

Salmon, T. N., Robertson, G. R. Jr., Tracy, N. H. Jr. and Hiatt, W. R.: Oral psoriasis, Oral Surg., *38*, 48, 1974.

Scofield, H. H., Werning, J. T. and Shukes, R. C.: Solitary intraoral keratoacanthoma. Review of the literature and report of a case, Oral Surg., *37*, 889, 1974.

Shafer, W. G.: Verrucous carcinoma, Int. Dent. J., *22*, 451, 1972.

Silverman, S., Jr., Sheline, G. E. and Gillooly, C. J. Jr.: Radiation therapy and oral carcinoma, Cancer, *20*, 1297, 1967.

Tomich, C. E. and Burkes, E. J.: Warty dyskeratoma (isolated dyskeratosis follicularis) of the oral mucosa, Oral Surg., *31*, 798, 1971.

Tomich, C. E. and Shafer, W. G.: Squamous acanthoma of the oral mucosa, Oral Surg., *38*, 755, 1974.

Waldron, C. A. and Shafer, W. G.: Leukoplakia revisited. A clinicopathologic study of 3,256 oral leukoplakias, Cancer, *36*, 1386, 1975.

Waldron, C. A. and Shafer, W. G.: Current concepts of leukoplakia, Int. Dent. J., *10*, 350, 1960.

White, D. K., Leis, H. J. and Miller, A. S.: Intraoral psoriasis associated with widespread dermal psoriasis, Oral Surg., *41*, 174, 1976.

Young, L. L. and Lenox, J. A.: Pachyonychia congenita. A long term evaluation of associated oral and dermal lesions, Oral Surg., *36*, 663, 1973.

Zegarelli, D. J.: Solitary intraoral keratocarcinoma, Oral Surg., *40*, 785, 1975.

Red Lesions

Buchner, A. and Begleiter, A.: Oral lesions in psoriatic patients, Oral Surg., *41*, 332, 1976.

Chaudhry, A. P., Mitchell, D. F. and Romano, A. D.: Pre-invasive epidermoid carcinoma of the oral cavity, Oral Surg., *10*, 84, 1957.

Collings, C. K. and Dukes, C. D.: Recurrent herpetic stomatitis treated by intradermal injections of influenza A and B virus vaccine, J. Periodont., *23*, 48, 1952.

Giansanti, J. S., Cramer, J. R. and Weathers, D. R.: Palatal erythema: another etiologic factor, Oral Surg., *40*, 379, 1975.

Kerr, D. A., McClatchey, K. D. and Regezi, J. A.: Idiopathic gingivostomatitis. Cheilitis, glossitis, gingivitis syndrome; atypical gingivostomatitis, plasma cell gingivitis, plasmacytosis of gingiva, Oral Surg., *32*, 402, 1971.

Kerr, D. A., McClatchey, K. D. and Regezi, J. A.: Allergic gingivostomatitis (due to gum chewing), J. Periodont., *42*, 709, 1971.

Millard, H. D. and Gobetti, J. P.: Nonspecific stomatitis—A presenting sign in pernicious anemia, Oral Surg., *39*, 562, 1975.

Schlesinger, S. L., Borbotsina, J. and O'Neill, L.: Petechial hemorrhages of the soft palate secondary to fellatio, Oral Surg., *40*, 376, 1975.

Shafer, W. G.: Oral carcinoma in situ, Oral Surg., *39*, 227, 1975.

Shafer, W. G. and Waldron, C. A.: Erythroplakia of the oral cavity, Cancer, *36*, 1021, 1975.

Shklar, G.: Oral lesions of erythema multiforme. Histologic and histochemical observations, Arch. Derm., *92*, 495, 1965.

Pigmentations

Bolden, T. E.: Histology of oral pigmentation, J. Periodont., *31*, 361, 1960.

Cheraskin, E.: Diagnosis of pigmentation of the oral tissues, J. Periodont., *31*, 375, 1960.

Dummett, C. O.: Oral pigmentation, J. Periodont., *31*, 356, 1960.

Dummett, C. O. and Borens, G.: Oromucosal pigmentation: an updated literary review, J. Periodont., *42*, 726, 1971.

Jackson, D. and Simpson, H. E.: Primary malignant melanoma of the oral cavity, Oral Surg., *39*, 553, 1975.

McCrea, M. W., Miller, A. S. and Rosenthal, S. L.: Intraoral blue nevi, Oral Surg., *25*, 590, 1968.

Marlette, R. H.: Generalized melanoses and non-melanotic pigmentations of the head and neck, J. Amer. Dent. Ass., *90,* 141, 1975.

Scofield, H. H.: The blue (Jadassohn-Tieche) nevus: a previously unreported oral lesion, J. Oral Surg., *17,* 4, 1959.

Teles, J. C. B., Cardoso, A. S. and Goncalves, A. R.: Blue nevus of the oral mucosa. Review of the literature and report of two cases, Oral Surg., *38,* 905, 1974.

Trodahl, J. N. and Sprague, W. G.: Benign and malignant melanocytic lesions of the oral mucosa. An analysis of 135 cases, Cancer, *25,* 812, 1970.

Troxell, M. A.: Syndrome of Peutz (melanoplakia and small intestinal polyposis), Arch. Derm., *70,* 488, 1954.

Volker, J. F. and Kenney, J. A., Jr.: The physiology and biochemistry of pigmentation, J. Periodont., *31,* 346, 1960.

Vesicles, Bullae, Erosions

Asboe-Hansen, G.: Blister-spread induced by finger-pressure, a diagnostic sign in pemphigus, J. Invest. Derm., *34,* 5, 1960.

Brooke, R. I.: The oral lesions of bullous pemphigoid, J. Oral Med., *28,* 36, 1973.

Cahn, L.: Virus disease of the mouth, Oral Surg., *3,* 1172, 1950.

Cooke, B. E. D.: The diagnosis of bullous lesions affecting the oral mucosa, Brit. Dent. J., *109,* 83, 1960 (Part I) and Brit. Dent. J., *109,* 131, 1960 (Part II).

Cooke, B. E. D.: Median rhomboid glossitis and benign glossitis migrans (geographical tongue), Brit. Dent. J., *112,* 389, 1962.

Cram, D. L. and Fukuyama, K.: Immunohistochemistry of ultraviolet-induced pemphigus and pemphigoid lesions, Arch. Derm., *106,* 819, 1972.

Eversole, L. R., Kenney, E. B. and Sabes, W. R.: Oral lesions as the initial sign in pemphigus vulgaris, Oral Surg., *33,* 354, 1972.

Giallorenzi, A. F. and Goldstein, B. H.: Acute (toxic) necrolysis, Oral Surg., *40,* 611, 1975.

Glickman, I. and Smulow, J. B.: Chronic desquamative gingivitis—its nature and treatment, J. Periodont., *35,* 397, 1964.

Hasler, J. F.: The role of immunofluorescence in the diagnosis of oral vesiculobullous disorders. Report of four cases, Oral Surg., *33,* 362, 1972.

Honeyman, J. F., Honeyman, A., Lobutz, W. C. Jr. and Storrs, F. J.: The enigma of bullous pemphigoid and dermatitis herpetiformis, Arch. Derm., *106,* 22, 1972.

McCarthy, P. L.: Benign mucous membrane pemphigoid, Oral Surg., *33,* 75, 1972.

Ossoff, R. and Giunta, J. L.: The staphylococcal scalded-skin syndrome versus erythema multiforme, Oral Surg., *40,* 126, 1975.

Perry, H. O. and Brunsting, L. A.: Pemphigus foliaceus, Arch. Derm., *91,* 10, 1965.

Pisanti, S., Sharav, Y., Kaufman, E. and Posner, L. N.: Pemphigus vulgaris: Incidence in jaws of different ethnic groups, according to age, sex, and initial lesion, Oral Surg., *38*:382, 1974.

Ramfjord, S. P.: Recurrent herpetic stomatitis treated with gamma-globulin, Oral Surg., *13,* 165, 1961.

Randell, S. and Cohen, L.: Erosive lichen planus. Management of oral lesions with intralesional corticosteroid injections. J. Oral Med., *29,* 88, 1974.

Russotto, S. B. and Ship, I. I.: Oral manifestations of dermatitis herpetiformis, Oral Surg., *31,* 42, 1971.

Shklar, G.: Erosive and bullous oral lesions of lichen planus, Arch. Derm., *97,* 411, 1968.

Shklar, G.: The oral lesions of pemphigus vulgaris: Histochemical observations, Oral Surg., *23,* 629, 1967.

Tagami, H. and Imamura, S.: Benign mucous membrane pemphigoid. Demonstration of circulating and tissue-bound membrane antibodies, Arch. Derm., *109,* 711, 1974.

Urbanek, V. E. and Cohen, L.: Benign mucous membrane pemphigoid. Management of an edentulous patient, Oral Surg., *31,* 772, 1971.

Weathers, D. R., Baker, G., Archard, H. O. and Burkes, E. J. Jr.: Psoriasiform lesions of the oral mucosa (with emphasis on "ectopic geographic tongue"), Oral Surg., *37,* 872, 1974.

Wooten, J. W., Katz, H. I., Hoffman, S. and Link, J. F.: Development of oral lesions in erythema multiforme exudativum, Oral Surg., *24,* 808, 1967.

Pustules

McCarthy, P. L. and Shklar, G.: A syndrome of pyostomatitis vegetans and ulcerative colitis, Arch. Derm., *88,* 913, 1963.

Ulcers

Abrams, A. M., Melrose, R. J. and Howell, F. V.: Necrotizing sialometaplasia. A disease simulating malignancy, Cancer, *32,* 130, 1973.

Buchner, A.: Hand, foot and mouth disease, Oral Surg., *41,* 333, 1976.

Graykowski, E. A., Barile, M. F., Lee, W. B. and Stanley, H. R. Jr.: Recurrent aphthous stomatitis, J.A.M.A., *196,* 637, 1966.

Hamilton, McD. K., Sherrer, E. L. and Schwartz, D. S.: Lethal midline granuloma: report of a case, J. Oral Surg., *23,* 514, 1965.

Kramer, I. R. H.: Ulceration of the mouth in children, Australian Dent. J., *12,* 83, 1967.

Lehner, T.: Autoimmunity and management of recurrent oral ulceration, Brit. Dent. J., *122,* 15, 1967.

McKinney, R. V.: Hand, foot and mouth disease: a viral disease of importance to dentists, J. Amer. Dent. Ass., *91,* 122, 1975.

Rapidis, A. D., Langdon, J. D. and Patel, M. F.: Recurrent oral and oculogenital ulcerations (Behçet's syndrome), Oral Surg., *41,* 457, 1976.

Ship, I. I., Brightman, V. J. and Laster, L. L.: The patient with recurrent aphthous ulcers and the patient with recurrent herpes labialis: a study of two population samples, J. Amer. Dent. Ass., *75,* 645, 1967.

Steiner, M. and Alexander, W. N.: Primary syphilis of the gingiva, Oral Surg., *21,* 530, 1966.

Tindall, J. P. and Callaway, J. L.: Hand-foot-and-mouth disease—It's more common than you think, Amer. J. Dis. Child., *124,* 372, 1972.

Weathers, D. R. and Griffin, J. W.: Intraoral ulcerations of recurrent herpes simplex and recurrent aphthae: two distinct clinical entities, J. Amer. Dent. Ass., *81,* 81, 1970.

Cysts and Cyst-like Lesions

Cataldo, E.: Mucoceles of the oral mucous membrane, Arch., Otolaryng., *91,* 362, 1970.

Meyer, I.: Dermoid cysts (dermoids) of the floor of the mouth, Oral Surg., *8,* 1149, 1955.

Standish, S. M. and Shafer, W. G.: The mucous retention phenomenon, J. Oral Surg., *17,* 15, 1956.

Hemorrhagic and Vascular Lesions

Conley, J. and Pack, G. T.: Melanoma of the mucous membranes of the head and neck, Arch. Otolaryng., *99,* 315, 1974.

Freeman, N. S. and Plezia, R. A.: Felty's syndrome, Oral Surg., *40,* 409, 1975.

Kramer, I. R. H.: Malignant lymphoma of children in Africa, Int. Dent. J., *15,* 200, 1965.

Leake, D. and Deykin, D.: The diagnosis and treatment of bleeding tendencies, Oral Surg., *32,* 852, 1971.

Little, J. W.: Detection and management of the potential bleeder in dental practice, J. Oral Med., *31,* 11, 1976.

Lynch, M. A. and Ship, I. I.: Initial oral manifestations of leukemia, J. Amer. Dent. Ass., *75,* 932, 1967.

Nalbandian, R. M., Henry, R. L., Kessler, D. L., Camp, F. R. Jr., and Wolf, P. L.: Consumption coagulopathy: Practice principles of diagnosis and management, Hum. Path., *2,* 377, 1971.

Roser, S. M. and Roxenbloom, B.: Continued anticoagulation in oral surgery procedures, Oral Surg., *40,* 448, 1975.

Southam, J. C. and Ettinger, R. L.: A histologic study of sublingual varices, Oral Surg., *38,* 879, 1974.

Tarsitano, J. J. and Cohen, S. M.: Revelation and initial diagnosis of mild hemophilia from dental findings: report of case, J. Amer. Dent. Ass., *76,* 823, 1968.

Walker, R. O. and Rose, M.: Oral manifestations of haematological disorders, Brit. Dent. J., *118,* 286, 1965.

Wintrobe, M. M.: *Clinical Hematology,* 7th Ed., Philadelphia, Lea & Febiger, 1974.

Yacabucci, J. E. and Kramer, H. S. Jr.: Platelet defects of importance in oral surgery, J. Oral Surg., *30,* 478, 1972.

Focal and Diffuse Soft Tissue Enlargements

Arons, M. S., Solitare, G. B. and Grunt, J. A.: The macroglossia of Beckwith's syndrome, Plast. Reconstr. Surg., *45,* 341, 1970.

Barber, J. W. and Burns, J. B.: Subcutaneous emphysema of the face and neck after dental restoration, J. Amer. Dent. Ass., *75,* 167, 1967.

Baughman, R. A.: Lingual thyroid and median rhomboid glossitis, M.S.D. thesis, Indiana University School of Dentistry, 1969

Bhaskar, S. N. and Jacoway, J. R.: Pyogenic granuloma—clinical features, incidence, histology and result of treatment: report of 242 cases, J. Oral Surg., *24,* 391, 1966.

Bochetto, J. F., Raycroft, J. F. and DeInnocents, L. W.: Multiple polyposis, exotosis and soft tissue tumors, Surgery, *177,* 489, 1963.

Bowers, D. G.: The serious implications of multiple mucosal neuromata, Plast. Reconstr. Surg., *56,* 554, 1975.

Chaudhry, A. P., Gorlin, R. J. and Mitchell, D. F.: Papillary cystadenoma of minor salivary gland origin, Oral Surg., *13,* 452, 1960.

Clark, D. C.: Prolonged trismus in chronic abscess of the pterygomandibular space, J. Oral Surg., *28,* 424, 1970.

Farman, A. G. and Uys, P. B.: Oral Kaposi's sarcoma, Oral Surg., *39,* 288, 1975.

Frable, W. J. and Elzay, R. P.: Tumors of minor salivary glands: a report of 73 cases, Cancer, *25,* 932, 1970.

Gambardella, R. J.: Kaposi's sarcoma and its oral manifestations, Oral Surg., *38,* 591, 1974.

Hall, H. D., Gunter, J. W. Jr., Jamison, H. C. and McCallum, C. A. Jr.: Effect of time of extraction on resolution of odontogenic cellulitis, J. Amer. Dent. Ass., *77,* 626, 1968.

Laskin, D. M.: Anatomic considerations in diagnosis and treatment of odontogenic infections, Oral Surg., *25,* 590, 1968.

Laymon, C. W.: Cheilitis granulomatosa and Melkersson-Rosenthal syndrome, Arch. Derm., *83,* 112, 1961.

Oberman, H. A. and Sullenger, G.: Neurogenous tumors of the head and neck, Cancer, *20,* 1922, 1967.

Shiffman, M. A.: Familial multiple polyposis associated with soft-tissue and hard-tissue tumors, J.A.M.A., *179,* 138, 1962.

Simpson, H. E., Howell, R. A. and Summersgill, G. B.: Oral manifestations of Crohn's disease, J. Oral Med., *29,* 49, 1974.

Spatz, S.: Angioneurotic edema of the maxillofacial region, Oral Surg., *18,* 256, 1964.

Spika, C. J.: Pathways of dental infection, J. Oral Surg., *24,* 111, 1966.

Standish, S. M. and Shafer, W.G.: Gingival reparative granulomas in children, J. Oral Surg., *19,* 367, 1961.

Steigman, A. J. *et al.*: Acute lymphonodular pharyngitis: a newly described condition due to Coxsackie A virus, J. Pediat., *61,* 331, 1962.

Stuteville, O. H. and Corley, R. D.: Surgical management of tumors of intra-oral minor salivary glands, Cancer, *20,* 1578, 1967.

Tomich, C. E. and Hutton, C. E.: Adenoid squamous cell carcinoma of the lip: report of cases, J. Oral Surg., *30,* 592, 1972.

Tomich, C. E. and Shafer, W. G.: Lymphoproliferative disease of the hard palate: a clinicopathologic entity, Oral Surg., *39,* 754, 1975.

Weathers, D. R. and Driscoll, R. M.: Darier's disease of the oral mucosa, Oral Surg., *37,* 711, 1974.

Weitzner, S. and Hentel, W.: Metastatic carcinoma in tongue, Oral Surg., *25,* 278, 1968.

Weitzner, S.: Adenoid squamous cell carcinoma of the vermilion mucosa of lower lip, Oral Surg., *37,* 587, 1974.

Varley, E. W. B.: Crohn's disease of the mouth, Oral Surg., *33,* 570, 1972.

Vellios, F. and Shafer, W. G.: Tumors of the intraoral accessory salivary glands, Surg. Gynec. Obstet., *108,* 450, 1959.

Chapter 15

Diseases of the Jaw Bones

Osteoid Osteoma
Chondroma
Hemangioma
Arteriovenous Aneurysm
Desmoplastic Fibroma of Bone, Fibroxanthoma
Central Neurogenic Tumors of the Jaws
Neuroectodermal Tumor of Infancy
Malignant Tumors
Osteosarcoma
Chondrosarcoma
Reticulum Cell Sarcoma of Bone
Fibrosarcoma of Bone
Ewing's Sarcoma
Multiple Myeloma
Carcinoma of the Antrum
Malignant Central Salivary Gland Tumors
Metastatic Bone Disease
Metabolic Disorders
Histiocytosis X Disease
Von Recklinghausen's Disease of Bone
Paget's Disease of Bone
Gaucher's Disease
Osteogenesis Imperfecta
Osteopetrosis
Osteoporosis
Caffey's Disease

DIFFERENTIAL DIAGNOSIS

The differential diagnosis of lesions of the jaw bones and odontogenic apparatus is predicated on an understanding of the biology of calcified tissues and a working knowledge of the spectrum of specific disorders affecting these tissues.

Evaluation of the physical and radiographic findings will generally suggest (1) the growth rate and pattern of the lesion, (2) the nature of the underlying basic pathologic process (e.g. developmental, neoplastic, inflammatory, metabolic, etc.), and (3) whether the disease is of odontogenic or non-odontogenic origin. Additionally, the presenting signs and symptoms; age and sex of the patient and distribution of the lesions; characterization of the radiographic lesion (radiolucent, radiopaque or combined lesion); anatomic site with reference to the teeth, marrow, cortex or other structures; and any pertinent laboratory findings and other systemic manifestations must be considered in arriving at a differential or provisional diagnosis. Frequently, the presenting clinical and radiographic features will be sufficiently characteristic for a definitive

diagnosis without further diagnostic tests or exploratory procedures. In difficult cases, the list of possible diagnoses can be further reduced by excluding the least likely possibilities.

In the following sections, these principles are discussed in further detail: (1) the reactions of bone to injury, (2) the significance of presenting signs and symptoms, (3) the evaluation of radiolucent, radiopaque and combined lesions of bone, (4) the significance of laboratory findings in bone disease, (5) lesions of bone which occur at particular anatomic sites, and (6) specific odontogenic and non-odontogenic diseases according to basic pathologic process.

REACTION OF BONE TO INJURY

As with all primary tissues of the body, bone reacts to injury in only a limited number of ways. With a given injury, whether it be developmental, infectious, traumatic, metabolic or neoplastic, bone will respond with (1) no discernible effect, (2) bone destruction, (3) bone formation, or (4) simultaneous bone destruction and formation. This response may then produce certain signs and symptoms which together with the radiographic findings are a reflection of the underlying disease process. Figure 15–1 presents the reaction of bone to injury in outline form.

CLINICAL EVIDENCE
OF BONE DISEASE

Pain is the most common overt symptom of disease involving the jaw bones and teeth (see. Chap. 10). Usually it can be related to pulpal or periodontal inflammation and infections; other sources of pain, such as tumors and fractures, may arise primarily in the jaw bones or from disease processes outside the jaws (*e.g.*, neuralgia, referred pain, metastatic bone disease, etc.). Neuritis secondary to acute inflammation, infection or post-herpetic neuralgia may account for the pain in some cases and thus may arise cen-

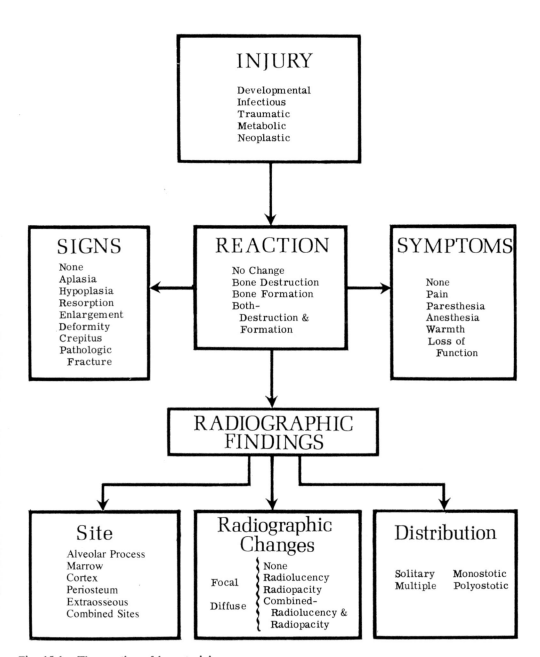

Fig. 15-1. The reaction of bone to injury.

trally within the bone or along nerve trunks supplying sensory function to the jaws. In this regard, *causalgia* is characterized by pain in the mucosa overlying an apparently healed extraction site. Pain in other bones is a fairly constant feature in multiple myeloma, Paget's disease of bone and metastatic carcinoma.

Paresthesia, hypesthesia, and anesthesia are uncommon symptoms of disease in the jaws. They may result from trauma, inflammation and infection or neoplastic disease. In every case of unexplained paresthesia, especially of the mandible, metastatic tumor to the jaw must be considered in the differential diagnosis and positive steps must be taken to confirm or rule out this possibility. Most commonly, the metastatic deposits will occur in the posterior body and ramus of the mandible as multiple, poorly defined radiolucencies, sometimes with intermixed radiopaque foci. Interrogation of the patient will often reveal a history of cancer treatment some years previously, although in some instances the metastatic jaw lesion may be the first clinical manifestation of malignancy elsewhere in the body. Prior trauma to the jaws with fracture, or tooth extraction with injury to the inferior alveolar nerve, may be associated with the onset of the paresthesia or anesthesia. Inflammatory and infectious processes in the bone may cause paresthesia of varying degrees, particularly if the reaction is acute or a proliferative (granulomatous) process impinging on major nerve trunks. In some cases, the paresthesia may be preceded by hyperesthesia and the inflammatory nature of the condition will be obvious.

Increased warmth of the bones is an uncommon symptom which has been described in acute inflammation and cellulitis of the jaws and Paget's disease of bone. In the latter, this symptom is noted most readily in long bones rather than the jaws.

Loss of function may be reported by the patient or observed by the examiner as mandibular deviation on opening, luxation or subluxation of the joint, inability to open the mouth (ankylosis or trismus) or inability to occlude the teeth.

Hypoplasia or failure of complete development of one or both jaws may signify a hereditary or familial tendency or indicate a disturbance in growth dating from early childhood. Retrognathia of the mandible is one manifestation of Pierre Robin syndrome or craniofacial dysostosis. Retrusion of the maxilla, seen in cleidocranial dysostosis, represents a disturbance of growth at the base of the skull rather than a significant underdevelopment of the maxilla. Acquired hypoplasia of the mandible usually is the result of injury to growth centers in the condylar region, often during childbirth, and sometimes results in temporomandibular joint ankylosis. If the injury involves only one condyle, unilateral hypoplasia results with deviation of the jaw on opening to the affected side.

Hyperplasia or generalized increased size of the jaws may also follow a familial pattern or appear in later life as an acquired condition. Radiographically, and histologically, the bone pattern is essentially normal. Mandibular prognathism is most commonly seen either as a familial trait or secondary to continued growth stimulus of the mandible. Condylar hyperplasia, either bilateral or unilateral, will produce mandibular prognathism or deviation of the jaw to the unaffected side, respectively. Generalized overgrowth of the mandible is seen in acromegaly and pituitary giantism (p. 253).

Enlargements of the jaws may be localized to one segment of the jaws or present as a generalized enlargement of one or both jaws. As used here and in contrast to hyperplasia, enlargement implies abnormal radiographic and histologic changes in the bone. Enlargement of a portion or segment of the jaw occurs in those conditions which involve the cortex by expansion, osteophyte formation or cortical reduplication. These include dentigerous cyst, ameloblastoma, Pindborg tumor, central cementifying fibroma, central giant cell granuloma, fibrous dysplasia, osteosarcoma, chondrosarcoma, Garre's osteomyelitis and Ewing's sarcoma. Conditions causing generalized enlargement of one or both jaws include Paget's disease of bone, familial fibrous dysplasia (cherubism), Hand-Schüller-Christian disease, chronic sclerosing osteomyelitis and infantile cortical hyperostosis (Caffey's disease).

Deformity of the jaws, resulting from gross anatomic deficiencies, is seen in cleft palate and following traumatic injury or radical surgery. Massive osteolysis ("disappearing bone"), a condition of unknown etiology, results in marked deformity of jaws due to progressive resorption of the alveolar process and basilar bone of the jaws.

Crepitus is a crackling sound heard when the segments of a fractured bone are moved against one another. The paper-thin cortical bone overlying a dentigerous cyst or other expansile lesion may also show crepitus.

Bruit, a murmur heard from a central lesion in bone with a stethoscope, generally indicates a hemangioma or vascular anomaly (A-V aneurysm).

Systemic signs often provide important clues in the diagnosis of lesions of the jaw bones. Certain syndromes with jaw lesions have associated systemic signs readily observable to the examiner: *Gardner's syndrome* with jaw osteomas, multiple supernumerary and impacted teeth, dermoid or sebaceous cysts of the skin and colon polyposis; *cleidocranial dysostosis* with hypoplasia of the maxilla, absence of the clavicles, wormian bones and other features; *Gorlin-Goltz syndrome* with odontogenic keratocysts, basal cell nevi, bifid ribs and other anomalies; *Papillon-Lefevre syndrome* with juvenile periodontosis and palmar and plantar hyperkeratosis; *osteogenesis imperfecta* with multiple long bone fractures, blue sclera and sometimes dentinogenesis imperfecta; *von Recklinghausen's disease of bone* with "bones, stones and abdominal groans," *i.e.* brown tumors, kidney stones and gastric ulcers (see also pp. 249–251).

Less specific systemic signs of disease, while not diagnostic, may also aid in supporting or excluding a particular diagnosis. Regional lymphadenopathy is seen in the inflammatory diseases whereas both local and distant lymph node metastasis is a late manifestation of malignant bone disease. Fever and malaise are also indicative of inflammation and infection; however, Ewing's sarcoma exhibits these features as well.

RADIOGRAPHIC EVIDENCE OF BONE DISEASE

The radiographic examination provides a major source of information in suspected bone disease and usually will permit a tentative clinical diagnosis on which to base further diagnostic studies.

The basic radiographic changes in bone are radiolucent, radiopaque or combined radiolucent-radiopaque reactions which may be focal, well-circumscribed with or without cortication, or diffuse and poorly outlined. Such lesions may also be solitary or multiple in a single bone (monostotic) or several bones (polyostotic).

The effect of disease arising centrally within bone upon the adjacent cortex may also provide important clues as to the nature of the process. The radiographic findings in lesions involving the cortex are cortical expansion and thinning, osteophyte formation, reduplication (onionskin) of the cortex, and cortical erosion. These reactions are discussed in some detail in the following sections since they provide guidelines to whether a given lesion is slow or fast growing, or even benign or malignant.

Radiolucent Lesions

The radiolucent lesions in the jaw bones may be unilocular or multilocular, focal or diffuse, confined to single bone or involving several bones.

A well-circumscribed radiolucency within the medullary cavity of bone suggests a relatively slow-growing lesion which is benign. The radiolucent area is sharply out-

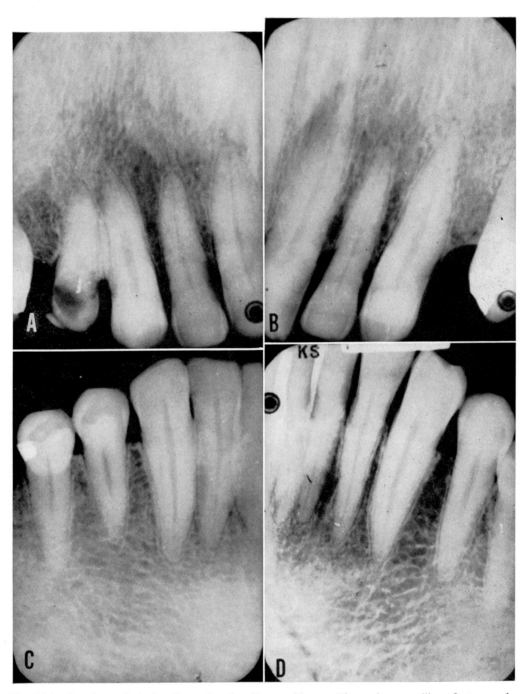

Fig. 15-2. Routine periapical radiographs of a 58-year-old man. The carious maxillary first premolar shown in *A* was extracted. (O'Shaughnessy, Oral Surg., *17,* 170, 1964.)

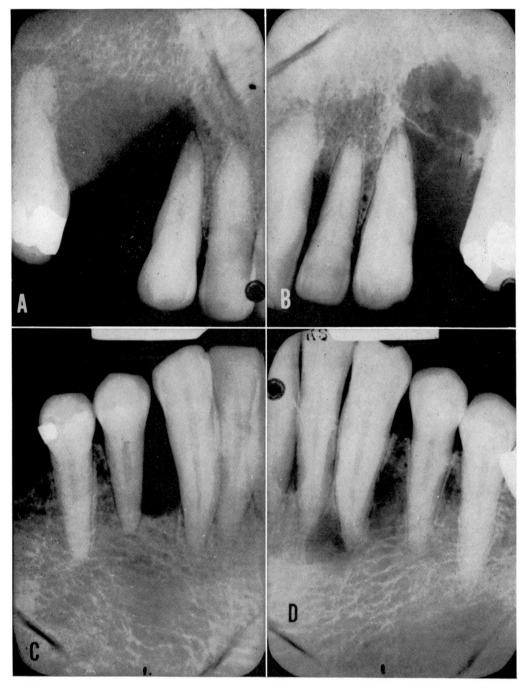

Fig. 15-3. *A–D,* Chronic lymphatic leukemia. Periapical radiographs of the same patient shown in Figure 15–2. The films in Figure 15–3 were taken 8 months later. Multiple destructive bone lesions are seen. (O'Shaughnessy, Oral Surg., *17,* 710, 1964.)

lined and surrounded by smooth bone which may or may not exhibit cortication. Although it has been suggested that a cortical border around a radiolucent defect is good evidence of cyst formation, a number of studies have established that cortication reflects only slow growth of the lesion with mild stimulus to the adjacent bone rather than the nature of the tissue present.

The most common discrete focal radiolucencies of the jaws are tooth-associated lesions such as the periapical granuloma, apical periodontal cyst and dentigerous cyst. The fissural cysts as well as certain central benign tumors also manifest themselves in this manner.

Radiolucencies without cortication and following an irregular outline may be seen in traumatic (hemorrhagic) bone cysts. Since clinically these lesions appear as fluid-filled or empty spaces without a lining, there seems to be little stimulus to the surrounding normal bone. The periphery of the lesions generally follows the path of least resistance and may extend around and between the roots of adjacent teeth.

A radiolucency showing a ragged appearance of the surrounding bone indicates a rapidly growing lesion which is infiltrating the adjacent marrow spaces (Figs. 15–2, 3). Although such reactions may be seen in acute infectious processes, a malignant neoplasm must be considered, especially if there are associated features of sudden onset, rapid growth, paresthesia or pain. Involvement of the cortex of bone with rapid perforation or pathologic fracture is strongly suggestive of malignant tumor (Fig. 15–4).

Multiple focal radiolucencies of the jaws not related to the tooth crown, periapex or periodontal tissue are suggestive of a generalized disease process such as histiocytosis X disease.

Multiple "punched-out" lesions central in bone are seen typically in multiple myeloma. These lesions show a well-circumscribed

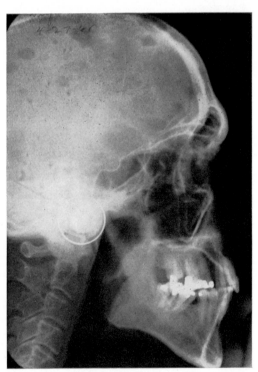

Fig. 15-5. Chronic lymphatic leukemia. Lateral head plate of the patient (Figs. 15-2 to 15-4) showing multiple "punched-out" lesions of the skull similar to that seen in multiple myeloma. Blood studies revealed the following: WBC—26,300/mm³ (polys, 19%; lymphocytes, 80%); Hbg—12.3 gm%; hematocrit—37%. (O'Shaughnessy, Oral Surg., 17, 170, 1964.)

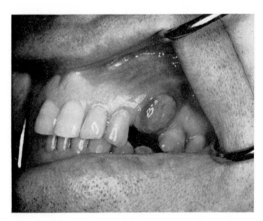

Fig. 15-4. Chronic lymphatic leukemia. Clinical photograph of the patient (Figs. 15-2, 15-3) showing a mass overlying the radiolucency seen in Figure 15-3B. This and a similar lesion on the opposite side of the mouth had been incised one week previously. No drainage occurred. (O'Shaughnessy, Oral Surg., 17, 170, 1964.)

radiolucency without evidence of reactivity of the adjacent bone (Fig. 15–5).

Multilocular radiolucencies are of two main types. The so-called multilocular cyst, characteristic of the ameloblastoma, classically shows a large number of communicating radiolucent cavities separated by long tortuous trabeculae. A second pattern seen is that of a reasonably well circumscribed radiolucency with delicate trabeculae extending from the outer borders and dividing the defect into a number of poorly outlined compartments. This latter reaction, sometimes described as having a soap-bubble appearance, is seen in varying degrees in odontogenic myxoma, central hemangioma, central giant cell granuloma and aneurysmal bone cyst.

A number of metabolic disturbances (endocrine and nutritional diseases, certain anemias and old age) exhibit a generalized reduction in the trabecular pattern of the bone (osteoporosis). Similar changes are seen in edentulous or non-functional dentulous areas.

Radiopaque Lesions

Radiopaque structures seen on routine radiographs must be evaluated on the basis of their density, configuration, growth pattern and distribution. They may be sharply circumscribed or diffuse and may be present as either solitary or multiple defects involving one or both jaws.

If teeth are present, the comparison of radiographic density with the relatively constant radiodense appearance of enamel and dentin provides a good guide to the quality of the film and permits an accurate estimate of the density of the object.

Generally, the relative density and configuration of the mass are sufficiently typical to identify those opacities that arise from teeth or tooth structure. For example, odontomas or retained root tips will contain varying amounts of enamel and dentin which may be compared with the density of other teeth in the radiograph. Metallic filling

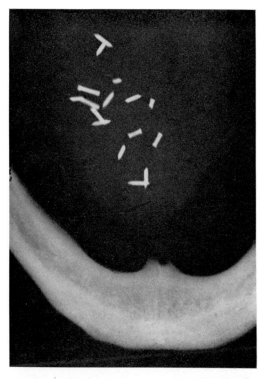

Fig. 15-6. Radon seeds in the tongue. Pellets or seeds of radon were used in radiation therapy of epidermoid carcinoma of the tongue. Since radon has a half-life of 3.8 days, the pellets are often left embedded in the tissues where they appear as radiopaque foreign bodies.

material or other foreign bodies may be identified by the unusual configuration or dense homogeneous pattern not typical of biologic structures. Fragments of glass will sometimes appear radiodense when they are embedded in the tissue. Other radiodense objects seen in routine dental radiographs include buckshot, bullets or substances which have been purposely implanted in the tissues, such as radon seeds and various kinds of submucosal implant materials (Figs. 15–6 and 7). Radiodense lesions composed chiefly of bone or calcified cartilage again may be compared with normal cortical bone seen in the radiograph.

Small, irregular radiodense lesions, or "bone scars," are frequently seen in edentulous mandibular molar areas. These foci of "sclerotic bone" are surrounded by normal

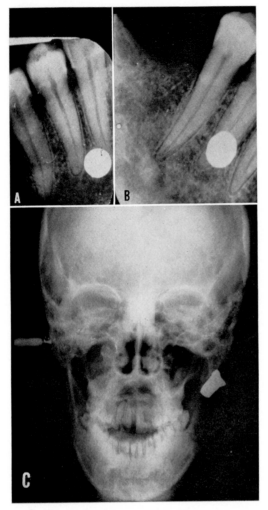

Fig. 15-7. Foreign bodies. *A* and *B*, Lead pellet
(BB) embedded in the cheek. It was discovered on
routine periapical radiographs where it appeared
superimposed over the apices of the teeth. The
absence of any bone reaction suggests it is located in the adjacent soft tissues. Radiographs
taken at different angles as shown indicate that
the object is located labially to the bone. *C*, Bullet
located in the cheek anterior to the mandibular
ramus. The mandible has been fractured. (*C*
courtesy of W. C. Baker.)

trabeculae and generally represent reactive
bone secondary to an earlier inflammatory
reaction. A similar but more productive reaction is seen in condensing osteitis (focal
sclerosing osteomyelitis).

Generalized increased bone density is seen
in osteopetrosis, characterized by inadequate
osteoclastic remodeling and reabsorption of
bone trabeculae.

Combined Radiolucent-radiopaque Lesions

Lesions which present alternate areas of
radiolucency and radiopacity can be grouped
into those that are well-circumscribed, solitary defects ("target lesions") and those
that are diffuse, poorly outlined single or
multiple lesions. An example of the former
is seen in the adenomatoid odontogenic
tumor which appears primarily as a radiolucency which is sharply outlined and may
exhibit radiodense shadows of considerably
less density than normal bone. Other target
lesions are the complex odontoma, osteoma,
osteoid-osteoma, Gorlin cyst, cementoma,
ameloblastic fibro-odontoma, ameloblastic
fibrodentinoma, cementoma and benign
cementoblastoma. In general, these appear
as well-circumscribed and rather homogeneously dense areas surrounded by a thin
radiolucent border representing a fibrous
connective tissue "capsule." The surrounding
bone generally shows a normal trabecular
pattern without cortication. Some lesions of
bone will appear as radiolucencies early
in their development and subsequently show
increasing amounts of calcification as they
mature. Examples of these include the
periapical cemental dysplasia (cementoma),
the developing odontoma, and the central
cementifying fibroma.

Among the diffuse reactions showing
simultaneous bone resorption and bone formation are such conditions as chronic diffuse
sclerosing osteomyelitis and Paget's disease
of bone (osteitis deformans). Bone enlargement is seen in both conditions but is most
prominent in Paget's disease. Both conditions may show varying proportions of bone
resorption and bone production, depending
upon the stage of the disease. For example,
Paget's disease may be primarily radiolucent
with scattered dense foci referred to as
cotton-wool or pumice bone. Chronic diffuse
sclerosing osteomyelitis is seen most fre-

quently in elderly individuals, usually women, and may affect one or both jaws.

Certain metastatic tumors to the jaws (most notably those from the prostate, breast and lung) may occasionally stimulate bone formation and appear as mixed radiolucent-radiopaque lesions, usually in the posterior mandible.

LABORATORY EVIDENCE OF BONE DISEASE

Clinical laboratory tests (Chap. 9) are ordinarily used to support or confirm the histologic diagnosis of bone disease; only rarely will routine laboratory studies call attention to the presence of a previously undiscovered bone disease.

Osseous and odontogenic disorders in which certain clinical laboratory tests are of diagnostic value are listed below:

Central giant cell lesions—serum calcium, phosphorus, alkaline phosphatase

Metastatic bone disease—serum calcium, phosphorus, alkaline phosphatase, LDH

Paget's disease of bone—serum alkaline phosphatase

Neuroectodermal tumor of infancy—vanillylmandelic acid

Specific infections of bone—bacterial smears, culture, antibiotic sensitivity tests

Multiple myeloma—total protein, electrophoresis, Bence-Jones protein

Blood dyscrasias involving bone—complete, differential blood count, bone marrow biopsy

Acromegaly, giantism—tests of pituitary function

Osteoporosis, osteomalacia—serum calcium, phosphorus, alkaline phosphatase

SITE-SPECIFIC LESIONS OF BONE

The anatomic site and shape of a given lesion often provide important clues for diagnosis and frequently may be so typical that a reasonably definitive diagnosis may be established. For example, the developmental or fissural cysts usually present a typical radiographic appearance at a specific site, and a working diagnosis can be established

on the basis of the radiograph alone. With certain exceptions, many odontogenic cysts and neoplasms can also be identified with reasonable accuracy, although histologic examination should be carried out in all cases.

In addition to those lesions that are anatomically related to fissural cysts, the odontogenic apparatus or the tooth-bearing areas of the jaws, radiographic defects which are located anatomically within the marrow cavity, associated with the bony cortex, or primarily periosteal in origin, should be distinguished. Further, contiguous extraosseous lesions may involve the adjacent periosteum and bone, resulting in bone remodeling or destruction.

Tooth-associated Lesions

Characteristically, the odontogenic lesions are associated with the teeth or tooth-bearing areas of the jaws. The non-odontogenic lesions, on the other hand, only coincidentally involve these structures. Thus, before a tentative diagnosis can be established, it is obviously necessary to decide whether a given lesion is more probably of odontogenic or non-odontogenic origin. Such a decision is made only after careful consideration of all the information collected in the examination procedure.

Crown-associated Lesions

Because of the neoplastic potential of the enamel organ, several odontogenic cysts and tumors are seen in association with the crowns of impacted teeth (Table 15–1).

Root-associated Lesions

As noted, non-odontogenic lesions arising centrally in the bone (see following section) may coincidentally involve the periapical or lateral radicular areas of the tooth and thus may simulate certain odontogenic disorders. More commonly, however, those lesions in direct continuity with the root or periodontal ligament space will be of odontogenic origin (Table 15–1).

TABLE 15-1. TOOTH-ASSOCIATED LESIONS OF THE JAWS

	Radiolucent Lesions	Radiopaque Lesions	Target Lesions	Loss of Lamina Dura	Widening of Periodontal Ligament
ROOT ASSOCIATED	Periapical granuloma	Hypercementosis	Periapical cemental dysplasia (intermediate and mature stages)	Hyperparathyroidism	Scleroderma
	Apical periodontal cyst	Condensing osteitis	Benign cementoblastoma	Paget's disease of bone	Osteosarcoma
	Lateral periodontal cyst		Odontoma	Chronic diffuse sclerosing osteomyelitis	
	Periodontitis			Sprue	
	Periodontosis			Cushing's syndrome	
	Juvenile periodontosis			Fibrous dysplasia	
	Periapical cemental dysplasia (osteolytic stage)				
	Fibrous healing defect				
CROWN ASSOCIATED	Dentigerous cyst		Adenomatoid odontogenic tumor		
	Odontogenic keratocyst (dentigerous cyst type)		Pindborg tumor		
	Mural ameloblastoma		Gorlin cyst		
	Ameloblastic fibroma		Ameloblastic odontoma		
			Ameloblastic fibrodentinoma		

Often subtle radiographic alterations of the lamina dura and/or the periodontal ligament space may precede the development of the root-associated lesions listed. Additionally, generalized structural changes in the lamina dura and periodontal ligament may be of diagnostic importance in certain reactive, dysplastic, neoplastic and metabolic disorders (Table 15–1).

Morphologic changes in the tooth roots in the vicinity of a pathologic process may also provide valuable diagnostic information. A benign, indolent process arising during some stage of root development will often cause *dilaceration* of the roots and permit the age of onset to be estimated by reference to standard tooth development charts. *Generalized hypercementosis* of the tooth is a feature of Paget's disease of bone. *Resorption* of tooth roots will generally indicate a chronic, inflammatory process or certain benign neoplastic processes. For example, some apical root resorption is often seen in long-standing periapical infections. Among the discrete radiolucencies, long-standing ameloblastoma often causes extensive root resorption whereas the central giant cell granuloma, aneurysmal bone cyst, traumatic bone cyst and odontogenic myxoma do not. Resorption of tooth roots in a destructive, poorly circumscribed radiolucency will generally indicate a benign process, probably inflammatory. While rapidly growing malignant tumors also cause extensive and poorly defined areas of bone destruction, they do not usually have time to induce the slower process of root resorption.

Central Lesions of Bone

Several lesions of the jaws show a predilection for characteristic sites along embryologic lines of closure (*e.g.* the fissural cysts) or centrally within bone. It should be emphasized, however, that other than the fissural cysts few if any of these conditions are invariably site-specific. However, a number do show a strong predilection for particular locations in the jaws. For example,

the traumatic bone cyst, ameloblastoma, odontogenic keratocyst, Pindborg tumor and tumor metastatic to the jaws are characteristically seen in the posterior mandible. Lesions which appear to arise within the mandibular canal are most probably neurofibromas or neurilemmomas.

Common *multilocular radiolucencies* in the posterior mandible are the ameloblastoma, the odontogenic myxoma, aneurysmal bone cyst and the traumatic bone cyst. Multilocular radiolucencies found anterior to the first and second molar teeth are commonly the central giant cell granuloma and the brown tumor of hyperparathyroidism. *Bilateral multilocular or diffuse radiolucencies* of the jaws are almost invariably those of familial fibrous dysplasia or Hand-Schüller-Christian disease.

Cortical and Periosteal Reactions

Infringement of a central lesion on the cortex of bone may result in thinning and expansion of the cortex. If the continuity of the cortex is preserved, a slow-growing and presumably benign lesion is suspected. Because of the simultaneous effort of the body to strengthen and buttress the cortex, a somewhat more rapidly growing central lesion may expand the cortex and stimulate periosteal osteophyte formation or even reduplication of the cortex. These latter periosteal reactions are analogous to the fracture callus and to the "hair-on-end" effect seen in the outer tables of the calvarium in Mediterranean and sickle-cell anemias, in which reactive hematopoietic tissue of the diploe apparently stimulates a periosteal response.

More rapidly growing central or extraosseous lesions adjacent to bone may perforate the cortex. In general, central lesions with a ragged border and cortical destruction are clearly indicative of a highly destructive process which is probably a malignant tumor. *Cortical expansion and thinning* are common findings with the dentigerous cyst, the odontogenic keratocyst and the central ce-

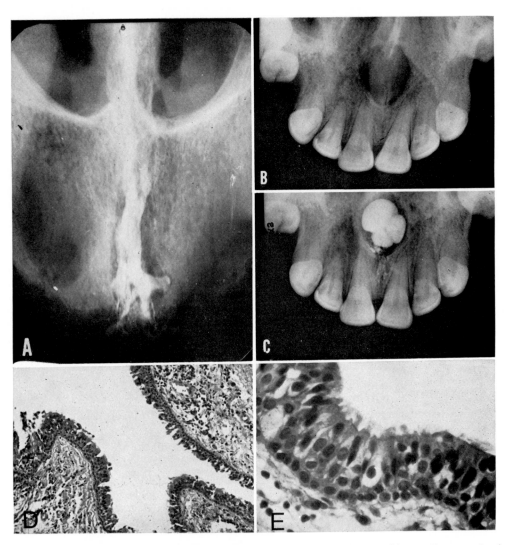

Fig. 15–8. *A*, Patent incisive canal and cyst. The radiolucency was injected with a radiopaque dye in order to determine its size and shape more clearly. (Courtesy of Grant Van Huysen.) *B*, Incisive canal cyst. *C*, Incisive canal cyst shown in *B* with radiopaque dye. *D*, Photomicrograph showing respiratory epithelium lining an incisive canal cyst. *E*, High-power photomicrograph of *D*.

mentifying fibroma if they are of long duration. Thinning and expansion of the cortex are also characteristic of the large multilocular radiolucencies (p. 447), features which indicate an aggressive but benign process.

Cortical osteophyte formation may occasionally occur in response to an underlying aggressive benign neoplasm; however, this "sunray" radiographic appearance mandates a provisional diagnosis of osteoblastic or juxtacortical osteosarcoma until proven otherwise.

Cortical reduplicaiton or onionskin cortex is characteristic of Garre's osteomyelitis in the young individual with an associated chronic pulpal infection. In the young child with central destructive bone lesions, the onionskin pattern is suggestive of Ewing's sarcoma. Bilateral cortical reduplication coupled with overlying soft tissue inflammation is indicative of infantile cortical hyperostosis (Caffey's disease).

Cortical erosion and perforation in association with a moth-eaten, ill-defined radiolucency are strongly suggestive of malignant disease or acute osteomyelitis. On the other hand, cortical destruction with alveolar bone loss surrounding one or more teeth in the young adult is most compatible with eosinophilic granuloma of bone.

Cortical "cuffing" of the edentulous alveolar process is characteristic of an overlying peripheral giant cell granuloma. Cupping out of the lower border of the mandible anterior to the angle is indicative of the submandibular salivary gland depression.

Extraosseous calcification of lesions in continuity with the periosteum may occur in the peripheral odontogenic (ossifying) fibroma, extraosseous Gorlin cyst and the extraosseous Pindborg tumor. Ossifying or calcifying lesions in adjacent soft tissue but not in continuity with the cortex are most probably calcified lymph nodes, phleboliths, myositis ossificans, calcinosis cutis or osseous choristomas.

DEVELOPMENTAL DISORDERS

Discrepancies in Jaw Size and Dental Arch Relationships

Gross variations in jaw size and dental arch relationships are discussed on pages 301–307. Both hypoplasia and hyperplasia of the jaws reflect disturbances in growth which may range from minor deviations from normal to severe and disfiguring discrepancies. Frequently, the latter are associated with other congenital anomalies and some comprise recognizable syndromes.

Fissural Cysts

The developmental or fissural cysts of the jaws are identified chiefly by their shape and characteristic location. They arise along lines of closure of embryonic processes of the jaws and are unrelated to the teeth. In some instances, a large cyst may appear to involve the periapex of an adjacent tooth, thereby suggesting the diagnosis of periapical granu-

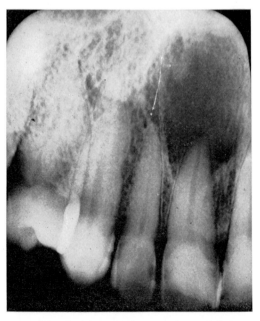

Fig. 15-9. Incisive canal cyst. The radiolucency is superimposed over the apex of the maxillary central incisor suggesting periapical disease. However, pulp vitality tests were normal. Additional radiographs taken at different angles are necessary.

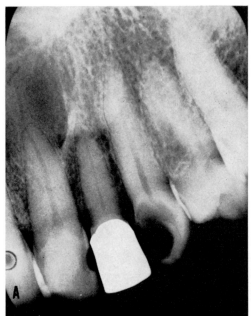

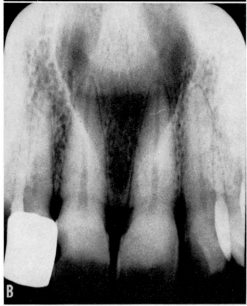

loma or apical periodontal cyst. By changing the angle of the radiograph, an intact lamina dura about the apex of the presumably involved tooth can usually be seen. Pulp vitality tests are of obvious value in such cases.

Nasopalatine Cyst

The nasopalatine (incisive canal, median anterior maxillary) cyst is presumed to arise from rests of epithelium of the embryonic nasopalatine duct (Fig. 15–8). It is usually diagnosed by its position in the midline of the anterior maxilla in the region of the incisive canal. In routine periapical radiographs, the cyst may be superimposed over apices of either or both of the central incisors suggesting a periapical lesion (Fig. 15–9). Changing the radiograph angle and the finding of normal pulp vitality usually establish the clinical diagnosis (Fig. 15–10). In most instances, surgical removal is not

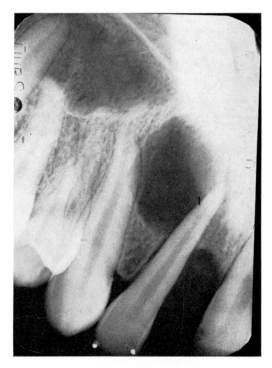

Fig. 15-10. Incisive canal cyst. *A,* The radiolucency is superimposed over the central incisor similar to the case shown in Figure 15-9. The intact periodontal membrane space and faint lamina dura visible in this case further suggest superimposition of images. *B,* Another view of the incisive canal cyst shown in *A.*

Fig. 15-11. Globulomaxillary cyst. A focal radiolucency is seen between the divergent roots of the maxillary canine and lateral incisor teeth. (Mitchell, *Practical Dental Monographs,* Jan. 1965, courtesy of Year Book Medical Publishers, Inc.)

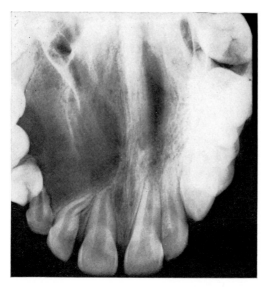

Fig. 15-12. Globulomaxillary cyst. The radio-lucent defect has caused divergence of the roots of the maxillary canine and lateral incisor teeth. Dilaceration of the lateral incisor tooth root is severe, indicating that the lesion has been present for many years.

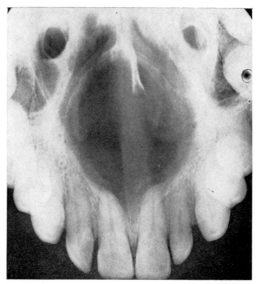

Fig. 15-13. Median palatal cyst. The radio-lucency is located in the midline of the palate.

indicated except in the very large cysts or those that are causing symptoms of pain or swelling and drainage.

Globulomaxilliary Cyst

The globulomaxillary cyst is typified by its position as a radiolucent lesion between the maxillary lateral incisor and canine teeth (Figs. 15–11 and 12). On frequent oc-casions, bilateral globulomaxillary cysts are seen. The neighboring teeth are vital and asymptomatic.

Median Palatal Cyst

The median palatal cyst arises from rem-nants of epithelium along the line of closure of the palatal processes of the maxillary processes (Fig. 15–13). These may reach a large size and cause bulging of the overlying palatal mucosa.

Median Mandibular Cyst

A median mandibular cyst has been re-ported but is of rare occurrence. It is located in the midline of the mandible between the roots of the central incisors which are vital and asymptomatic. In some instances, these cysts have been lined by ciliated epithelium.

Median Alveolar Cyst

The median alveolar cyst is found in the alveolar process of the maxilla anterior to the incisive canal. Although it has certain histologic factors suggesting fissural origin, it could very well represent a primordial cyst arising at the site of an unformed mesiodens.

Other Developmental Defects

Cleft Palate

Cleft palate is discussed on pages 60, 83 and 302.

Submucous Cleft

Submucous cleft refers to a partial bony cleft of the palate in which the overlying mucous membrane is intact. For this reason, the condition may not be recognized early in life or even until the child learns to talk, when he may develop hypernasal speech. The condition may be accompanied by bifid

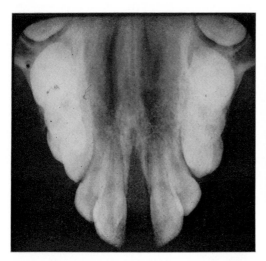

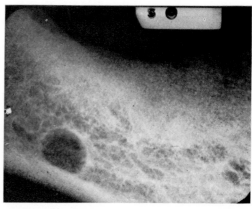

Fig. 15-15. Mandibular salivary gland depression. A focal radiolucency with a crescent-shaped border is shown. These lesions are often bilateral and are found at or near the lower border of the mandible.

Fig. 15-14. The median maxillary anterior alveolar cleft. (Gier and Fast: Oral Surg., *24*, 496, 1967.)

uvula, a midline notching of the posterior bony palate and midline muscle separation.

Median Maxillary Anterior Alveolar Cleft

This minor anomaly, estimated to be present in about 1 percent of the population, appears as a midline separation of anterior maxillary alveolus which is unrelated to cleft lip and palate (Fig. 15–14). It is usually first recognized in routine radiographs. No specific treatment of the cleft is required although the central incisors on either side may show mesial axial inclination.

Mandibular Salivary Gland Depression
(Latent Bone Cyst, Stafne Cyst, Idiopathic Bone Cavity, Static Bone Cyst)

Found typically at or near the lower border of the mandible anterior to the angle, the mandibular salivary gland depression represents a developmental defect associated with the formation of the submaxillary gland. It is seen radiographically as a sharply defined, focal radiolucency with a crescent-shaped cortical border (Fig. 15–15). Since the defect in most cases is actually a concavity on the lingual aspect of the mandible, the cortical outline is crescent shaped and

will vary in density depending upon the angulation used in taking the radiograph. If the mandible is thin at the lower border, the defect will "burn" through on the radiograph and appear as a distinct notching, again with the crescent-shaped cortical border along its superior aspect. Unfortunately, it is difficult or impossible to palpate the defect in this location and the lesion will be frequently interpreted as a central lesion in the bone (Fig. 15–16). Bilateral defects are not uncommon and, when present, are highly suggestive of the diagnosis. Surgical exploration results in perforation into the defect and

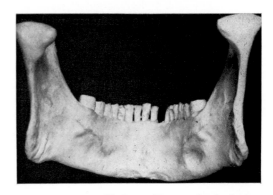

Fig. 15-16. Mandibular salivary gland depression. (Courtesy of Grant Van Huysen from Shafer, Hine and Levy, *Oral Pathology*, courtesy of W. B. Saunders Co.)

thus into the floor of the mouth. Soft tissue obtained from the area consists of an essentially normal submaxillary gland lobule around which the mandible presumably formed during development. Occasional cases have been reported in which the salivary gland is apparently entirely enclosed within bone. On very rare occasions, this tissue may give rise to salivary gland neoplasms, notably mucoepidermoid carcinoma (p. 354).

Fibrous Dysplasia of Bone

Several varieties of fibrous dysplasia are recognized: monostotic fibrous dysplasia, polyostotic fibrous dysplasia, and familial fibrous dysplasia (cherubism).

The several recognized types of fibrous dysplasia are rather arbitrarily categorized here as developmental disorders inasmuch as these conditions, of unknown etiology and pathogenesis, arise early in life and one form (cherubism) has a familial pattern. As the name implies, these conditions are dysplastic processes which have been described as "disturbances in bone-forming mesenchyme." Since fibrous dysplasia has many features in common with other bone lesions composed of fibrous connective tissue and osseous tissue, it is also broadly categorized with the "fibro-osseous lesions" of bone.

Both monostotic and polyostotic fibrous dysplasia present a similar radiographic appearance which may vary from a radiolucent lesion if the tissue present is predominantly fibrous to one somewhat more radiopaque if there is a significant amount of abnormal bone formation. Delicate "Chinese-character" trabeculae of bone seen microscopically produce the typical "ground-glass" radiographic appearance in those cases of an admixture of connective tissue and bony trabeculae.

Monostotic Fibrous Dysplasia

The monostotic variety of fibrous dysplasia of bone characteristically involves only one bone and appears radiographically as a distinct radiolucent or "ground-glass" lesion which frequently blends gradually into the adjacent normal bone. Often there is associated cortical expansion (Fig. 15–17). In the mandible, the lesion may create eroded "bays" in the thicker cortex, giving a multilocular appearance. It must be distinguished from central cementifying fibroma of the bone by histologic examination (Fig. 15–45).

Polyostotic Fibrous Dysplasia

At least two varieties of polyostotic fibrous dysplasia are recognized: Albright's syndrome and Jaffe's type. In Albright's syndrome, bone lesions are found in nearly all bones in the skeleton and, in addition, café-au-lait spots are seen on the skin. There is precocious sexual development in the female as well as other endocrine disturbances. In Jaffe's type of fibrous dysplasia fewer bones are involved and, while the patient may exhibit café-au-lait spots, no endocrine disturbances are noted.

Familial Fibrous Dysplasia (Cherubism)

Cherubism (familial fibrous dysplasia) is a unique, familial form of fibrous dysplasia characterized by bilateral fullness of the cheeks giving the child a cherubic appearance. Commonly, involvement of the mandible occurs initially in the rami and molar regions. The maxilla may or may not show similar changes. Radiographically, there is expansion of the cortical plates and marked radiolucency of the jaw. Since the onset of cherubism is prior to 6 years of age, the formation of the teeth is disturbed or aborted completely. Those teeth that have erupted become loose and have to be extracted. Except for control of secondary infection which may involve certain of the erupted teeth, no specific treatment is available. Generally, these children become completely edentulous and require artificial dentures. The chief differential diagnoses are Hand-Schüller-Christian disease and infantile cortical hy-

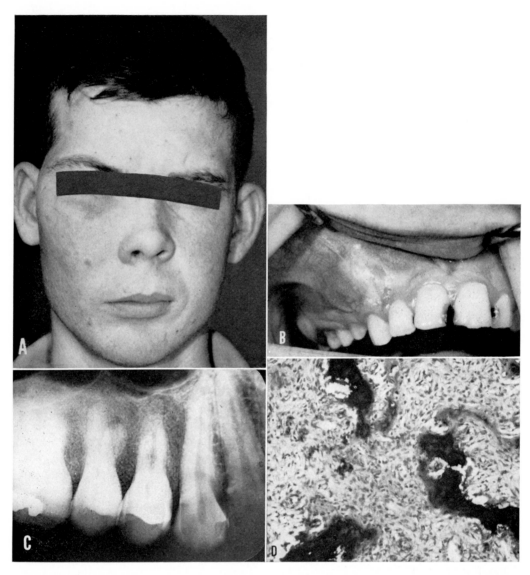

Fig. 15-17. Fibrous dysplasia of bone. *A*, Deformity of the face had gradually developed in this boy over a period of several years. *B*, Intraoral examination showed a bony enlargement of the right maxilla. *C*, Periapical radiographs shows a "ground glass," "orange-peel" or "smoke-screen" trabeculation with an indistinct lamina dura around the associated teeth. *D*, "Chinese-character" trabeculae of bone devoid of osteoblasts show a random distribution in a fibrous connective tissue stroma.

perostosis (Caffey's disease). The disease appears to be self-limiting at about the time of puberty. The "cherubic" appearance becomes less obvious as the patient grows older, although some roundness of the face can still be detected in the adult.

INFLAMMATORY AND REACTIVE DISORDERS

Fibrous Healing Defect

Following extraction of a tooth, the socket sometimes fills in with dense fibrous connective tissue rather than new bone. This is typically seen in the maxillary lateral incisor area when there was perforation of both the labial and palatal cortices of bone due to periapical disease and/or apicoectomy. The radiograph shows a circumscribed radiolucency without cortication similar to a residual granuloma or cyst (Fig. 15–18).

Osteoporotic Bone Marrow Defect

Normal bone marrow occurs in the jaws of the adult in greatest amounts in the molar

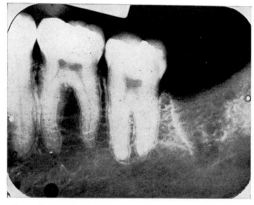

Fig. 15-19. Periapical radiograph of the mandibular molar area showing a third molar extraction site. Small focal radiolucencies are seen which represent bone marrow spaces. Bone marrow spaces are also seen in the bifurcation area of the first molar.

region and angle of the mandible. In some instances, diffuse, poorly defined areas of radiolucency are seen in edentulous spaces in the mandible that may simulate specific disease processes such as osteoporosis, focal osteomyelitis and metastatic tumor. Diagnosis of these poorly defined radiolucencies is difficult, and frequently the dentist elects to biopsy the region (Fig. 15–19). If the "lesions" are bilateral, he may decide to follow a given case by reexamination and additional radiography. Microscopic examination of many of these reveals hematopoietic and fatty marrow. In some instances, these defects are seen in the regions of previous extractions. If earlier radiographs are available for comparison, it may be noted that no change has occurred over a long period of time. Unfortunately, a clinical diagnosis cannot be made with any assurance and biopsy is indicated in those cases in which the basic nature of the disease is questioned.

Traumatic (Hemorrhagic, Extravasation) Cyst

Seen most commonly in young adult males, the so-called traumatic cyst appears clinically as an asymptomatic radiolucency, usually in the mandibular molar region.

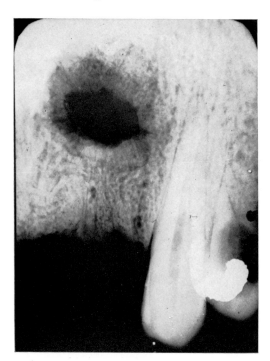

Fig. 15-18. Fibrous healing defect.

Typically, the radiolucency is focal, without cortication, and located superior to the mandibular canal; it may extend around and between the roots of the teeth (Fig. 2–33). Although it is presumed to arise following physical trauma and associated intramedullary hemorrhage, a positive history of a blow to the jaw cannot always be obtained. Aspiration of the defect has yielded a bloody fluid on occasion (Fig. 6–2C). Electrophoretic analysis of this aspirate will usually show normal serum proteins. Surgical exploration has revealed an "empty cavity" according to several reports. The latter is unexplainable, unless diligent evacuation at the moment of surgical entry has displaced the contents revealing the "empty" cavity (p. 115). Vigorous curettage of the space produces only a few strands of connective tissue and a few slender trabeculae of bone and associated bone marrow from the osseous wall. Since the lesion is not a true cyst, epithelium is not found. The defect fills in with new bone after surgical exploration and the creation of a new blood clot.

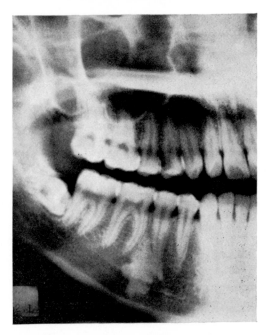

Fig. 15-20. Condensing osteitis. A low-grade inflammatory process arising near the apex of the mandibular second premolar tooth has stimulated bone formation rather than bone destruction.

Surgical Ciliated Cyst

This unusual cyst is found high in the maxillary alveolar ridge in the canine-premolar regions. A history of previous extraction with antrostomy (Caldwell-Luc) operation for removal of a root tip in the maxillary sinus is almost invariably obtained. Radiographically, a focal radiolucency which does not communicate with the sinus is seen. Quite often the lesion will be interpreted as the floor of the maxillary sinus or as a residual apical periodontal cyst. Aspiration and injection of the radiolucency with radiopaque media will usually demonstrate that it is separate from the sinus. Histologic examination reveals respiratory epithelium lining a cystic space.

Condensing Osteitis (Chronic Focal Sclerosing Osteomyelitis)

Low-grade chronic inflammation of the marrow spaces frequently induces reactive bone formation and increased density in a focal area. Condensing osteitis represents such a process and is characteristically seen at the apices of lower first molar teeth in young individuals (Fig. 15–20). Quite often the tooth is carious and some pulpal involvement may be presumed. Radiographically these areas are somewhat diffuse in their early stages but become more dense and discrete in severe cases.

Similar small sclerotic areas in the jaws are sometimes referred to as "bone scars" or "sclerotic bone" and are usually seen in edentulous areas. It is presumed that these represent foci of bone production that occurred secondarily to low-grade inflammation sometime previously. They are of no clinical significance.

Acute Suppurative Osteomyelitis

Acute infectious processes in the jaws most often arise secondarily to pulp or

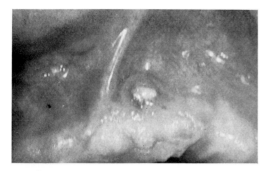

Fig. 15-21. Sequestrum. Surgical removal and control of infection are indicated.

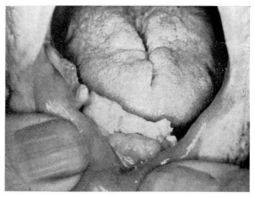

Fig. 15-22. Osteoradionecrosis. A large section of exposed, necrotic, alveolar bone is shown. The patient had received heavy radiation therapy for epidermoid carcinoma of the floor of the mouth.

periodontal infection. Fracture or other wounds, or the hematogenous spread from other infectious foci, account for some cases. The patient experiences pain in most cases and shows signs of an infectious process including fever, elevated white blood cell count and regional lymphadenopathy. In the initial stages, radiographic changes in the bone may not be seen. Later, diffuse foci of radiolucency appear with loss of trabeculation in irregular fashion. Bone sequestra appear as islands of bone within areas of radiolucency giving the appearance of a combined radiolucent-radiopaque lesion even though it is in fact a bone destructive process.

The overlying mucosa becomes reddened and drainage of suppurative material is seen. Culture of the organisms commonly reveals staphylococci, streptococci or mixed infections. Mycotic infections (*e.g.* actinomycosis or blastomycosis), tuberculosis, syphilis and other specific infections may give rise to osteomyelitis. Antibiotic control, surgical removal of sequestra and other general supportive measures are required (Fig. 15-21).

Osteoradionecrosis

Osteoradionecrosis is a form of osteomyelitis which may occur months or even years following radiation therapy in the vicinity of the jaws. The mandible is characteristically affected. Severe pain may be present and sequestra similar to those seen in other forms of osteomyelitis may develop (Fig. 15–22). The radiographic appearance shows patchy sclerotic areas, foci of bone surrounded by diffuse areas of radiolucency and, in advanced cases, pathologic fracture (Fig. 15–23). Preradiation extraction of the teeth with careful removal of all sharp spicules of bone, the use of supravoltage (cobalt 60) therapy and the prevention of subsequent denture injury and infection are important preventive measures.

Chronic Diffuse Sclerosing Osteomyelitis (Sclerotic Cemental Masses, Florid Osseous Dysplasia)

A low-grade infectious process, this form of osteomyelitis is characterized by periods of exacerbation and remission of the infection. It is seen quite often in elderly, edentulous patients (Fig. 15–24). The radiographs show extensive involvement of the jaw, usually the mandible, with a somewhat moth-eaten appearance of radiolucent areas intermixed with diffuse, radiopaque areas of bone production. These features are quite similar to those seen in Paget's disease of bone. At times of acute exacerbation, the patient experiences mild pain and suppuration. The treatment is conservative with antibiotic support during the acute phases.

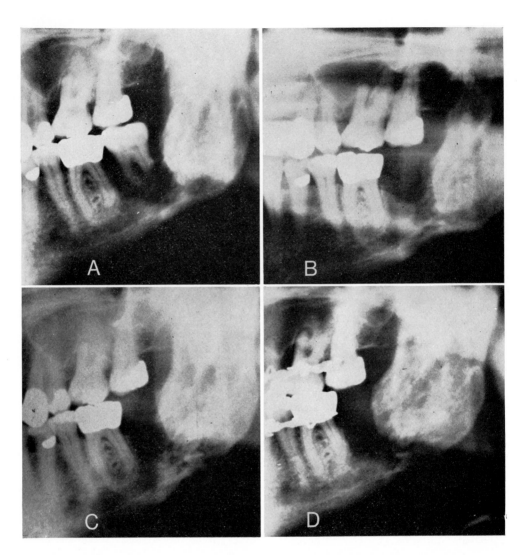

Fig. 15-23. Osteoradionecrosis. *A*, Severe pain and swelling developed around the loose second molar approximately 8 years following heavy therapeutic radiation for a carcinoma of the tonsillar region. *B*, Radiographic appearance 3 weeks following extraction of the second molar. *C*, Radiographs taken 3 weeks later showing progression of the bone necrosis and pathologic fracture despite intensive antibiotic therapy. *D*, Appearance of fracture site approximately 1 month later. Note the fracture splint used to immobilize the jaws. (Courtesy of Dr. Paul Jurgens.)

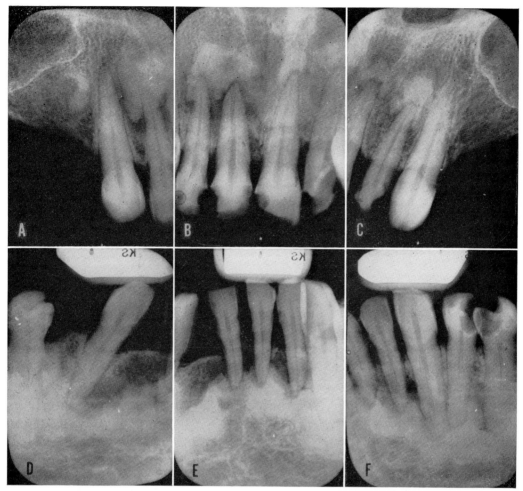

Fig. 15-24. *A–F*, Chronic diffuse sclerosing osteomyelitis. Periapical radiographs showing multiple diffuse radiopaque and radiolucent areas. The patient experienced moderate bone pain with occasional periods of suppuration. The differential diagnoses include condensing osteitis (focal sclerosing osteomyelitis) or sclerotic bone, cementoma and Paget's disease of bone (see Figs. 15–58 and 15–59).

Garre's Proliferative Periostitis (Chronic Non-suppurative Sclerosing Osteitis, Chronic Osteomyelitis with Proliferative Periostitis, Periostitis Ossificans)

This unusual form of osteomyelitis is characterized by periosteal thickening and extracortical bone formation overlying a relatively chronic infectious process. Seen typically in the mandible of a young individual, infection arising from a tooth perforates the cortex, elevates the periosteum and stimulates new bone formation. Facial asymmetry may be marked and occlusal radiographs show new bone formation of surprisingly uniform trabeculation and apparent reduplication of the cortex. Occasionally, the point of perforation of the original bony cortex by the infection can be seen. Removal of the involved tooth results in slow remodeling of the bony enlargement over a period of several months.

Central Giant Cell Granuloma

The central giant cell granuloma of bone presents a somewhat irregular radiolucency which may be focal or multilocular with occasional delicate bony trabeculae extend-

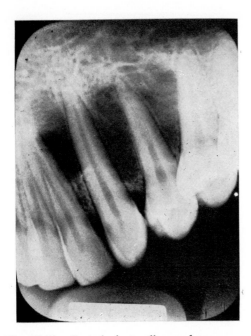

Fig. 15-25.   Central giant cell granuloma.

ing into the lesion from the outer bony wall (Fig. 15–25). The radiolucent defect, quite extensive in some instances, has no constant association with the teeth. Frequently, however, it causes displacement and/or root resorption of adjacent teeth. Expansion and eventual perforation of the cortex are seen in advanced cases. The majority of cases have been reported in young adults with some predilection for females. The distribution of lesions is approximately equal between the maxilla and mandible. The diagnosis is made by histologic examination which shows large numbers of multinucleated giant cells distributed within a somewhat vascular and granulomatous stroma. The diagnosis of a central giant cell lesion of bone necessitates additional study to rule out the existence of hyperparathyroidism (Fig. 9–19, p. 249).

Aneurysmal Bone Cyst

An uncommon lesion of bone, the aneurysmal bone cyst presents a number of radiographic, clinical and microscopic features similar to the central giant cell granuloma.

In many instances, there is thinning and expansion of the cortex presenting the classical "blown-out" appearance characteristic of such lesions in the long bones. The nature of the supporting stroma and the large numbers of multinuclear giant cells are essentially the same; however, large sinusoidal spaces filled with blood and rimmed by osteoid are the principal differentiating features. Inasmuch as only a few cases have been reported in the jaws, the natural history of the disease has not been completely defined. However, experience to date suggests that it behaves like the central giant cell granuloma and should be treated by relatively conservative curettage.

"Vanishing Bone" Disease (Massive Osteolysis, "Phantom Bone," Progressive Osteolysis, Gorham's Syndrome)

This rare and unusual condition is characterized by progressive lysis of bone and replacement by fibrous connective tissue for no apparent reason. The reported cases have been in teenagers and young to middle-aged adults and involved essentially every individual bone in the body, including the mandible and maxilla. Slowly progressive resorption of the bone occurs over a protracted period and eventuates in pathologic fracture. The radiographic changes begin as a patchy osteoporosis which coalesces producing large defects. The histologic features are non-specific but "hemangiomatous" changes have been described. This resorption may subside but bone regeneration does not occur.

Radiation therapy, resection of the involved bone and replacement with bone grafts, and treatment with a variety of drugs and vitamins have proved unsuccessful in most cases.

ODONTOGENIC CYSTS AND TUMORS

The odontogenic cysts and neoplasms arise mainly within bone in association with the odontogenic apparatus or its cellular remnants. Most of them show a wide range of radiographic and clinical features which nevertheless are often distinctive. For this reason they are discussed separately from the non-odontogenic cysts and tumors.

The most common odontogenic lesions are the apical periodontal cyst and the dentigerous cyst, both of which by definition are tooth associated (see pp. 449–451). A number of the other odontogenic cysts and tumors also show a predilection for specific sites or age groups. It should be noted that a few lesions of odontogenic origin are found in extraosseous or ectopic sites. The gingival cyst and Bohn's nodules occur in the gingiva. The calcifying and keratinizing odontogenic cyst (Gorlin cyst) is found extraosseously in about 25 percent of cases (p. 470). On rare occasions, the adenomatoid odontogenic tumor, calcifying epithelial odontogenic tumor, extraosseous ameloblastoma and hamartomatous odontongenic lesions arise in the gingiva. Ectopic odontogenic neoplasms include the pituitary ameloblastoma (craniopharyngioma) and the tibial adamantinoma, although the latter is believed by some to represent an angioblastoma.

Odontogenic Cysts

The odontogenic cysts are differentiated by their location, association with the teeth or tooth-bearing areas, and their pathogenesis.

In most instances a reasonably accurate diagnosis can be made from the clinical findings, radiographic appearance and gross features noted at surgery.

However, a number of other disease processes of the jaws may, at times, simulate the odontogenic cysts clinically and radiographically. Further, certain of the odontogenic cysts may give rise to odontogenic neoplasms not apparent on gross examination. For these reasons it is good practice to confirm the clinical diagnosis by histologic examination.

Other than the gingival cyst, cysts of odontogenic origin typically are found at the root apex of pulpless teeth (apical periodontal cyst), along the lateral root surface of

vital teeth (lateral periodontal cyst), enclosing the crown of an unerupted tooth (dentigerous cyst), or occurring in the place of a tooth (primordial cyst). The so-called keratocyst of the jaws is of considerable clinical significance since the recurrence rate appears to be higher than for the usual dentigerous cyst. Further, multiple keratocysts are associated with the basal cell nevus-bifid rib syndrome (Fig. 4–4, p. 310).

Apical Periodontal (Periapical, Radicular, Root End) Cyst

The most common cyst of the jaws, the apical periodontal cyst, appears most often as an asymptomatic, circumscribed radiolucency at the apex of a tooth which is invariably non-vital (Figs. 15–26 and 27). In most instances the pulp underwent necrosis following carious pulp exposure or, occasionally, after a traumatic accident. Uncom-

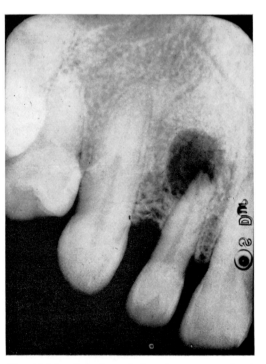

Fig. 15-26. Apical periodontal cyst associated with an upper lateral incisor with a small dens in dente. This developmental anomaly is often associated with a built-in pulp exposure causing the necrotic pulp and periapical reaction.

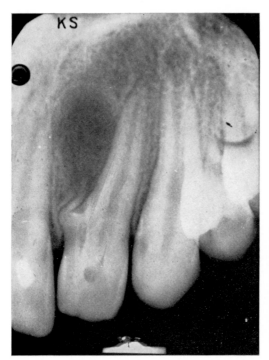

Fig. 15-27. Apical periodontal cyst associated with a more bizarre dens in dente. (Courtesy of Samuel Patterson.)

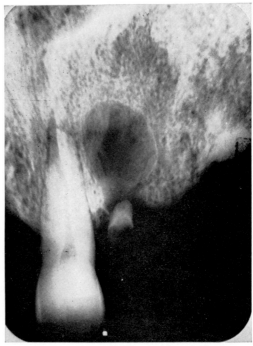

Fig. 15-28. Apical periodontal cyst associated with a nearly exfoliated root tip. This illustrates how the residual cyst may be left in place after tooth extraction or exfoliation.

monly, there may be marked bone enlargement with clinically apparent expansion and crepitus of the cortical plate. While the apical periodontal cyst and the periapical granuloma cannot be differentiated on radiographic evidence alone, aspiration of the former usually reveals clear yellow fluid and gross examination of the surgical specimen will show a central lumen sometimes with masses of cholesterol crystals. Positive diagnosis depends upon the identification of a central lumen lined by stratified squamous epithelium (or, rarely, respiratory epithelium in lesions adjacent to the nose or maxillary sinus) by microscopic examination.

Residual (Post-extraction) Cyst

This term refers to a cyst (usually periapical) which was left in position after extraction of the associated tooth (Fig. 15–28). Preextraction radiographs are usually helpful in determining whether the cyst is a residual apical periodontal, lateral perio-

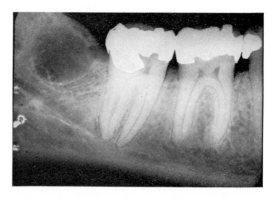

Fig. 15-29. Extraction site. This radiolucency distal to the second molar resembles a residual cyst but could conceivably be a primordial cyst. In fact, the extraction wound after removal of an impacted third molar was filled with petrolatum inadvertently left in place for 5 years. The bone remodeled most efficiently around the mass and literally enclosed it with a "lamina dura." (Stafne, *Oral Roentgenographic Diagnosis*, courtesy of the W. B. Saunders Co.)

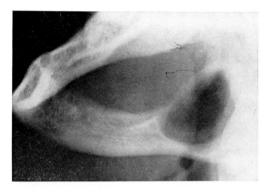

Fig. 15-30. Residual cyst. Without preextraction records, it would not be possible to tell whether this is a residual dentigerous cyst or a primordial cyst.

dontal or dentigerous cyst since these present a similar, if not identical, histologic appearance. Similarly, the primordial cyst occurring in an edentulous area of the jaws ordinarily cannot be differentiated from the other cysts without preextraction records and an accurate history (Figs. 15–29 and 30).

Lateral Periodontal Cyst

This uncommon cyst is found typically in the mandibular cuspid-bicuspid regions in association with neighboring vital teeth (Fig. 15-31 *A* to *C*). It appears as a smoothly outlined radiolucency between or superimposed over the lateral aspect of the tooth root. Generally, the lamina dura is not present adjacent to the radiolucent defect, suggesting continuity of the periodontal membrane with the wall of the cyst. An origin from epithelial cell rests of Malassez in the periodontal membrane seems most likely in view of its direct continuity. Nevertheless, it is microscopically indistinguishable from the primordial cyst and may in fact represent such a cyst arising from a supernumerary tooth follicle (Fig. 15—31).

Dental Lamina Cyst of the Newborn (Epstein's Pearls, Bohn's Nodules, Gingival Cyst of the Newborn)

Keratin cysts or Bohn's nodules, seen on the alveolar ridge of newborn infants, ap-

pear as multiple white nodules which are soon exfoliated. Epstein's pearls are clinically similar nodules found on the palates of newborns. The former are probably derived from remnants of the dental lamina, whereas the latter are believed to arise from mucous gland elements.

Gingival Cyst of the Adult

The gingival cyst appears clinically as a small fluid- or keratin-filled bleb on the free or attached gingiva. It is lined by flattened squamous epithelium derived from remnants of the dental lamina or so-called glands or rests of Serres. No radiographic changes in the underlying bone are seen although the larger gingival cysts may cause superficial erosion of the adjacent cortex. If a circumscribed radiolucency associated with the lateral root surface of a vital tooth is present, the lesion is probably a lateral periodontal rather than a gingival cyst. The gingival cyst has some clinical similarity to the mucocele but it should be remembered that accessory salivary glands are not found on the free or attached gingiva.

Primordial Cyst

This rare cyst develops from the follicle of a tooth which fails to form. Most cases are encountered in the region of the lower third molar. The diagnosis depends upon clear evidence that the missing tooth did indeed fail to form, as well as upon microscope confirmation (Fig. 15-30).

Dentigerous (Follicular) Cyst

The dentigerous cyst is seen as a well-defined radiolucency surrounding the crown of the tooth, usually an unerupted lower third molar (Fig. 15-32). It arises from the dental follicle and occasionally is found around the crowns of other teeth, especially the maxillary canines, or, in rare instances, around odontomas. The dentigerous cyst may give rise to ameloblastoma and for this reason should always be submitted for microscope examination. Additionally, a

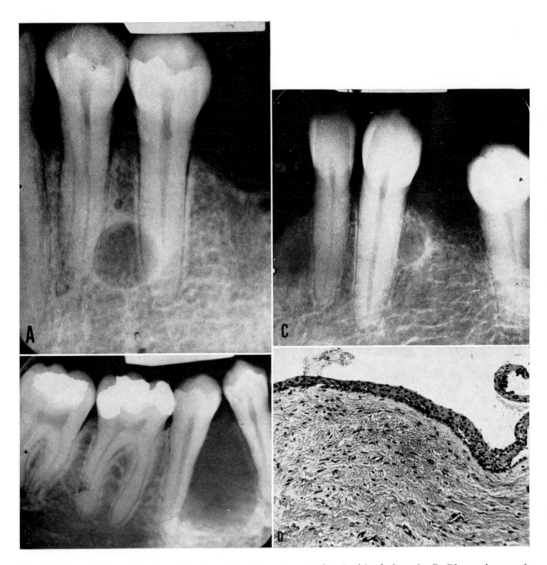

Fig. 15-31. *A, B,* and *C* show lateral periodontal cysts, associated with vital teeth. *D,* Photomicrograph of a lining epithelium of a lateral periodontal cyst. (Standish and Shafer, J. Periodont., *29,* 27, 1958.)

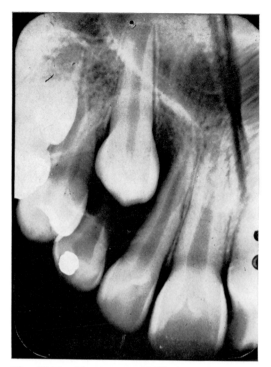

Fig. 15-32. Dentigerous (follicular) cyst around crown of unerupted permanent canine tooth.

some instances the cyst expands bone and may perforate through the bone into the soft tissue or maxillary sinus. While the cyst may occur at any age, most studies indicate a mean age of occurrence at about 35 years with some predilection for males. The cysts appear radiographically as sharply defined radiolucencies with cortication and multiloculation (Figs. 4–4, 15–33). Multiple cysts are seen, especially in patients with the nevoid basal cell carcinoma syndrome (p. 310).

From a radiographic and clinical standpoint, several types of odontogenic keratocysts are recognized: primordial, lateral periodontal, dentigerous, those associated with the syndrome and, rarely, the radicular cyst type. Although a large proportion of the cysts are of the dentigerous cyst type, unlike the dentigerous cyst the lumen does not actually contact the associated impacted tooth.

The chief clinical differential diagnosis is the ameloblastoma, which it simulates in

number of other neoplasms are known to arise on rare occasions in association with impacted teeth and presumably from the wall of dentigerous cysts, namely, adenomatoid odontogenic tumor, Gorlin cyst, epidermoid carcinoma, mucoepidermoid carcinoma (p. 425) and, very probably, the Pindborg tumor.

Another form of dentigerous cyst is the so-called eruption cyst which occurs in the mucosa overlying an erupting tooth. The soft tissue is elevated, boggy and a bluish-red color. Radiographs show an underlying tooth which is partially erupted through the alveolar bone.

Odontogenic Keratocyst

The odontogenic keratocyst occurs most commonly (approximately 80 percent) in the mandible, usually in the third molar and ramus areas (Fig. 15–33). Both the maxillary and mandibular cysts generally are found posterior to the premolar teeth. In

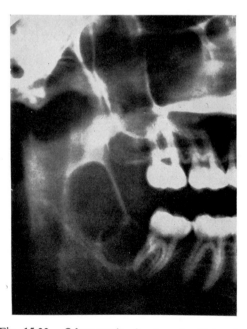

Fig. 15-33. Odontogenic keratocyst. Note the multilocular radiolucency with cortication involving the third molar region and a portion of the ramus.

most clinical and radiographic respects (see p. 471). Since the cystic contents of the keratocyst have been shown to have a lowered soluble protein content, it has been suggested that aspiration (Fig. 6–2) and electrophoretic examination of the cyst fluid may be diagnostic. The diagnosis is clearly established by histologic examination.

Histologically, the odontogenic keratocyst consists of a thin, corrugated lining of stratified squamous epithelium with a keratin or parakeratin surface. The lumen may be filled with keratin, epithelial squames or opaque fluid. Satellite cysts are common in the cyst wall.

Once the diagnosis of odontogenic keratocyst is established the patient should be medically evaluated for the possibility of the nevoid basal cell carcinoma syndrome. It should also be recognized that recurrence rates of 35 percent or higher can be expected after surgical removal and that the patient should be followed post-operatively 5 years or longer.

Keratinizing and Calcifying Odontogenic Cyst (Calcifying Epithelial Odontogenic Cyst, Gorlin Cyst)

While this lesion tends to behave as a benign cystic process, its unusual histologic pattern would justify its inclusion with the odontogenic neoplasms as well. It occurs typically in adults and predominately in the mandible. As noted earlier, about one-fourth of the cases have been reported at extraosseous sites in the gingiva. Radiographically, the Gorlin cyst appears as a well-circumscribed target lesion with flecks or even large masses of calcification distributed throughout the radiolucency. It may be associated with an odontoma, impacted tooth or, more rarely, the ameloblastic fibro-odontoma. The bizarre histologic features of a cystic lesion composed of cuboidal or columnar lining, proliferating epithelial cells resembling stellate reticulum and ghost cells which show keratinization and calcification have suggested a resemblance to the cuta-

neous epithelioma of Malherbe (p. 324). The lesion may slowly enlarge, sometimes reaching several centimeters in diameter.

Odontogenic Tumors, Benign

These tumors exhibit considerable variation in clinical behavior and therefore their treatment also varies. While a definitive diagnosis of most is dependent upon microscopic examination, a number of tumors of this group demonstrate clinical and radiographic features which are useful in establishing a differential diagnosis. Even though the odontogenic tumors are not necessarily restricted to the tooth-bearing regions of the jaws (nor are all intrabony tumors of these areas odontogenic), tumors showing slow growth and an intimate association with the teeth or tooth-like structures are most likely to be odontogenic.

The recognized odontogenic lesions differ markedly in their incidence. The cementoma and odontoma can be considered relatively common in comparison to the calcifying epithelial odontogenic tumor and cyst, adenomatoid odontogenic tumor, odontogenic myxoma and ameloblastoma. The remainder of the tumors are encountered even more rarely.

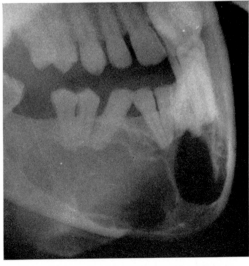

Fig. 15-34.   Extensive ameloblastoma of the mandible. Note the multilocular appearance.

Ameloblastoma (Adamantinoma)

The classical multilocular radiographic appearance of the simple ameloblastoma is seen chiefly in comparatively advanced cases and reflects the characteristic infiltrative growth pattern of this lesion (Fig. 15–34). On the other hand, the early ameloblastoma

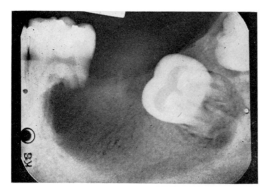

Fig. 15-35. Ameloblastoma arising within a pre-existing dentigerous cyst. Note the root resorption of the first permanent molar tooth.

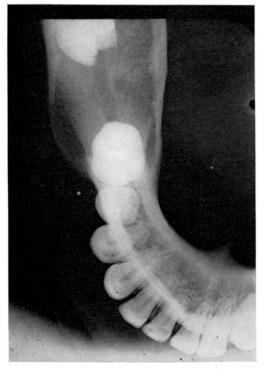

Fig. 15-36. An occlusal view of the lesion shown in Figure 15-35.

may appear as a discrete radiolucent defect resembling a residual cyst. As noted previously, the dentigerous cyst may give rise to an ameloblastoma which may be identified only by microscopic detection of the neoplastic proliferation in the wall of the cyst (Figs. 15–35 and 36). The ameloblastoma should be strongly considered in the large dentigerous cyst or one exhibiting radiolucent compartments.

The majority of ameloblastomas are discovered during the fourth decade (average age 35 years) and most are in the posterior mandible, although they may occur at any age or site in the jaws. The definitive diagnosis of ameloblastoma must be established by histologic examination (Fig. 15–37).

Several histologic variants are recognized: follicular (simple), plexiform, basal cell,

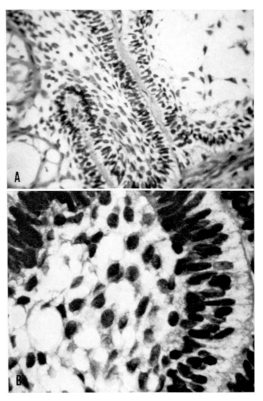

Fig. 15-37. Ameloblastoma. *A*, Ameloblast-like cells are arranged about central areas resembling stellate reticulum. *B*, Higher magnification shows typical columnar cells and stellate reticulum.

acanthomatous and granular cells. The histologic type appears to have little bearing on predicting the behavior of the lesion although it should be noted that several case reports of metastasis of granular cell ameloblastoma have appeared in the literature.

Extraosseous ameloblastoma represents an unusual variant found entirely outside the cortex of the jaw bone and thus is presumably derived from surface epithelium or from remnants of the dental lamina. Another associated odontogenic lesion is the *odontogenic gingival epithelial hamartoma* which represents a small, asymptomatic nodular excrescence of the alveolar ridge or gingiva, usually in adults. It consists of islands and cords of odontogenic epithelium distributed in a mature fibrous stroma, often with inductive changes. The treatment is by surgical excision. Other related ectopic neoplasms are the *pituitary ameloblastoma (craniopharyngioma, Rathke's pouch tumor)* and the *adamantinoma of long bones (tibial adamantinoma).* While the latter has some histologic similarity to the ameloblastoma, it probably represents a malignant angioblastoma.

The treatment of ameloblastoma is largely a matter of clinical judgment once the histologic diagnosis has been established. A tumor confined to the lumen or wall of a dentigerous cyst might require no further treatment other than careful follow-up over several years. Larger tumors might require local block resection provided that the lower border of the mandible remained intact. The ameloblastoma is a "persistent, not malignant" tumor and it might be reasoned that the patient is entitled to one or more recurrences before jaw resection is undertaken.

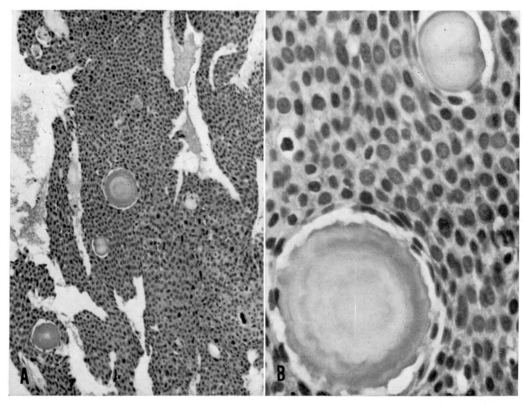

Fig. 15-38. Calcifying epithelial odontogenic tumor. *A,* Photomicrograph showing broad sheets of epithelial cells and foci of calcification (Liesegang calcifications). *B,* High-power photomicrograph showing calcifications and polyhedral epithelial cells. Bizarre nuclear forms are often found.

On the other hand, jaw resection seems indicated in massive tumors in which the lesion has broken out of bone into adjacent soft tissue.

The prognosis of the treated ameloblastoma depends chiefly upon the size of the lesion at the time of discovery and the adequacy of excision.

Calcifying Epithelial Odontogenic Tumor (Pindborg Tumor)

First described by Pindborg in 1956, this unusual tumor is seen most frequently in the premolar and molar regions of the mandible in adults of middle age. Occasional tumors of this type may also arise on the gingiva. Its radiographic appearance may be that of the simple ameloblastoma although most are mixed radiolucent-radiopaque with central densities described as "driven snow." Approximately half of the cases are associated with an impacted tooth. Sheets of pleomorphic polyhedral epithelial cells (derived from the stratum intermedium of the enamel organ), foci of Liesegang calcifications and amyloid deposits make up the distinctive histologic features of this unique tumor (Fig. 15–38). The clinical behavior and treatment are essentially identical to that of the simple ameloblastoma.

Adenomatoid Odontogenic Tumor (Adenoameloblastoma)

This unusual neoplasm occurs most commonly in children and adolescents and almost always anterior to the molar teeth (Fig. 15–39). The maxilla and mandible are affected with nearly equal frequency. It appears radiographically as a sharply circumscribed radiolucency and is often seen in association with an unerupted tooth. In such cases it may be mistaken for dentigerous cyst; however, the central portion of the radiolucency may demonstrate faint "snowflake" areas of radiopaque material. The lesion is characterized histologically by tube-like structures giving it the characteristic adenoid appearance (Fig. 15–39C and D). Simple enucleation is the treatment of choice. The prognosis is excellent.

Central Odontogenic Fibroma

This rare central tumor of the jaws is seen most frequently in the mandible of children, often in association with impacted or unerupted teeth. It is composed of a delicate connective tissue stroma comparable to the tissue of the dental papilla. Scattered epithelial cells may be present and, although these are not considered an essential part of the tumor, they may suggest the odontogenic origin of the lesion. These lesions should be differentiated clinically and histologically from the simple enlarged dental follicle with which they are commonly confused. Radiographically, the tumor appears as a circumscribed radiolucency and is sometimes expansile and multilocular, much like the ameloblastoma.

Peripheral Odontogenic Fibroma

This lesion, presumed to be derived from the periodontal ligament and therefore of odontogenic origin (p. 427), appears clinically as focal swelling of the gingiva with a pedunculated or sessile base. Cundiff, in his study of 365 cases, reported a peak incidence at 13 years of age with a predilection for females.

Generally seen anterior to the first molar teeth, the lesion may be of normal mucosa color or red according to the degree of fibrosis present. Ulceration may be present. Since the peripheral odontogenic fibroma clinically resembles the peripheral giant cell granuloma and the pyogenic granuloma, a definitive diagnosis must be based on histologic examination of the excised specimen. It is distinguished by the presence of calcifications (resembling dystrophic calcification, acellular cementum or bone) distributed in a cellular connective tissue stroma (Fig. 15–40). Focal areas of multinucleated giant cells may also be present.

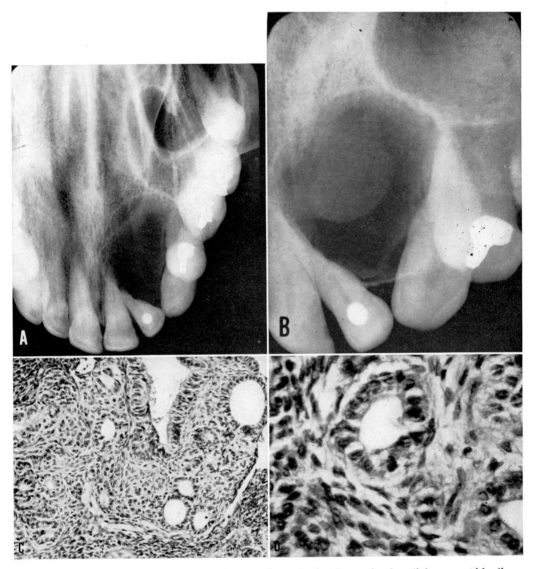

Fig. 15-39. Adenoameloblastoma. *A*, Occlusal radiograph showing a focal radiolucency with divergence of the tooth roots similar to that seen in globulomaxillary cyst. *B*, Periapical radiograph showing a central density within the radiolucency. *C*, Low-power photomicrograph showing the gland-like pattern. *D*, Higher magnification of one of the "ductal" structures. (Courtesy of Charles Redish.)

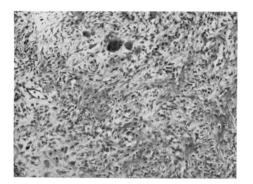

Fig. 15-40. Peripheral odontogenic fibroma. A few foci of amorphous calcifications are present near the top of the field.

Occasional recurrences are noted following excision; however, extraction of adjacent teeth is not indicated.

Odontogenic Myxoma

This uncommon tumor appears to be native to the jaw bones. A central radiolucency of the bone is seen with delicate trabeculae radiating from the somewhat scalloped outer border (p. 451). Grossly, it is composed of a mucoid, delicate stroma said to resemble Wharton's jelly. Histologically, loosely arranged, stellate-shaped cells are distributed in a poorly staining stroma. In some, transition of the myxomatous tissue into more fibrous connective tissue may be seen. Although these are benign tumors, their clinical behavior seems to be somewhat more aggressive, with a greater recurrence rate, when they occur within the maxilla. On the other hand, myxomas in the mandible are generally controlled by simple surgical excision.

Periapical Cemental Dysplasia (Cementoma, Ossifying Periapical Fibroma, Periapical Fibrous Dysplasia)

Periapical cemental dysplasia, commonly known as the cementoma, occurs adjacent to the apices of the lower anterior teeth in adults. Women seem to be affected more

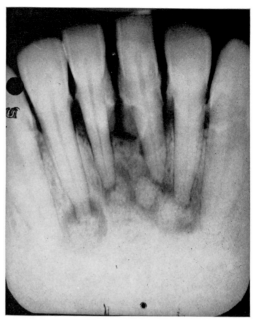

Fig. 15-41. Multiple cementomas (ossifying periapical fibromas). The associated teeth are vital and there are no associated symptoms. Note the severe periodontal disease and calculus unrelated to the periapical lesions.

frequently than men, and Negroids are more commonly affected than Caucasoids. Inasmuch as they are asymptomatic, most cases are discovered on routine radiographic examination (Figs. 15–41 to 44).

In its initial osteolytic (fibrous) state, it is a somewhat poorly circumscribed radiolucency adjacent to the apices of one or more teeth (Fig. 15–44A). At this stage it resembles a periapical granuloma; however, the pulps of the associated teeth are vital. The cementoblastic stage shows beginning calcification in the central portion of the defect (Fig. 15–42A to C). If several teeth are involved, both osteolytic and cementoblastic stages may be seen simultaneously (Fig. 15–44B). At its mature stage, the lesion appears as a radiopacity which may be outlined by a thin radiolucent border. The cementoblastic stage must be differentiated from focal sclerosing osteomyelitis (con-

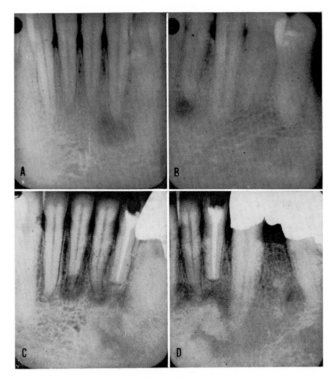

Fig. 15–42. Cementomas. *A* and *B* show two different views of one lesion (periapical fibroma) at the apex of a lateral incisor. This tooth was treated endodontically at the time because it was assumed that the lesion was a common form of pathosis associated with a necrotic pulp. *C* and *D*, Fourteen years later, two views of the same region show two more periapical fibromas associated with the central incisors and demonstrate the changes taking place in the lateral and cuspid apical areas. All but the treated tooth are vital.

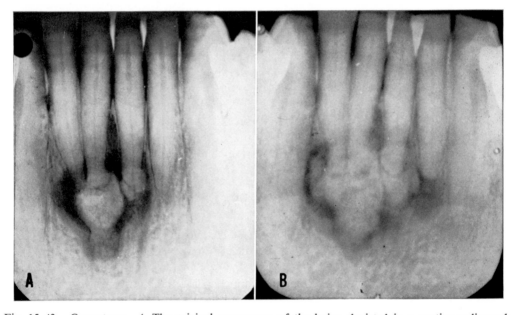

Fig. 15–43. Cementoma. *A,* The original appearance of the lesion depicted in a routine radiograph. There were no symptoms and the associated teeth were vital. *B,* The same lesion 12 years later. No treatment has been given. The teeth are vital and asymptomatic.

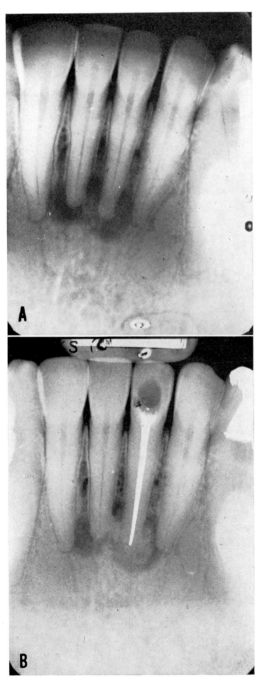

Fig. 15-44. Cementomas. *A,* A young adult female. The left central incisor was mistakenly treated endodontically. *B,* Same lesions 6 years later. Note the tendency for calcification.

densing osteitis). This latter condition is seen more frequently in the posterior mandible, often in association with the apices of the first molar tooth (p. 450). Both conditions may persist within the jaw without remodeling even though the teeth are extracted. With resorption of the alveolar ridge, the bony mass may fail to resorb and project above adjacent bone where it may interfere with an overlying appliance.

Central Cementifying Fibroma

This lesion appears as a central radiolucency, usually in the body of the mandible, with varying degrees of radiopacity depending upon the amount of calcification present (Fig. 15–45). Expansion of the cortical plate is frequent and divergence or dilaceration of the roots of adjacent teeth is often seen. It is characterized by multiple scattered areas of amorphous calcification distributed in a fibrous connective tissue stroma (Fig. 15–45C and D). Inasmuch as these foci of calcification resemble cementum and its counterpart is not seen in the long bones, there is good reason to classify this lesion with the odontogenic tumors. Comparable lesions, which also may arise from periodontal structures, are the *cemento-ossifying fibroma* and the *ossifying fibroma*.

Benign Cementoblastoma (True Cementoma)

This rare lesion shows considerable potential for proliferation and behaves more like a true neoplasm. Attached to the involved tooth root as an overgrowth of cementum resembling a massive hypercementosis, it may reach an extremely large size with expansion of the adjacent cortical plates (Fig. 15–46A to D). Because of this growth potential, surgical removal has been advocated upon recognition.

Dentinoma

This rare neoplasm is composed of a dense, radiopaque mass made up entirely of dentin and clinically and microscopically resembling the odontoma. The diagnosis de-

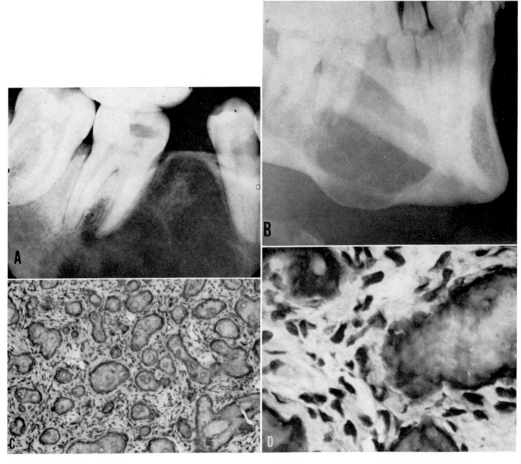

Fig. 15-45. Central cementifying fibroma. *A*, Periapical radiograph showing a large focal radio-lucency. The molar tooth is carious and shows a small periapical radiolucency which is unrelated to the larger defect. *B*, Lateral jaw radiograph showing the extent of the radiolucency. The cortical plate is thin and expanded but intact. Divergence of the adjacent tooth roots would also suggest a benign process of long duration. *C*, Photomicrograph showing calcification. *D*, Higher magnification showing amorphous calcifications. A distinct osteoblastic layer is not present. (Courtesy of C. E. Hopkins.)

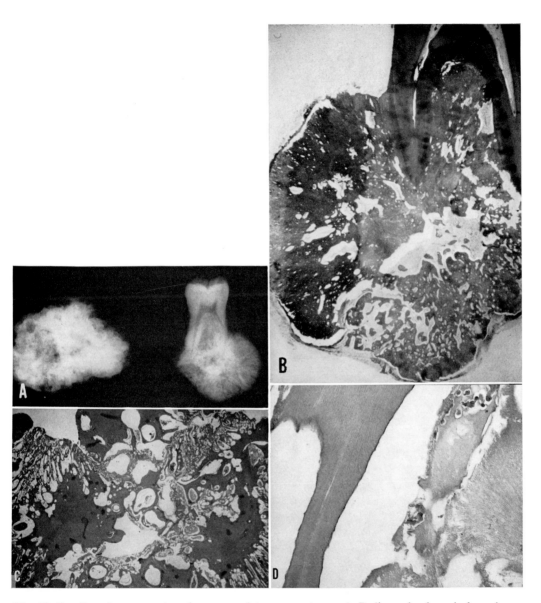

Fig. 15-46. Complex composite odontoma and true cementoma. *A,* Radiograph of surgical specimens. *B,* Photomicrograph of true cementoma attached to root of the molar. *C,* Photomicrograph of the odontoma shown on the left in *A.* Most of the dark tissue is dentin and many of the spaces were filled with enamel. (Courtesy of Ayoub Amer.) *D,* Photomicrograph showing disorganized arrangement of dentin on the left and remnants of enamel matrix on the right in a complex composite odontoma.

pends upon the histologic demonstration of dentin without evidence of enamel formation. Clinical behavior and treatment are similar to those of the odontoma.

Ameloblastic Fibroma

This uncommon lesion represents a true mixed odontogenic tumor consisting of epithelial and mesenchymal elements. It is seen in children and adolescents (average age 17 years) but exhibits no particular sex predilection. Radiographically, it appears as a well-defined radiolucent defect which may cause expansion of cortical plates of bone or separation of adjacent teeth. Most cases occur in the mandible and generally are asymptomatic. They are composed of primitive connective tissue resembling the dental papilla interspersed with cords of odonto-

genic epithelium (Fig. 15–47). Surgically, these tumors tend to shell out of the bone readily and recurrence is not expected.

Ameloblastic Fibro-odontoma

This mixed odontogenic tumor exhibits features of the ameloblastic fibroma with a significant element of more mature calcified tooth structure present. The lesions are well-circumscribed radiolucencies often in association with a radiodense mass resembling an odontoma. They are treated conservatively, and do not tend to recur.

Odontoma

The odontoma is composed of a mass made up of all the tissues which combine to form a tooth. The complex composite odontoma is made up of dentin, enamel and pulp in an irregular pattern, whereas the

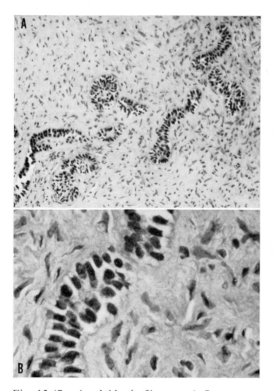

Fig. 15-47. Ameloblastic fibroma. *A*, Low-power photomicrograph showing strands of odontogenic epithelium (comparable to dental lamina) in a primitive connective stroma (comparable to dental papilla). *B*, Higher magnification of one of the epithelial cords shown in (*A*).

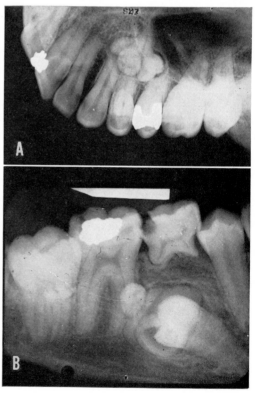

Fig. 15-48. *A*, Compound composite odontoma. *B*, Unusual odontoma associated with the crown of an unerupted lower second bicuspid.

compound composite odontoma is composed of multiple anomalous teeth sufficiently characteristic to be identified radiographically. Such lesions may be located between the roots of teeth causing malocclusion or interfering with the eruption of adjacent teeth. The radiographic appearance of the compound composite odontoma is characteristic, since the miniature teeth usually can be recognized (Fig. 15–48A). The complex composite type may be identified with reasonable accuracy if sufficient enamel is present in the lesion to permit comparison with the density of the other teeth in the mouth (Fig. 15–48B). The radiodense mass may be surrounded by a radiolucent capsule, producing a target lesion, and on occasion the odontogenic epithelium may proliferate to produce a dentigerous cyst. Such cases should be examined histologically. Surgical treatment is conservative and the prognosis is excellent.

Ameloblastic Odontoma

Of rare occurrence, the ameloblastic odontoma is composed of ameloblastomatous tissue together with more mature elements of tooth structure as in an odontoma. Radiographically, it is seen as a combined radiolucent-radiopaque area which is poorly circumscribed. On the basis of the few reported cases, the tumor can be expected to behave like a simple ameloblastoma with considerable likelihood of recurrence.

Ameloblastic Fibrodentinoma

In this rare variant of dentinoma, neoplastic epithelial strands are present along with dentin or dentinoid material. Treatment is by surgical excision and curettage.

Ameloblastic Hemangioma

A simple ameloblastoma with a significant hemangiomatous element, the so-called ameloblastic hemangioma, may represent a true mixed odontogenic tumor, a collision tumor, or a simple ameloblastoma which is highly vascular. Its clinical behavior and management are the same as those of the simple ameloblastoma.

Odontogenic Tumors, Malignant

The malignant odontogenic tumors are extremely rare lesions. Nevertheless, the dentist should be aware of the recognized variants and the broad spectrum of neoplasms which characterize the odontogenic apparatus.

Odontogenic Fibrosarcoma

This highly malignant tumor is presumed to arise from the mesenchymal components of the odontogenic apparatus; however, it does not differ substantially from the non-odontogenic central fibrosarcoma of bone. Like most sarcomas, it appears as a highly destructive, fleshy tumor and there is often associated pain. It is composed of sheets and fascicles of malignant fibroblasts in a fibrous stroma. Wide resection of the tumor is the treatment of choice.

Malignant Ameloblastoma

Rarely, metastasis of ameloblastoma to the lungs is seen. Even more rarely, ameloblastoma has been identified in lymph nodes as well. In such cases, the pulmonary lesion is identical to the primary tumor in the jaws and is presumed to represent truly malignant behavior. On the other hand, some reported cases of metastatic ameloblastoma are thought to represent aspiration of tumor cells at the time of surgery.

Ameloblastic Carcinoma

This term implies that malignant transformation of the epithelium in an ameloblastoma has occurred, resulting in metastatic deposits which differ from the benign-appearing primary tumors (cf. Malignant Ameloblastoma).

Primary Intra-alveolar Epidermoid Carcinoma

This rare central epidermoid carcinoma arises from entrapped epithelium or remnants of odontogenic rests. In the cases reviewed by Shear, most appeared in the mandible of elderly males. The tumor produces marked destruction extending into the oral soft tissues. The tumor has a histologic resemblance to odontogenic epithelium of the basal cell type. Treatment is by wide surgical resection.

Ameloblastic Fibrosarcoma

The few rare examples of this tumor appear to represent an ameloblastic fibroma in which the primitive mesenchymal component is malignant. It occurs in young adults and causes marked bone destruction, pain and loosening of the teeth. The cure rate is extremely poor.

NEOPLASTIC AND NEOPLASTIC-LIKE LESIONS (NON-ODONTOGENIC)

Benign Tumors (Non-odontogenic)

Exostoses and Mandibular and Palatal Tori

The exostoses appear as nodular excrescences of bone on the labial and buccal aspects of the alveolar process (Fig. 15–49). These are of little clinical significance except when dentures are to be constructed.

The mandibular tori are easily identified clinically as protuberances of bone covered by smooth mucosa located on the lingual aspect of the mandible in the premolar region (Fig. 15–50). Palatal tori are found in the

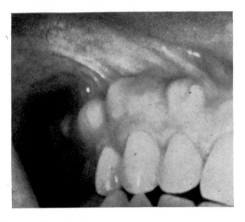

Fig. 15-49.   Multiple exostoses.

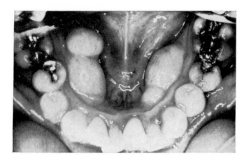

Fig. 15-50.   Mandibular tori.

palatal vault at the midline. Both may take a variety of forms ranging from smooth to lobulated. The tori are radiodense masses (Fig. 2–39). Seen in adults, they are of little clinical significance except in patients for whom dentures need to be constructed. On occasion, traumatic injury to the thin covering mucosa results in an ulcer and sequestration of a portion of the rather avascular torus.

Osteoma

This is a slow-growing benign tumor found centrally in the bone (Fig. 10–13). It is rare in the jaws. The osteoma appears radiographically as a circumscribed radiopaque mass with a thin radiolucent outline. Differentiation from some varieties of complex odontoma is difficult or impossible radiographically.

Multiple osteomas of the jaws and facial skeleton are characteristic of *Gardner's syndrome*. Other features of the syndrome include skin lesions (epidermal inclusion cysts, dermoids, lipomas, other fibrous tumors) and intestinal polyposis of the colon and rectum. The polyps have a significant potential for malignant transformation.

Benign Osteoblastoma (Giant Osteoid Osteoma)

The benign osteoblastoma is found chiefly in children or young adults but differs from the osteoid osteoma in that it is generally larger (greater growth potential) and not as painful. It is a fairly well-circumscribed radiopaque lesion composed of disorganized spicules and trabeculae of calcified matrix and osteoid with bizarre osteoblasts. It is being recognized with increasing frequency in jaws.

Osteoid Osteoma

A painful lesion seen typically in the long bones of adolescents and young adults, the osteoid osteoma is extremely rare in the jaws. It is seen radiographically as a compact, central nidus of calcifying osteoid sharply demarcated from an outer sclerotic border.

Chondroma

This benign cartilaginous tumor is surprisingly rare in the jaws. Radiographically, it appears as a radiolucent or mixed lesion, usually in the anterior maxilla, posterior mandible or near the temporomandibular joint. The histologic differentiation from chondrosarcoma is often difficult.

Hemangioma

The central hemangioma of bone is an extremely rare but serious condition that should be considered in the differential diagnosis of any unexplained radiolucent lesion. It most frequently occurs in the mandible as a solitary radiolucency which sometimes exhibits delicate trabeculae at vertical angles to the periphery and coursing through the center of the radiolucency giving a "soap-bubble" effect. The presenting symptoms are often not remarkable although unexplained hemorrhage of the overlying mucosa or around the teeth is sometimes present. Aspiration of the radiolucency with a large-gauge needle will usually confirm its vascular nature. Patients with suspected hemangioma or other vascular anomalies of bone should be hospitalized since, upon surgical exploration, massive hemorrhage may occur.

Arteriovenous Aneurysm (AV Fistula, AV Malformation)

The congenital AV aneurysm, which has many features in common with the heman-gioma, is composed of anomalous shunts or connections between the arterial and venous system which have persisted after development of the vascular network. Most cases do not become clinically evident until the teens or even adulthood. Depending upon the local hemodynamics, additional AV shunts may become patent with time, thereby resulting in a gradual increase in size of the defect. It may occur in the oral soft tissues (p. 417) as well as in bone and in some instances may arise following trauma with atypical repair of the vascular bed.

The radiographic features of the central AV aneurysms of bone range from a honeycomb appearance to a completely lytic lesion. When a tooth-bearing area of the jaw is involved, mobility of the teeth and a dusky discoloration of the gingiva with spontaneous bleeding may be present. Pain is uncommon but the patient may report a throbbing sensation, pulsation or a "swishing" noise, especially at night. A bruit or thrill may be detected with the use of a stethoscope over the area. Needle aspiration will produce copious amounts of arterial blood which is often under pressure. Obviously, attempts at surgical exploration at this time may lead to disastrous hemorrhage. Angiography must be performed to help confirm the diagnosis as well as to establish the extent of the lesion. Various treatment modalities have been employed with varying success, including surgical resection, x-ray therapy, embolization with plastic spheres, sclerosing agents and ligation of major vessels.

Desmoplastic Fibroma of Bone, Fibroxanthoma (Fibrous Histiocytoma of Bone)

The benign, non-odontogenic fibrous connective tissue lesions of bone are relatively rare. Like their counterparts in the skin (e.g. nodular fasciitis, aggressive fibromatosis or extra-abdominal desmoid, proliferative myositis, etc.), these tumors are locally aggressive and may be confused with the well-differentiated fibrosarcoma. The differentiation of this broad spectrum of cellular lesions, composed chiefly of histiocytes or facultative fibroblasts, is primarily histologic with few distinguishing radiographic or other clinical features. For the most part, the fibrous histiocytoma and desmoplastic fibroma of bone occur in children and young adults, often with rapid local growth with bone destruction. Definitive treatment requires wide surgical excision or resection. While metastasis is unlikely, recurrences are common.

Central Neurogenic Tumors of the Jaws

The peripheral nerve tumors are of rare occurrence in the jaws. They appear as radiolucencies, often in the body or ramus of the mandible and sometimes in continuity with the mandibular canal (Fig. 15–51). In this latter location, the early benign tumors (neurofibroma, neurilemmoma) often are characterized by a fusiform enlargement of the canal. Growth is slow but persistent and some cases may reach considerable size with expansion or perforation of the cortex and facial deformity. In the latter instance, the radiographic appearance is suggestive of ad-

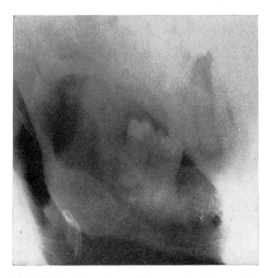

Fig. 15-51. Central neurilemmoma of bone. The fusiform enlargement of the mandibular canal is strongly suggestive of the diagnosis, which must be established histologically (see also Fig. 14-39).

vanced ameloblastoma or even malignancy. Intraosseous neurofibromas may be found in some cases of von Recklinghausen's disease of skin (Fig. 14–38).

The amputation (traumatic) neuroma occurs intraosseously on rare occasions following traumatic injuries such as jaw fracture or tooth extraction. Pain or paresthesia (in contrast to the typically asymptomatic neurilemmoma and neurofibroma) occurs in addition to the small focal radiolucency.

The neurogenic sarcoma is extremely rare in the jaws.

Neuroectodermal Tumor of Infancy

Once classified with the odontogenic neoplasms, this rare tumor occurs chiefly in the maxilla of female infants and is found clinically as a dark pigmented mass with destruction of the underlying alveolar process. One or more developing deciduous teeth are characteristically seen floating in the protuberant soft tissue mass. It should be differentiated clinically from the congenital epulis of the newborn which may also be present at birth. The latter lesion is not pigmented and has an entirely different histologic pattern (p. 423). The melanotic neuroectodermal tumor is composed of alveoli of cuboidal cells containing rod-shaped melanin and central collections of small dark round cells. Despite its ominous clinical appearance, this lesion is treated by rather conservative surgery and does not tend to recur.

Malignant Tumors (Non-odontogenic)

Osteosarcoma

The osteosarcoma of the jaw bones occurs chiefly in the mandible in the second and third decades of life. Those that are predominantly bone producing exhibit areas of radiolucency with irregular radiopaque masses and the classical "sunray" appearance of the cortex (Fig. 15–52). The osteolytic types of osteosarcoma will show relatively larger areas of radiolucency. In either

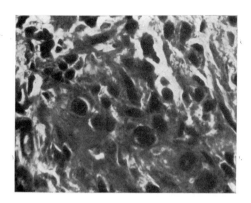

Fig. 15-52. Osteosarcoma. Malignant osteoblasts and small focus of tumor osteoid are shown.

type, the reaction is that of a destructive, rapidly growing and malignant disease which is accompanied by other ominous signs as pain or paresthesia and loosening of the teeth. Prompt diagnosis by histologic examination followed by radical surgery or combined surgery and irradiation is essential if cure is to be accomplished.

Chondrosarcoma

Chondrogenic tumors are very uncommon. The chondrosarcoma ordinarily occurs in a somewhat older age group (30 to 50 years) than the osteosarcoma and generally has a considerably poorer prognosis. The

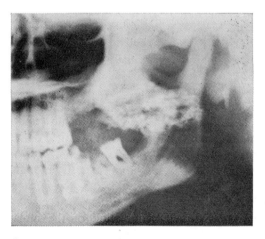

Fig. 15-53. Chondrosarcoma. Portion of a Panorex radiograph showing a proliferating radiolucent-radiopaque mass.

clinical signs are usually those of an expanding growth in the jaws which may or may not be painful. The radiographic features are quite variable with diffuse osteolytic areas intermixed with foci of calcification, often with periosteal involvement (Fig. 15–53).

Reticulum Cell Sarcoma of Bone

Primary reticulum cell sarcoma of bone generally exhibits local bone pain and enlargement with gradual loosening of the teeth over a period of several weeks or months. Radiographically, the advanced tumor appears as a destructive, poorly defined radiolucency. In the early lesions, the changes may be indistinct with a general loss of trabeculation density inconsistent with the patient's complaints. Because of its better prognosis, reticulum cell sarcoma should be distinguished from its soft tissue counterpart (see pp. 340–341).

Fibrosarcoma of Bone

Fibrosarcoma arising primarily in the jaw bone is of rare occurrence. Most cases are seen in the third to fifth decades although both young children and older adults may be affected. Histologic diagnosis is often difficult since it may resemble odontogenic fibrosarcoma (p. 482), desmoplastic fibroma of bone (p. 483) and fibroblastic osteosarcoma (p. 484). It is important to note that some cases of fibrosarcoma have followed irradiation of fibrous dysplasia of bone (p. 457). The prognosis of fibrosarcoma, dependent upon the degree of histologic differentiation, is generally better than other soft tissue sarcomas.

Ewing's Sarcoma (Endothelial Myeloma)

Ewing's sarcoma is a highly malignant neoplasm seen most commonly in the long bones of children and young adults, generally less than 25 years of age. Other bones, including the jaws, may also be affected. Bone pain, often accompanied by fever and leukocytosis, may suggest an infectious process. The bone lesions appear as diffuse radiolucencies, sometimes with a cortical onionskin reaction (p. 453). The histologic findings consist of necrotic foci and broad sheets of round cells which must be differentiated from lymphosarcoma of bone. Although the tumor is radiosensitive, the prognosis is poor.

Multiple Myeloma

This malignant neoplasm arises primarily in bone, revealing the classic "punched-out" radiolucency without a distinct cortical border. The disease occurs predominantly in males, usually in the fourth decade or later. The chief presenting symptom is bone pain and, occasionally, pathologic fracture. Most cases at the time of diagnosis exhibit multiple lesions in various bones of the body, particularly the skull, spine, ribs and long bones. The mandible is involved with considerable frequency.

In some cases, a solitary radiolucency may be discovered (plasmacytoma, solitary plasma cell myeloma). Unfortunately, the prognosis of the solitary lesion cannot be predicted with any certainty since some patients subsequently develop additional bone lesions, while others will be cured following local removal of the lesion. The extramedullary plasmacytoma occurs as a solitary soft tissue lesion and has a considerably better prognosis than the bone tumor.

The diagnosis of plasma cell myeloma of bone is established by biopsy. Whether a given lesion is solitary or multiple must be determined by skeletal radiographic survey (Fig. 15–54). Bence-Jones protein in the urine is found in approximately three-fourths of the patients with multiple myeloma. Therefore, absence does not rule out the diagnosis. The total serum proteins are elevated and characteristic globulin fractions are shown by electrophoresis (p. 225). The albumin/globulin ratio is reversed. Bone marrow aspirates (sternal puncture) will often show myeloma cells.

Essentially the same diagnostic procedures are followed in the case of the solitary

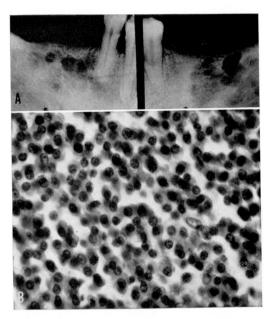

Fig. 15-54. Plasma cell myeloma. *A,* Routine periapical radiographs in this 44-year-old man showed multiple "punched-out" radiolucencies of the jaws. *B,* Bone biopsy showing sheets of plasma cells. Skull films revealed additional lesions of the calvarium and other laboratory studies confirmed the diagnosis.

plasma cell myeloma and extramedullary plasmacytoma. Even though the radiographic and laboratory findings are negative, the patient must be followed at regular intervals inasmuch as additional lesions may develop later.

Treatment of multiple myeloma is usually by irradiation although chemotherapeutic agents are sometimes used. Death generally occurs within 2 or 3 years.

Carcinoma of the Antrum

Antral carcinoma is included with tumors of the jaw bones since it frequently invades the maxilla, producing a swelling on the lateral aspect of the hard palate, in the mucobuccal fold, or superiorly in the infraorbital region. Often the swelling or, occasionally, loosening or migration of the molar teeth is the first clinical sign, even though the tumor may be far advanced. Radiographically, destruction of the maxillary process and a large communication with the sinus are seen. Antral carcinoma, seen chiefly in older males, is usually treated by radical surgery which may be supplemented by radiation therapy. However, the prognosis is poor.

Malignant Central Salivary Gland Tumors

Malignant salivary gland tumors arising centrally within the jaw bones are almost invariably mucoepidermoid carcinomas, with most of these found posterior to the first molar teeth of the mandible. It has been postulated that these tumors arise from enclaved salivary gland tissue in the jaw, ectopic salivary glands as in the static bone cyst (p. 456), or the pluripotential lining epithelium of odontogenic cysts. The radiographic features of the reported cases have resembled ameloblastoma or dentigerous cyst. For the most part, the age range and clinical behavior of these tumors have paralleled the soft tissue tumors. Rare examples of adenoid cystic carcinoma and malignant mixed tumor have been reported centrally in the jaws.

Metastatic Bone Disease

A number of malignant neoplasms have a tendency to metastasize to bones, including the jaws (Fig. 15–55). Since lesions of this type are disseminated by way of the bloodstream, the metastatic lesion is most apt to occur in areas of hematopoietic tissue. In the jaw bones, residual bone marrow is found at the angle of the mandible, in the mandibular molar area and in the maxillary tuberosity; however, some hematopoietic tissue may be found in other regions (see p. 459).

Primary malignant tumors in other organs which have metastasized to the jaw include those of breast, prostate, thyroid, lung, kidney, colon, testes and adrenal. Although most metastatic lesions are radiolucent, tumors of the prostate, breast and lung occasionally stimulate bone formation at the secondary site, resulting in a combined radiolucent-radiopaque lesion (p. 448). For the

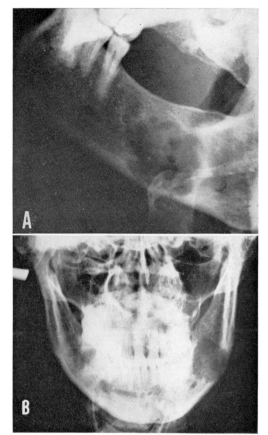

Fig. 15-55. Carcinoma of the breast metastatic to the mandible. *A,* The lateral jaw radiograph shows a large, poorly defined radiolucency with several other focal radiolucent areas. Paresthesia of the lower lip was present. *B,* The PA radiograph shows perforation of the bone cortex. The diagnosis of metastatic tumor was made upon histologic examination. A history of carcinoma of the breast treated 5 years previously was obtained.

most part, they are diffuse and poorly defined, although sharply outlined focal lesions are found occasionally.

Associated symptoms of metastatic tumor to the jaw bones may include paresthesia and unexplained loosening of the teeth. The clinical importance of these signs and symptoms cannot be overemphasized.

The history of a previous diagnosis of malignant disease in some other organ is extremely helpful in evaluating an unknown radiolucency of the jaw. It should be noted that the patient is unlikely to volunteer, and may even deliberately withhold, such information since he is unaware of the possible relation of malignant disease in another part of the body with his oral symptoms. In other instances, the presence of a malignant tumor in some other organ or tissue may not be known. Once the microscopic diagnosis of probable metastatic tumor to the jaw is established, the patient must be referred immediately for complete physical examination to establish the primary site and detect other possible secondary sites. The diagnosis of metastatic tumor to the jaw is not justified until the entire case has been evaluated.

METABOLIC DISORDERS

Histiocytosis X Disease

The term histiocytosis X is applied to three related conditions characterized chiefly by proliferation of reticuloendothelial cells. Sometimes referred to as the non-lipid reticuloendothelioses, these conditions are Letterer-Siwe disease, Hand-Schüller-Christian disease and eosinophilic granuloma. While they have several features in common, the age of onset and the prognosis are considerably different.

Letterer-Siwe disease behaves as a malignant histiocytoma or malignant lymphoma. It arises in infants and young children generally less than 2 years of age and is almost invariably fatal. The principal pathologic features are related to generalized involvement of the reticuloendothelial system resulting in hepatomegaly and lymph node, skin, lung and bone marrow involvement. Because of the rapid course of the disease, radiologically distinct bone lesions are not usually encountered.

Hand-Schüller-Christian disease occurs at a somewhat later age than Letterer-Siwe disease, usually in children up to the early teens. The classical triad of symptoms, namely, exophthalmos, bone lesions, and diabetes insipidus, are fairly common manifestations of the disease but are not neces-

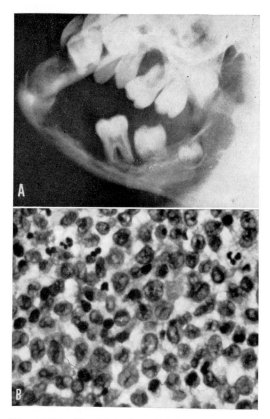

Fig. 15-56. Hand-Schüller-Christian disease. *A,* Lateral jaw radiograph showing extensive bone loss in an 11-year-old boy. Eventually all his teeth were lost and full dentures were constructed. *B,* Uniform sheets of pale-staining histiocytes with scattered eosinophils (dark cells in photomicrograph) are characteristic histologic findings.

sary for the diagnosis. Exophthalmos and diabetes insipidus indicate histiocytic cell proliferation in the orbit and the pituitary gland respectively. Because of its more chronic nature, Hand-Schüller-Christian disease produces marked bone changes, particularly of the facial bones and the jaws. Radiographs of the jaws show extensive resorption of the alveolar bone (Fig. 15–56). The teeth loosen and have to be removed. It is not uncommon for children that survive to require full dentures once the disease is under control.

Eosinophilic granuloma occurs most commonly in young adults, generally males. There is common involvement of the jaw

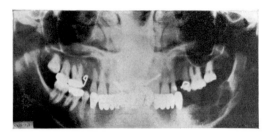

Fig. 15-57. Panorex radiograph showing an extensive radiolucency of the mandibular molar region. A loose molar tooth had been extracted 2 years previously with a clinical diagnosis of "pyorrhea." The extraction site never completely healed and the patient was finally referred for consultation with a preoperative diagnosis of ameloblastoma. A biopsy was obtained and a diagnosis of eosinophilic granuloma established.

bones, especially of the alveolar process around the teeth (Fig. 15–57). The radiolucency is poorly defined and may present the clinical appearance of advanced periodontal disease involving a single tooth or two adjacent teeth. Both the clinical and radiographic impression is that the tooth is "floating in soft tissue." The associated inflammation and secondary infection may create local symptoms suggesting disease of periodontal or pulpal origin. In most instances, there is no reason to suspect pulpal infection and the pulps test vital. Likewise, periodontal disease can be tentatively ruled out since the bony support of other teeth in the arch is generally adequate (Fig. 15–58). The rule for investigation of unexplained loosening of a tooth applies and the

tissue curetted from the radiolucency along with the extracted tooth should be submitted for histologic examination. Once the diagnosis is established, additional steps should be taken. Since eosinophilic granuloma may be either solitary or multiple, skeletal radiographs should be obtained to determine whether other similar bone lesions are present.

As to prognosis, Letterer-Siwe disease is almost invariably fatal whereas Hand-Schüller-Christian disease may show eventual spontaneous recovery, respond to irradiation, or undergo transition to Letterer-Siwe disease and ultimately be fatal. Eosinophilic granuloma has an excellent prognosis and responds to local surgical curettage or irradiation.

Von Recklinghausen's Disease of Bone

Lesions of the jaw bones in hyperparathyroidism may manifest themselves as "brown tumors" (osteitis fibrosa cystica), loss of lamina dura or a generalized decrease in bone density approaching a ground-glass appearance. These and other aspects of the disease are discussed on pages 249–251.

Paget's Disease of Bone

Of unknown etiology, Paget's disease of bone affects chiefly males past the age of 40. It is quite likely that a significant number of cases remain undiagnosed since the disease has an insidious onset and an indolent course. The majority of cases are discovered coincidentally on radiographs taken for other purposes (Fig. 15–59). In some instances, the patient may seek professional advice because of bone pain, deformity, fracture, increased warmth or other associated symptoms (Fig. 15–1). The dentist may recognize the disease through oral radiographs inasmuch as the maxilla is commonly involved (seldom the mandible). The striking "cotton-wool" appearance of the bone in radiographs is characteristic of Paget's disease. This effect is produced by the areas of alternating bone resorption and bone formation

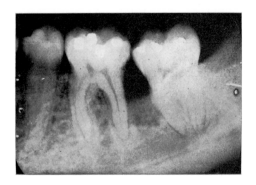

Fig. 15-58. Eosinophilic granuloma of bone.

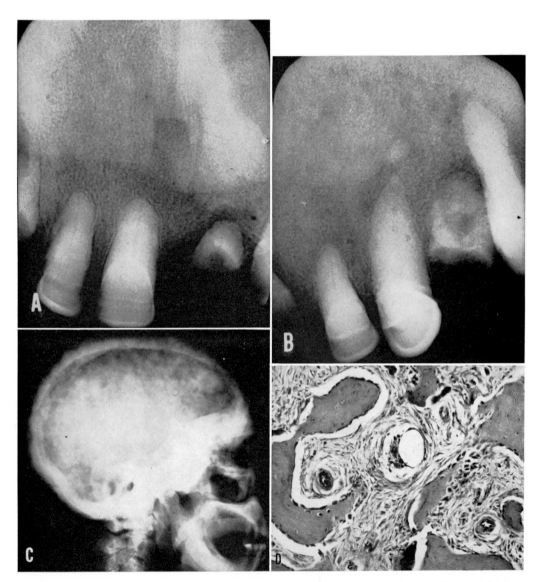

Fig. 15-59. Paget's disease of bone. *A* and *B*, Periapical radiographs showed generalized involvement of the maxilla with alteration in the trabecular pattern. The osteoblastic activity was quite uniform in this area of the jaw giving a ground-glass appearance. *C*, A lateral head-plate demonstrates the classical "cotton-wool" appearance in the calvarium. *D*, Photomicrograph shows areas of both osteoblastic and osteoclastic activity.

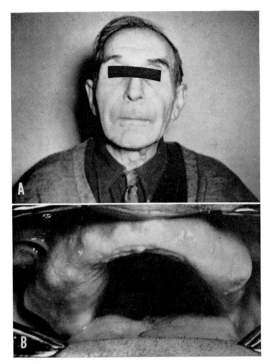

Fig. 15-60.   Paget's disease of bone. *A,* Enlargement of the maxilla is evident by the tense appearance of the upper lip. This patient was stoopshouldered and complained of mild bone pain. *B,* The edentulous maxilla was markedly enlarged. Radiographs showed the typical "cottonwool" bone.

characteristic of this disease. Accordingly, a radiograph may vary from one which is predominantly radiolucent to one which is characteristically radiopaque in a mottled pattern, depending upon the stage of the disease. In addition to the cotton-wool appearance of the jaw bone, marked deformity is seen, usually enlargement of the maxilla. Hypercementosis and ankylosis of the teeth have been reported. The distribution of the lesions may be confined to one or many bones of the body.

Patients with Paget's disease present a classical clinical appearance caused by the bone enlargement and deformity. They tend to be stoop-shouldered with a sunken chest, curved back, bowed legs, and a simian appearance (Fig. 15-60). Classically, the head size gradually increases over a period

of time and, if the patient is edentulous, the dentures become too tight and must be remade.

It has been noted the radiographs may vary considerably in their pattern with areas of sclerosis, areas of radiolucency or combinations of both. Even in the same patient, all of the affected bones may not show the same radiographic stage of the disease (cf. Fig. 15–59*A* and *C*). The diagnosis is made on the basis of clinical and radiographic features and confirmed by histologic and laboratory findings. Serum calcium and phosphorus values are normal, but there is a markedly elevated serum alkaline phosphatase.

The associated bone pain and radiographic changes are similar to those seen in chronic diffuse sclerosing osteomyelitis. The possibility of a primary or metastatic tumor to the bone must also be considered inasmuch as some malignant tumors of this variety may be bone producers. If only periapical radiographs are available, radiolucent or radiopaque lesions in the vicinity of apices of the teeth may suggest periapical granulomas or focal sclerosis, respectively.

No definitive treatment for Paget's disease is available although some success has been obtained with fluoride therapy. The chief complications of Paget's disease of bone are pathologic fracture, anemia, neurologic disturbances such as blindness or deafness and, in approximately 10 to 15 percent of reported cases, osteosarcoma in bone.

Gaucher's Disease

This hereditary disorder of sphingolipid metabolism is classified as one of the lipid reticuloendothelioses. (Others of this group are Niemann-Pick disease, Tay-Sachs disease, Fabry's disease, metachromatic leukodystrophy, etc.).

Gaucher's disease occurs in both infantile and adult forms although the adult form is the more common. In the infantile form, the infant rarely survives beyond the second year whereas in the adult the disease has a long, protracted course. The latter is characterized by hepatosplenomegaly, pancytopenia, weakness, pingueculae (yellow, wedge-shaped areas of the conjunctiva) and yellow skin pigmentation, chiefly on the lower extremities. Jaw radiographs show osteoporotic defects with enlargement and thinning of the cortex, especially in the mandible where there may be root resorption. Biopsy of bone marrow or other reticuloendothelial organs (*e.g.* spleen, liver) shows Gaucher's cells (reticuloendothelial cells packed with kerasin). Laboratory studies show a pancytopenia and elevated serum acid phosphatase. There is no specific treatment for this condition.

Osteogenesis Imperfecta ("Brittle Bones," Lobstein's Disease)

This disorder is characterized by marked fragility of the bones with multiple fractures, blue sclera of the eyes and, usually but not invariably, dentinogenesis imperfecta. Those cases present *in utero* or at birth are extremely severe and the infant is often stillborn. Cases becoming manifest later in childhood (tarda type) involve numerous bone fractures following even minor stress or trauma. As a consequence, marked deformities of limbs and interference with growth centers results.

Osteopetrosis

This disease is characterized by increased density and brittleness of the bones believed due to inadequate osteoclastic bone resorption (Fig. 15–61). Of unknown etiology, a hereditary factor is undoubtedly present in most cases. Radiographically, the bones exhibit marked thickening of the cortex and trabeculae with reduction of the marrow spaces. With reduction in the volume of hematopoietic tissue, myelophthisic anemia occurs. No significant changes in serum calcium, phosphorus, or serum alkaline phosphatase are found. In some instances, the failure of bone resorption and remodeling causes reduction of the size of nerve fora-

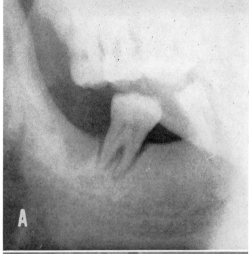

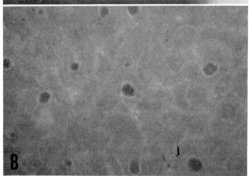

Fig. 15-61. Osteopetrosis. *A*, Trabecular thickening is generalized with resultant reduction in the size of the marrow spaces and reduced blood supply. The mandibular canal is partially obliterated. The tooth is loose due to periodontal disease. *B*, Tetracycline antibiotics were administered 4 days prior to extraction of the tooth shown in *A*. Fluorescence microscopy of a rib biopsy (ground section) shows labeling of active osteogenesis around Haversian canals as a yellow fluorescent line. The continual bone production has obliterated the marrow cavity.

mina and resultant neurologic problems such as blindness or deafness. The entire skeleton including the jaws is affected.

In addition to the delayed eruption of the teeth, the most serious complications arise upon extraction of the teeth. Even though the bone is denser than usual, it tends to be somewhat more brittle and fracture of the teeth or jaws may occur. Because of the reduced vascularity of the bone (essential for normal inflammation and repair), these patients exhibit a marked tendency to develop postoperative osteomyelitis.

No specific treatment for osteopetrosis is known.

Osteoporosis

In addition to the simple atrophy of the alveolar process following loss of teeth, reduced bone density may be associated with aging and certain endocrine disturbances, chiefly menopause. Postmenopausal women may show a generalized osteoporosis brought about by reduced estrogen activity. In most instances, however, such changes in the bone are quite subtle and recognized only after consideration of technical factors which influence the density of the radiograph, size of the jaws and body build, and comparison with other bones.

Alterations of the orientation of alveolar bone trabeculae (stepladder pattern) have also been described in certain anemias (p. 409).

Caffey's Disease

This unusual condition occurs in early infancy, usually about 10 weeks to 6 months of age, and is characterized by pain and often symmetrical soft tissue swelling over one or several bones. Subperiosteal cortical thickening of the bones, particularly the mandible and long bones, may be seen radiographically. Additional symptoms of fever and irritability suggest a preliminary diagnosis of a generalized infectious process or allergy. Laboratory studies show an elevated sedimentation rate, elevated serum alkaline phosphatase and leukocytosis with a relative eosinophilia.

Aside from the involvement of the mandible and the facial swelling, the dentist's responsibility in arriving at a diagnosis is largely to rule out acute pyogenic infection arising from the teeth or alveolar processes. The differential diagnoses, based largely upon the bone changes, are osteomyelitis, scurvy, vitamin A intoxication, congenital syphilis and subperiosteal hematoma. The bilateral swelling of the face may suggest mumps although it should be noted that the very young infant will probably still have maternal antibodies to this disease. Familial fibrous dysplasia (cherubism) is not easily recognized in the infant and does not affect bones other than the jaws.

Although the disease exhibits certain features of infection, traumatic injury, allergy, nutritional disturbance or endocrine disease, a specific causative factor has not been established. In view of its unknown nature, treatment is largely symptomatic. The steroids are generally helpful.

The prognosis of Caffey's disease is excellent since the infants recover without specific treatment and are left with no residual effects other than some bowing of the limbs which corrects itself in time by remodeling.

BIBLIOGRAPHY

Differential Diagnosis

Curtis, A. B.: Childhood leukemias: osseous changes in jaws on panoramic dental radiographs, J. Amer. Dent. Ass., 83, 844, 1971.

Eversole, L. R. and Rovin, S.: Differential radiographic diagnosis of lesions of the jawbones, Radiology, 105, 277, 1972; Dent. Radiogr. Photogr., 46, 71, 1973.

Henrikson, C. O., Nordenram, A. and Nyborg, H.: Radiopaque areas in human jaws, Sartryck ur Odontölögisk Tidskrift, 71, 373, 1963.

Hinds, E. C.: Noninflammatory bone disease, J. Oral Surg., 38, 37, 1970.

Jayne, E. H., Hays, R. A. and O'Brien, F. W. Jr.: Cysts and tumors of the mandible: their differential diagnosis, Amer. J. Roentgen., 86, 292, 1961.

Lichtenstein, L.: Tumors of periosteal origin, Cancer, 8, 1060, 1955.

Lilly, G. E.: Differential diagnosis of lesions of the jawbones, J. Oral Surg., 28, 65, 1970.

Merrell, R. A. and Yanagisawa, E.: Radiographic anatomy of the paranasal sinuses (parts I-IV), Arch. Otolaryng., 87, 88 and 100, 1968 and 87, 97 and 109, 1968.

Mourshed, F. and Tuckson, C. R.: A study of the radiographic features of the jaws in sickle-cell anemia, Oral Surg., 37, 812, 1974.

Poyton, H. G.: Methodical approach to radiographic interpretation, J. Canad. Dent. Ass., 32, 354, 1966.

Stern, M. H. and Cole, W. L.: Radiographic changes in the mandible associated with leukemic cell infiltration in a case of acute myelogenous leukemia, Oral Surg., *36*, 343, 1973.

Updegrave, W. J.: Normal radiodontic anatomy, myelogenous leukemia, Oral Surg., *36*, 343, 1973.

Developmental Disorders

Abrams, A. M., Howell, F. V. and Bullock, W. K.: Nasopalatine cysts, Oral Surg., *16*, 306, 1963.

Choukas, N. C. and Toto, P. D.: Etiology of static bone defects of the mandible, J. Oral Surg., *18*, 16, 1960.

Christ, T. F.: The globulomaxillary cyst: An embryologic misconception, Oral Surg., *30*, 515, 1970.

D'Eramo, E. M. and Poidmore, S. J.: Developmental submandibular gland defect of the mandible. Review of the literature and report of a case, Oral Surg., *39*, 14, 1975.

Jonck, L. M.: Facial asymmetry and condylar hyperplasia, Oral Surg., *40*, 567, 1975.

Lilly, G. E.: Differential diagnosis of lesions of the jawbones, J. Oral Surg., *28*, 65, 1970.

Lucchesi, F. J. and Topazian, D. S.: Multilocular median developmental cyst of the mandible: report of case, J. Oral Surg., *19*, 64, 1961.

Miller, A. S., Greelay, J. N. and Catena, D. L.: Median maxillary anterior alveolar cleft: report of three cases, J. Amcr. Dent. Ass., *79*, 896, 1969.

Miller, A. S. and Winnick, M.: Salivary gland inclusion in the anterior mandible. Report of a case with a review of the literature on aberrant salivary gland tissue and neoplasms, Oral Surg., *31*, 790, 1971.

Standish, S. M. and Shafer, W. G.: Focal osteoporotic bone marrow defects of the jaws, J. Oral Surg., *20*, 123, 1962.

Uemura, S., Fujishita, M. and Fuchihata, H.: Radiographic interpretation of so-called developmental defect of mandible, Oral Surg., *41*, 120, 1976.

Inflammatory and Reactive Disorders

Barker, B. F., Jensen, J. L. and Howell, F. V.: Focal osteoporotic bone marrow defects of the jaws, Oral Surg., *38*, 404, 1974.

Beasley, J. D. III: Traumatic cyst of the jaws: report of 30 cases, J. Amer. Dent. Ass., *93*, 145, 1976.

Biewald, H. F.: A variation in the management of the hemorrhagic, traumatic, or simple bone cyst, J. Oral Surg., *25*, 427, 1967.

Gothberg, K. A. T,. Little, J. W., King, D. R. and Bean, L. R.: A clinical study of cysts arising from mucosa of the maxillary sinus, Oral Surg., *41*, 52, 1976.

Gregory, G. T. and Shafer, W. G.: Surgical ciliated cysts of the maxilla: report of cases, J. Oral Surg., *16*, 251, 1958.

Hansen, L. S., Sapone, J. and Sproat, R. C.: Traumatic bone cysts of jaws. Report of sixty-six cases, Oral Surg., *37*, 899, 1974.

Jacobsson, S., Hallen, O., Hollender, L., Hansson, C.-G. and Lindström, J.: Fibro-osseous lesion of the mandible mimicking chronic osteomyelitis, Oral Surg., *40*, 433, 1975.

Keen, E. G., Sammartino, C. A. and Johnson, E. S.: Chronic sclerosing osteomyelitis of the mandible: report of case, J. Amer. Dent. Ass., *76*, 597, 1968.

Mainous, E. G. and Boyne, P. J.: Healing of mandibular osteomyelitis in a narcotics addict following hyperbaric oxygen: case report, Milit. Med., *140*, 196, 1975.

Marchetta, F. C., Sako, K. and Holyoke, E. D.: Treatment of osteoradionecrosis by intraoral excision of the mandible, Surg. Gynec. Obstet., *125*, 1003, 1967.

Melrose, R. J., Abrams, A. M. and Mills, B. G.: Florid osseous dysplasia, Oral Surg., *41*, 62, 1976.

Meyer, I.: Infectious diseases of the jaws, J. Oral Surg., *28*, 17, 1970.

Rubin, R. L. and Doku, H. C.: Therapeutic radiology—the modalities and their effects on oral tissues, J. Amer. Dent. Ass., *92*, 731, 1976.

Shafer, W. G.: Chronic sclerosing osteomyelitis, J. Oral Surg., *15*, 138, 1957.

Spilka, C. J.: Pathways of dental infections, J. Oral Surg., *24*, 111, 1966.

Waldron, C. A.: Fibro-osseous lesions of the jaws, J. Oral Surg., *28*, 58, 1970.

Waldron, C. A., Giansanti, J. S. and Browand, B. C.: Sclerotic cemental masses of the jaws (so-called chronic sclerosing osteomyelitis, sclerosing osteitis, multiple enostosis and gigantiform cementoma), Oral Surg., *39*, 590, 1975.

Waldron, C. A. and Shafer, W. G.: The central giant cell reparative granuloma of the jaws, Amer. J. Clin. Path., *45*, 437, 1965.

Odontogenic Cysts

Altini, M. and Farman, A. G.: The calcifying odontogenic cyst. Eight new cases and a review of the literature, Oral Surg., *40*, 751, 1975.

Attenborough, N. R.: Recurrence of an odontogenic keratocyst in a bone graft: report of a case, Brit. J. Oral Surg., *12*, 33, 1974.

Browne, R. M.: The odontogenic keratocyst. Histological features and their correlation with clinical behavior, Brit. Dent. J., *131*, 249, 1971.

Chen, S–Y. and Miller, A. S.: Ultrastructure of the keratinizing and calcifying odontogenic cyst, Oral Surg., *39*, 769, 1975.

Fast, T. B and Mitchell, D. F.: Production of macroscopic cysts by autogenous epithelial implants, J. Dent. Res., *45*, 1242, 1966.

Freedman, P. D., Lumerman, H. and Gee, J. K.: Calcifying odontogenic cyst. A review and analysis of seventy cases, Oral Surg., *40*, 93, 1975.

Fromm, A.: Epstein's pearls, Bohn's nodules and inclusion-cysts of the oral cavity, J. Dent. Child., *34*, 275, 1967.

Gorlin, R. J., Pindborg, J. J., Redman, R. S., Williamson, J. J. and Hansen, L. I.: The calcifying odontogenic cyst—a new entity and possible analogue of the cutaneous calcifying epithelioma of Malherbe, Cancer, *17*, 723, 1964.

Gorlin, R. J., Yunis, J. J. and Tuna, N.: Multiple nevoid basal cell carcinoma, odontogenic keratocysts and skeletal anomalies, a syndrome, Acta Dermatovener, *43*, 39, 1963.

Keith, D. A.: Macroscopic satellite cyst formation in the odontogenic keratocyst, Oral Surg., *35*, 21, 1973.

Lile, H. A., Rogers, J. F. and Gerald, B.: The basal cell nevus syndrome, Amer. J. Roentgen., *103*, 214, 1968.

McClatchey, K., Batsakis, J. G., Hybels, R. and VanWieren, C. R.: Odontogenic keratocysts and nevoid basal cell carcinoma syndrome, Arch. Otolaryng., *101*, 613, 1975.

Panders, A. K. and Hodders, H. N.: Solitary keratocysts of the jaws, J. Oral Surg., *27*, 931, 1969.

Payne, T. F.: An analysis of the clinical and histopathologic parameters of the odontogenic keratocyst, Oral Surg., *33*, 538, 1972.

Sauk, J. J. Jr.: Calcifying and keratinizing odontogenic cyst, J. Oral Surg., *30*, 893, 1972.

Stafne, E. C.: *Oral Roentgenographic Diagnosis*, 4th Ed., Philadelphia, W. B. Saunders Co., 1975.

Standish, S. M. and Shafer, W. G.: The lateral periodontal cyst, J. Periodont., *29*, 27, 1958.

TenCate, A. R.: The epithelial cell rests of Malassez and the genesis of the dental cyst, Oral Surg., *34*, 956, 1972.

Toller, P. A.: Protein substances in odontogenic cyst fluids, Brit. Dent. J., *128*, 317, 1970.

Weathers, D. R. and Waldron, C. A.: Unusual multilocular cysts of the jaws (botryoid odontogenic cysts), Oral Surg., *36*, 235, 1973.

Wysocki, G. P. and Sapp, J. P.: Scanning and transmission electron microscopy of odontogenic keratocysts, Oral Surg., *40*, 494, 1975.

Odontogenic Tumors

Abrams, A. M. and Howell, F. V.: Calcifying epithelial odontogenic tumors: report of four cases, J. Amer. Dent. Ass., *74*, 1231, 1967.

Abrams, A. M., Kirby, J. W. and Melrose, R. J.: Cementoblastoma. A clinicopathologic study of seven new cases, Oral Surg., *38*, 394, 1974.

Anneroth, G., Isacsson, G. and Sigurdsson, Å.: Benign cementoblastoma (true cementoma), Oral Surg., *40*, 141, 1975.

Bhaskar, S. N.: Adenoameloblastoma: its histogenesis and report of 15 new cases, J. Oral Surg., *22*, 218, 1964.

Cataldo, E., Nathanson, N. and Shklar, G.: Ameloblastic sarcoma of the mandible, Oral Surg., *16*, 953, 1963.

Chambers, K. S.: The adenoameloblastoma, Brit. J. Oral Surg., *10*, 310, 1973.

Changus, G. W., Speed, J. S. and Stewart, F. W.: Malignant angioblastoma of bone. A reappraisal of adamantinoma of long bone, Cancer, *10*, 540, 1957.

Chaudhry, A. P., Spink, J. H. and Gorlin, R. J.: Periapical fibrous dysplasia (cementoma), J. Oral Surg., *16*, 483, 1958.

Corio, R. L., Crawford, B. E. and Schaberg, S. J.: Benign cementoblastoma, Oral Surg., *41*, 524, 1976.

Couch, R. D., Morris, E. E. and Vellios, F.: Granular cell ameloblastic fibroma, Amer. J. Clin. Path., *37*, 398, 1962.

Courtney, R. M. and Kerr, D. A.: The odontogenic adenomatoid tumor, Oral Surg., *39*, 424, 1975.

DeLathouwer, C. and Verhest, A.: Malignant primary intraosseous carcinoma of the mandible, Oral Surg., *37*, 77, 1974.

Dunlap, C. L. and Fritzlen, T. J.: Cystic odontoma with concomitant adenoameloblastoma (adenoameloblastic odontoma), Oral Surg., *34*, 450, 1972.

Eversole, L. R., Tomich, C. E. and Cherrick, H. M.: Histogenesis of odontogenic tumors, Oral Surg., *32*, 569, 1971.

Forest, D.: Compound composite odontoma associated with keratinizing masses, J. Canad. Dent. Ass., *33*, 487, 1967.

Frissell, C. T. and Shafer, W. G.: Ameloblastic odontoma, Oral Surg., *6*, 1129, 1953.

Giansanti, J. S., Someren, A. and Waldron, C. A.: Odontogenic adenomatoid tumor (adenoameloblastoma, Oral Surg., *30*, 69, 1970.

Gorlin, R. J., Chaudhry, A. P. and Pindborg, J. J.: Odontogenic tumors: classification, histopathology and clinical behavior in man and domesticated animals, Cancer, *14*, 73, 1961.

Gorlin, R. J., Meskin, L. H. and Brodey, R.: Odontogenic tumors in man and animals: pathologic classification and clinical behavior—a review, Ann. New York Acad. Sci., *108*, 722, 1963.

Goldberg, S. J. and Friedman, J. M.: Ameloblastoma: review of the literature and report of a case, J. Amer. Dent. Ass., *90*, 432, 1975.

Hamner, J. E. III, Gamble, J. W. and Gallegos, G. J.: Odontogenic fibroma, report of two cases, Oral Surg., *21*, 113, 1966.

Hartman, K. S.: Granular-cell ameloblastoma, Oral Surg., *38*, 241, 1974.

Hooker, S. P.: Ameloblastic odontoma, an analysis of 26 cases. Presented at the Twenty-First Annual Meeting of the American Academy of Oral Pathology, Miami Beach, Florida, April 5–9, 1967.

Hornova, J.: Adenoameloblastoma in the wall of a dentigerous cyst, Oral Surg., *19*, 508, 1965.

Ikemura, K., Tashiro, H., Fujino, H., Ohbu, D. and Nakajima, K.: Ameloblastoma of the mandible with metastasis to the lungs and lymph nodes, Cancer, *29*, 930, 1972.

Johnson, R. H. and Topazian, R. G.: The management of variants of ameloblastoma, Plast. Reconstr. Surg., *41*, 356, 1968.

Kalnins, V.: Calcification and amelogenesis in craniopharyngiomas, Oral Surg., *31*, 366, 1971.

Krolls, S. O. and Pindborg, J. J.: Calcifying epithelial odontogenic tumor. A survey of 23 cases and discussion of histomorphologic variations, Arch. Path., *98*, 206, 1974.

Large, N. D., Niebel, H. H. and Fredricks, W. H.: Myxoma of the jaws, Oral Surg., *13*, 1462, 1960.

Leider, A. S., Nelson, J. F. and Trodahl, J. N.: Ameloblastic fibrosarcoma of the jaws, Oral Surg., *33*, 559, 1972.

Meenaghan, M. A., Appel, B. N. and Greene, G. W. Jr.: Amyloid-containing odontogenic tumors of man, Oral Surg., *34*, 908, 1972.

Miller, A. S., Lopez, C. F., Pullon, P. A. and Elzay, R. P.: Ameloblastic fibro-odontoma, Oral Surg., *41*, 354, 1976.

Naji, A. F., Murphy, J. A., Stasney, R. J., Neville, W. E. and Chrenka, P.: So-called adamantinoma of long bones, report of a case with massive pulmonary metastasis, J. Bone Joint Surg., *46–A*, 151, 1964.

Oehlers, F. A. C.: So-called adenoameloblastoma, Oral Surg., *19*, 252, 1961.

Oliver, R. T., McKenna, W. F. and Shafer, W. G.: Hemangioameloblastoma, J. Oral Surg., *19*, 245, 1961.

Perzik, S. L.: Management of advanced odontogenic mandibular tumors in children, Arch. Surg., *83*, 816, 1961.

Pindborg, J. J.: A calcifying epithelial odontogenic tumor, Cancer, *11*, 838, 1958.

Pindborg, J. J.: Ameloblastic sarcoma in the maxilla, Cancer, *13*, 917, 1960.

Pindborg, J. J.: The calcifying epithelial odontogenic tumor—review of literature and report of an extraosseous case, Acta Odont. Scand., *24*, 419, 1966.

Pullon, P. A., Shafer, W. G., Elzay, R. P., Kerr, D. A. and Corio, R. L.: Squamous odontogenic tumor. Report of six cases of a previously undescribed lesion, Oral Surg., *40*, 616, 1975.

Regezi, J. A., Courtney, R. M. and Kerr, D. A.: Keratinization in odontogenic tumors, Oral Surg., *39*, 447, 1975.

Shafer, W. G.: Ameloblastic fibroma, J. Oral Surg., *13*, 317, 1955.

Shafer, W. G. and Frissell, C. T.: The melano-blastoma and retinal anlage tumors, Cancer, *6*, 360, 1953.

Shatkin, R. and Hoffmeister, F. S.: Ameloblastoma: a clinico-pathological appraisal, Oral Surg., *20*, 421, 1965.

Shear, M.: The unity of tumours of odontogenic epithelium, Brit. J. Oral Surg., *2*, 212, 1965.

Seward, G. R., Beales, S. J., Johson, N. W. and Sita Lumsden, E. G.: A metastasing ameloblastoma associated with renal calculi and hypercalcaemia, Cancer, *36*, 2277, 1975.

Simpson, H. E.: Basal-cell carcinoma and peripheral ameloblastoma, Oral Surg., *38*, 233, 1974.

Small, I. A. and Waldron, C. A.: Ameloblastomas of the jaws, Oral Surg., *8*, 281, 1955.

Solomon, M. P., Vuletin, J. C., Pertschuk, C. O., Gormley, M. B. and Rosen, Y.: Calcifying epithelial odontogenic tumor. A histologic, histochemical, fluorescent and ultrastructural study, Oral Surg., *40*, 522, 1975.

Soni, N. N. and Simpson, T. H.: Compound composite odontoma, Oral Surg., *25*, 556, 1968.

Spouge, J. D.: Odontogenic tumors, Oral Surg., *24*, 392, 1967.

Stimson, P. G., Luna, M. A. and Butler, J. J.: Seventeen-year history of calcifying epithelial odontogenic (Pindborg) tumor, Oral Surg., *25*, 104, 1968.

Topazian, R. G. and Simon, G. T.: Adenoameloblastoma, report of three cases, Oral Surg., *13*, 1038, 1960.

Trodahl, J. N.: Ameloblastic fibroma, Oral Surg., *33*, 547, 1972.

Tsukada, Y., de la Pava, S. and Pickren, J. W.: Granular-cell ameloblastoma with metastasis to the lungs, Cancer, *18*, 916, 1965.

Vap, D. R., Dahlin, D. C. and Turlington, E. G.: Pindborg tumor: the so-called calcifying epithelial odontogenic tumor, Cancer, *25*, 629, 1970.

Vickers, R. A. and Gorlin, R. J.: Ameloblastoma: delineation of early histopathologic features of neoplasia, Cancer, *26*, 699, 1970.

Waldron, C. A., Thompson, C. W. and Conner, W. A.: Granular-cell ameloblastic fibroma, report of two cases, Oral Surg., *16*, 1202, 1963.

Wesley, R. K., Wysocki, G. P. and Mintz, S.: The central odontogenic fibroma. Clinical and morphologic studies, Oral Surg., *40*, 235, 1975.

White, D. K., Chen, S–Y, Mohnac, A. M. and Miller, A. S.: Odontogenic myxoma, Oral Surg., *39*, 901, 1975.

Yazdi, I. and Nowparast, B.: Extraosseous odontogenic tumor with special reference to the probability of the basal-cell layer of oral epithelium as a potential source of origin, Oral Surg., *37*, 249, 1974.

Non-odontogenic Tumors, Tumor-like Lesions (Benign)

Baum, S. M., Pochaczevsky, R., Sussman, R. and Stoopack, J. C.: Central hemangioma of the maxilla, J. Oral Surg., 30, 885, 1972.

Bernier, J. L. and Bhaskar, S. N.: Aneurysmal bone cysts of the mandible, Oral Surg., 11, 1018, 1958.

Bhoweer, A. L. and Shirwatkar, L. G.: Central hemangioma of mandible, J. Oral Med., 30, 111, 1975.

Breitenecker, G. and Wepner, F.: A pleomorphic adenoma (so-called mixed tumor) in the wall of a dentigerous cyst, Oral Surg., 36, 63, 1973.

Bryant, W. M. and Maull, K. I.: Arteriovenous malformation of the mandible. Graduated surgical management, Plast. Reconstr. Surg., 55, 690, 1975.

Cherrick, H. M., King, O. H. Jr., Lucatorto, F. M. and Suggs, D. M.: Benign cementoblastoma, Oral Surg., 37, 54, 1974.

Dorfman, H. D., Steiner, G. C. and Jaffe, H. L.: Vascular tumors of bone, Human Path., 2, 349, 1971.

Eversole, L. R.: Central benign and malignant neural neoplasms of the jaws: a review, J. Oral Surg., 27, 716, 1969.

Foss, E. L., Dockerty, M. B. and Good, A.: Osteoid osteoma of the mandible: report of a case, Cancer, 8, 592, 1955.

Ghosh, B. C., Huvos, A. G., Gerold, F. P. and Miller, T. R.: Myxoma of the jaw bones, Cancer, 31, 237, 1973.

Goodsell, J. O. and Hubinger, H. L.: Benign chondroblastoma of mandibular condyle: report of a case, J. Oral Surg., 22, 73, 1964.

Hamner, J. E., Scofield, H. H. and Cornyn, J.: Benign fibro-osseous jaw lesions of periodontal membrane origin, Cancer, 22, 861, 1968.

Kent, J. N., Castro, H. F. and Girotti, W. R.: Benign osteoblastoma of the maxilla: case report and review of the literature, Oral Surg., 27, 209, 1969.

McComb, R. J. and Trott, J. R.: Spontaneous oral hemorrhage: Arteriovenous aneurysm, an unusual case, Brit. Dent. J., 128, 239, 1970.

Nutter, P. D. and Lu, M.: Unilateral multiple chondromatosis of the temporomandibular joint (a case report), Plast. Reconstr. Surg., 27, 69, 1961.

Oliver, L. P.: Aneurysmal bone cyst. Report of a case, Oral Surg., 35, 67, 1973.

Samter, T. G., Vellios, F. and Shafer, W. G.: Neurilemmoma of bone, report of 3 cases with a review of the literature, Radiology, 75, 215, 1960.

Sherman, R. S. and Wilner, D.: The roentgen diagnosis of hemangioma of bone, Amer. J. Roentgen., 86, 1146, 1961.

Waldron, C. A. and Giansanti, J. S.: Benign fibro-osseous lesions of the jaws: a clinical-radiologic-histologic review of sixty-five cases, Oral Surg., 35, 340, 1973.

Walker, D. G.: Benign non-odontogenic tumors of the jaws, J. Oral Surg., 28, 39, 1970.

Non-odontogenic Tumors, Malignant

Albright, R. L., Finkelman, A., Doner, J. M. and Beaubien, J.: Multiple myeloma with manifestation of a maxillary lesion and plasmacytoma, Oral Surg., 26, 167, 1968.

Bennett, J. E., Tignor, S. P. and Shafer, W. G.: Osteogenic sarcoma of the facial bones, Amer. J. Surg., 116, 538, 1968.

Blakemore, J. R. and Stein, M.: Primary Ewing's sarcoma of the mandible: report of a case, J. Oral Surg., 33, 376, 1975.

Boyer, C. W., Brickner, T. J. Jr. and Wratten, G. P.: The treatment of osteogenic sarcoma of the mandible, Amer. J. Roentgen., 49, 326, 1967.

Browand, B. C. and Waldron, C. A.: Central mucoepidermoid tumors of the jaws, Oral Surg., 40, 631, 1975.

Chaudhry, A. P., Robinovitch, M. R., Mitchell, D. F. and Vickers, R. A.: Chondrogenic tumors of the jaws, Amer. J. Surg., 102, 403, 1961.

Eversole, L. R., Sabes, W. R. and Rovin, S.: Aggressive growth and neoplastic potential of odontogenic cysts with special reference to central epidermoid and mucoepidermoid carcinomas, Cancer, 35, 270, 1975.

Garrington, G. E., Scofield, H. H., Cornyn, J. and Hooker, S. P.: Osteosarcoma of the jaws, analysis of 56 cases, Cancer, 20, 377, 1967.

Hardt, N. P.: Metastatic neuroblastoma in the mandible, report of a case, Oral Surg., 41, 314, 320, 1976.

Marano, P. D. and Hartman, K. S.: Central mucoepidermoid carcinoma arising in a maxillary odontogenic cyst, J. Oral Surg., 32, 915, 1974.

O'Shaughnessy, P. E.: Chronic lymphatic leukemia suggestive of multiple myeloma, Oral Surg., 17, 170, 1964.

Shear, M.: Primary intra-alveolar epidermoid carcinoma of the jaw, J. Oral Path., 97, 645, 1969.

Metabolic Disorders

Bender, I. B.: Dental observations in Gaucher's disease, Oral Surg., 12, 546, 1959.

Booksaler, F. and Miller, J. E.: Infantile cortical hyperostosis, J. Pediat., 48, 739, 1956.

Cherrick, H. M., King, O. H. Jr. and Dorsey, J. N. Jr.: Massive osteolysis (disappearing bone, phantom bone, acute absorption of bone) of the mandible and maxilla, J. Oral Med., 27, 67, 1972.

Collins, E. M., Schmale, J. and Kiersch, T. A.: Chronic disseminated histiocytosis X treated with vinblastine sulfate and prednisone, Oral Surg., 38, 388, 1974.

Dedolph, T., Chaudhry, A. P. and Mitchell, D. F.: Eosinophilic granuloma, J. Oral Surg., 15, 247, 1957.

Esposito, W. J. and Berne, A. S.: Polyostotic bone sarcoma associated with osteitis deformans, Amer. J. Roentgen., 83, 698, 1960.

Gerrard, J. W., Holman, G. H., Gorman, A. A. and Morrow, I. H.: Familial infantile cortical hyperostosis, J. Pediat., 59, 543, 1961.

Johnson, R. P. and Mohnac, A. M.: Histiocytosis X: report of 7 cases, J. Oral Surg., 25, 7, 1967.

Jones, J. C., Lilly, G. E. and Marlette, R. H.: Histiocytosis X, J. Oral Surg., 28, 461, 1970.

McDonald, R. E. and Shafer, W. G.: Disseminated juvenile fibrous dysplasia of the jaws, Amer. J. Dis. Child., 89, 354, 1955.

McKelvy, B. D., Sanders, B., Cox, R. L. and Arnett, G. W.: Chronic disseminated histiocytosis X of adulthood clinically mimicking subacute osteomyelitis, J. Oral Med., 30, 73, 1975.

Phillips, R. M., Bush, O. B. Jr. and Hall, H. D.: Massive osteolysis (phantom bone, disappearing bone). Report of a case with mandibular involvement, Oral Surg., 34, 886, 1972.

Porretta, C. A., Dahlin, D. C. and Janes, J. M.: Sarcoma in Paget's disease of bone, J. Bone Joint Surg., 39–A, 1314, 1957.

Reitzik, M. and Lownie, J. F.: Familial polyostotic fibrous dysplasia, Oral Surg., 40, 769, 1975.

Rothstein, J. P.: Panographic surveys of selected metabolic bone diseases, Oral Surg., 26, 173, 1968.

Silverman, S., Ware, W. H. and Gillooly, J. C.: Dental aspects of hyperparathyroidism, Oral Surg., 26, 184, 1968.

Steinbach, H. L.: Some roentgen features of Paget's disease, Amer. J. Roentgen., 86, 950, 1961.

Walsh, R. R. and Karmiol, M.: Oral roentgenographic findings in osteitis fibrosa generalisata associated with chronic renal disease, Oral Surg., 28, 273, 1969.

Section IV

Analysis of Findings, Planning Therapy and Patient Management

This section provides an overview of the management of the individual patient's needs in terms of appropriate planning for the effective delivery of dental care and certain corollary aspects of dental practice, including emergency treatment and the legal aspects of professional life. Specifically, the section is designed to: (1) guide the reader in the synthesis of the diagnostic findings leading to a logical approach to treatment (Chap. 16), (2) develop an understanding of the diagnosis and management of the common dental and less common systemic emergencies (Chaps. 17 and 19), and (3) provide a brief review of forensic dentistry and the legal ramifications of dental practice (Chap. 18).

Chapter 16

Analysis of Diagnostic Findings and Treatment Planning

Except in emergency care, a written plan of treatment should be developed prior to instituting definitive therapy. Usually even in emergency management some thought at least should be given to the patient's long-range dental health.

GENERAL PRINCIPLES

There are three basic types of treatment plans: comprehensive, limited, and provisional or tentative.

A *comprehensive treatment plan* is the most thorough and is established only after a comprehensive examination and an analysis of all diagnostic data have been accomplished. Comprehensive or *total patient care* takes into account the patient's general and oral health, psychic makeup, dental I.Q., and attitudes, socioeconomic status and expectations. It is related strictly to the patient's long-range needs and involves all the skills and techniques covered in previous chapters of this textbook.

A *limited plan* is one developed for the treatment of only one or several limited disease entities, as might be done by an endodontist, orthodontist, oral surgeon or other specialist. Even a limited plan must be developed with the total long-range care of the patient in mind.

A *provisional* or *tentative treatment plan* is developed when all necessary information is not available for the development of a comprehensive plan. For example, a patient may have a questionable periodontal prognosis, or may appear disinterested in his oral health. In this event it is wise to develop a tentative plan, institute therapy and watch the response of the patient as well as the tissues. It is unwise to provide extensive periodontal or prosthetic treatment for a disinterested or uncooperative patient; to do so would probably result in failure. It is wise at times to first test the patient's ability to cooperate, and his motivation, and then to develop a more comprehensive plan.

Many dentists develop and present to their patients a *preferred* and an *alternative* plan of therapy using different techniques and materials, both of which are acceptable without compromising principles of quality of care.

In all planning, the patient's general health and projected longevity should be

17

considered. Given specific similar dental findings, a plan for an 18-year-old would vary from that for an 81-year-old.

One of the most important facets of a treatment plan is the follow-up. Patients should be advised at the outset of the importance of regular examinations after the completion of treatment. Likewise, patients with periodontal disease, rampant caries, or other progressive or recurrent forms of pathosis should understand the nature of their condition and should be impressed with the importance of maintenance.

THE GENERAL PATTERN OF MOST TREATMENT PLANS

The dentist has a fourfold obligation to manage the problems of his patient, more or less in the following order:

1. *Elimination of Pain and Disease:* Infection or other pathoses are removed. This is the absolute minimum of treatment. Biopsy and other diagnostic procedures outside the common realm should be performed.
2. *Restoration of Function:* This is the next most important phase of treatment and includes all procedures necessary to provide the patient with adequate masticatory ability.
3. *Acquisition of Proper Esthetics:* While this phase often seems to be of primary importance to the patient, it is of lesser importance with respect to his overall health. The dentist must, however, be lenient in his demands for function before esthetics, as it would be unwise, for example, to let a patient go for long periods of time without anterior teeth while posterior occlusion is being restored. Often it is possible to construct immediate or temporary prostheses which will provide improvement in esthetics and encourage the patient to view the functional phase of treatment with greater interest.
4. *Maintenance Phase:* If properly carried out, this phase protects the patient against future gross changes in his oral condition, and helps prevent misunderstanding between patient and dentist. The patient will then enjoy optimum oral health at a minimum of expense, and undesirable changes usually can be intercepted before they become major complications.

FEES

Charges for treatment should be based on several factors: (1) the skill and ability necessary to furnish the therapy, (2) the responsibility taken by the dentist in performing the treatment, (3) the importance of the treatment to the patient's general health, and (4) the dentist's operating expense and use of auxiliary personnel (overhead). If these are considered carefully, a fee which is fair to the patient and the dentist can be determined.

Patients who question the fees that a dentist charges should be reminded of the above factors, and advised that when they have treatment in a dental office they are in effect in a private dental hospital where all of the facilities for treatment are maintained and paid for by the dentist through his fees. Many patients have little knowledge of the cost of dental equipment and they should not be told; however, it may be useful to point out that when they are treated in a hospital they pay the physician and the hospital. If the patient understands these facts and the benefit of the treatment he is about to receive, he will usually have no further questions as to the acceptability of the fees excepting the adequacy of his personal finances. In regard to this matter, the dentist must be aware of financial plans, insurance and other facets of dental economics.

SPECIAL CONSIDERATIONS OF THE AGE OF THE PATIENT

With current advances in medical care, the average life span has increased to more than 70 years, and many elderly patients need dental care. People of advanced age often have chronic ailments and certain precautions are necessary when administering dental treatment. Those in good health often may be treated as though they were younger, except that appointments should be shortened. There is no strict formula to follow since all patients are individuals and should be analyzed individually. For a very elderly patient in poor health, it is the dentist's obligation to eliminate sources of infection and if possible to provide occlusion adequate for mastication.

Occasionally, it is impossible to provide any but the minimum of care. Obviously, not all loose teeth need be removed in a very ill or very elderly patient, especially if consultation with the patient's physician reveals that a serious risk would be involved. Extensive crown and bridge procedures can be supplanted by removable prostheses or frequent periodontal therapy to control infection in some cases. Morning appointments are desirable for the elderly, as well as for children. Explanations of treatment plans and diagnoses also must be varied, depending upon the age of the patient as well as his educational background and appreciation of dental treatment.

It is wise to discuss the proposed treatment with the patient's nearest of kin when treating a child or an elderly patient. Gerodontics someday in the future may reach the proportions of the practice of pedodontics at present. The dentist must learn by experience how to manage and treat the elderly. Often geriatric patients are easily agitated and complain of vague pains and other problems. These should be dealt with promptly in a straightforward manner. Elderly and young patients, if properly managed, can be very good patients.

In general, pedodontics involves patients with high susceptibility to caries, whereas gerodontics involves more periodontal disease and prosthodontics. Malocclusion is important to the young, but less to the aged. Many physiologic and pathologic factors vary with age, such as salivary flow, vascularity, tissue wound healing and susceptibility to neoplasia, and systemic diseases with their varied oral manifestations.

SPECIAL CONSIDERATIONS OF THE HANDICAPPED PATIENT

People with handicaps of mind and/or body make up an increasing number of patients in today's dental practice. Each treatment plan should be geared to the patient's physical and emotional ability to withstand the procedure, as well as to his individual needs. Often certain procedures can be delayed until a later date when the patient will be better able to tolerate dental treatment.

Patients who are highly irritable or nervous can be given premedication using one of a variety of sedatives. Those with severe local or systemic infections may need prophylactic antibiotics. Neuromuscular diseases, such as multiple sclerosis or muscular dystrophy, call for special management since such patients often are unable to control their movements. Patients subject to seizures are poor risks for removable prostheses because of the danger of aspiration during an attack. Patients with cardiovascular disease should be treated only after consultation with their physicians. The treatment plan should be as simple as possible with short appointments to reduce stress.

Patients with certain endocrine disturbances such as adrenal cortical insufficiency, hyperthyroidism or diabetes mellitus should be treated with extreme caution after consultation with a physician. Adrenal and thyroid crises or insulin shock may occur during dental care.

Many other systemic conditions as well as medications taken by patients may complicate dental treatment. Again, if a complete medical history is taken and all medications are identified, most patients can and should be given at least a minimum of treatment. It is the dentist's duty to provide such minimum care for the handicapped patient and counsel him regarding preventive measures.

Institutionalized patients should be furnished toothbrushes and taught oral hygiene procedures. Attendants and nurses on the staffs of mental institutions, general hospitals, prisons and other infirmaries should be encouraged to assist patients in the care of their mouths. At the very least, emergency dental care should be available to all such patients. In many institutions extensive dental care is available and may be limited only by the degree of cooperation of the patient.

Patients with Terminal Illnesses

Patients in need of dental care who have terminal systemic illnesses or those with oral diseases which might terminate fatally should be handled with care and understanding. Often it is wise to consult the patient's family or his physician or clergyman to determine the best way to discuss the findings and/or recommendations with the patient. Good doctor-patient rapport is very important in these cases. The Foundation of Thanatology is dedicated to the study of death and its associated medical and behavioral phenomena, and the reader is referred to their publications for further information.*

OUTLINE FOR FORMULATING A TREATMENT PLAN FOR THE AGED OR HANDICAPPED

The dentist should obtain and completely understand the patient's past and present medical history. Consultation with a physician should be obtained when there is suspicion of systemic disease. A textbook of medicine or the *Merck Manual* is a handy reference for such matters. The nature of any illness the patient may have should be reviewed before the treatment plan is completed.

Medications

All drugs taken by the patient (past and present) should be known and identified, and the reasons for taking these drugs should be known, along with their side effects. The problem of possible interaction of systemic medications with those to be used in dental treatment should be considered. The *Physician's Desk Reference* or

* Archives of the Foundation of Thanatology, 630 West 168th Street, New York, New York 10032

a textbook of pharmacology will help in these determinations.

Psychic Makeup

The patient's attitudes toward dental treatment, his fears and anxieties, and an estimate of his mentality should be determined. The retarded child or disturbed patient may present problems of management.

Physical Makeup

Any physical problems which might alter the treatment plan should be noted. The palsied or paralyzed may have poor motor control; the aged patient may not need as extensive procedures as the younger patient.

Functional and Esthetic Requirements

It is obvious that esthetics play a more important part in the treatment of a young woman than in that of a 75-year-old man. This is not to say that esthetics should not be considered in the older patient, just that it is of lesser importance. In all cases a maximum of function should be sought; however, it would be foolish to construct dentures for a patient who could not control his jaws, unless for esthetic purposes only.

General Prognosis

In general, the more extensive treatment would be given the younger patient and extensive procedures should be avoided in patients whose life expectancy is very short, except conceivably as a morale builder.

Financial Status

This is an important consideration in any treatment plan, and often the handicapped patient has had many expenses and has a limited income. Regardless of the patient's ability to pay, the dentist still is obligated to relieve pain and eliminate disease.

Oral Examination

Insofar as possible, the examination should be conducted in the thorough manner provided for any other patient.

Professional Ability

All dentists should recognize their weaknesses and the limitations of their facilities. When a practitioner sees that procedures are indicated which are impractical for him, he should refer the patient elsewhere or call in a consultant.

Consultation and Referral

Referral of patients to physicians or dental specialists is becoming commonplace in today's general practice. With the tendency toward centralization of health treatment facilities, referral of patients from one practitioner to another and consultation with members of the many specialty disciplines are becoming simpler, and patients benefit from the thoroughness of such examinations and treatment.

The general practitioner should be the focal point from which all consultations are sought and referrals are made. The patient then will not feel lost, because the doctor-patient relationship will be maintained. The patient may be referred for consultation regarding a diagnostic problem, and/or for treatment. In each case, as much information about the patient as possible should be forwarded to the consultant. The referring dentist should be honest in assessing his own knowledge and capabilities, and in a situation where the dentist is unsure of his diagnosis or feels unable to treat the patient adequately he should obtain help. Referred patients should understand the reasons why they are being sent elsewhere. This will not detract from their respect for the general practitioner.

Occasionally, patients will prefer to have the general dentist perform a procedure which he, the dentist, feels incapable of performing. In these instances, the patient should be thanked for his confidence and then told that if he truly has that much confidence in his dentist, he knows that his dentist is directing him in the best way.

A patient should not be referred to an oral surgeon, for example, because the general dentist "does not have the instruments for removing a third molar." The patient should be told that he is being referred for removal of this third molar to "someone who is able to perform more competently and with a background of more experience."

Medical Consultation. If a patient has signs or a history suggestive of a systemic disease, the dentist should refer him to his family physician, requesting consultation regarding any possible systemic pathoses. Specific reasons for the referral should be included, preferably in writing, and a proper reply can then be expected. The patient should be advised *in general* as to the reason for this request for medical consultation. The results of the consultation should be obtained before dental treatment is instituted unless there is a dental emergency. Occasionally it is necessary for the dentist to refer a patient directly to a medical specialist, but it is usually better to work through the patient's family physician. Pages 2 and 3 list the specialties approved by the American Medical Association.

Dental Consultation. Patients requiring difficult procedures beyond the scope of the general practitioner should be referred to a specialist. The dentist should be familiar with nearby representatives of the eight approved specialties of the American Dental Association. Such referral saves time and results in better care for more patients. It also provides better overall treatment for the patients by the general practitioner. No one dentist can possibly know and master all facets of dentistry completely. This is why the dental specialties have developed. They should be used.

Most dental schools have departments of oral diagnosis or oral medicine to which patients may be referred for diagnostic consultation and special treatment. The general dentist who uses consultants also benefits because it helps him broaden his own knowledge. Also it allows him to share the responsibility for difficult cases with another interested individual. Often specialists can be used for advice in establishing a treatment plan when there is some doubt as to the prognosis of a particular condition.

Care should be taken neither to minimize nor exaggerate the reasons for referral. If a patient is referred to an oral surgeon for the removal of an impacted tooth, the patient should not be told that this will be an extremely difficult operation. He should be told that it may be a difficult extraction and that further details will be explained by the oral surgeon. Likewise, the referring dentist should not put the consultant at a disadvantage by trying to describe in detail the procedure that will be performed. For example, it is improper to refer a patient to a specialist to have an operation "under general anesthesia"—the selection of the anesthetic is up to the consultant.

It is best to send a referral letter to the specialist. Telephone conversations may suffice on occasion; however, the written word, including the salient features of the patient's medical and dental history, clinical findings and specific questions involved, is better. In addition, it may be prudent to furnish radiographs, diagnostic casts, diagnostic test reports or other materials. The consultant should be told whether he is expected to treat the patient or merely answer the questions. If this is done, the referring dentist can rightfully expect a written reply, not only thanking him but also explaining the findings, treatment and outcome. Proper consultation and referral help establish good working relationships between practitioners of the different disciplines of dentistry.

Referring a patient for consultation regarding a condition does not obligate the dentist to accept any recommendation obtained. Consultation implies advice from other sources, and the resultant diagnosis and/or treatment plan might best be chosen from even another source.

A good way to learn how to write consultation and referral notes is to study hospital charts of patients on the medicine service. Here requests for consultations are frequent and usually in proper form. There are special consultation sheets on which the requests are answered by the consultant, and these are usually filled out completely (Fig. 16-1). If the dentist will follow a similar form, he will find that cooperation and rapport among the many disciplines of the health sciences will improve greatly.

The referring dentist should be complimentary toward the practitioner to whom he is referring the patient. It should be noted that fee splitting between the referring dentist and the consultant is unethical. When the general dentist is consulted by a physician or other dentist, the above conduct also applies. He should expect to receive all pertinent information and materials from the referring practitioner. He is then obligated to make his examination or provide the necessary treatment and then return a written report to the referring practitioner, following a format similar to that sent to him originally.

With an increasing understanding of the importance of dentistry to general health, more physicians are requesting dental consultation for patients both in and out of the hospital. Thus, the dentist should be well versed in such office and hospital procedures. If he will apply himself, he will continue to learn daily many interesting things, and he will appreciate more the services he renders his patients.

HOSPITAL DENTISTRY

In past years, most hospital dentistry has been confined to oral surgical services, such as multiple tooth extractions, serious dental infections, fractures of the jaws, and reconstructive jaw surgery. Today with increasing emphasis on the importance of oral health to total health, the scene is changing. Dental restorative procedures often are needed by hospital patients for whom general anesthesia is advisable. The dentist and hospital anesthetist can furnish such needed service.

CONSULTATION REQUEST
HOSPITAL AND CLINICS

Consultation Requested:	Medicine
Requested By:	Dentistry – Dr. Gregory Smith
Date of Previous Consultation none	Walk __X__ Stretcher_____ Wheelchair_____ Bedside_____

Pertinent History and Findings:	Provisional Diagnosis:
History of congestive heart failure – myocardial infarction – 1965	Reason for Consultation and Specific Questions: Evaluation of cardiac status – needs several extractions and restorative dental care (fillings)
Medications Influencing Findings: taking digitoxin:.1 mg daily	

CONSULTANT'S REPLY:

BP 140/80; pulse 80; Ht.6 feet; wt. 190 lbs; temp. 98.6°F.

Physical exam reveals well compensated post MI patient with no ECG changes since last physical one year ago. Chest clear, no evidence of pedal edema. Performs normal activities without limitation.

Rec: 1.) Continue digitoxin as above

2.) No contraindications to Oral Surgery or routine dental care

Thank you,

W.C. Borman M.D.

W. C. Borman, M.D.

WHITE-Chart Copy, YELLOW-Department Copy, PINK-Professional Fee Copy   15-0305

Fig. 16-1. Reproduction of an actual request for medical consultation and a brief consultation report. Many consultation requests and reports are much more elaborate.

Many hospitals have dental departments with well-trained dental staffs consisting of specialists and general practitioners. These departments enjoy parity with other medical services in the hospital. In less developed hospitals, however, the dental service often is a subservice of one of the medical departments.

A dentist interested in applying for admission to a hospital staff should obtain information from the hospital administrator not only as to the procedures for applying for hospital privileges, but also as to the organization of the hospital staffs. The hospital administrator usually is responsible to a governing body consisting of members of the staff. The clinical staff, which is made up of physicians and dentists, develops bylaws that determine the status of the dental or any other service in the hospital. Anyone practicing in the hospital is bound by staff rules and regulations, as well as by those of his department. The governing body usually selects staff members and occasionally analyzes their clinical efforts and records.

The function of a hospital is concerned with administrative, consultative, clinical and educational efforts. For a dentist to qualify for staff membership, he must be a graduate of an accredited dental school, have membership in the American Dental Association or National Dental Association or be eligible for same, and be an ethical practitioner.

In applying for staff membership, the dentist should obtain an application and a copy of the rules and bylaws from the administrator's office and complete the application form. The application is processed through the staff secretary and the credentials committee. This committee makes recommendations to the governing body, which takes the necessary action. It is common for privileges to be granted on an annual basis at first; after reevaluation of the staff member at a later date, permanent staff privileges may be extended.

Staff appointments usually are made in the following categories. *Active staff*: the member usually has been on the staff in a different capacity, but now has the privileges of using the hospital as well as certain duties in the management of the hospital. *Consulting staff*: these consultants are recognized specialists, and they also may be active staff members. *Associate staff*: these individuals use the hospital infrequently and are less experienced; they are on probation before consideration for an active staff appointment. *Courtesy staff*: these members may use the hospital but they have no administrative rights or responsibilities. *Honorary staff*: these persons usually are well recognized in their fields and usually are active staff members given this recognition because of their status in their specialty. *Interns and residents*: these are graduates of accredited medical or dental schools and are in training in specialty services in the hospital.

Nowhere in the health sciences is teamwork more organized toward one purpose than in the general hospital. All of the services and facilities are directed and coordinated to care for the patient. A dentist who has had experience in a hospital has seen the overall function of the hospital and appreciates its importance to the total health of the patient. If he has admitting privileges, he usually is allocated a certain number of beds or otherwise limited facilities, barring unforeseen emergencies.

Elective procedures are scheduled with the hospital administration well in advance. The patient should not be admitted as an emergency unless a true emergency exists. Most hospitals require that, regardless of staff status of the dentist, the patient must have a complete physical examination by a physician within 24 hours after admission. This is a good ruling. For the same reasons, many smaller hospitals require that the patient be admitted by a physician and then transferred to the dental service. This is unnecessary when the dentist is adequately trained in the procedures of the hospital.

It is important for the dentist to be a hospital staff member and to understand how the hospitals in his area function, how their emergency wards operate, and how to use their operating room facilities, so that when the need arises he will be able to serve in an efficient manner compatible with other staff members.

Excellent handbooks are available, including *A Guide to Hospital Dental Procedure* published by the American Dental Association and sponsored by the Council on Hospital Dental Services. In addition, most of the following information will be found in the rules and bylaws published by the hospital and should be known and understood by all staff members.

In cities where there are hospital-trained dental specialists, the general practitioner may refer patients for hospital admission to them, unless he has had hospital training himself. In any community, however, it is important for the general practitioner to understand and use the hospital for patients who would benefit by it, and the only way he can learn this is to have a good relationship with the local physicians.

Hospital status for the practicing dentist aids in establishing rapport between the dentist and the physician, and soon an understanding is forthcoming which is beneficial for all concerned. The dentist should not be discouraged from using the hospital unless he is uninterested or incapable of using the privileges properly.

When a staff dentist wishes to admit a patient for a dental procedure, he should first call the admitting office and ask for a bed for his patient. Next he calls in or, preferably, writes orders for the patient's care and requests a routine physical examination by a physician whom he has already alerted. He must then write a complete medical history of his patient which should be included in the material sent with the patient to the hospital. On the routine admitting orders, it should be remembered that a diet for the patient should be specified.

as well as a request for a history and physical examination. Likewise, any supportive, presurgical, or other special care should be specified in the doctor's orders. The orders should state whether or not the patient may be ambulatory *ad libitum,* with bathroom privileges. Special orders for medications or other therapy should be included. The usual procedure is to order a complete blood count and routine urinalysis so that these can be accomplished before the physician conducts the physical examination.

Ordinarily, the patient is admitted in the morning and should be seen by his dentist soon thereafter. Each time the patient is visited, "progress notes" should be entered in the patient's chart on the proper form. These should be kept up-to-date and complete so that at the end of hospitalization they can be summarized on the discharge note.

Should the patient be admitted for surgical purposes, arrangements should be made prior to admission for use of the operating room and a discussion with the anesthesiologist should take place.

Many large hospitals publish a formulary listing all the drugs and medications they carry in their pharmacy and most of the orders written for medications should be for those within this document. Most hospital wards have treatment rooms where any special treatment necessary can be accomplished. The day before surgery, the patient should be prepared psychologically as well as physically for the procedure and the preanesthetic and presurgical orders should be entered under "doctor's orders."

Some hospitals have a cut-off date for narcotic prescriptions. Thus, a narcotic prescription written in the "doctor's orders" will not hold for more than 24 to 48 hours in some instances.

When a dentist is called to a hospital for consultation, he need only go to the ward, greet the nurse and tell her why he is there, review the patient's chart, examine the patient, and record his findings and recommendations on the special consultation sheet provided at the nursing station.

The dentist can perform many other important functions as a consultant in the hospital, such as advising nurses, giving short courses in care of the dental patient, and teaching preventive dentistry in the hospital.

The dentist should be well aware of the methods for using hospital emergency rooms. He should know the facility and how to transport his patient there if necessary. Likewise, he should know the hospital fees and insurance forms involved in the emergency ward as well as in other areas of the hospital.

Some hospitals have facilities for the care of dental outpatients. With the advent of Medicare and other insurance programs, and the increasing number of geriatric patients needing the care of a dentist, it becomes more important for the dentist to understand and use the hospital for patient care. The future of dentistry in the hospital is very bright for dentists who recognize the needs and limitations within this facility.

BIBLIOGRAPHY

Bernstein, A.: *Intern's Manual,* Chicago, The Year Book Medical Publishers, Inc., 1961.

Christen, A. G., Meffert, R. M., Cornyn, J. and Tiecke, R. W.: Oral health of dentists: analysis of panoramic radiographic survey, J. Amer. Dent. Ass., *75,* 1167, 1967.

Douglas, B. L. and Casey, G. J.: *A Guide to Hospital Dental Procedure,* Chicago, American Dental Association, 1965.

Elfenbaum, A.: Dent. Clin. North America, March, 1968.

Francis, L. E.: Dent. Clin. North America, March, 1968.

Gier, Ronald E.: Management of neurogenic and psychogenic problems, Dent. Clin. North America, March, 1968.

Hollander, L. N.: *Modern Dental Practice,* Philadelphia, W. B. Saunders Co., 1967.

Kutscher, A. H. *et al.: Death and Bereavement,* Springfield, Charles C Thomas, 1970.

Levy, S.: *Dentist's Handbook of Office and Hospital Procedures,* Chicago, Year Book Medical Publishers, Inc., 1963.

Shock, N. W.: Current concepts of the aging process, J.A.M.A., *175,* 654, 1961.

Chapter 17

Management of Common Emergencies

An emergency problem requires an attempt at immediate diagnosis and therapy. Emergencies which confront the dentist include those of an oral-dental nature, such as toothache, acute oral infection and excessive hemorrhage; emergencies of a systemic nature, such as fainting or drug reactions which might occur during dental treatment; and general emergencies outside of the dental office, such as accidental injuries. The dentist should be well versed in methods of caring for such situations and eager to do all within his professional capabilities to alleviate them. If the dentist is confronted with a serious emergency of a medical nature, he should be able to provide supportive care until medical assistance can be obtained. It is advisable, for example, for every dentist to have a small emergency kit in his automobile as well as in his home and office. This emergency kit should include not only materials for treating toothache and other dental problems, but also materials and equipment for treating general systemic emergencies.

Pain (fear of pain) is the oldest and still one of the primary reasons for patients seeking dental care. Brief, careful interrogation of the patient will reveal the anatomic distribution of the pain, its nature, and the means by which it can be induced or relieved. At the same time, some indication of the emotional status of the patient should be noted.

In the mind of the dentist, the term "toothache" most often is associated with a severe pulpitis; however, patients use this term for many different painful conditions. A periapical or lateral periodontal abscess, fracture or avulsion of teeth, severe necrotizing gingivitis, pericoronitis, dry socket and other conditions are often termed "toothache" by the patient. The differential diagnosis of such conditions has been discussed previously (Chap. 10).

In some instances, the administration of a local anesthetic will give temporary relief, but it should be remembered that any diagnostic tests which depend on the response to induced pain (*e.g.* pulp test) should be performed before the induction of anesthesia. Once temporary relief is obtained, the examination should be completed to provide a sound basis for definitive treatment.

PAINFUL PULPITIS

Painful pulpitis is almost invariably the result of pulp exposure and concomitant infection. After detecting the offending tooth and demonstrating the exposure, the dentist places cotton dampened with eugenol over the exposure. Relief may occur within a moment, and the tooth may be temporarily restored with a zinc oxide and eugenol dressing. When this is done without the aid of an anesthetic, the effect can be noted readily. When anesthesia is used, its effect must subside before one can be sure that relief has been obtained. The patient should be warned that relief of pain by this method is temporary and that definitive treatment must be performed as soon as possible to prevent an exacerbation.

PAINFUL ABSCESS

Drainage is the method of choice in relieving an abscess. If the abscess is periapical, this may be done through an opening into the pulp chamber. If it is periodontal, insertion of the periodontal pocket probe may release the suppuration. If gross submucosal fluctuation is palpable, incision may be chosen. Drainage should be maintained by inserting a drain, or in the case of a periapical abscess by keeping the opening into the pulp chamber patent. Suction by the patient and rinses with warm saline solution will promote drainage.

The painful periodontal pocket which has not reached the proportions of an abscess may be relieved by drainage or by lavage and the application of eugenol.

PAINFUL PERIODONTAL CONDITIONS

Necrotizing ulcerative gingivitis is best treated by local debridement and supportive therapy. If it is severe enough, systemic antibiotics and analgesics are warranted. Good supportive home care, dietary regulation, gross debridement and gingival stimulation are advisable as soon as the patient is able to tolerate this regimen. Mouth rinses, such as hydrogen peroxide or urea peroxide in glycerin, help to improve oral hygiene. Topical application of a compound containing vancomycin hydrochloride has been found useful in treating Vincent's infection (Fig. 7-43).

Pericoronitis is most often found around the incompletely erupted mandibular third molar, and is best treated locally by irrigating under the flap with saline solution or hydrogen peroxide solution, and then placing a small drain saturated with eugenol under the operculum. If an opposing tooth is traumatizing the tissue, it can be removed or reduced with a diamond stone. Once the acute condition has been alleviated, the flap or the tooth should be removed.

AVULSION OF TEETH

A totally avulsed tooth may be reimplanted immediately after performing root canal therapy and thoroughly cleansing the tooth surface with a mild soap solution. In the past, such teeth invariably have become ankylosed and eventually suffered root resorption. This must be taken into consideration before reimplantation is performed. Recently it has been shown that freshly removed teeth with attached periodontal membrane fibers are more likely to endure than are those from which the membrane has been scraped before being reimplanted. The tooth should be properly positioned and the alveolar bone compressed labiolingually. The teeth should be splinted for several days.

If immediate root canal therapy was not performed, later tests for vitality should be made. It is not uncommon for a partially avulsed tooth to test non-vital for several weeks following repositioning, and later to respond to the pulp vitality test. However, final decisions on endodontic therapy should be made after a few weeks' waiting period as often chronic pulpitis develops followed by internal resorption or calcific metamorphosis, thus complicating later endodontic instrumentation.

FRACTURED TEETH

If the pulp is involved, it may be wise to extirpate the pulp initially, but it is often useful to do a pulp capping procedure with calcium hydroxide and then cover the tooth with a temporary crown for several weeks to see if the pulp survives. Permanent restoration depends upon the judgment of the practitioner, the age of the patient and the overall treatment plan. Fractures exposing dentin only should be covered with a zinc oxide and eugenol dressing inside a temporary crown.

DRY SOCKET (FOCAL OSTEOMYELITIS, POST-EXTRACTION ALVEOLITIS)

Treatment consists of cleansing the socket by irrigation and placing a drain saturated with eugenol or other obtundent dressing material lightly in the socket to relieve the pain. If severe cellulitis is present, antibiotics are indicated and analgesics often are necessary. The obtundent dressing should be replaced daily for several days until the symptoms subside and healing is apparent. When the dressing ceases to emit an objectionable odor of necrosis, healing has usually begun.

APHTHOUS, HERPETIC AND OTHER ULCERATIONS

These lesions, often of uncertain origin, are best treated by covering them with an agent such as Orabase or tincture of benzoin. If the cause is known (*e.g.* traumatic), it should be eliminated. Occasionally other supportive care is indicated, such as Dyclone mouth washes or other topical anesthetics just prior to mealtime so that the patient can eat comfortably. The patient should be advised to force fluids so as not to become dehydrated (an isotonic solution such as Gatorade is useful), and dietary instructions are in order.

LUXATION (MANDIBULAR DISLOCATION)

Luxation of the mandible is due to a malposition of the head of the condyle anterior to the articular eminence. The patient is unable to close his mouth and the dental relationship at this time is Class III. This may occur following prolonged dental treatment, or following trauma or even yawning. After condylar fractures have been ruled out, the treatment is to reposition the mandible in its proper position. The patient should first be reassured that nothing serious has occurred, and then asked to relax. Massaging the tissues in the preauricular region often causes the mandible to fall back into position. If not, the mandible should be grasped by placing the thumbs on the posterior teeth with the rest of the fingers outside the mouth and below the border of the mandible. The mandible should then be gently forced downward and backward to

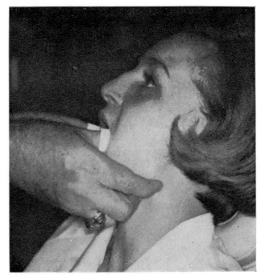

Fig. 17-1. Reduction of mandibular luxation. The patient should be seated in an upright position. The thumbs of the dentist should be heavily wrapped with gauze and placed over the occlusal surfaces of the mandibular teeth. The mandible should be grasped from the occlusal surface and inferior border and gently forced inferiorly and then posteriorly so that the condyles slip back into their glenoid fossae. (Courtesy of Ralph E. Beatty.)

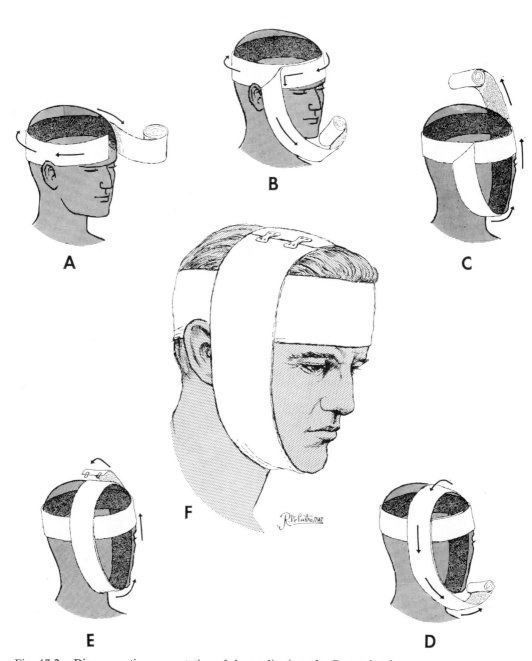

Fig. 17-2. Diagrammatic representation of the application of a Barton bandage.

allow the condyles to drop back into the fossae. The thumbs should be protected by heavy gauze wraps because the teeth may close sharply when the condyles snap back into position (Fig. 17-1). Following reduction, it is advisable to place the patient on a muscle relaxant such as Equanil or Robaxin for several days to help avoid muscle spasms, and to warn him not to open his mouth widely.

FRACTURES

The dentist's responsibility in diagnosing and treating fractures of the facial skeleton, particularly of the jaws, is assuming increasing importance. This area of knowledge is decidedly within the realm of dentistry, since the dentist best understands the occlusion of the teeth which is so often involved. With the increase in automobile accidents, the number of fractures of the jaws is on the increase and patients should be counseled regarding such safety measures as seat belts—this is good preventive dentistry.

Fractures are usually accompanied by pain, edema, ecchymosis, deformity, limitation of movement and, if major nerves are injured, paresthesia. Manipulation of the fractured parts may cause a grating sound (crepitation) and pain. If the jaws are fractured, there are usually discrepancies of the occlusion of the teeth. Selected radiographs often reveal breaks in the continuity of the cortical plate—provided the radiograph is taken in the correct plane and provided there is some displacement. It is useful to place a stethoscope head on one side of a suspected fracture line and then tap the mandible on the other side with a finger. If a sharp report is heard, it suggests that the mandible is intact. A muffled sound may indicate a fracture.

Emergency treatment of fractures involves immobilization of the segments, often with a Barton bandage (Fig. 17-2). This technique is also useful on a temporary basis for acute temporomandibular pain following trauma. If teeth are present, this is useful until a definite reduction of the fracture can be performed. The patient should be checked for any neurologic damage by a physician prior to being given any narcotics for pain. A thorough knowledge of the patient's health and past medical history also is mandatory. The patient should be placed on a high caloric, high protein, full liquid diet supplemented with vitamins. It is best to do the final reduction as soon as practical. If it must be delayed, the patient should have ice packs placed on the face to help prevent swelling. Generally, it is believed that cold packs should be used for the first 24 hours after trauma and heat thereafter. After surgical reduction the process should be repeated, with cold again being used first.

A greenstick fracture is an incomplete break best described by that word. Simple fractures are those in which the break is clean, but no bone is exposed to the oral cavity or the outside environment. Compound fractures have their segments exposed to the outside environment. Comminuted fractures are those with multiple fragmentation (Fig. 17-3).

Treatment of fractures may be classified into two categories. *Closed reduction* refers to immobilization by applying arch bars to the teeth and tying the teeth (or dentures) in occlusion. *Open reduction* involves an incision and direct manipulation of the segments into apposition, and fixation by wiring or other devices. One of the prime considerations is to obtain and maintain the proper occlusion. Fractures are usually treated by the oral surgeon.

OTHER LOCAL TRAUMA

Any patient who reports that he has had trauma to the face should be carefully examined. Occasionally cracks in teeth are difficult to detect clinically. If a dye such as Merthiolate or a disclosing solution is applied to the tooth surface and then wiped away, the fracture line may become apparent. The teeth should be tested for vitality and mobility. The other intra- and extraoral

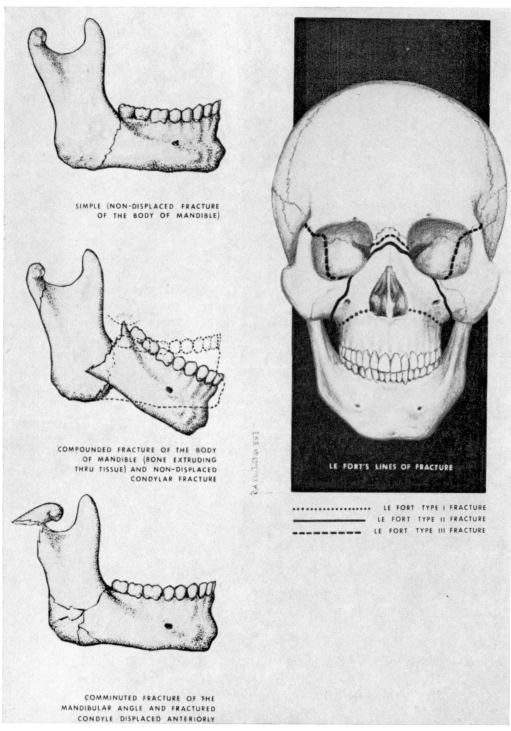

SIMPLE (NON-DISPLACED FRACTURE
OF THE BODY OF MANDIBLE)

COMPOUNDED FRACTURE OF THE BODY
OF MANDIBLE (BONE EXTRUDING
THRU TISSUE) AND NON-DISPLACED
CONDYLAR FRACTURE

LE FORT'S LINES OF FRACTURE

•••••••••••••••••••   LE FORT TYPE I FRACTURE
———————   LE FORT TYPE II FRACTURE
— — — — — —   LE FORT TYPE III FRACTURE

COMMINUTED FRACTURE OF THE
MANDIBULAR ANGLE AND FRACTURED
CONDYLE DISPLACED ANTERIORLY

Fig. 17-3. Diagrammatic representation of common maxillary and mandibular fractures. The more common locations and types of fractures of the maxilla and mandible are shown. Many combinations of these fractures are seen and the classification is strictly for descriptive purposes. In these types of fractures, the patient's occlusion often is affected and therefore responsibility for treatment belongs to the dentist.

tissues should be checked for damage and the presence of embedded foreign bodies. Palpation, probing and radiography are useful. Ice packs to prevent swelling may be advisable.

Factitial injuries, iatrogenic injuries, gunshot wounds, drug burns, toothpick and toothbrush injuries, sucker-stick trauma and surgical accidents are some of the many possible causes of traumatic injury. After specific oral diseases have been ruled out, traumatic ulcers should be treated by covering them with a bland ointment, and they then should be observed periodically until they heal. Any suspected self-induced injuries should be explained to the patient.

Lacerations of the mucosa due to the dental bur or other surgical causes should be carefully debrided and irrigated before they are sutured closed. Occasionally, systemic antibiotics are indicated if infection is probable or if the injury enters one of the fascial spaces. If a patient should swallow or aspirate any object, he should be so advised and medical consultation with a gastroenterologist, or laryngologist, should be sought.

HEMORRHAGE

In all cases where excessive oral hemorrhage is present, the site of bleeding should be located. Often this necessitates cleaning away poorly formed clots and debridement with gauze sponges moistened in normal saline. Usually local pressure with sponges held in place for 30 minutes will allow for the reestablishment of a normal clot, after which the patient should be advised against vigorous rinsing with any solution which will break down the clot again. Large or deep lacerations should be debrided, irrigated and sutured. If the wound is from a foreign body,

a tetanus booster should be suggested to the patient's physician.

EXPOSED DENTIN

This of course is seldom an emergency, but management of this discomfort is included here for purposes of completeness. Dentin exposed from caries should be covered with zinc oxide and eugenol until the tooth is permanently restored. Painful exposed cervical dentin may often be treated by burnishing a 10 percent stannous fluoride solution into the exposed dentinal tubules; however, several treatments are often necessary to get optimum results. There are several other methods of treating cervical hypersensitivity, but none is universally successful. To relieve the symptom, it is occasionally necessary to prepare and restore the area with an appropriate material. The topical application of water-soluble corticoids has shown promise, and strontium-containing toothpastes, as well as those containing formalin and stannous fluoride, seem to help.

BIBLIOGRAPHY

Berlove, I. J.: *Dental-Medical Emergencies and Complications*, Chicago, Year Book Medical Publishers, Inc., 1963.

Cheraskin, E.: The control of bleeding, J. Amer. Dent. Ass., *58*, 17, 1959.

Compton, D. E. and Mitchell, D. F.: Pharmacologic treatment of painful pulpitis: A five-year report, J. Dent. Res., *49*, 183, 1970.

Gardner D. E., Mitchell, D. F. and McDonald, R. E.: Treatment of pulps of monkeys with vancomycin and calcium hydroxide, J. Dent. Res., *50*, 1273, 1971.

Kutscher, A. H., Zegarelli, E. V. and Hyman, G. A.: *Pharmacotherapeutics of Oral Disease*, New York, McGraw-Hill Book Co., 1964.

McCarthy, F. M.: *Emergencies in Dental Practice*, Philadelphia, W. B. Saunders Co., 1967.

Sherman, P.: Intentional replantation of teeth, J. Dent. Res., *47*, 1066, 1968.

Chapter 18

Dentistry and the Law

As a health practitioner, the dentist must be aware of his responsibilities to his patients and their responsibilities to him. He must know how to prevent legal problems and protect his rights in his doctor-patient relationships, and he must know the business mechanics of operating a practice. In addition, the dentist can provide valuable aid to law enforcement officials in identifying bodies and causes of death. This chapter deals with these topics.

It goes without stating that the dentist should always attempt to provide the best and most thorough diagnostic and therapeutic services for his patient. Nonetheless, under our system of law, anyone can sue anyone else for real or imagined injuries. The dentist's knowledge of the law can help prevent claims and reduce the possibility of a malpractice lawsuit.

Even though the dentist attempts to provide diagnostic service and dental treatment to the best of his ability, this is not enough. He must keep complete records and see that his patient is well informed, and he must be sure that his business and legal affairs are in good condition and up-to-date. It behooves the new dentist, especially, to consult an attorney before making major purchases and establishing purchasing contracts for dental equipment, and for other important legal matters.

At the first sign of any legal problem with a patient or other individual with whom he deals, the dentist should seek advice from his attorney. He should say nothing to the patient from which any inference of negligence might be drawn and upon which any action might be predicated. If the claim is the result of dental treatment or injury in a dental office, the dentist should contact his insurance company representative and he will arrange for an attorney to advise and defend the dentist if necessary.

The astute dentist should be familiar with all his rights and responsibilities, and he should read the literature on dental jurisprudence for more complete information.

PREVENTION OF LEGAL PROBLEMS

It is a cardinal rule in dentistry not to criticize the work of another dentist. The dentist should remember that the circumstances under which earlier dental treatment was given may have been much different from what they are now and that criticism is therefore not only unfair but also unsound legally. If the patient chooses to sue his former dentist, the criticizing dentist, in some jurisdictions, could be compelled to testify as to his reasons for the adverse criticism regarding the dental treatment administered. In addition, the dentist who was criticized could sue the other dentist for defamation of character.

Good diagnostic treatment and financial records must be maintained and the patient must be kept well informed of the fees. Misunderstandings regarding fees between the patient and the dentist lead to many lawsuits.

A good up-to-date medical history is mandatory for each patient. If a systemic disease is detected, or if a disease develops during extended dental treatment, the dentist should obtain medical consultation to determine if the disease or its treatment has bearing on the oral condition or treatment procedure. Although it may be a verbal consultation, the information obtained should be kept in writing in the patient's chart for future reference It is best, however, for such consultation to be done through correspondence.

Consultation is good in difficult cases, and although the use of consultants does not reduce the responsibility of the referring dentist to his patient, it does give the dentist a better basis for sound judgment. The dentist is not bound by the suggestions of the consultant. Although a dentist seldom is convicted of malpractice for an incorrect diagnosis, he must always use the same reasonable care as other dentists, under the same or similar circumstances, in order to establish a correct diagnosis and before beginning treatment. Any difficulty in making a final diagnosis should be reported to the patient and the patient should always be kept informed as to what the dentist is planning and any possible untoward se-

quelae of the diagnosis or treatment. This information should be related to the patient in terms he can understand, and an entry indicating that this was done should be placed in the patient's chart. This includes postsurgical instructions and advice.

When an examination or dental treatment is contemplated, it is necessary to obtain consent from the patient. For consent to be valid, the patient must understand the procedures and reasonable sequelae to be expected. When the patient is a minor, or otherwise legally incompetent, consent should be obtained from the parent or legal guardian. Consent forms are good only if they are specific; however, for most adult patients they are not necessary because of the doctrine of implied consent. This states that when a patient comes to a dentist, he consents by implication to an examination and dental treatment. Failure to obtain written consent or at least verbal consent before treating a minor could result in difficulty in collecting the fee for the service rendered or other more serious legal problems, such as being prosecuted for technical assault. Written consent (Fig. 18-1) is most important in the case of the particularly troublesome patient or unusual case.

A contract is an agreement between two individuals and usually does not have to be in written form to be legally binding. Contracts used by dentists include those with patients who need extensive dental treatment; those for purchasing of dental offices and equipment, and for rental of office space; and those between two or more dentists who are establishing associateships or partnerships. These contracts should be written when possible. Most contracts between papatient and dentist are verbal. Recognize, however, that a contract binds both parties; the dentist must abide by the contract just as stringently as must the patient.

The dentist, after obtaining his dental license, should carefully review the dental practice act for his state. Many states have specialty laws preventing dentists from list-

CONSENT FOR DENTAL TREATMENT

by

John Doe, D.D.S.

Case No._____   Name_____

    I hereby grant permission to the dentist in charge of the case of the patient whose name appears above to administer anesthetics and to employ such operative or technical procedures as may be deemed necessary or advisable in the diagnosis or treatment of this case.

Treatment includes:_____

Exceptions:_____

Signature of Patient:_____

Signature of Parent or Guardian:_____
(If patient is minor or unable to sign)

Relation to Patient:_____

                                                Date_____

Witness of the signature of parent or guardian:

_____

_____

Fig. 18-1.   Sample form for written consent.

ing themselves as specialists unless they have specialty board status or specified types of formal training. Likewise, it is considered unethical to misrepresent oneself to the public in this way.

    The dentist obviously should always exercise care in his examination and treatment so as not to cause undue injury to his patient (Figs. 18-2, 18-3). He should not guarantee the results of treatment, not only because this is unethical, but also because the courts have held that either a direct or an implied guarantee constitutes a contract and the patient can sue the dentist should the results not be up to the standards of the guarantee. Likewise, the dentist should be careful not to specify completion times of prostheses or dental treatment, as occasionally it is necessary to delay completion times because of

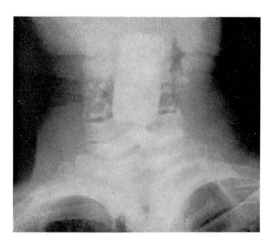

Fig. 18-2.   Bite-wing radiograph in pharynx. In the course of taking a bite-wing radiograph on this mentally retarded patient, the film suddenly disappeared. The dentist wisely located it in the patient's pharynx with this radiograph. He then retrieved the film with a curved hemostat.

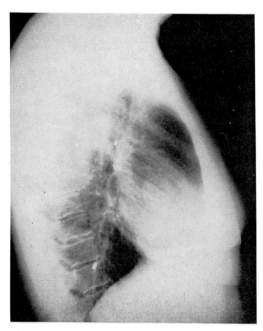

Fig. 18-3. Aspiration of root canal file. This lateral chest plate reveals a root canal file which was swallowed by the patient. It is located in the lower esophagus. Had a rubber dam been used, this accident might not have occurred.

special problems. With no real or implied contract, the dentist may be tested in court only as to the reasonableness of a result.

If a patient should be injured accidentally in the dental office, for example, receive a laceration from a rotary instrument, the dentist should make no statement to the patient other than that an injury has occurred. He should not excuse himself or say "I'm sorry" because he could later be forced to admit saying these things on the witness stand, and thus appear to be guilty of malpractice. The courts recognize that even with reasonable caution injuries do occur in the dental office.

Once a patient has been accepted for treatment and an agreement has been reached regarding the form of treatment and the fee, it is the duty of the dentist to complete the treatment in a reasonable time. Thus, before activating a lengthy treatment plan, the dentist must understand the patient's response to his plan and ascertain

his ability to cooperate during the treatment. It would be unfortunate if the dentist agreed on a difficult treatment plan for a specified fee only to find later that the patient was very difficult to treat because of some psychic or physical factor. The dentist would then be obligated to treat this patient at the predetermined fee even if it were unreasonably low under the circumstances.

Following the examination and completion of treatment, the disposition should be noted in the patient's chart. If the treatment has been completed, or if further treatment is necessary, the patient should be so informed. This includes recalls and reexaminations.

If any surgical or other procedures are performed which might require post-operative instructions, the patient should be given adequate instruction, preferably in writing, and a notation made in the chart. This also is true for pulpitis or other conditions in which there is a question as to the prognosis. When a patient is given a sedative prior to treatment, he should be informed as to the effects of that sedative and the length of time that its effects will last. The same is true for nitrous oxide analgesia and general anesthesia. He should be cautioned specifically not to drive a care or engage in any activity requiring his best judgment. The dentist should not release the patient until he has regained complete control of his faculties or is placed under the care of a responsible adult. It is wise when giving patients a prescription for a potentially dangerous drug to request the pharmacist to place special instructions as to the nature and dangers of this drug on the label. The dentist should also give these instructions to his patient verbally.

The dentist who declares or implies that he is a specialist owes his patients a greater degree of skill and ability than does the average practitioner; the courts have held this to be true. Any dentist must meet the standards of a reasonably prudent dentist. If he represents himself as a specialist he must meet the standards of a reasonably prudent specialist, which are higher standards. Therefore, when a patient is told that he is being treated by a specialist, either by way of professional cards or office signs, he can reasonably expect a higher degree of skill in diagnosis and treatment.

If a needle breaks accidentally or a tooth is aspirated into a lung, it is the duty of the dentist and/or specialist to inform the patient and to refer him for proper treatment. Courts have held that it is the duty of the dentist to refer his patient to another practitioner when a similarly trained dentist in that community would have done likewise.

In the course of an examination, it is often important for the dentist to take full-mouth radiographs. Some attorneys feel that it is the legal responsibility of a prudent dentist to take diagnostic radiographs as part of an examination. These films should be retained by the dentist; they are not the property of the patient. The dentist should be careful not to send a statement to the patient specifically for x-ray films, lest the courts take this to mean that the films belong to the patient. In fact, the radiographs are part of the diagnostic procedure and the patient pays a fee for the diagnosis. The good oral diagnostician tells his patient only that there is a fee for the examination which includes the use of x-ray films and other diagnostic measures. Ordinarily films and other records should be lent only to other practitioners, not to patients.

The dentist is legally responsible for the acts of any of his agents, such as his assistant, hygienist and office manager. If an assistant or another auxiliary should slip with a retractor or do anything else that injures the patient, the patient would have legal recourse against the assistant or the dentist or both. This responsibility has even extended to an incident in which an auxiliary person was instructed to go to a given place as part of her job and was involved in an automobile accident.

The dentist as an employer should be aware of his responsibilities and liabilities to his employees and should understand the workman's compensation law.

If a partnership between dentists exists, it should be recognized that in some states each member of the partnership is legally responsible for the acts of the other, and the two can be jointly sued for the act of one.

If the dentist wishes to use photographs of a patient in a scientific publication, he should secure a release in writing. Otherwise, he could be sued for invasion of the patient's privacy.

The dentist should be fully aware of the prescription laws, control drugs and laws concerning the inventory of narcotics and barbiturates. He should write his prescriptions carefully and indicate his registration number on each prescription for narcotics.

He should carry malpractice and liability insurance and should report any threats of lawsuits to his attorney and his insurance company. He should consult with his attorney to establish general guidelines for taking actions against patients regarding non-payment of fees.

GUIDELINES FOR PREVENTING LEGAL PROBLEMS

1. Keep the patient informed of the diagnosis, treatment procedures, and fees.
2. Make sure that the patient understands the possible results of treatment (good and bad) before starting.
3. Do not guarantee results.
4. Make agreements and contracts in writing when indicated.
5. Obtain consent in writing when indicated.
6. Practice thorough and careful dentistry and do not allow the patient to dictate the type of treatment.
7. Avoid specifying completion dates.
8. Do not abandon the patient after starting treatment.
9. Keep good records.
10. Use radiographs when indicated and retain the films.
11. Know your state's dental act and your limitations.
12. Carefully regulate the duties of your auxiliaries.

13. Have periodic legal and insurance reviews.
14. Advise patients of the effects and side effects of drugs prescribed.
15. Prescribe prophylactic antibiotics whenever the medical history indicates it should be done.
16. Use consultants effectively.
17. Give written post-operative instructions to patients.
18. Get a written release before publishing photographs of a patient.
19. If threatened with a lawsuit, make no statements until you have consulted an attorney or your insurance company.

FORENSIC DENTISTRY

Forensic odontology may be defined as: the study of the teeth as they relate to, or are used in the courts of law for the identification and assistance in determining the cause of death. The principles here are the same as those used in anthropology and paleontology.

According to law, a person cannot be certified as dead until his body has been found and identified, or until an extended period of time has elapsed since he became missing. Death from fires, airplane accidents and other multiple death catastrophes, drowning, or death with advanced decay of the human body often makes positive identification of that body difficult. Murderers sometimes mutilate their victims by burning the remains, using chemicals, removing limbs, or using other methods to prevent identification. In most of these cases, the teeth and jaws remain intact. The oral diagnostician is in an unusual position to aid the authorities in identification.

Methods of Identification

Various methods are used in identification. The least reliable are those utilizing visual identification by persons who knew the deceased or clothing or personal effects (e.g. credit cards) which may have been found on the body. More scientific methods of identification (fingerprints, dental records, chest or long bone x-rays, serology, autopsy findings) are based on comparisons of postmortem and antemortem records.

The teeth are a unique means of identification in that they are highly resistant to destruction. Secondly, it is highly improbable that any two individuals will have identical sets of teeth. The number of combinations of missing teeth, caries and restorations that can be used to distinguish one individual from another is almost infinite. If radiographs of the teeth and jaws are also considered, numerous additional features characteristic of that individual can be added—root and pulp chamber morphology, stage of tooth eruption, bone trabeculation patterns, nutrient canals, bone "scars" and various pathologic processes.

A corpse may be unidentified for a long time. The police department, however, has access to missing persons files and usually suspects the corpse to be the remains of one of several persons. If good diagnostic dental records are available, the remains of the victim can be compared with the records and identification made.

If the dentist is asked to assist in the identification of an unknown body he should

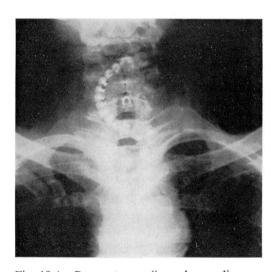

Fig. 18-4. Postmortem radiograph revealing upper denture in pharynx as cause of death. Occasionally patients aspirate or swallow dental appliances, and the dentist would be wise to consider this possibility before constructing a dental prosthesis.

carry out a thorough oral examination, recording not only fillings, caries and missing teeth but the state of oral hygiene, occlusion, wear facets, gingival health, etc. Radiographs and diagnostic models should also be obtained since the data which will be important in a later comparison of records cannot be known in advance. It is wise to have two dentists examine the corpse to ensure accuracy. If the body is in a state of rigor mortis and difficulty is encountered in opening the jaws, the examination can be delayed a few hours until the rigor subsides, or the forensic pathologist conducting the autopsy can assist in freeing the jaws at the time he opens the cranium for examination. If the body is partially decomposed or badly burned and thus cannot be viewed at the funeral, the jaws can even be removed.

Radiographs, study models and photographs are valuable, and in some countries patients receiving dental treatment have a standard chart completed for identification purposes. This is an additional reason for using and maintaining a standard charting system and complete dental radiographs for each patient. The armed forces and other federal services have used dental identification charts for their members for many years.

Even if identification is not made immediately, the dentist can usually discover certain information about the corpse that may prove valuable later. It can be assumed that, if the person had had good dental care with many gold restorations, he must have been of at least moderate financial means. Occasionally the type of dental treatment performed can be associated with a particular dental school, dentist or dental laboratory and further investigation will lead to the identification. Morphology of the teeth and intra-oral pigmentation are sometimes helpful in determining national origin or race. The head shape and size can sometimes be estimated roughly from the size of the teeth. The presence of orthodontic bands or prostheses may help in identification. In the young individual, the presence of unerupted teeth in various stages of development is helpful in determining the age at the time of death. Occasionally the occupation of the individual can be surmised from the dentition. Notching of a maxillary central incisor suspected to be due to the habitual opening of bobby pins might suggest the sex of the corpse, or conceivably indicate a male carpenter who held nails between his teeth. Even if the information is not sufficient for a court of law, it might lead the police toward ultimate identification or turn their attention to other possibilities.

Determination of Age

A person's age can be estimated with reasonable accuracy, especially if he was less than 21 years old, through assessment of dental development and eruption stages (Appendix, Table 2). Certain principles also help in deciding the age at the time of death. Root formation most often begins as active eruption starts, and approximately two years elapse before the root is completed. Microscopic examination of ground sections of teeth is helpful in determining whether death came before or after birth. There have been cases in which the presence of a neonatal line in the teeth of an infant resulted in prosecution for murder rather than for criminal abortion. Since mineralization of the lower first permanent molars starts somewhat later in males, a neonatal line will be found in only about one-half of the boys whereas essentially all girls will show this feature in first molar teeth.

Determination of age in the adult is more difficult. Several criteria which are related largely to aging have been described by Gustafson: attrition, height of periodontal attachment, secondary dentin formation, thickness of root cementum, apical closure and root transparency. These factors are assigned scores and the age estimated by reference to a previously prepared regression line.

Determination of Sex

Determination of the sex of a corpse strictly from dental findings is difficult. However, when coupled with findings from the skull, it is possible. The following factors are helpful: (1) female jaws and skull structure are smoother, and males have rougher bone at sites of muscle attachment; (2) the maxillary sinuses of the male are larger and the maxillae over the cuspid and bicuspid regions are more prominent; (3) the incisal index is greater in the male (the incisal index is defined as the width of the upper second incisor divided by the width of the upper first incisor times 100); (4) male teeth are thicker faciolingually; (5) young males have everted mandibular angles and shallow sigmoid notches with blunt coronoid processes, while females have smooth, rounded mandibular angles and deep sigmoid notches with high pointed coronoid processes; (6) zygomatic arches of males are thicker and less smooth; (7) supraorbital ridges are more prominent in the male; and (8) skull differences between male and female are greatest between the ages of 17 and 45. After menopause, the female skull becomes more masculinized.

Fluorescent histologic methods for the demonstration of the male Y chromosome in cells of the tooth pulp, as well as other cell types, may be useful in sex determination. Buccal cytologic smears are commonly utilized to determine the sex of newborn infants by identifying the female X chromosome or Barr body (pp. 71, 208).

Acquired Characteristics

Extreme occlusal wear suggestive of tobacco chewing or bruxism might be useful for identification. Certain wear patterns and stains associated with pipe smoking and habits which result in tooth movement may cause characteristic changes. Evidence of cheek chewing, scars acquired during seizures, Dilantin gingival hyperplasia, intrinsic dental stains due to fluorosis or tetracycline drug administration should be considered.

A general idea of the occupation of an unknown corpse can sometimes be gleaned from the dental structures. A body with missing maxillary anterior teeth usually can be assumed not to be that of a salesman or other person involved in meeting the public. Evidence of bruxism suggests an occupation in which there is a great deal of stress.

Developmental Characteristics

It is sometimes possible to identify the race and even the nationality of the individual. The American Indians (mongoloid) and Negroid people tend to have a high rate of shovel-shaped maxillary incisors which are large compared to the Caucasoid. Indians also have a protostylid on the deciduous second molar and permanent first and sometimes second mandibular molars. Central European whites usually have wide based prominent cinguli on the incisors rather than smooth rolled cinguli. East Indian, Mediterranean, European, and American populations have smaller rounded incisors with smoother surfaces. The most important tooth morphologically is the first permanent molar. Any changes in its shape are usually duplicated to a lesser extent in the second molar. Arch length tends to be more adequate in the non-Caucasoid. The shape of the palatal rugae is characteristic for each individual, and soft tissue pigmentation may be helpful.

Bite Marks

The evaluation and identification of bite marks are difficult and challenging tasks in forensic dentistry which often require much ingenuity on the part of the dentist. He may be of assistance in the investigation of bite marks found at the scene of a crime, in foodstuffs (or other inanimate objects) or in human tissues. The proper handling of the evidence in such cases may be critical to the successful prosecution of cases of robbery, assault, murder or other criminal activity.

Bite marks in foodstuffs or other perishable substances may be of evidential value provided they can be adequately documented by close-up photography or even impressions. Generally, substances of firm consistency such as apples provide well-defined profiles comparable to "tool marks," and are useful in identification if the teeth of the suspect are malaligned or have characteristic fractures or diastemas. Since marks in food will undergo marked dimensional changes from drying, shrinkage or decomposition, the material should be photographed immediately, impressions taken whenever possible and the specimen preserved by freezing whenever appropriate.

Human bites in human tissue may occur either in the victim or the assailant in a crime and thus may be inflicted in self-defense or sadistically by either party. In some instances, the mark will be self-inflicted when the assailant forces the victim's own hand or arm into his mouth to stifle outcries. The psychotic or mentally deranged person may also bite himself as a form of self-inflicted punishment. Dead bodies which remain undiscovered for a period of time may be fed upon by dogs, rodents and other predators and thus carry animal bites. Attacks on a living person by vicious dogs or other animals commonly leave characteristic marks.

Although human flesh is a poor impression material, some bite marks, particularly those produced sadistically, may be sufficiently distinctive to warrant legal action against a suspect or eliminate a possible suspect. It must be recognized, however, that bite marks in human tissue are frequently distorted by the elasticity of the tissue, changes in body position and postmortem changes in the body, or by normal healing or secondary infection if the victim survives. The bite mark evidence must be fully documented even if there is no suspect at the time of the examination.

Blood group (ABO) substances may be identified in various body secretions (sweat, urine, semen, saliva) in a large percentage of the population. Swabs should therefore be obtained of all bite marks before taking impressions or washing the wound. Control swabs should also be obtained from other areas on the victim's skin.

Numerous color and black and white photographs of the mark should be obtained, using various types of lighting. Often strong side lighting will demonstrate texture and shadow patterns of indentations not visible with flat lighting. The camera should be positioned at right angles to the skin surface whenever possible to minimize parallax distortion. Since most bite marks occur on curved skin surfaces, such as the breast, face or arm, multiple photographs are necessary. A ruler should be included in the picture to illustrate actual dimensions; however, identical pictures should be taken without the scale since some courts may rule that the ruler constitutes an alteration of the evidence.

Impressions of the bite mark are then taken, using silicone, rubber base or similar materials. Stone models of the mark with a wide margin of surrounding skin are prepared. These models may be duplicated in polyvinyl latex to simulate the resilient skin of the living person. From these photographs and models, various measurements, photograms and tracings may be prepared for later comparison with dental casts from any suspects. If the victim is deceased, the bite mark can even be removed at autopsy and preserved in the frozen state. If the bite is on the face and it is expected that the body will be viewed at the funeral, it would of course not be possible to excise the bite mark and surrounding skin.

Evaluation of the bite mark evidence should initially be made objectively and without reference to the dental casts of any suspects. With bite marks of good quality, certain dental characteristics of the assailant can be deduced, such as arch form and length, malposed teeth, diastemas, fractures, etc. Similar evaluations are then made of the dental characteristics of available suspects and, finally, comparisons are made of any concordant or inconsistent or negative points that would implicate or exclude a suspect.

The dentist, particularly if he has had no prior experience in this field, should refer to the literature on this subject for additional details.

Forensic Dentistry Kit

The following is a list of equipment and supplies suggested for use in an identification bag by a dentist when examining a corpse for the police or other authorities.

1. An official dental chart.
2. 2 × 2 inch gauze.
3. Chloroform or other organic solvent.
4. Rubber gloves.
5. Scissors, tissue forceps and scalpel.
6. Hemostat and tongue blades.
7. Chisel, mallet or portable hand drill.
8. Flashlight.
9. Mouth prop.
10. Mirror and explorer.
11. Impression material and plaster.

The dentist as a good citizen should be willing to assist and use his ingenuity in examining the dead for forensic purposes.

BIBLIOGRAPHY

Aitchison, J.: Sex differences in teeth, jaws and skulls, Dent. Pract., *14*, 52, 1963.
——: Some racial differences in human skulls and jaws, Brit. Dent. J., *116*, 25, 1964.
Calonius, P. E. B., Lunin, M. and Stout, F.: Histologic criteria for age estimation of the developing human dentition, Oral Surg., *29*, 869, 1970.
Cameron, J. M. and Sims, B. G.: *Forensic Dentistry*, Edinburgh, Churchill Livingstone, 1973.
Cleland, J. B.: Teeth and bites in history, literature, forensic medicine and otherwise, Aust. J. Dent., *48*, 107, 1944.
Dahlberg, A. A.: Dental traits as identification tools, Dent. Prog., *3*, 155, 1963.
Emery, G. T.: Dentistry in forensic archaeology, Brit. Dent. J., *122*, 26, 1967.
Furness, J.: A new method for the identification of teeth marks in cases of assault and homicide, Brit. Dent. J., *124*, 261, 1968.

Furuhata, T. and Yamamoto, K.: *Forensic Odontology*, Springfield, Charles C Thomas, 1967.
Gustafson, G.: *Forensic Odontology*, New York, American Elsevier Publishing Co., 1966.
Haines, D. H.: Dental identification in the Stockport air disaster, Brit. Dent. J., *123*, 336, 1968.
Hanihara, K.: Racial characteristics in the dentition, J. Dent. Res., Supplement No. 5, *46*, 923, 1967.
Harmeling, B. L., Schuh, E. and Humphreys, H. S.: Dental identification of bodies in a major disaster, S. C. Dent. J., *26*, 4, 1968.
Harvey, W.: *Dental Identification and Forensic Odontology*, London, Henry Kimpton, 1976.
Jerman, A. C.: Denture identification, J. Amer. Dent. Ass., *80*, 1358, 1970.
Johnson, C. C.: Transparent dentine in age estimation, Oral Surg., *25*, 834, 1968.
Keiser-Nielsen, S.: Forensic odontology, Int. Dent. J., *18*, 668, 1968.
Lalonde, E. R.: The role of the dentist in identification of unknown corpses, J. Kentucky Dent. Ass., *20*, 19, 1968.
Luntz, L. L. and Luntz, P.: *Handbook for Dental Identification. Techniques in Forensic Denitstry*, Philadelphia, J. B. Lippincott Co., 1973.
Miles, A. E. W. and Fearnhead, R. W.: Postmortem color changes in teeth, J. Dent. Res., *33*, 735, 1954 (abstract).
Mitchell, D. F.: A history of aviation dentistry, Ann. Dent. *5*, 1, 1946.
Nash, R. B.: An evaluation of the dental identification records: report of a case, J. Amer. Dent. Ass., *43*, 209, 1951.
Sarner, H.: *Dental Jurisprudence*, Philadelphia, W. B. Saunders Co., 1963.
——: *The Business Management of Dental Practice*, Philadelphia, W. B. Saunders Co., 1966.
Sarner, H. and Lassiter, H. C.: *Insurance for the Doctor*, Philadelphia, W. B. Saunders Co., 1967.
Sopher, I. M.: *Forensic Dentistry*, Springfield, Charles C Thomas, 1975.
Standish, S. M. and Stimson, P. G. (Eds.): *Forensic Dentistry: Legal Obligations and Methods of Identification for the Practitioner*, Dent. Clin. North America, January, 1977.
Sussman, L. N.: *Blood Grouping Tests, Medicolegal Uses*, Springfield, Charles C Thomas, 1968.
Suzuki, K., Suzuki, H. and Hadano, K.: Criminal case reports of bite marks, Bull. Tokyo Dent. Coll., *11*, 33, 1970.
Taylor, R. M. S.: Variation in form of human teeth: I. An anthropologic and forensic study of maxillary incisors, J. Dent. Res., *48*, 5, 1969.
Vale, G. L.: The dentist's expanding responsibilities: forensic odontology, J. S. Calif. Dent. Ass., *37*, 248, 1969.
Zander, H. A. and Hurzeler, B.: Continuous cementum apposition, J. Dent. Res., *37*, 1035, 1958.

NOTES

NOTES

NOTES

NOTES

NOTES

Chapter 19

Diagnosis and Management of Medical Emergencies

It is recommended that study be supplemented with practice in cardiopulmonary resuscitation using a mannequin and that knowledge be updated periodically by restudy of this chapter and by additional training in basic life support and emergency procedures. A list of additional manuals, equipment and materials is included at the end of this chapter.

This chapter has been specially designed to aid in your study of this vital subject. The educational goal and behavioral objectives of the chapter are provided below, and should be reviewed prior to reading. Questions are posed throughout the text material so that each concept or subunit of material may be mentally reviewed. The answers are at the end of the chapter.

Educational Goal

To develop an orderly and confident approach to the diagnosis and **supportive care** of a person who becomes acutely ill and whose life is endangered.

Objectives

At the conclusion of your study, you should be able to:
1. List and describe significant emergency preventive measures.
2. Describe emergency preparedness in a dental office.
3. Recognize signs or symptoms of impending emergencies.
4. Recognize that an emergency situation exists.
5. Classify the emergency into one or more groups or categories.
6. List steps of action when a medical emergency arises in a dental office.
7. Describe minor and major respiratory emergencies and their management.
8. Describe mild and severe cardiovascular emergencies and their management.
9. Describe treatment of anaphylactic shock, hemorrhagic problems and acute hypertension.
10. Recognize the cause, signs, symptoms and treatment of common specific emergency conditions.
11. List emergency equipment which should be available in a dental office.

12. List the basic drugs for use in emergencies including dosage, routes of administration, actions, and indications for usage of stimulants and vasopressors, coronary dilators, anticonvulsants, sedatives, analgesics, antihistamines, antistress and antiasthmatic drugs.

13. Describe and/or demonstrate the following techniques:
    a. cardiopulmonary resuscitation
    b. mouth-to-mouth breathing
    c. pulse and blood pressure determination
    d. use of bag and mask
    e. parenteral administration
    f. endotracheal intubation
    g. Heimlich maneuver

TABLE OF CONTENTS

GENERAL CONSIDERATIONS

Responsibilities of Dentist

Serious medical life-threatening emergencies seldom occur in a dental office but, when they do, as the dentist you have an implied legal and certainly a moral responsibility to provide adequate care regardless of whether the patient is in the process of being treated or in your waiting room. Laws are not specific regarding the dentist's responsibilities, but it must be assumed that the principle of "standard of care" would apply. Considering only your responsibilities to support life and prevent serious physiologic damage to your patient (or friend) in a crisis, the courts would expect you to act prudently and with a level of skill equivalent to other dentists in a similar situation. The court might reasonably expect at least minimal emergency equipment to be available in your office and a type of prearranged emergency plan to be in effect.

> **Q–1 If you have no emergency equipment and no prearranged emergency plan established in your office, you are on weak ground legally? TRUE OR FALSE (Refer to p. 560 for answer.)**

Prevention

1. A medical history indicating allergies, previous cardiac disease, paroxysmal nocturnal dyspnea (P.N.D.), orthopnea or other forms of dyspnea, asthma, fainting spells, diabetes, hemorrhagic tendencies, or a multitude of other medical problems should alert the dentist to the possibility of trouble.

2. Judicious use of sedatives and TLC (tender loving care) along with good doctor-patient rapport can often allay the stress and fear which precipitate many emergencies. Anxiety is probably as damaging to the sick patient as is any specific dental procedure.

3. Be familiar with any medications which the patient is taking, their contraindications and side effects.

4. Make some prearrangements with a nearby physician and have his phone number at hand. Also, be familiar with the nearest hospital emergency ward and how to use it correctly.

5. Consult with the patient's physician, by phone or preferably in writing, when this is indicated by a questionable history.

6. When administering a local anesthetic, use an aspirating syringe.

7. When a patient has a morning appointment, make sure he has eaten breakfast; this does not apply if a general anesthetic is to be used.

Prepare for an emergency in advance. All equipment must be available and in working order, and your staff should be trained and ready to go into action. Prearranged duties for each assistant are helpful. Practice "dry runs."

When an emergency occurs, the important diagnosis is that there is an emergency. For example: If an injection of a local anesthetic is given and the patient loses consciousness, it is important to recognize that he is in shock which should be treated promptly along with any respiratory problems which might arise; time should not be wasted trying to determine whether the reaction was allergic, idiosyncratic or toxic.

Q–2 Which is the most important emergency prevention measure?
  (1) Make use of an aspirating syringe.
  (2) Make patient eat before appointments because fear causes release of endogenous epinephrine which in turn causes increased burning of glucose and results in hypoglycemia.
  (3) Know all medications a patient is taking, the reasons why, and the side effects.
  (4) Take and interpret the patient's medical history.

Q–3 You should prepare for emergencies in advance, *i.e.*, practice "dry runs" with your auxiliaries? TRUE OR FALSE.

Q–4 A patient loses consciousness. It is important to immediately determine the cause (etiology)? TRUE OR FALSE.
(Check answers on p. 560.)

Most serious emergencies fall into one of the following groups: (1) Respiratory—dyspnea, apnea, obstruction, sighing, asthmatic breathing, etc., (2) cardiovascular (circulatory)—shock, strokes (CVA), coronaries, cardiac arrest, fainting, etc., and (3) hemorrhagic—postsurgical bleeding, traumatic injuries and hemorrhagic diseases, etc.

PHYSICAL SIGNS AND SYMPTOMS OF TROUBLE OR IMPENDING TROUBLE

1. Skin and mucosal pallor
2. Cold sweating
3. Pupils dilated and non-responsive to light
4. Hemorrhage
5. Malaise

6. Emesis
7. Unusual pains or sensations
8. Apnea or dyspnea, hemoptysis, cyanosis
9. Pulse slow, rapid or weak
10. Blood pressure elevated or depressed

Q–5 **From memory list the three groups of serious emergencies and give examples. (Check answers on p. 560.)**

Q–6 **List the ten signs and symptoms of trouble or impending trouble. (Check answer on page 560.)**

WHAT TO DO WHEN AN EMERGENCY ARISES

1. Get immediate medical assistance; use office girl to summon assistance.
2. Check for adequate respiration; secure a patent airway and support respiration if indicated.
3. Determine whether patient has adequate circulation by checking level of consciousness, blood pressure, pulse and/or pupils, when practical. Usually circulation improves with good ventilation.
4. Once the patient has been stabilized, consider a more specific diagnosis and supplemental treatment. Avoid emergency drugs until you are sure what is needed.

REMEMBER THAT ANY ONE OF THE THREE LISTED SYSTEMS (GROUPS)
CAN FAIL AND LEAD TO FAILURE OF THE OTHER, OR ALL THREE
CAN FAIL AT ONCE. ABOVE ALL, "KEEP 'EM BREATHING."

Q–7 **Organize the following four general steps in managing an emergency into the proper sequence?**
   (1) Determine circulation adequacy.
   (2) Determine specific etiology and definitive treatment.
   (3) Get medical assistance.
   (4) Check adequacy of respiration.
           (Check answer on p. 560.)

Respiratory Difficulties

Minor Difficulties

Psychic (anxiety, hysteria)—often associated with dental treatment, pre- and post-injection, and pre- and postsurgical care. Usually characterized early by sighing or deep inhalations. Treat early to prevent further difficulties such as primary or neurogenic shock (fainting).

Management

1. Ask patient questions to distract him. Don't look disturbed. Reassure patient.
2. TLC (tender loving care)—reassure patient and tell him to relax and breathe deeply and regularly.
3. Check pulse.
4. Shock position—head down, feet above level of head.

Additional treatment may be needed if signs of syncope develop:

1. Cold cloth to forehead
2. Spirits of ammonia—inhalant
3. Oxygen
4. Blood pressure and pulse check

Further complications include apnea and/or deepening circulatory depression. Treat as indicated under the section on major respiratory difficulties which follows.

When patient begins to feel better and responds well, have him relax and give him a cola drink or coffee (which acts as a stimulant). It is best to discontinue dental treatment. Consideration should be given to the use of sedative premedication prior to the next appointment.

> **Q–8 Your healthy 35-year-old patient looks frightened, is sighing deeply and has pale clammy skin. What would you do? (Check answer on p. 560.)**

Mild dyspnea (air hunger) may occur from fainting, mild asthmatic attacks, acute congestive heart failure, coronary occlusion or angina pectoris. Often the cause is not known initially. Give oxygen and get immediate medical assistance. If the patient has asthma and has his own medication with him, let him use it. If the patient has trouble breathing in a reclining position, let him sit upright.

> **Q–9 A patient becomes dyspneic. What action would you take first? (1) Give oxygen, (2) get medical help, (3) administer aminophyllin IV, or (4) strike the patient sharply between scapulae and institute the Heimlich maneuver. (Check answer on p. 560.)**

Major Difficulties

Partial or complete obstruction of the respiratory passages can result from aspiration of a foreign body (teeth, gauze, vomitus), laryngospasm or laryngeal edema. Consequences if left untreated can be general hypoxia, circulatory depression, cerebral hypoxia, unconsciousness and/or convulsions, cardiac arrest, death.

Signs

1. Choking and coughing, wheezing, gasping.
2. Straining and extremely violent attempts to breathe with depression in the supraclavicular region during the inspiratory cycle (from negative pressure).
3. Cyanosis (of nail beds, lips and mucosa).
4. Rales (abnormal breath sounds), heard with a stethoscope.
5. Dyspnea, apnea.

Management

1. Attempt to dislodge or remove the foreign body, if present, by inverting patient and hitting him sharply between the scapulae, using your fingers to remove the obstruction, instituting the Heimlich manuever or using a laryngoscope and forceps (see Special Techniques, p. 559).
2. Aspirate the patient's airway with a tonsil suction or suction catheter.

3. Place oral airway and give oxygen, or place S-tube and give mouth-to-mouth resuscitation.

4. If unable to inflate lungs, perform a cricothyrotomy with a 10-gauge (or larger) needle.

5. If apnea develops, aspirate respiratory passages, place airway or obtain patent airway by cricothyrotomy, if necessary, and give positive-pressure resuscitation by any of the acceptable methods, if the apnea still exists.

KEEP PATIENT'S MANDIBLE IN A PROTRUDED POSITION TO AID IN MAINTAINING OF PATENCY.

Q–10 You are removing a fixed bridge when it slips out of your fingers back into the patient's throat. He coughs violently, strains, and his face becomes flushed as he grabs his throat. He then becomes semiconscious and makes a "crowing" sound with his labored shallow breathing. He is becoming increasingly cyanotic. In what order would you perform the following four actions? (1) Give positive pressure oxygen, (2) bend the patient's head between his knees and strike him sharply between the scapulae, (3) stick your finger behind his tongue and attempt to scoop out the foreign body and/or perform the Heimlich manuever, or (4) call your lawyer.

Q–11 Your patient apparently faints but isn't breathing. What would your first two steps be?

(Check answers on p. 560.)

Circulatory Difficulties

Mild Circulatory Depression

Signs and Symptoms

1. Cold sweat and feeling of lightheadedness (vertigo)
2. Weak, thready pulse, rapid rate
3. Decreased blood pressure (depends on normal for patient)
4. Pallor of nails, lips, skin and mucosa
5. Nausea
6. Malaise
7. Cyanosis

Management

1. Shock position (head down, feet up); to raise cerebral blood pressure by autotransfusion of blood from the legs and splanchnic area to the head
2. TLC (tender loving care); reassurance
3. NH_3 pearl inhalants; to act as a respiratory and circulatory stimulant and raise cerebral blood pressure
4. Oxygen by inhalation
5. Cola, coffee or other stimulants after patient is completely aroused
6. Instruction for patient to eat before next appointment
7. Premedication prior to next appointment

Q–12   From memory, list the signs and symptoms of mild circulatory depression.

Q–13   Give two methods of treating lowered cerebral blood pressure and reasons.

Q–14   Why is oxygen given for shock?

Q–15   Why the TLC and coffee?
(Check answers on pp. 560, 561.)

More Severe Circulatory Depression

Signs

Lower blood pressure than in mild depression, a weak pulse, unconsciousness, deepening cyanosis.

Management

1. Treat as mild depression and, if not satisfactory, do as follows:
2. If infusion equipment is available, tape patient's arm to an arm board and start an IV infusion with 500 cc of 5% D&W (dextrose and water), using an 18-gauge or larger needle. The flow rate should be adjusted to 14 to 16 drops per minute. This technique provides an opening into the circulatory system for possible later use in giving IV medications (vasopressors or blood). If patient goes into severe shock, it is very difficult to do a venipuncture. The medication chosen may then be given directly through the rubber receptacle on the infusion set, or mixed with the D&W and administered in the infusion to regulate blood pressure (see Special Techniques, p. 555.)
3. If (2) is not done, medications used must be given by the slower intramuscular, intratracheal, or subcutaneous route (see Special Techniques, p. 556). If patient is hypertensive or has cardiac disease, use mephentermine sulfate (Wyamine) 15 to 30 mg for mild circulatory depression, or 20 mg metaraminol (Aramine) or methoxamine (Vasoxyl) for a severe circulatory depression. These should be given subcutaneously and the patient's pulse should be checked along with the blood pressure for 15 minutes before readministering. Epinephrine can also be used if patient has no cardiac problems. These drugs may also be given intralingually or intratracheally (see Special Techniques, p. 557).
4. Support respiration and other systems as indicated.

Q–16   What is the most normal blood pressure? (1) 160/90, (2) 100/60, (3) 120/80, (4) 110/85, or (5) depends on patient.

Q–17   Your 45-year-old patient loses consciousness, becomes cyanotic, his blood pressure is 80/40 and he does not respond to ammonia inhalants, shock position, or oxygen therapy. What would you do? As far as you know, he is healthy.

Q–18   Your 45-year-old female patient is acutely hypotensive and has a history of MI (myocardial infarction). Her blood pressure is 60/30 presently; normally it is 160/100. What would you do?
(Check answers on p. 561.)

Very Severe Depression (Anaphylaxis or Anaphylactoid Reactions)

Anaphylaxis is an antigen-antibody reaction resulting in complete loss of vasomotor tone.

Signs

1. Usually occurs in seconds up to 2 hours postinjection of the antigen (most patients have a history of allergies).
2. First signs often are asthmatic breathing, urticaria and angioedema. Shock may then follow, or may occur immediately. The angioedema may occur in the tongue or larynx, making a cricothyrotomy necessary.

Management

1. Place patient in shock position and tape on stethoscope diaphragm and sphygmomanometer.
2. Take blood pressure and pulse.
3. Support respiration according to previously stated principles.
4. If cardiac arrest occurs, treat by external cardiac compression.
5. Give 0.5 cc of 1:1000 epinephrine intralingually, intratracheally or subcutaneously and wait, then retake blood pressure. Readminister in 15 minutes if necessary. Other vasopressors may be used. It is wise to start an IV drip; however, since the vessels have collapsed, this is often nearly impossible and the other routes must be used. DO NOT GIVE EPINEPHRINE IV UNLESS DILUTED.
6. Once blood pressure has been stabilized, 50 mg of diphenhydramine HCL (Benadryl) should be given IV slowly over a 3-minute period as an antihistamine (supportive therapy).
7. Hydrocortisone sodium succinate (Solu-Cortef, 100 mg—50 IM and 50 IV) should also be given as supportive therapy to prevent recurrence of shock.
8. If no response occurs to the above and venipuncture is not possible, a venous cutdown should be performed and the IV route maintained by use of a drip infusion. A vasopressor can be added to the D&W and titrated into the patient to support the blood pressure.

THE ABOVE PROCEDURES REPRESENT THE MOST DESIRABLE METHODS AND SEQUENCE OF TREATMENT OF THIS CONDITION. ACTUAL TREATMENT DEPENDS UPON THE FACILITIES, THE PERSONNEL AND THE MATERIALS AVAILABLE.

> **Q–19 Describe signs of anaphylactic shock and its etiology.**
>
> **Q–20 How would you treat a severe drop in blood pressure such as anaphylactic shock?**
>
> **(Check answers on p. 561.)**

Hypertensive Reactions

Cause

1. Fear in patients with arteriosclerotic heart disease.
2. Intravascular injections of vasopressors (usually transient).

CHART ON DIAGNOSIS AND TREATMENT OF COMMON MEDICAL EMERGENCIES

Although it is not necessary to diagnose the specific condition or disorder prior to instituting emergency support therapy (only the system failure), it is helpful to recognize the more common problems. Following is a chart which you should study and then use for future reference.

Condition	Cause	Signs and Symptoms	Treatment
Syncope	Cerebral hypoxia	Skin is pale and moist; pulse rapid at first, then slow and weak; blood pressure falls	Oxygen therapy, elevation of feet, spirits of ammonia
Angina pectoris	Diminished blood supply to the cardiac muscle	Substernal pain of short duration; (pain may radiate to left arm, neck or jaws); blood pressure rises; pulse remains strong	Oxygen therapy, amyl nitrite inhalant or nitroglycerin tablets sublingually
Coronary occlusion	Obstruction of blood supply to part of the myocardium, usually due to thrombosis	Crushing substernal pain of long duration; skin cold, clammy and cyanotic; dyspnea, weak rapid pulse, often irregular; lowered blood pressure	Oxygen therapy; patient in semireclined position; morphine sulfate, 10 to 15 mg IM.
Heart failure	Improper emptying of ventricle (due to fatigue of the cardiac muscle)	Stressed feeling in the chest; dyspnea and cough; peripheral and/or pulmonary edema; cyanosis; distention of cervical veins	Oxygen therapy; patient semireclined; morphine sulfate, 10 to 15 mg IM
Cerebral vascular accident	Hemorrhage, embolism, thrombosis, or spasm of a cerebral artery	Mild dizziness to unconsciousness; varying degree of paresis or paralysis; possible aphagia; headache, nausea and vomiting	Oxygen for impaired respiration; head elevated; don't move patient; no narcotics
Diabetic coma	Faulty carbohydrate metabolism caused by lack of insulin	A gradual loss of consciousness; face flushed, skin dry, eyeballs soft and sunken in sockets; mouth dry; breath with fruity odor; headache, apathy, weakness, abdominal pain, nausea, vomiting	Recognize early in course and obtain medical care; may give sugar to distinguish from insulin shock

Condition	Cause	Symptoms	Treatment
Insulin shock	Hypoglycemia	Profuse sweating and nervousness; headache, dizziness, and mental confusion; transient unconsciousness, convulsions and coma	Glucose orally, sublingually, or intravenously
Epilepsy (grand mal)	Usually idiopathic	Warning aura and cry; unconsciousness; convulsions and coma	Oxygen; firm pad between teeth; loosened clothing
Asthma	Bronchial spasm; may be associated with allergy	Difficult wheezing expiration, cyanosis and productive cough	Oxygen therapy, isoproterenol spray; 1:1000 epinephrine, 0.3 cc sub-Q, or aminophylline, 0.5 gm IV
Anaphylactic shock	Antigen-antibody reaction to drug or foreign protein	Sudden pallor, dyspnea and cyanosis; marked fall in blood pressure; pulse weak or imperceptible	Epinephrine (1:000), 0.5 cc; oxygen; other supportive therapy
Epinephrine reversal reaction	Reflex vasodilation following injection of small doses of epinephrine	Tachycardia, malaise, unconsciousness; fall in blood pressure, usually transient	Oxygen; general reassurance and supportive therapy.

Toxic Reactions (often caused by intravascular injections)

Epinephrine: Patient feels as if he is "flying apart" and has a tachycardia and CNS stimulation
  Treatment: TLC, oxygen—is transient and passes in several minutes

Benzoic acid derivatives (procaine, tetracaine, etc.): Starts with CNS stimulation and then severe depression and convulsions
  Treatment: Support systems as failure occurs and treat convulsions with barbiturates (IV) if indicated

Anilides (Carbocaine, Xylocaine and Citanest): No stimulation, just depression
  Treatment: Support systems as above and use barbiturates for convulsions as needed

Management

1. Keep patient quiet and retake blood pressure.
2. If blood pressure is elevated significantly above normal for the patient, give him a barbiturate and get him to the hospital (get medical advice).
3. If there is anginal pain, treat accordingly (technique covered later).

SPECIFIC DRUGS USED TO LOWER BLOOD PRESSURE ARE DANGEROUS AND SHOULD BE USED ONLY UNDER HOSPITAL CONDITIONS WITH PROPER MEDICAL SUPERVISION.

Hemorrhagic Emergencies (Intraoral)

Causes

Tooth extraction, periodontal treatment, trauma from burs or other surgery, fractures and other accidents can cause hemorrhage. These problems can be further complicated if the patient has systemic hemorrhagic tendencies. The latter possibility emphasizes the importance of a thorough medical history.

Management

1. Most local hemorrhage can be controlled by placing gauze pressure packs over the bleeding surface.
2. Suture tightly over wounds or lacerations, including suturing packs in place and suturing absorbable sponges into extraction wounds.
3. Ruptured vessels (spurters and pumpers) can be clamped with a hemostat and tied off, if in soft tissue. If this occurs in bone, bone wax may be forced into the vessel area or the bone over the area may be crushed, thereby obliterating the vessel opening.
4. Tannic acid and other chemicals are sometimes placed over areas of hemorrhage to help clot formation.
5. Most bleeding from large vessels can be controlled by local pressure. If this will not stop the bleeding, the hospital should be alerted to the possibility that carotid ligation might be necessary and the patient should be taken to the hospital for treatment.
6. Hemorrhage caused by capillary defects or defects in the clotting mechanism (hemophilia, etc.) should be controlled by local measures and the patient should then be taken to a physician for further treatment.

NOTE: (1) Most intraoral hemorrhage is mixed with saliva and looks worse than it really is. (2) With intraoral bleeding, the clots and other debris should be cleared from the mouth so that the exact location of the bleeding can be determined prior to attempts to control same. (3) Once bleeding has been controlled, the patient should be kept quiet and placed in a sitting position. He should not be allowed to rinse his mouth.

Q–21 How would you manage a patient with an acute hypertensive episode and severe chest pain?

Q–22 What is the best emergency method for controlling hemorrhage, regardless of the cause?

**Q–23 How would you control a "spurter" or "pumper" in bone?
(Check answers on p. 561.)**

EQUIPMENT AND DRUGS FOR EMERGENCY USE

Respiratory Equipment

1. Oral airways (selected sizes) (Fig. 19–1)
2. Several suction catheters
3. Tapered 3-way connector (to connect catheter to suction tube; open end closed with finger when in use)
4. Disposable plastic oxygen masks (selected sizes)
5. Resuscitube (S-tube)
6. Oxygen tank, pressure valve and flowmeter with tank stand
7. A self-inflating bag, plus 3 selected size masks (small, medium and large) for use in positive-pressure resuscitation (Figs. 19–2, 19–3)
8. Tracheostomy or cricothyrotomy kit. This should consist of a 10-gauge or larger needle, or an emergency tracheostomy needle (Fig. 19–4)

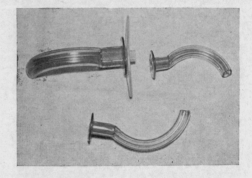

Fig. 19-1. Oral airways and Resuscitube. When respiratory obstruction occurs in an unconscious patient because of the tongue lying against the posterior oral pharynx, an artificial airway may be placed to keep the airway patent.

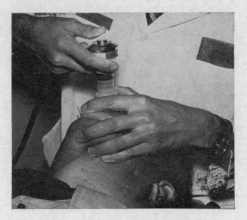

Fig. 19-2. Manually triggered resuscitation unit. An appropriately size mask is selected to cover the nose and mouth. It is positioned as shown and held in place with the thumb and first finger over the mask and the third, fourth and fifth fingers supporting the mandible and extending the head. Oxygen is delivered to the patient by depressing the valve button with the right thumb, as shown.

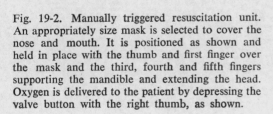

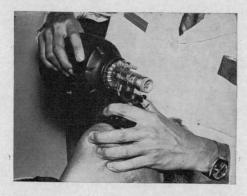

Fig. 19-3. Self-inflating bag. The mask is positioned over the patient's face, as in Fig. 19-2. The self-inflating bag is squeezed to deliver oxygen or air to the patient's lungs.

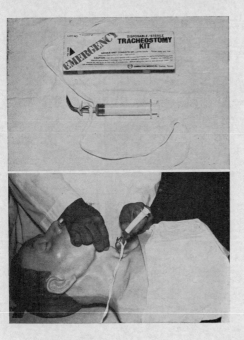

Fig. 19-4. Tracheostomy kit. In the event of an upper respiratory obstruction, when all other measures fail, an emergency tracheostomy should be performed. A small incision through the skin should be made just over the cricothyroid ligament. The tip of the lancet-needle should then be forced through the cricothyroid ligament. As the trachea is entered, air can be aspirated from the syringe. The tip should then be directed inferiorly in such a way that it does not damage the posterior wall of the trachea. The ribbons are secured around the patient's neck to hold the needle in place. Mouth-to-needle resuscitation may be used or oxygen may be directed into the opening, if necessary.

Optional

9. Endotracheal tubes of selected sizes, connectors, mouth prop
10. Anesthetic spray (for vocal cords) and atomizer
11. Laryngoscope and McGill forceps

Cardiovascular Equipment

1. Needles: six each of: 18-, 20- and 25-gauge
2. Syringes: two each of: 1-cc, 5-cc, and 10-cc sizes
3. Sphygmomanometer and stethoscope (diaphragm head) and 1-inch tape
4. Two 500-cc bottles of 5% D&W or lactated Ringer's solution and a venoclysis set.
5. Venous cutdown set; 3-0 silk suture, #15 blades (Bard Parker) and handle, curved mosquito hemostat, rubber gloves and gauze 2 × 2, 14-gauge needle and plastic tubing or Intracath.

Q–24 A self-inflating bag is used for delivering air or oxygen to a patient's lungs artificially? TRUE OR FALSE.

Q–25 A 12-gauge needle inserted through the cricothyroid ligament will provide an adequate airway? TRUE OR FALSE.

Q–26 The purpose of spraying the cords with an anesthetic prior to intubation procedures is to keep then open? TRUE OR FALSE.

Q–27 As the gauge number increases, the outer diameter of a needle decreases? TRUE OR FALSE.

Q–28 McGill forceps are used to hold the tongue during intubation? TRUE OR FALSE.

Q–29 Venous cutdown refers to stripping a vein? TRUE OR FALSE.

(Check answers on pp. 561, 562.)

Stimulants and Vasopressors

NOTE: Emergency drugs should only be used as directed and their indications, the precautions and side effects should be reviewed by reading the brochures accompanying the packages (Fig. 19–5).

Mephentermine Sulfate (Wyamine Sulfate)

Used to correct moderate drops in blood pressure. Works by increasing force of contraction of heart (positive inotropic effect). Good in shock associated with myocardial

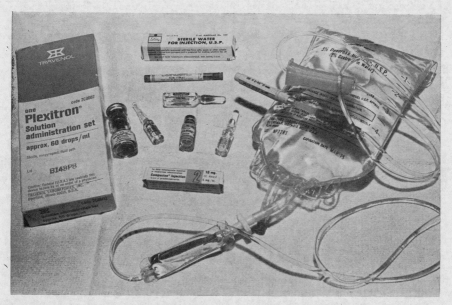

Fig. 19-5. Selected emergency drugs and syringes. A minimum number of selected drugs and syringes should be available in any emergency kit. Single- or multiple-dose vials of most of the drugs covered in this chapter are readily available from pharmacies and hospital or medical supply companies, as are needles, syringes, intravenous solutions and solution administration sets. Always read accompanying directions.

infarction, obstetrics, surgical and spinal anesthesia, mental illness, etc., and has a unique antiarrhythmic action.

Dose: 30 to 45 mg direct IV or IM or 20 cc (30 mg/cc) can be added to 500 cc 5 percent D&W and titrated in IV infusion (drip) to elevate blood pressure.

Metaraminol (Aramine)

Used as a potent vasopressor to increase blood pressure for prolonged duration without tissue slough. Has a direct beneficial effect on myocardium in coronary shock, with few renal effects. No hyperglycemic effects. Can give direct IV or IM. Takes up to 10 minutes to act. Use with care in heart, diabetic, hyperthyroid and hypertensive patients. Because the response is somewhat delayed, care should be taken not to give additional doses too soon, lest the blood pressure be raised too high.

Dose: IM 2 to 10 mg; IV infusion 15 to 100 mg/500 cc of 5 percent D&W slowly and titrated to blood pressure needs; in dire emergency, 5 mg direct IV. Supplied in ampules of 10 mg/cc.

Methoxamine (Vasoxyl)

A prompt, potent vasopressor without cardiac stimulation such as tachycardia or cardiac arrhythmias. For use during spinal anesthesia, to restore blood pressure. Good for shock associated with myocardial infarction.

Dose: 15 mg IM or, if blood pressure below 60 mm, 5 mg IV followed by IV infusion containing 35 mg/250 cc 5 percent D&W. Use with care in hypertensives and hyperthyroids. Overdose may give headaches, vomiting, urinary retention, etc., as with other vasopressors. Good for epinephrine reversal reactions, and relatively safe. Supplied in 20 mg/cc ampules or 10 mg/cc, 10-cc ampules.

Adrenalin (Epinephrine 1:1000)

A very potent vasopressor which produces peripheral vasoconstriction and stimulates the heart, increasing the cardiac output. Specifically indicated in severe allergic reactions, anaphylaxis, severe asthma and shock. Contraindicated in hyperthyroidism, heart disease and in patients taking phenothiazine derivatives and monoamine oxidase inhibitors (MAOI).

Dose: 0.2 to 0.5 cc of 1:1000 solution, intralingually, subcutaneously, or diluted and injected intratracheally. Do not use IM and use IV cautiously only after diluting. May be repeated after checking results and blood pressure, every 15 to 30 minutes.

Aromatic Spirits of Ammonia Inhalant (2-cc Pearls)

A mild respiratory and circulatory stimulant for use in syncope or other mild hypotensive reactions. Slowly approach the nostrils with the broken pearl to prevent a violent response, especially when the patient is still conscious.

Q–30 List four cardiovascular stimulants, their average dosage and routes of administration.

Q–31 Which vasopressor is best for anaphylaxis and asthma and what are the precautions?

Q–32 In shock associated with possible myocardial infarction, which vasopressors would you use?

Q–33 Match the following:

Usual Dosage

a) 35 mg IV
b) 5 mg IV
c) 0.5 cc of 1:1000

Generic Name

a) metaraminol
b) mephetermine sulfate
c) epinephrine
d) methoxamine

Dosage	Trade Name	Generic Name
_____	Vasoxyl	_____
_____	Adrenalin	_____
_____	Aramine	_____
_____	Wyamine	_____

Coronary Dilators (for Angina Pectoris)

Glyceryl Trinitrate (Nitroglycerin) 0.4 mg (1/150 grains)

Used in the prevention and treatment of angina pectoris. The patient will usually give a history of this condition. Placed sublingually and may be used up to 10 times a day. Overdosage will cause a fall in blood pressure.

Amyl Nitrite Inhalant (Pearls)

A coronary dilator for use in angina pectoris and has short duration of action. Also useful in acute asthmatic attacks.

Anticonvulsants and Sedatives

Secobarbital or pentobarbital sodium (Seconal Sodium or Nembutal Sodium) Injectable (50 mg/cc): A sedative, hypnotic and a good anticonvulsant. Care should be used in persons with liver damage or those in extreme pain (produces excitement). For convulsions, give IV or IM at a dosage sufficient to control.

Dose: 100 to 200 mg, given slowly IV or IM (oral route not practical here)

NOTE: Ideally a more rapid acting barbiturate would be desirable but their aqueous solutions are unstable and have a limited shelf life.

Analgesics (Narcotics)

Meperidine (Demerol)

An excellent analgesic midway between codeine and morphine in potency. Also antispasmodic, antisialogogic and has sedative effects. Little effect on blood pressure and respiratory rate or cardiac function. Good for use in pain of myocardial infarction and other types of severe pain. Care should be used in unconscious patients or those with head injuries.

Dose: 100 mg IM or orally (every 4 hours).

Morphine Sulfate

A very good analgesic for use in severe pain. Some tendency to produce nausea and decreased respiratory rate and depth. Good for use in myocardial infarction or other severe pain. Do not use in presence of unconsciousness or head injuries or when there is respiratory distress.

Dose: 8 to 15 mg orally or IM.

NOTE: Narcotics depress respiration and increase cerebrospinal fluid pressure.

Antihistamine, Antistress and Antiasthmatic Drugs

Diphenhydramine HCl (Benadryl)

For use in allergic reactions such as urticaria, or in support of therapy for anaphylaxis. Also good for nausea, and as a sedative for emotional disturbances especially in children. USE WITH CARE IN PATIENTS WITH HYPERTENSION AND DO NOT INJECT SUBCUTANEOUSLY OR PERIVASCULARLY. Use IV or IM.

Dose: 50 to 100 mg given slowly IV or IM or half and half.

Hydrocortisone Sodium Succinate (Solu-Cortef)

For use in status asthmaticus and severe allergic drug reactions, or as an adjunct to standard therapy in anaphylactic reactions. Also used in patients with a history of previous steroid therapy or who have acute adrenocortical insufficiency such as that produced by stress in patients with Addison's disease.

Dose: 100 mg IV or IM or half and half. Also, 100 mg may be added to 250 or 500 cc of 5 percent D&W and used in an IV infusion. Methyl prednisolone and some other corticoids may be substituted, but dosage varies with the product.

Aminophylline

An excellent drug for use in acute asthmatic attacks when other measures fail. It acts to relax smooth muscles and as a diuretic and cardiac stimulant. It may give some degree of CNS stimulation.

Dose: 500 mg IV very slowly.

Epinephrine (Adrenalin)

A very potent antiasthmatic and antiallergic drug. Also a potent vasopressor. Refer to previously detailed information.

Q–34 Why is the oral route of barbiturate administration impractical for control of convulsions? (1) Hard to give oral medication to convulsing patient, (2) patient might get obstructed from capsule, (3) therapeutic blood level is obtained slowly.

Q–35 How does a barbiturate control convulsions?

Q—36 Morphine sulfate is more potent than meperidine, dose for dose, but care should be exercised in using both for patients with head injuries because: (1) patient may become nauseous, (2) euphoria produced may mask a more serious injury, (3) narcotics increase cerebrospinal fluid pressure.

Q—37 Nitroglycerin is a dilator of the coronary artery and is usually administered IM? TRUE OR FALSE?

Q—38 Benadryl is an antihistamine which is also a sedative and antiemetic. It should be given slowly IV? TRUE OR FALSE.

Q—39 Solu-Cortef or other corticoids are used in emergencies to reduce inflammation? TRUE OR FALSE.

Q—40 Aminophyllin is a choice over epinephrine for acute severe asthmatic attacks or other allergies of a sudden severe nature? TRUE OR FALSE.

(Check answers on p. 562.)

SPECIAL EMERGENCY TECHNIQUES
Cardiopulmonary Resuscitation (Figs. 19-6, 19-7)

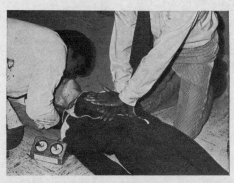

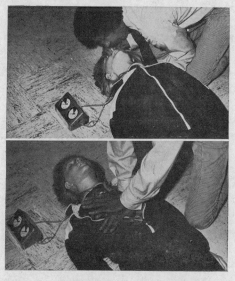

Fig. 19–6. Cardiopulmonary resuscitation with two rescuers. *Cardiac compression:* the heel of the right hand is placed over the lower one-half of the sternum (not including the xiphoid process). The left hand is then placed over the right hand, as shown. Both arms are kept straight. The rescuer leans forward depressing the sternum 1½ to 2 inches 60 to 80 times/minute. Care should be taken to keep the fingertips away from the rib cage so as not to fracture ribs during compression. *Mouth-to-mouth breathing:* The airway is first cleared. With the right hand the neck is supported and with the left hand the nostrils are held closed and head extended. The rescuer inflates the mannequin (patient's) lungs at the end of every fifth chest compression cycle. If the two activities are coordinated properly, there is no need for hesitation in either case.

Fig. 19-7. Cardiopulmonary resuscitation with one rescuer. Initially, in the event of cardiac arrest or ventricular fibrillation, a quick karate chop type of blow with no follow through, directly to the lower half of the sternum, may reestablish normal sinus rhythm. If this fails then: *above,* start by ventilating the patient with four quick breaths, *lower,* provide 15 compressions at a rate of 60 to 80 per minute followed by two more quick breaths. Thenceforth, maintain a rate of 15 compressions followed by two quick breaths followed by 15 more compressions, etc.

Diagnosis of cardiac arrest based on apnea, cyanosis, lack of pulse and dilated, non-responsive pupils.

1. Place victim flat on his back on a hard surface
2. If unconscious, open airway
   a. lift neck
   b. push forehead back
   c. clear out mouth if necessary
   d. observe for breathing
3. If not breathing, begin artificial breathing by administering *four* quick full breaths to the victim.
4. Check carotid pulse
5. If pulse absent, begin artificial circulation by depressing sternum 1½ to 2 inches, using heel of hand on lower half of sternum.
   a. one rescuer: 15 compressions at a rate of 80/min followed by 2 quick breaths.
   b. two rescuers: 5 compressions at a rate of 60/min followed by 1 quick breath.
6. Continue uninterrupted until victim responds or advanced life support is available.

NOTE: If it is known that arrest has been present for over 10 minutes, cardiac compression is not likely to be successful. However, resuscitation should be attempted if there is any doubt.

Mouth-to-Mouth Breathing or Ventilation

1. Tilt head all the way back and protrude mandible
2. Clear airway and place artificial airway if needed
3. Pinch victim's nostrils closed and completely seal victim's mouth with yours
4. Take deep breaths and blow into the victim's mouth at the rate of 12 times per minute. Watch for victim's chest to rise

SUPPLEMENT THIS WITH PRACTICE ON MANNEQUINS AND ADDITIONAL STUDY. PROGRAMS ARE AVAILABLE THROUGH THE AMERICAN HEART ASSOCIATION AND OTHER AGENCIES (see list at end of chapter).

> Q—41 Which findings indicate cardiac arrest or ventricular fibrillation? (1) Pupillary constriction, (2) apnea, (3) cyanosis, (4) convulsions.
>
> Q—42 When performing external cardiac massage, you should depress the sternum? (1) 1 to 1½ inches, (2) 1½ to 2 inches, (3) 2 to 2½ inches.
>
> Q—43 Mouth-to-mouth breathing (only) should be at a rate of . . .? (1) 8 times per minute, (2) 12 times per minute, (3) 18 times per minute.
>
> Q—44 Protruding the mandible prevents the patient from swallowing his tongue? TRUE OR FALSE.
>
> (Check answers on p. 562.)

Use of Bag and Mask (Figs. 19-2, 19-3)

A self-filling bag is recommended.
Apneic Patient

1. Secure a patent airway.

2. Select mask of sufficient size to fit over nose and mouth.

3. Attach mask to connector on bag.

4. Open tank valve and set flowmeter 3 to 4 liters per minute or to a rate which will keep enough oxygen in bag to meet demands of patient.

5. Place mask over patient's face, with connector between thumb and first finger and with third and fourth fingers supporting mandible in a protruded position. STAND BEHIND PATIENT FOR THIS PROCEDURE.

6. Compress bag with free hand to inflate patient's lungs and raise chest. This should be repeated every 3 to 4 seconds.

NOTE: Leaks around the mask usually occur between nose and eyes of the patient. This usually can be corrected by repositioning the mask, by using a smaller mask, or by adjusting the pressure in a more inferior direction.

Assisting Respiration

This technique is used when a patient is breathing, but the depth of inspiration is insufficient. The technique is the same as for the apneic patient except that the bag is compressed with each inspiration of the patient, assisting same and increasing the inspiratory volume.

Oxygen for the Breathing, Conscious Patient

Here the above procedure is adhered to with the exception that the patient is allowed to inspire the oxygen without assistance from bag and mask.

NOTE: Most resuscitation equipment comes with instructions. It is essential that you practice resuscitation under qualified supervision in order to become adept.

Cricothyrotomy (Tracheostomy)

1. The cricothyroid ligament is located by palpating the thyroid cartilage (Adam's apple) and the cricoid cartilage which lies just inferior. The C-T ligament is located between the two. A 10-gauge or larger needle is then forced through the skin and C-T ligament and secured in place, care being taken not to damage the posterior tracheal wall (Fig. 19—4). ADDITIONAL STUDY, INCLUDING PRACTICAL DEMONSTRATIONS, IS HIGHLY RECOMMENDED.

2. Alternatively, a midline incision is made from above the thyroid cartilage to just below the cricoid and the edges of the incision are retracted laterally. The C-T ligament is then noted and a transverse incision is made through this ligament, thereby entering the trachea. The opening is dilated with a suitable instrument. A compressible bivalve cannula or other suitable hollow obturator (tracheostomy needle) is used to maintain the opening. This is held in place with tape or string. WHEN ENTERING THE TRACHEA, CARE MUST BE TAKEN NOT TO DAMAGE THE POSTERIOR WALL OF THE TRACHEA.

3. *Adequate suction* should be available all during this procedure to secure a clear, visible field.

4. After the airway is secured, an oxygen supply should be either attached or placed in close proximity to the opening. (Mouth-to-stoma artificial resuscitation may be required if oxygen equipment is not readily accessible.)

5. Other indicated emergency measures should be continued as indicated.

Q–45 Describe the use of oxygen and a bag and mask to artificially ventilate an apneic patient.

Q–46 The most frequent leak around a mask (which is of proper size for the patient can be corrected by . . .? (1) adjusting pressure and repositioning, (2) moving mask more inferiorly.

Q–47 Assisting respirations is accomplished by compressing the bag at beginning of the patient's inspiratory cycle?

Q–48 Describe the use of a 10-gauge needle to open an obstructed airway?

Q–49 Describe the surgery involved in a cricothyrotomy (tracheostomy)?

Intubation

This is a special skill requiring practical experience.

1. If all equipment is available and *the patient is unconscious,* this is a valuable procedure in certain emergencies.

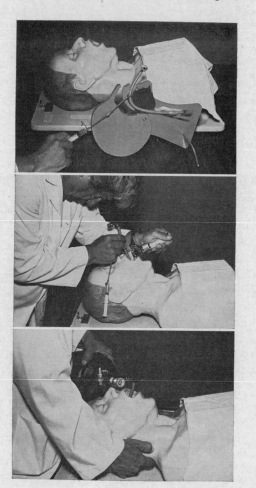

Fig. 19-8. Intubation procedure. *Upper,* the cuffed endotracheal tube is overlying the space it will occupy when the mannequin (patient) is intubated. *Middle,* the blade of the laryngoscope is used to displace the tongue and epiglottis anteriorly, exposing the cords and allowing the passage of the endotracheal tube tip beyond that opening. *Lower,* the cuff is then inflated with the syringe, the connecting tube clamped with a hemostat and an oxygen delivery system attached.

2. The unconscious, apneic patient is placed in Trendelenburg position, and the oral pharynx is aspirated free of mucus, vomitus, and foreign matter.

3. The head is extended and the mandible is held in a protruded position. The blade of a laryngoscope is placed posterior to the tongue, which is then retracted anteriorly (Fig. 19–8).

4. The vocal cords are then visualized and sprayed with 0.5 cc of local anesthetic.

5. A suitably sized endotracheal tube with a connector and a cuff is then inserted into the trachea.

6. The cuff is inflated by use of a syringe filled with air and attached to the tube cuff. The tube to the cuff is clamped with a hemostat.

7. Oxygen is forced into the endotracheal tube to assure that it is placed properly (the chest will rise).

8. The apparatus is attached to self-filling bag (or other positive-pressure device) and resuscitation is begun. BE SURE TO PLACE BITE BLOCK BETWEEN TEETH TO PREVENT PATIENT FROM CLAMPING DOWN ON TUBE, OBSTRUCTING IT.

9. When patient begins to breathe on his own and cough violently, the tube may be removed by deflating the cuff (releasing the hemostat), placing the rubber suction catheter down the center of the endotracheal tube, and pulling both out of the patient's mouth simultaneously. THIS LATTER TECHNIQUE REQUIRES A HIGH DEGREE OF SKILL AND PREVIOUS EXPERIENCE AND IS PRESENTED ONLY AS A REVIEW FOR USE BY THOSE WITH PREVIOUS TRAINING AND EXPERIENCE.

Parenteral Administration (Routes and Techniques)

NOTE: Only drugs marked as such should be given parenterally.

Venipuncture (for Direct Injection or for Starting IV Infusion)

1. Use 18-gauge 1½-inch needle preferably (especially if infusion), in case blood is to be given later (Fig. 19–9).

2. Force solution to end of needle to clear out air bubbles.

3. Locate large vein in antecubital area or on back of hand. If doing infusion, tape arm to board with 1-inch tape.

4. Place tourniquet above vessel to be entered.

5. Slap area sharply over vein and/or let arm hang below level of rest of body to create distention of the vein.

6. Wipe area over vein with alcohol sponge.

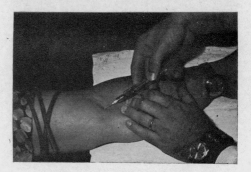

Fig. 19-9. Venipuncture technique as described in text. Note that fourth finger is pulling back on syringe plunger, producing a negative pressure so that when the vein is entered blood will appear. The tourniquet is then released.

7. Insert needle with bevel up, through the skin, about ⅛-inch lateral to vein and parallel to same.
8. Pull skin with inserted needle over vein with thumb of left hand.
9. Enter vein with tip of needle and thread needle a short distance into the vein.
10. Release tourniquet.
11. Check to see if in vein by aspirating (if using infusion set, squeeze rubber connector to get blood back up in the tube). If blood rushes back into the syringe without effort in aspirating, you may be in an artery. In that case, withdraw needle and apply pressure over the site of injection.
12. Place a piece of tape over needle just below the hub and adjust the stopcock to 14 to 16 drops per minute if using infusion (drip). Otherwise, if injecting a drug directly, do so very *slowly*.
13. When removing needle, do so rapidly and hold piece of alcohol cotton under pressure over puncture site.
14. If venipuncture is unsuccessful and a hematoma begins to develop, constant pressure and/or cold packs will often prevent its progression. Don't worry about this, however, if there is an emergency.

Intramuscular Injections (Slower Absorption)

A 1-inch, 20- to 22-gauge needle should be used. The insertion should be made perpendicular to the surface and deep into the muscle. The best sites are either the deltoid muscle or the upper, outer quadrant of the buttocks. Always aspirate prior to injection and do not inject more than 2 cc in any one site. Do not give epinephrine by this route as muscle necrosis may occur (Fig. 19–10).

Venous Cutdown

To be used when a venipuncture cannot be accomplished because of collapsed veins, etc.
1. Locate the vein to be cannulated (a branch of the saphenous goes through a groove on the medial surface of the ankle).
2. Make incision through the skin with a scalpel beside and parallel to vein.
3. Use a curved mosquito hemostat and blunt dissection, with a gauze sponge to keep field dry and clear. Locate the vein and isolate it.
4. Place two separate pieces of 3-0 silk suture under the vein and tie off the vein at its most distal point with one of the sutures.

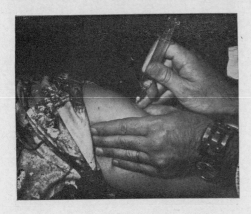

Fig. 19-10. Intramuscular injection technique as described in text. Needle should be inserted into muscle in a quick dart-like fashion using the fourth and fifth fingers as a stop.

Fig. 19-11. Intralingual injection technique as described in text.

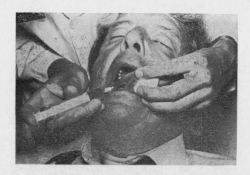

5. Enter vein just proximal to tie-off with a large-bore needle (18-gauge) and tie other suture around vein and needle. A venous cannula may be used if available.
6. Tape needle down carefully and close incision later, if necessary.
7. Aspirate blood through needle and then attach administration set after clearing the tubing of air.
8. Set drip rate for 14 to 16 per minute, by opening the stopcock on the tubing.
9. To administer direct IV drugs, use a syringe with a 25-gauge needle, close stopcock and inject through the gum rubber connector. Then reopen stopcock to original rate.
10. If dripping stops at any time, carefully move the needle to assure that it is not obstructed by the wall of the vein and attempt to reestablish the patency of the system.

Intralingual Injection (for Vasopressors)

A ½-inch, 25-gauge needle should be used and the injection should be made into the musculature of the tongue on its inferior surface. Absorption into the bloodstream by this method is quite rapid and, because of the good circulation, necrosis should not occur, even if 1:1000 epinephrine is given (Fig. 19–11).

Intratracheal Injection (Diluted Epinephrine Only)

Using a 5-cc syringe and an 18-gauge or larger needle, withdraw ½ cc of 1:1000 epinephrine. Then dilute with saline or sterile water. Locate the cricothyroid ligament and

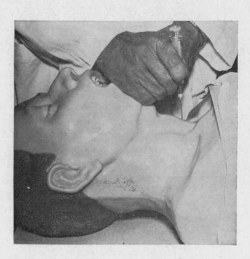

Fig. 19-12. Intratracheal injection technique as described in text.

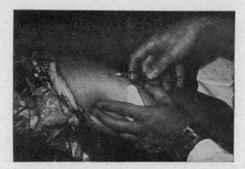

Fig. 19-13. Subcutaneous injection. Barrel of syringe should be closely parallel to surface of skin so that needle enters at an acute angle and does not go too deeply.

force needle through skin and this ligament; then aspirate. Aspiration of air indicates needle is in trachea. Inject solution. Patient will usually cough and solution will spray into the respiratory tree where it will be rapidly absorbed. This is a good alternative route for acute asthma and anaphylactic shock (Fig. 19–12).

Subcutaneous Injections (for Vasopressors)

A ½-inch, 25-gauge needle should be used. The deltoid region is a good location. The solution is deposited just beneath the skin. Always aspirate prior to injection to prevent intravascular injection (Fig. 19–13).

THE DEVELOPMENT AND MAINTENANCE OF SKILLS IN PARENTERAL ADMINISTRATION COMES FROM SUPERVISED PRACTICE.

MISCELLANEOUS SPECIAL TECHNIQUES

Vomiting Patient

1. Remove trap from cuspidor to prevent overflowing.
2. Help patient hold head over cuspidor to vomit.
3. After patient begins to feel better, give cola drink or antiemetic medication such as Compazine (See *Physicians' Desk Reference*).

Suspected Coronary Occlusion

Characterized by severe precordial pain often radiating to left arm, neck and jaws. Also frequently accompanied with dyspnea and shock.

Treatment: Get immediate medical assistance. Place patient in semireclining position and keep him calm and comfortable. Loosen constrictive clothing and give oxygen. Upon advice of physician, give patient morphine sulfate 8 to 15 mg IM. Institute other supportive procedures as indicated in the specific instance. Get patient to nearest emergency ward as soon as possible.

Acute Hypoglycemic Reactions

Occurs usually in the morning. Often patient has not had breakfast and is quite anxious and weak. Here loss of consciousness is associated with a strong pulse and much sweating. This can occur in non-diabetics as well as in diabetics who have taken an overdose of insulin.

Treatment: Shock position, oxygen and other supportive therapy. After patient responds well, give candy or sugar to help elevate the blood glucose level. IV glucose may be given.

Epinephrine Reversal Reactions

Small amounts of epinephrine (such as those in local anesthetic solutions) may cause a reflex fall in blood pressure. This usually occurs shortly after injection of a local anesthetic containing epinephrine. It is difficult to diagnose this condition accurately or to differentiate it from other causes of shock.

Treatment: Shock position and other supportive measures as needed and described earlier for shock.

Toxic Reactions to Local Anesthetics (from Intravascular Injections)

Benzoic acid derivatives (procaine, etc.) produce a stimulation followed by depression while amide derivatives (Xylocaine, Carbocaine, etc.) initially produce depression.

Prevention: Use aspirating syringe.

Treatment: Barbiturates (IV) for convulsions and other indicated supportive therapy.

Heimlich Maneuver

Acute airway obstruction from dentures, food and foreign bodies of all kinds is not uncommon.

Treatment: Attempts to dislodge foreign bodies by inverting the individual and administering a sharp blow between the scapulae or by using the fingers sometimes fail. Prior to performing a cricothyrotomy the Heimlich maneuver should be attempted. This consists of: (Fig. 19—14)

1. Standing behind the victim and wrapping your arms around his chest.
2. Making a fist with one hand and clasping it with the other hand against the victim's upper abdomen. With the victim drooped forward, give a quick inward

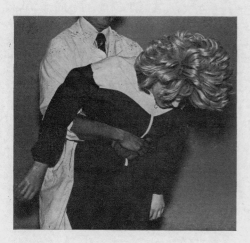

Fig. 19-14. Heimlich maneuver as described in text.

thrust at about the level of the diaphragm. This compresses air trapped in the lungs and will often dislodge a foreign body. If successful, other supportive measures should be performed. (If results are not obtained and obstruction persists, laryngoscopy or cricothyrotomy is indicated.)

ANSWER KEY (with Feedback)

A-1　TRUE is probably correct: You should have at least a minimum of equipment, drugs and know-how, plus a prearranged emergency plan. It would be advisable to practice dry runs so your auxiliaries also know what they should do. The moral issue of responsibility to your fellow man, however, certainly far overrides any legal responsibility imposed upon you. If you answered FALSE, you must be thinking that no law explicitly requires any particular obligation for you toward your patient. However, you should certainly feel the moral obligation.

A-2　(1)　Partially correct
　　　　(2)　Partially correct
　　　　(3)　Partially correct
　　　　(4)　Correct. A good medical history encompasses most conditions which might lead to an emergency.
　　　　If you had trouble, reread the text information.

A-3　TRUE is correct. Nice going, but this was a gift.

A-4　FALSE is correct. Don't waste time on specific etiology. Diagnose the system failure and give supportive therapy, then consider specific etiology.

A-5　Refer to text page 536.

A-6　Refer to text page 536.

A-7　The correct order is 3, 4, 1, 2; however, medical assistance could be in any position. If you didn't check respiration and circulation first and second or second and third, however, your answer was incorrect.

A-8　Check answer with text preceding the question.

A-9　Your first concern should be with getting oxygen to the patient's lungs. If you interpreted the question to indicate mechanical obstruction, (4) would be appropriate; if you were not considering obstruction, (1) could be correct; if you considered the patient to have a severe asthmatic attack, (3) could be correct depending on your competency. (2) would be correct only if a physician was immediately available in person or by phone or if you had already assumed initial respiratory support and were considering more definitive therapy.

A-10　(2) and (3) first or second; if dislodge, then (1); if obstruction remains, you may still attempt to force oxygen, but be careful not to force the foreign body further down the throat. You might use a 10-gauge needle for a cricothyrotomy. Get assistance fast.

A-11　(1) Aspirate oral pharynx (obtain patency), and give positive-pressure resuscitation. (2) Check for circulatory deficiency.

A-12　Refer to text page 539.

A—13 (1) Shock position: Lets pooled blood in legs and splanchnic area flow by gravity to head. (2) NH_3 inhalants: Stimulates circulation.

A—14 Oxygen is given to provide a maximum concentration of this gas in the inspired air. Since circulation is poor, only minimum oxygen is picked up in the lungs and carried to the brain; if there is a higher concentration of oxygen in the inspired air, theoretically more will get into the bloodstream and hence to the brain, even without improved circulation.

A—15 To relax the patient and to stimulate respiration and circulation.

A—16 (5) is the most correct; however, (3) and (4) would certainly be considered within normal range. Normalcy, however, depends on the patient and you should have a base-line blood pressure under normal conditions. Extremes such as diastolic over 100 or systolic under 100 are usually considered abnormal. It is possible for a patient to be in shock with a blood pressure of 120/80, if his *usual* blood pressure is very high. The mean figure or normal is 120/80.

A—17 (1) Continue oxygen therapy and shock position. (2) Administer (a) 1:1000 epinephrine 0.5 cc subcutaneously, intratracheally, or intralingually or (b) mephentermine (Wyamine) IM, subcutaneously or intralingually if patient has a history of heart disease. (3) Recheck blood pressure and repeat, if necessary. (4) Get medical assistance.

A—18 (1) Maintain airway and support respiration. (2) Attempt to start an IV drip with 5 percent D&W or lactated Ringer's solution, then slowly titrate a vasopressor (Vasoxyl or Aramine) to elevate the blood pressure. (3) Use an alternate route of administration if veins are collapsed.

A—19 (1) A true antigen-antibody reaction resulting in tissue release of histamine and a generalized vasodilatation. (2) Usually occurs soon after antigen administration (penicillin, local anesthetic, bee sting, etc.). (3) Starts with asthmatic breathing, then urticaria and laryngeal edema followed by decreased blood pressure and ultimately cardiac arrest. (4) Shock possibly occurring immediately without the intermediate signs.

A—20 (1) Maintain adequate ventilation. (2) Shock position of patient. (3) Give 1:1000 epinephrine 0.5 cc subcutaneously, intralingually, diluted intratracheally or intravenously, or (4) start IV if possible, and give diluted vasopressors, slowly into rubber receptacle on the infusion set or diluted in the solution. (5) Follow-up with diphenhydramine HCl (Benadryl) and hydrocortisone sodium succinate (Solu-Cortef). (6) If can't get IV started, do 1, 2, and 3, then do venous cutdown. (7) Administer CPR if cardiac arrest occurs.

A—21 (1) Keep patient quiet. (2) Get medical assistance. (3) Consider use of barbiturates and nitroglycerin. (4) Obviously, maintain adequate ventilation.

A—22 Pressure over bleeding site.

A—23 (1) Force bone wax into vessel channel, or (2) crush bone over channel opening.

A—24 TRUE. This bag has a spring-back ability and can be used with or without connection to an oxygen source.

A—25 FALSE. It has been shown that a 10-gauge or larger needle (preferably 8-gauge) inserted into the trachea through the cricothyroid ligament will provide an adequate airway.

A–26 TRUE. This anesthetizes the recurrent laryngeal and other efferent nerves to the cords, preventing closure of the cords during intubation. As you know, the vocal cords close in response to anything foreign in the area, as a protective mechanism.

A–27 TRUE. Therefore, a 10-gauge needle has a larger diameter than an 18-gauge. You might be interested to know that in general an 18-gauge is considered minimal size for aspiration or administration of blood; therefore, it is wise to start an IV infusion with this or a larger needle in case blood is needed later.

A–28 FALSE. McGill forceps are used to grasp and slide the endotracheal tube past the cords and into the trachea. The cords are viewed during this procedure through a laryngoscope.

A–29 FALSE. Venous cutdown refers to surgically exposing and cannulating a vein.

A–30 Check your answer with the text material.

A–31 Adrenalin (epinephrine) 1:1000, 0.5 cc subcutaneously, intralingually or intra-tracheally, and IV if diluted and titrated while monitoring the blood pressure. Caution in hyperthyroids, existing heart disease and patients on phenothiazide and MAOI medication as reactive effects might occur.

A–32 (1) Wyamine Sulfate—moderate potency, (2) Aramine or (3) Vasoxyl.

A–33

b	Vasoxyl	d
c	Adrenalin	c
b	Aramine	a
a	Wyamine	b

A–34 (1), (2) and (3).

A–35 Decreases the irritability of the cerebral cortex.

A–36 (3) is the best answer, but (1) and (2) are also true. Narcotics may complicate a head injury by further elevating CSF pressure, causing further brain damage or death.

A–37 FALSE. Given by sublingual tablet.

A–38 TRUE. You should be careful not to infiltrate perivascularly since it is irritating to tissues.

A–39 FALSE. They are used because of their remarkable antistress activities and in adrenal insufficiency. Since they act more slowly, they should be used after more immediate treatment has been instituted.

A–40 FALSE. Adrenalin (epinephrine) would be the treatment first, then later aminophylline in refractory cases of asthma.

A–41 (2) and (3) are correct.

A–42 (2) is correct.

A–43 (2) is correct.

A–44 TRUE. In essence, however, you really cannot swallow your tongue. Obviously, this refers to the tongue falling back against the posterior oral pharynx blocking the airway. Protruding the mandible unblocks the airway because the tongue is attached to the lingual surface of the mandible at the genial tubercles. Placement of an artificial airway also helps.

A–45   Check the text.

A–46   (1) and (2).

A–47   FALSE. Just as the inspiratory cycle ends.

A–48   Check the text.

A–49   Check the text.

SUMMARY

No final chapter questions have been provided because further instruction is indicated in order to assure competency in the procedures described. It is suggested that the objectives listed at the beginning of this chapter now be reviewed.

This chapter has covered the principles and techniques necessary to recognize, diagnose and provide supportive care for patients in an emergency life-threatening situation. It is highly recommended that this chapter be supplemented with additional study and practice using mannequins and simulations.

Special courses, brochures, manuals, pamphlets, discussion guides, movies, videotapes and other study information are readily available from the American Dental Association, the American Medical Association, the American Heart Association, the National High Blood Pressure Education Program and other sources. A partial list is included herein.

AUDIOVISUAL AND OTHER INSTRUCTIONAL PROGRAMS

Slide—Audiotape Programs

1. *Cardiopulmonary Resuscitation,* 30 min, Dr. Thomas B Fast, Box J-425, MSB, University of Florida, College of Dentistry, Gainesville, Florida, 32610.
2. *Cricothyrotomy,* 20 min, Dr. Thomas B Fast.
3. *Drug Administration* (Parts I, II, III), 75 min, Dr. Thomas B Fast.

16-mm Films

1. *Pulse of Life,* 30 min, American Heart Association, 44 East 23rd St., New York, New York, 10010.
2. *Life in Balance,* 25 min, American Heart Association.
3. *Prescription for Life,* 25 min, American Heart Association.
4. *Emergency Airway,* 20 min, Department of Audiovisual Education, Kansas University Medical Center, Kansas City, Kansas 66103.
5. *Dental Office Emergencies* (Parts I, II, III, IV), 60 min, Veterans' Administration Central Office Film Library, 810 Vermont Ave., N. W., Washington, D. C. 20409
6. *Endotracheal Intubation,* 20 min, Medical Skills Library, ROCOM Division of Hoffmann-LaRoche Inc., Nutley, New Jersey 07110.
7. *Venous Cutdown,* 20 min, Medical Skills Library.
8. *Tracheostomy,* 20 min, Medical Skills Library.

Texts and Manuals

1. Henderson, J., *Emergency Medical Guide*, 3rd Ed., McGraw-Hill Book Co., 1221 Avenue of the Americas, New York, New York 10020.
2. *Standards for Cardiopulmonary Resuscitation and Emergency Cardiac Care*, J.A.M.A., Vol. 227, No. 7, February 18, 1974. Reprints of this supplement are available from the American Heart Association, 44 East 23rd St., New York, New York 10010.
3. *Cardiopulmonary Resuscitation: A Manual for Instructors*, American Heart Association, (EM-408E), 1967.
4. *The Dentist's Role in Cardiopulmonary Resuscitation*, American Heart Association, (EM-407A), 1968.
5. *Emergency Measures in Cardiopulmonary Resuscitation*, American Heart Association, (EM-376A, rev. PE), 1969.
6. *Definitive Therapy in Cardiopulmonary Resuscitation*, American Heart Association, (EM-377A, rev. PE), 1971.
7. *Recommendations for Human Blood Pressure Determination by Sphygmomanometers*, American Heart Association, (EM-34, rev. PE), 1967.

Specialists in Emergency Equipment and Training Aids

1. Laerdal Medical Corporation
   1 Labriola Ct.
   Armonk, New York 10504
2. All Florida Rescue
   990 Old Dixie Highway
   Lake Park, Florida 33403
3. Medical Supply Company
   1027 West State Street
   Rockford, Illinois 61101
4. Healthfirst Corporation
   P.O. Box 279
   Edmonds, Washington 98020
5. Para Medical Devices, Inc.
   1893 Grand Ave.
   Baldwin, New York 11510
6. Robert J. Brady Company
   Bowie, Maryland 20715

BIBLIOGRAPHY

Berlove, I. J.: *Dental-Medical Emergencies and Complications*, 2nd Ed., Chicago, Year Book Medical Publishers, 1963.

Eiseman, B., Spencer, F. and Dachi, S. F.: The role of the dentist in the diagnosis and prevention of cerebrovascular accidents, Oral Surg., *16*, 1174, 1963.

Jude, J. R., Kouwenhoven, W. B. and Knickerbocker, G. G.: *Essentials of External Cardiopulmonary Resuscitation*, Philadelphia, Smith, Kline & French Laboratories, 1962.

Management of Dental Problems in Patients with Cardiovascular Disease, report of a working conference jointly sponsored by the American Dental Association and American Heart Association, J. Amer. Dent. Ass., *68*, 333, 1964.

The Merck Manual, 12th Ed., West Point (Pa.), Merck, Sharp & Dohme Research Laboratories, 1972.

Parnell, A. G.: Adrenal crisis and the dental surgeon, Brit. Dent. J., *116*, 294, 1964.

Physicians' Desk Reference, 31st Ed., Oradell (N.J.), Medical Economics, Inc., 1977.

Appendix

Table 1. Normal Laboratory Values*

Blood Plasma or Serum Values

Determination	Material Used	Normal Value
Acetoacetate plus acetone	Serum	0.3–2.0 mg%
Amylase	Serum	80–150 Somogyi units/100 ml
Ascorbic acid	Blood	0.4–1.5 mg%
Bilirubin (van den Bergh test)	Serum	One minute: 0.4 mg% Direct: 0.4 mg% Total: 0.7 mg% Indirect is total minus direct
Blood volume		8.5–9.0% body weight in kg
Bromsulphalein (BSP)	Serum	Less than 5% retention
Calcium	Serum	8.5–10.5 mg% (slightly higher in children)
Carbon dioxide content	Serum	50–70 vol% 26–28 mEq/liter, 20–26 mEq/liter in infants as (HCO_3)
Cephalin flocculation	Serum	2+ or less in 48 hrs
Chloride	Serum	100–106 mEq/liter
Cholesterol	Serum	150–280 mg%
Congo-red test	Serum	More than 60% retention in serum
Creatine phosphokinase (CPK)	Serum	0–4 units
Creatinine	Serum	0.7–1.5 mg%
Cryoglobulins	Serum	0
Dilantin (diphenylhydantoin)	Serum	Therapeutic level, 1–11 μg/cc
Glucose	Blood	Fasting: 70–100 mg%
Hydrogen ion concentration	Blood, serum or plasma	pH 7.3–7.5
Icteric index	Serum	4–6 units
Iodine (protein bound)	Serum	3.5–8.0 μg%
(butanol extractable)	Serum	3–6.5 μg%
Iron	Serum	50–100 μg/100 ml (higher in males)

* Adopted in part from Indiana University Medical Center Laboratories and from values compiled by staff members of the Massachusetts General Hospital (see New England J. Med., *276*, 167, 1967). See also Wintrobe: *Clinical Hematology*. 7th Ed., Philadelphia, Lea & Febiger, 1974.

Blood Plasma or Serum Values (Continued)

Determination	Material Used	Normal Value
Lactic dehydrogenase	Serum	200–600 units/ml
Lipase	Serum	Under 2 units/cc
Phosphatase (acid)	Serum	Male—Total: 0.13–0.63 Sigma units/cc Female—Total: 0.01–0.56 Sigma units/cc Prostatic: 0–0.7 Fishman-Lerner units/100 cc
Phosphatase (alkaline)	Serum	2.0–4.5 Bodansky units/cc (infants to 14 units; adolescents to 5 units). 5–10 King-Armstrong units 0.8–2.3 Bessey-Lowry units (children 3.4–9 units)
Phosphorus (inorganic)	Serum	3.0–4.5 mg% (infants in 1st year up to 6 mg%)
Potassium	Serum	3.5–5.0 mEq/liter
Protein: Total	Serum	6–8 gm%
Albumin	Serum	4–5 gm%
Globulin		2–3 gm%
Paper electrophoresis:	Serum	Percent of total protein
Albumin		50–60%
Globulin:		
Alpha$_1$		5–8%
Alpha$_2$		8–13%
Beta		11–17%
Gamma		15–25%
Albumin-globulin ratio		1.5–2.5: 1
Sodium	Serum	136–145 mEq/liter
Thymol:		
Flocculation	Serum	Up to 1+ in 24 hrs
Turbidity		0–4 units
Transaminase (SGOT)	Serum	10–40 units/cc
Urea nitrogen (BUN)	Blood or serum	8–25 mg%
Uric acid	Serum	3–7 mg%

Urine Values

Determination	Normal Value
Acetone plus acetoacetate (quantitative)	0
Ammonia	20–70 mEq/liter
Calcium	Under 150 mg/day
Catecholamines	Epinephrine: under 10 μg/day. Norepinephrine: under 100 μg/day
Creatine	Under 100 mg/day or less than 6% of creatinine. In pregnancy: up to 12%. In children under 1 yr.: may equal creatinine. In older children: up to 30% of creatinine.
Creatinine	15–25 mg/kg/day
Cystine or cysteine	0
Hemoglobin and myoglobin	0

Urine Values (Continued)

Determination	Normal Value
Homogentisic acid	0
5-Hydroxyindoleacetic acid	0
Phenolsulfonphthalein (PSP)	At least 25% excreted by 15 min; 40% by 30 min; 60% by 120 min
Phosphorus (inorganic)	Varies with intake; average 1 gm/day
Pituitary gonadotropins	6–12 rat units/24 hrs for normal men and women; over 25 rat units/24 hrs postmenopausal
Protein:	
Quantitative	0
Electrophoresis	0
Steroids:	

17-ketosteroids (per day)

Age	Males	Females
10	1–4 mg	1–4 mg
20	6–21	4–16
30	8–26	4–14
50	5–18	3–9
70	2–10	1–7

Determination	Normal Value
17-hydroxysteroids	2–7 mg/day (women lower than men)
Sugar:	
Quantitative glucose	0
Identification of reducing substances	
Fructose (quantitative)	0
Pentose (quantitative)	0
Titratable acidity	20–40 mEq/day

Hematologic Values

Determination	Normal Value
Coagulation factors:	
Bleeding time	
Duke's method	Below 5 min
Clotting time	
Capillary tube method	1–7 min
Kruse & Moses method	2.5–5 min
Lee & White method	5–10 min
Clot retraction time	
Quantitative	80–90%
Qualitative	begins 1–6 hrs complete 24 hrs
Factor V assay	75–125%
Factor VIII (antihemophilic globulin) assay	50–200%
Factor IX (plasma thromboplastin component) assay	75–125%
Factor X (Stuart factor) assay	75–125%
Fibrinogen	0.15–0.30 gm%
Fibrinolysins (whole-blood clot lysis time)	No clot lysis in 24 hrs
Partial thromboplastin time (cephalin time)	35–45 sec

Hematologic Values (Continued)

Determination	*Normal Value*
Coagulation factors:	
Prothrombin consumption	Over 80% prothrombin consumed in 1 hr
Prothrombin content	100%
Specific prothrombin assay	75–125%
Erythrocyte sedimentation rate	Less than 0.4 mm/min (corrected for hematocrit) or less than 20 mm/hr
Hematocrit	Males: 42–50% Females: 40–48%
Hemoglobin	Males: 13–16 gm% Females: 12–14 gm%
Osmotic fragility of red cell	Increased if hemolysis occurs in over 0.5% NaCl; decreased if hemolysis is incomplete in 0.3% NaCl
Platelet count	250,000/cu mm (average)
Red cell count	
(millions/mm^3 blood)	
Children	
1st year	6.1–4.5
2–10 years	4.6–4.7
11–15 years	4.8
Adults	
Males	4.6–6.2
Females	4.2–5.4
Red-cell corpuscular values (adults):	
Mean corpuscular volume (MCV)	80–90 cuμ
Mean corpuscular hemoglobin (MCH)	27–32 pg
Mean corpuscular hemoglobin concentration (MCHC)	33–38%
White cell count	
(cells/mm^3 of blood)	
Infants	8,000–16,500
4–7 years	6,000–15,000 (average 10,700)
8–18 years	4,500–13,000 (average 8,300)
Adults	5,000–10,000 (average 7,000)
Differential white cell count	
Adults:	
Myelocytes	0%
Metamyelocytes	0–1%
Band cells	4–8%
Adult neutrophils	54–62%
Lymphocytes	25–33%
Monocytes	3–7%
Eosinophils	1–5%
Basophils	0–1%

Children:

The newborn infant exhibits a neutrophilia immediately after birth along with high eosinophil, basophil and monocyte values. Neutrophils gradually subside to a 25–50% level during the first two weeks (with associated lymphocytosis) and then gradually rise to 40–60% during the next few months. Stable neutrophil levels are not reached until about 12 years of age. Immature red and white cells are frequently seen in infants and children.

Table 2.   Normal Chronological Development of the Teeth*

Deciduous Teeth	Initiation (wks in utero)	Calcification Begins (mos in utero)	Crown (mos) Completed	Eruption (mos)	Root Formation Complete (yr)	Root Resp. Begins (yr)	Tooth Shed (yr)
Central incisors	7	4–5	2–4	6–9	1½–2	5–6	7–8
Lateral incisors	7	4–5	2–5	7–10	1½–2	5–6	7–9
Canines	7½	6	9	16–20	2½–3	6–7	10–12
1st molars	8	5	6	12–16	2–2½	4–5	9–11
2nd molars	10	6	10–12	20–30	3	4–5	11–12

Permanent Teeth	Initiation (mos)	Calcification Begins	Crown (yr) Completed	Eruption (yr)	Root Formation Complete (yr)
Maxillary					
Central incisors	5–5¼ in utero	3–4 mo	4–5	7–8	10
Lateral incisors	5–5¼ in utero	1 yr	4–5	8–9	11
Canine	5½–6 in utero	4–5 mo	6–7	11–12	13–15
1st premolar	Birth	1½–1¾ yr	5–6	10–11	12–13
2nd premolar	7½–8	2–2½ yr	6–7	10–12	12–14
1st molar	3¼–4 in utero	Birth	2½–3	6–7	9–10
2nd molar	8½–9	2½–3 yr	7–8	12–13	14–16
3rd molar	3¼–4 yr	7–9 yr	12–16	17–25	18–25
Mandibular					
Central incisors	5–5¼ in utero	3–4 mo	4–5	6–7	9
Lateral incisors	5–5¼ in utero	3–4 mo	4–5	7–8	10
Canine	5½–6 in utero	4–5 mo	6–7	9–11	12–14
1st premolar	Birth	1¾–2 yr	5–6	10–12	12–13
2nd premolar	7½–8	2¼–2½ yr	6–7	11–12	13–14
1st molar	3¼–4 in utero	Birth	2½–3	6–7	9–10
2nd molar	8½–9	2½–3 yr	7–8	11–13	14–15
3rd molar	3½–4 yr	8–10 yr	12–16	17–25	18–25

* Logan, W. H. G. and Kronfeld, R.: Development of the human jaws and surrounding structures from birth to the age of 15 years, J. Amer. Dent. Ass., 20, 379, 1933. Schour, I. and Massler, M.: Studies in tooth development. The growth pattern of human teeth, J. Amer. Dent. Ass., 27, 198, 1940.

Index

Page numbers followed by f indicate figures; those followed by t indicate tables